Evidence-Based Practice for Public Health Emergency Preparedness and Response

Ned Calonge, Lisa Brown, and Autumn Downey, *Editors*

Committee on Evidence-Based Practices for Public Health Emergency Preparedness and Response

Board on Health Sciences Policy

Board on Population Health and Public Health Practice

Health and Medicine Division

A Consensus Study Report of

The National Academies of

SCIENCES · ENGINEERING · MEDICINE

THE NATIONAL ACADEMIES PRESS

Washington, DC

www.nap.edu

THE NATIONAL ACADEMIES PRESS 500 Fifth Street, NW Washington, DC 20001

This activity was supported by a contract between the National Academy of Sciences and the Centers for Disease Control and Prevention (Contract #200-2011-38807, Task Order 60). Any opinions, findings, conclusions, or recommendations expressed in this publication do not necessarily reflect the views of any organization or agency that provided support for the project.

International Standard Book Number-13: 978-0-309-67038-8
International Standard Book Number-10: 0-309-67038-1
Digital Object Identifier: https://doi.org/10.17226/25650
Library of Congress Control Number: 2020943124

Additional copies of this publication are available from the National Academies Press, 500 Fifth Street, NW, Keck 360, Washington, DC 20001; (800) 624-6242 or (202) 334-3313; http://www.nap.edu.

Printed in the United States of America

Suggested citation: National Academies of Sciences, Engineering, and Medicine. 2020. *Evidence-based practice for public health emergency preparedness and response*. Washington, DC: The National Academies Press. https://doi.org/10.17226/25650.

The National Academies of
SCIENCES • ENGINEERING • MEDICINE

The **National Academy of Sciences** was established in 1863 by an Act of Congress, signed by President Lincoln, as a private, nongovernmental institution to advise the nation on issues related to science and technology. Members are elected by their peers for outstanding contributions to research. Dr. Marcia McNutt is president.

The **National Academy of Engineering** was established in 1964 under the charter of the National Academy of Sciences to bring the practices of engineering to advising the nation. Members are elected by their peers for extraordinary contributions to engineering. Dr. John L. Anderson is president.

The **National Academy of Medicine** (formerly the Institute of Medicine) was established in 1970 under the charter of the National Academy of Sciences to advise the nation on medical and health issues. Members are elected by their peers for distinguished contributions to medicine and health. Dr. Victor J. Dzau is president.

The three Academies work together as the **National Academies of Sciences, Engineering, and Medicine** to provide independent, objective analysis and advice to the nation and conduct other activities to solve complex problems and inform public policy decisions. The National Academies also encourage education and research, recognize outstanding contributions to knowledge, and increase public understanding in matters of science, engineering, and medicine.

Learn more about the National Academies of Sciences, Engineering, and Medicine at **www.nationalacademies.org**.

The National Academies of

SCIENCES • ENGINEERING • MEDICINE

COMMITTEE ON EVIDENCE-BASED PRACTICES FOR PUBLIC HEALTH EMERGENCY PREPAREDNESS AND RESPONSE

BRUCE (NED) CALONGE (*Chair*), President and Chief Executive Officer, The Colorado Trust

DAVID M. ABRAMSON, Associate Professor and Director, Program on Population Impact Recovery and Resilience (PiR2), New York University School of Global Public Health

JULIE CASANI, Medical Director of Student Health Services, North Carolina State University

DAVID EISENMAN, Professor in Residence, David Geffen School of Medicine and Fielding School of Public Health, Division of General Internal Medicine and Health Services Research, University of California, Los Angeles

FRANCISCO GARCÍA, Deputy County Administrator and Chief Medical Officer, Pima County, and Professor Emeritus of Public Health, University of Arizona

PAUL HALVERSON, Founding Dean and Professor, Richard M. Fairbanks School of Public Health, Indiana University

SEAN HENNESSY, Professor of Epidemiology and of Systems Pharmacology and Translational Therapeutics, Perelman School of Medicine, University of Pennsylvania

EDBERT HSU, Associate Professor, Department of Emergency Medicine and Associate Director, Office of Critical Event Preparedness and Response, Johns Hopkins University

NATHANIEL HUPERT, Associate Professor of Medicine and Population Health Sciences, Weill Medical College, and Co-Director, Cornell Institute for Disease and Disaster Preparedness, Cornell University

REBECCA A. MAYNARD, University Trustee Chair Professor of Education and Social Policy, University of Pennsylvania

SUZET McKINNEY, Executive Director and Chief Executive Officer, Illinois Medical District

JANE P. NOYES, Professor of Health and Social Services Research and Child Health, School of Health Sciences, Bangor University, United Kingdom

DOUGLAS K. OWENS, Henry J. Kaiser Jr. Professor, Professor of Medicine and Director, Center for Health Policy and Center for Primary Care and Outcomes Research, Stanford University

SANDRA QUINN, Professor, Department of Family Science, School of Public Health, University of Maryland

PAUL SHEKELLE, Founding Director, Southern California Evidence-Based Practice Center, RAND Corporation

ANDY STERGACHIS, Professor of Pharmacy and Global Health, Associate Dean, School of Pharmacy, Director, Global Medicines Program, University of Washington

MITCH STRIPLING, National Director, Emergency Preparedness and Response, Planned Parenthood Federation of America

STEVEN M. TEUTSCH, Adjunct Professor, Fielding School of Public Health, University of California, Los Angeles; and Senior Fellow, Leonard D. Schaeffer Center for Health Policy and Economics, University of Southern California

TENER GOODWIN VEENEMA, Professor of Nursing and Public Health, School of Nursing and Bloomberg School of Public Health, Johns Hopkins University

MATTHEW WYNIA, Director, Center for Bioethics and Humanities, University of Colorado

National Academy of Medicine Fellow

MAHSHID ABIR, Director, Acute Care Research Unit, and Associate Professor, Department of Emergency Medicine, University of Michigan; and Senior Physician Policy Researcher, RAND Corporation

Study Staff

LISA BROWN, Study Co-Director
AUTUMN DOWNEY, Study Co-Director
MEGAN KEARNEY, Associate Program Officer (*from November 2019*)
LEAH RAND, Associate Program Officer (*until August 2019*)
MATTHEW MASIELLO, Research Associate (*until August 2019*)
ALEX REPACE, Senior Program Assistant
REBECCA MORGAN, Senior Research Librarian
KATHLEEN STRATTON, Senior Scholar, Board on Population Health and Public Health Practice
ANDREW M. POPE, Senior Director, Board on Health Sciences Policy

Consultants

LGND, Graphic Design Team
RONA BRIERE, Senior Editor, Briere Associates, Inc.
SGNL Solutions, Science Writer

Commissioned Paper Authors

ETHAN BALK, Center for Evidence Synthesis in Health, Brown University
JEREMY GOLDHABER-FIEBERT, Stanford University
JENNIFER HORNEY, University of Delaware
KARLI KONDO, Portland VA Evidence Synthesis Program
JULIE NOVAK, Wayne State University
SNEHA PATEL, Columbia University
IAN SALDANHA, Center for Evidence Synthesis in Health, Brown University
PRADEEP SOPORY, Wayne State University
MARCIA TESTA, Harvard University

Public Health Emergency Preparedness and Response Subject-Matter Consultants

JESSICA CABRERA-MARQUEZ, Puerto Rico Department of Health
CARINA ELSENBOSS, Public Health Seattle and King County
STEVEN HULEATT, West Hartford-Bloomfield Health District
CHRISTIE LUCE, Florida Department of Health
PATRICK LUJAN, Guam Department of Public Health and Social Services
DAVID NEZ, Navajo Department of Health
PAUL PETERSON, Tennessee Department of Health
LOU SCHMITZ, American Indian Health Commission for Washington State
EDNA QUINONES-ALVAREZ, Puerto Rico Department of Health

Evidence Review Methodology Subject-Matter Consultant

HOLGER SCHÜNEMANN, McMaster University

Reviewers

This Consensus Study Report was reviewed in draft form by individuals chosen for their diverse perspectives and technical expertise. The purpose of this independent review is to provide candid and critical comments that will assist the National Academies of Sciences, Engineering, and Medicine in making each published report as sound as possible and to ensure that it meets the institutional standards for quality, objectivity, evidence, and responsiveness to the study charge. The review comments and draft manuscript remain confidential to protect the integrity of the deliberative process.

We thank the following individuals for their review of this report:

RICHARD N. ASLIN, Haskins Laboratories, Yale University
JEANNE MARIE GUISE, Oregon Health & Science University
SHELDON H. JACOBSON, University of Illinois at Urbana-Champaign
HARRY B. JEFFRIES, JR., Georgia Department of Public Health (retired)
YASMIN KHAN, University of Toronto
CHRISTOPHER NELSON, RAND Corporation
ALONZO PLOUGH, Robert Wood Johnson Foundation
JEFFREY SCHLEGELMILCH, National Center for Disaster Preparedness, The Earth Institute, Columbia University
HILARY THOMSON, University of Glasgow
W. CRAIG VANDERWAGEN, East West Protection, LLC
CHRIS J. WIANT, Caring for Colorado (retired)
STEPHANIE ZAZA, American College of Preventive Medicine

Although the reviewers listed above provided many constructive comments and suggestions, they were not asked to endorse the conclusions or recommendations of this report, nor did they see the final draft before its release. The review of this report was overseen by **ENRIQUETA C. BOND,** Burroughs Wellcome Fund, and **LINDA C. DEGUTIS,** Henry M. Jackson Foundation. They were responsible for making certain that an independent examination of this report was carried out in accordance with the standards of the National Academies and that all review comments were carefully considered. Responsibility for the final content rests entirely with the authoring committee and the National Academies.

Preface

In 1946 the federal government created the Communicable Disease Center to address the spread of malaria in the United States. Building on prior state and local activities to address infectious disease outbreaks through the development of public health laboratories, coordinated quarantine and isolation efforts, and national efforts that included the creation of the Public Health Service, this early version of what would become the Centers for Disease Control and Prevention (CDC) was initially created in response to what today would be called a "public health emergency."

Infectious disease control remained a core element of public health practice, and as the nation experienced ongoing challenges with seasonal influenza and other new threats began to emerge, CDC funded a small number of state health departments to develop planning around pandemic influenza and bioterrorism preparedness in the late 1990s. The terrorist attacks of September 11, 2001, followed by the anthrax letters the following month, brought into sharp focus the need for a more substantial commitment to preparing for those emergencies that involve a public health response. The Public Health Security and Bioterrorism Preparedness and Response Act was passed in 2002, and the Center for Preparedness and Response at CDC was created in 2003, with unprecedented new funding for states to support preparedness efforts. Since then, the number of events requiring a public health response has been impressive, and not limited to infectious diseases. These events have involved West Nile virus; severe acute respiratory syndrome; the federal smallpox vaccination program; monkeypox; the 2004–2005 influenza vaccine shortage; the H1N1 virus (swine flu); Hurricanes Katrina and Harvey; Midwest and Rocky Mountain West floods; California wildfires; several regional national food recalls for *E. coli* O157, *Salmonella*, and *Listeria*; and Ebola virus—just to name those that reached national attention.

Policy makers have recognized the need for rigor in public health's emergency planning and response activities, but while investments have been made in research, this funding has been sporadic, not well coordinated, and not always focused on the needs of public health practitioners. The result has been a relatively sparse evidence base for public health emergency preparedness and response (PHEPR) practices, reflecting broad variation in research design, implementation, reporting, synthesis, and translation.

Recognizing the substantial benefit for human health that could be realized through an evidence-based approach to identifying those practices that warrant being recommended to PHEPR practitioners, leaders from CDC's Center for Preparedness and Response commissioned the National Academies of Sciences, Engineering, and Medicine to undertake a study focused on developing an evidence synthesis methodology specific to PHEPR practices and piloting that methodology by evaluating a number of practices important to practitioners in the field. Bringing together experts in research methods and evidence synthesis and leaders and researchers in PHEPR, the study committee created a customized evidence review and synthesis and evidence-to-recommendation methodology that recognizes the value of and utilizes the full body of available research. Creating this methodology thus entailed applying synthesis methods created for both quantitative and qualitative data, as well for more novel evidence categories that encompassed parallel evidence (i.e., evidence regarding the same or similar intervention but in different contexts), mechanistic evidence (i.e., evidence based on an identifiable causal link or pathway, generally previously established in other fields), and case reports and after action reports (prepared as a standard practice in review and evaluation of public health emergency response).

The committee applied this methodology in formulating recommendations and guidance for specific practices in four of CDC's 15 Preparedness and Response Capabilities[1]: engaging with and training community-based partners to improve the outcomes of at-risk populations (falls under Capability 1, Community Preparedness); activating a public health emergency operations center (Capability 3, Emergency Operations Coordination); communicating public health alerts and guidance with technical audiences during a public health emergency (Capability 6, Information Sharing); and implementing quarantine to reduce or stop the spread of a contagious disease (Capability 11, Non-Pharmaceutical Interventions). The process by which these four diverse practices were selected was designed in such a way as to ensure that the committee's evidence synthesis methodology can be applied to other practices that fall under all 15 Capabilities. It was not, however, a prioritization process based on importance; all 15 Capabilities are critical to the preparation for and response to a public health emergency. As it is applied to other practices, the committee is confident its methodology will continue to evolve to provide public health leaders with guidance based on the best available evidence—the key tenet of evidence-based practice.

A NOTE ON COVID-19

In the final weeks of the committee's work, a public health emergency of international concern emerged with the outbreak of the novel coronavirus responsible for the COVID-19 pandemic. We recognized that each of the practices we had evaluated with our methodology, which were selected roughly 2 years prior to the emergence of this disease, were operative to some extent in the response to this emergency: working with community-based organizations

---

[1] The other 11 Capabilities are Community Recovery (Capability 2), Emergency Public Information and Warning (Capability 4), Fatality Management (Capability 5), Mass Care (Capability 7), Medical Countermeasure Dispensing (Capability 8), Medical Materiel Management and Distribution (Capability 9), Medical Surge (Capability 10), Public Health Laboratory Testing (Capability 12), Public Health Surveillance and Epidemiological Investigation (Capability 13), Volunteer Management (Capability 14), and Responder Safety and Health (Capability 15), as defined in CDC (Centers for Disease Control and Prevention). 2018. *Public health emergency preparedness and response capabilities: National standards for state, local, tribal, and territorial public health.* https://www.cdc.gov/cpr/readiness/00_docs/CDC_PreparednesResponseCapabilities_October2018_Final_508.pdf (accessed March 11, 2020).

to address the needs of at-risk populations (Chapter 4); activation of an emergency operation center (Chapter 5); communication with health care providers and other technical audiences (Chapter 6); and, of particular note, quarantine (Chapter 7). Although our reviews were not conducted in response to the COVID-19 pandemic, the likely applicability of many of our findings is noteworthy. For example, while it is too soon to conclude definitively whether quarantine is effective at reducing and stopping transmission of this novel coronavirus, the findings from the qualitative evidence synthesis (discussed in Chapter 7) regarding the psychological and financial harms of this practice will undoubtedly be just as relevant to the current quarantine experience as they are to past outbreak scenarios. Given the rapid and evolving nature of the COVID-19 pandemic and the speed at which new studies are being published on non-peer-reviewed, preprint servers, it was not possible at this time to update the committee's evidence reviews to incorporate studies examining the implementation of the four PHEPR practices reviewed for this study as applied to COVID-19. However, it will be important to expand and update these reviews once the field has rigorously collected, analyzed, and published the relevant data and information.

The emergence of COVID-19 has highlighted critical evidence gaps and lost opportunities to expand the evidence base for these and other PHEPR practices. The lack of interoperable and harmonized data and capacity for local-level monitoring impedes both evidence-based research and response. It reinforces the critical, ongoing need to have processes and programs in place to perform research and evaluation, even in real time, to better inform future decisions. Without these systems in place before, during, and after the unfolding of a disaster, it will be extremely difficult to build the PHEPR evidence base prospectively and retrospectively.

The release of this report in the context of the COVID-19 pandemic puts the challenges of limited research to support evidence-based PHEPR practices in bold relief. The committee's recommendations around adequate stable funding, robust design and conduct of research studies, development of the research workforce and programs, and a commitment to collaboration between public health practitioners and experienced researchers all are vital to ongoing support of the knowledge development for and implementation of interventions that will better protect the public's health and minimize the impact of the broad spectrum of emergencies that have and will certainly continue to threaten the security of the nation. The unprecedented costs of COVID-19 show that the nation cannot afford to ignore the calls for these critical investments in public health that have been made by this committee and many others before.

Ned Calonge, *Chair*
Committee on Evidence-Based Practices for
Public Health Emergency Preparedness and Response

Contents

Boxes, Figures, and Tables

BOXES

FIGURES

TABLES

Acronyms and Abbreviations

AAR	after action report
AHRQ	Agency for Healthcare Research and Quality
ASPR	Assistant Secretary for Preparedness and Response
ASTHO	Association of State and Territorial Health Officials
CASP	Critical Appraisal Skills Programme
CBP	community-based partner
CDC	Centers for Disease Control and Prevention
CERQual	Confidence in the Evidence from Reviews of Qualitative Research
COE	certainty of the evidence (of effectiveness)
CPHP	Center for Public Health Preparedness
CPSTF	Community Preventive Services Task Force
DECIDE (project)	Developing and Evaluating Communication Strategies to Support Informed Decisions and Practice Based on Evidence
DHS	U.S. Department of Homeland Security
DoD	U.S. Department of Defense
DOI	U.S. Department of the Interior
EBM	evidence-based medicine
EOC	emergency operations coordination/center
EtD	Evidence to Decision (framework)
FEMA	Federal Emergency Management Agency
GRADE	Grading of Recommendations Assessment, Development and Evaluation
HPP	Hospital Preparedness Program

HSDL	Homeland Security Digital Library
NACCHO	National Association of County & City Health Officials
NIEHS	National Institute of Environmental Health Sciences
NSF	National Science Foundation
PAHPA	Pandemic and All Hazards Preparedness Act
PERLC	Preparedness and Emergency Response Learning Center
PERRC	Preparedness and Emergency Response Research Center
PHAB	Public Health Accreditation Board
PHEOC	public health emergency operations center
PHEPR	public health emergency preparedness and response
PPHR	Project Public Health Ready
RCT	randomized controlled trial
RoB	risk of bias
ROBINS-I (tool)	Risk of Bias in Non-Randomized Studies of Interventions
SLTT	state, local, tribal, and territorial
USPSTF	U.S. Preventive Services Task Force
WHO	World Health Organization
WWC	What Works Clearinghouse

Abstract

Preparing for and responding to public health emergencies requires scientific evidence to save lives, prevent disruption to the social fabric of society, and mitigate unprecedented damages and costs. Public health emergencies are becoming increasingly common and complex—a trend that is likely to continue. State, local, tribal, and territorial public health agencies play a vital role in responding to these emergencies. They must do so effectively, and as in other fields, effectiveness requires scientific evidence. The Centers for Disease Control and Prevention (CDC) recognizes the need to provide clear guidance on evidence-based practices to those public health emergency preparedness and response (PHEPR) practitioners routinely required to make difficult decisions about how to respond effectively to a wide range of public health threats. Accordingly, CDC charged the National Academies of Sciences, Engineering, and Medicine with developing the methodology for and conducting a systematic review and evaluation of the evidence for selected PHEPR practices that fall within the 15 PHEPR Capabilities defined in CDC's *Public Health Emergency Preparedness and Response Capabilities: National Standards for State, Local, Tribal, and Territorial Public Health*[1] and to make recommendations for future research needed to address critical gaps in evidence-based PHEPR practices, as well as processes to improve the overall quality of evidence in the field. As described in this report, the committee found that despite the investments that have been made in PHEPR research over the past two decades, **the science underlying the nation's system of response to public health emergencies is seriously deficient, hampering the nation's ability to respond to emergencies most effectively to save lives and preserve well-being.** The lack of a clear, progressive research agenda and sporadic funding, among other things, has resulted in a sparse and uneven evidence base reflecting broad variation in research design, implementation, reporting, synthesis, and translation.

[1] CDC (Centers for Disease Control and Prevention). 2018. *Public health emergency preparedness and response capabilities: National standards for state, local, tribal, and territorial public health.* https://www.cdc.gov/cpr/readiness/00_docs/CDC_PreparednesResponseCapabilities_October2018_Final_508.pdf (accessed March 11, 2020).

To address this deficiency, this report aims to move the PHEPR field forward in terms of identifying and using evidence-based practices. The committee provides herein eight overarching recommendations (summarized in the four points below)[2] that, if implemented, would transform the infrastructure, funding, and methods of PHEPR research and enhance the nation's capacity for comprehensive and effective response to public health emergencies:

1. **An enduring national science framework is needed for PHEPR.** CDC, in collaboration with relevant agencies, researchers, and practitioners, should develop a National PHEPR Science Framework to ensure a coordinated approach to the development and implementation of a unified PHEPR research agenda (Recommendation 3). CDC and its partners should create the infrastructure necessary to support the production of high-quality PHEPR research (Recommendation 4).
2. **Improving and expanding PHEPR research will require incentives for both researchers and public health agencies.** CDC and other relevant funding agencies should use funding requirements to drive improvements in the conduct and reporting of effectiveness and implementation research for PHEPR practices (Recommendation 5). CDC should convene an expert panel to advance a process for quality improvement in the PHEPR arena and enhance the quality and utility of postincident after action reports as tools for evaluating effectiveness (Recommendation 6).
3. **The research and other evidence driven by the proposed National PHEPR Science Framework needs to be translated into clear evidence-based practices for public health agencies through an ongoing evidence review process.** CDC should support an independent group charged with reviewing all relevant research and distilling it into evidence-based practice guidelines for the benefit of practitioners, further developing the PHEPR evidence review methodology developed by the committee (see below), and identifying evidence gaps (Recommendation 1). CDC should establish the infrastructure necessary to support this group and ensure a sustained process for conducting these evidence reviews (Recommendation 2).
4. **It is essential to get these evidence-based practices into the hands of the public health practitioners who most need them.** CDC should use a multipronged dissemination approach to ensure that evidence-based practice recommendations achieve broad reach and become the standard of practice of the target audience(s) (Recommendation 8). Working with professional and academic organizations across relevant disciplines, CDC should develop the workforce capacity development programs necessary to both ensure the conduct of quality PHEPR research and improve the implementation capacity of public health agencies (Recommendation 7).

In conducting this study, the committee developed a fit-for-purpose evidence review methodology, drawing on the elements of existing frameworks to carry out a systematic review and evaluation of the evidence for four PHEPR practices that fall within the 15 PHEPR Capabilities and to understand the associated benefits and harms. To ensure that the methodology would be applicable to practices from across the full range of PHEPR Capabilities (see Box 1-2 in Chapter 1), the criteria and process for selecting the four review topics (depicted in Figure 3-1 in Chapter 3) were developed with the aim of yielding a set of diverse PHEPR practices for which the evidence base would be expected to differ in nature. Applying its

[2] The numbering of the recommendations reflects the order in which they are presented in the report chapters. Recommendations are presented out of sequence in the bullets in this abstract to support a focus on the committee's proposed National PHEPR Science Framework.

methodology, the committee reviewed the available evidence and provides in this report evidence-based practice recommendations and/or implementation guidance relating to

- engaging with and training community-based partners to improve the outcomes of at-risk populations[3] after public health emergencies (falls under Capability 1, Community Preparedness);
- activating a public health emergency operations center (Capability 3, Emergency Operations Coordination);
- communicating public health alerts and guidance with technical audiences during a public health emergency (Capability 6, Information Sharing); and
- implementing quarantine to reduce or stop the spread of a contagious disease (Capability 11, Non-Pharmaceutical Interventions).

This report and the committee's recommendations show that implementing strategies to build the foundations for a robust scientific evidence base in the PHEPR field is feasible, and that an investment in PHEPR research and an evidence review system has the potential to yield significant public benefits in terms of preventing the needless loss of lives and disruption to communities in future public health emergencies. As the PHEPR research field continues to evolve and mature, the committee asserts that such an evidence base should be the foundation for future changes in both policy and practice.

[3] For the purposes of this report, the committee defined at-risk populations as comprising individuals with social and/or structural vulnerabilities whose access and functional needs may not be fully met by traditional service providers or who feel they cannot comfortably or safely use the standard resources offered during preparedness, response, and recovery efforts. A more comprehensive description of at-risk populations is provided in Box 4-1 in Chapter 4.

Summary[1]

Communities across the nation are facing increasingly complex public health emergencies that are responsible for loss of life, disruption of the social fabric of society, and unprecedented damages and costs. State, local, tribal, and territorial (SLTT) public health agencies routinely make difficult decisions about how to respond effectively to a wide range of public health threats (e.g., infectious disease epidemics, natural and human-made disasters) and prepare for worst-case scenarios, including chemical, biological, radiological, and nuclear events. Yet, the existing scientific evidence base that informs the actions of SLTT public health agencies in preparing for and responding to these emergencies is sparse and uneven, and fails to meet the needs of public health emergency preparedness and response (PHEPR) practitioners for clear and accessible guidance. This deficiency impedes the efforts of these dedicated professionals who work tirelessly to protect the lives and health of the people of this country and threatens the nation's health security. This report calls for a transformation in the infrastructure, funding, and methods of PHEPR research to ensure that PHEPR practice is grounded in robust evidence for what works, where, why, and for whom.

ABOUT THIS REPORT

Study Charge

In the aftermath of September 11, 2001, and the subsequent anthrax bioterrorism attacks, the Centers for Disease Control and Prevention (CDC) and other governmental and nongovernmental organizations together invested billions of dollars and immeasurable human capital to develop and enhance PHEPR infrastructure, systems, and science. Since 2011, 15 foundational Capabilities—defined in CDC's *Public Health Emergency Preparedness and Response Capabilities: National Standards for State, Local, Tribal, and Territorial Public*

[1] This Summary does not include references. Citations for the discussion presented in the Summary appear in the subsequent report chapters.

Health—have guided public health agencies in building and sustaining robust systems to prevent, protect against, quickly respond to, and recover from public health emergencies. The PHEPR Capabilities alone do not constitute the PHEPR system; rather, the system comprises the interactions among the Capabilities and the context in which they are operationalized. As a result, those PHEPR practices[2] that fall within the PHEPR Capabilities are often complex, are generally implemented simultaneously with an array of other practices, and may target multiple levels (i.e., individual, community, organizational, or systems levels). Thus, it is critical to understand and appreciate the underlying characteristics and relationships of the PHEPR system and to apply this understanding to the design and evaluation of PHEPR practices.

As the nation approaches two decades since the events of September 11, 2001, this is an opportune time to take stock of the state of the evidence on PHEPR practices and the improvements necessary to move the field forward and to strengthen the PHEPR system. Therefore, CDC charged the National Academies of Sciences, Engineering, and Medicine with developing the methodology for and conducting a systematic review[3] and evaluation of the evidence for selected PHEPR practices that fall within CDC's 15 PHEPR Capabilities. The committee was also charged with making recommendations for future research needed to address critical gaps in evidence-based PHEPR practices, as well as processes needed to improve the overall quality of evidence within the field. The full charge to the committee is presented in Chapter 1 of this report.

How This Report Is Organized and Intended to Be Used

Throughout this report, the committee seeks to guide practitioners, researchers, policy makers, funding organizations, and other stakeholders in understanding and using the available evidence to inform their decision making. It also seeks to demonstrate for methodologists and other researchers interested in the field of evidence synthesis and guideline development the application of a mixed-method approach to evidence synthesis and the challenges associated with evaluation of complex interventions, such as those the committee reviewed.

The report is organized around the two distinct aspects of the committee's charge, each of which comes with its own set of recommendations: (1) recommendations for evidence-based PHEPR practices based on reviews of the evidence for their effectiveness, carried out using the committee's customized methodology; and (2) recommendations for future research needed to address critical gaps in evidence-based PHEPR practices and processes to improve the overall quality of evidence within the field. The latter set of recommendations, which will be of greatest interest to **policy makers** and **researchers,** is presented in Chapter 8, which considers the role that funders, researchers, and practitioners can play in advancing the evidence base. For the four selected PHEPR practices reviewed by the committee, evidence-based practice recommendations and implementation guidance are presented in Chapters 4–7, respectively. These four chapters are oriented to **practitioners** and include high-level evidence summaries for the four PHEPR practices; each of these chapters opens with a two-page action sheet pro-

[2] In PHEPR, in contrast to clinical medicine, there is seldom a discrete "intervention"; therefore, the committee defined PHEPR practice broadly as a type of process, structure, or intervention whose implementation is intended to mitigate the adverse effects resulting from a public health emergency on the population as a whole or a particular sub-group within the population. PHEPR practices fall within the 15 PHEPR Capabilities.

[3] Although the term "comprehensive review" was used in the committee's Statement of Task (see Box 1-1), the committee uses the field-accepted term "systematic review" throughout this report. The committee applied a mixed-method approach to its systematic review.

viding key takeaways for practitioners. For those audiences seeking additional, more detailed information, each of these four chapters has an associated appendix (see Appendixes B1–B4) containing a comprehensive description of the evidence base for the respective PHEPR practice. To facilitate the linkage between the evidence summaries in the four chapters and the detail in the corresponding appendixes on the body of studies from which the chapter findings were generated, each of the four chapters references specific numbered sections in the respective appendix. Chapter 3 describes the committee's proposed methodology for reviewing and evaluating the evidence for PHEPR practices and is likely to be most relevant for **methodologists** and others interested in applying or adapting the methodology.

This Summary and the preceding Abstract are oriented to policy makers who will be responsible for implementing the committee's recommendations. To facilitate a focus on the key policy issues, the recommendations in the Abstract and Summary are presented in a different sequence from that used in the report chapters. Specifically, Recommendations 1 and 2 are presented after Recommendation 7 in this Summary.

IMPROVING AND EXPANDING THE EVIDENCE BASE FOR PHEPR

State of the Evidence and Underlying Reasons

The findings from the committee's four PHEPR practice evidence reviews (described below) and a broader scoping review of the evidence for the PHEPR Capabilities (discussed in Chapter 2) are generally consistent with previously published reviews of the PHEPR research landscape. Despite an increase in published empirical studies over the past two decades, attributable in part to the investments made in preparedness and response research centers after September 11, 2001, and the subsequent anthrax attacks, the body of PHEPR research remains overwhelmingly descriptive, lacking in objective evaluations using validated measures that are capable of supporting conclusions on practice effectiveness. Existing PHEPR research also is notably uneven across the 15 Capabilities, with few (and in some cases no) impact studies for the majority of PHEPR practices evaluated in the committee's commissioned scoping review. The picture that emerges is that of a field based on long-standing rather than evidence-based practice.

Currently, the PHEPR field is relying on fragmented and largely uncoordinated research efforts. PHEPR research funding, and the field as a whole, moves from one disaster to the next with little continuity, and with investments generally inversely proportional to the time since the last event. The lack of stable funding for PHEPR research creates inefficiencies as the field rebuilds and then deconstructs its research infrastructure and workforce capacity with each new emergency. Moreover, research investments related to mitigating the effects of public health emergencies have been skewed toward more traditional biomedical research. For example, annual federal investments in research and development for medical countermeasures have ranged from \$1.6 to \$1.8 billion since 2004. In contrast, total 10-year research funding (2008–2017) for the Medical Countermeasure Dispensing and Administration Capability was estimated at just over \$100,000 in one recent study. This extreme imbalance positions public health emergency response for failure, as practitioners lack fundamental knowledge regarding how to best distribute the countermeasures the nation invested billions of dollars to produce.

Overall, the committee concluded that the science underlying the nation's response to public health emergencies is seriously deficient, hampering the nation's ability to respond to emergencies most effectively to save lives and preserve well-being. Significant advances are needed to improve and expand the evidence base for PHEPR practices.

Developing a National PHEPR Science Framework

In the absence of a system to support coordination and collaboration in the conduct of PHEPR research, academic researchers will continue to face numerous barriers to the conduct of this research, and much of the evidence base for PHEPR practices will continue to reflect a series of one-off studies that lack the comparability necessary to address knowledge gaps important to policy makers and practitioners. Addressing those knowledge gaps will require sustained lines of research, with multiple studies addressing similar research questions in different contexts and populations. An enduring national framework is needed to establish goals and objectives for improving coordination, integration, and alignment among existing but often fragmented PHEPR research efforts, and specifically to direct and coordinate available research funding to address prioritized PHEPR knowledge gaps most effectively (see Figure S-1). Through the development of such a national framework, the com-

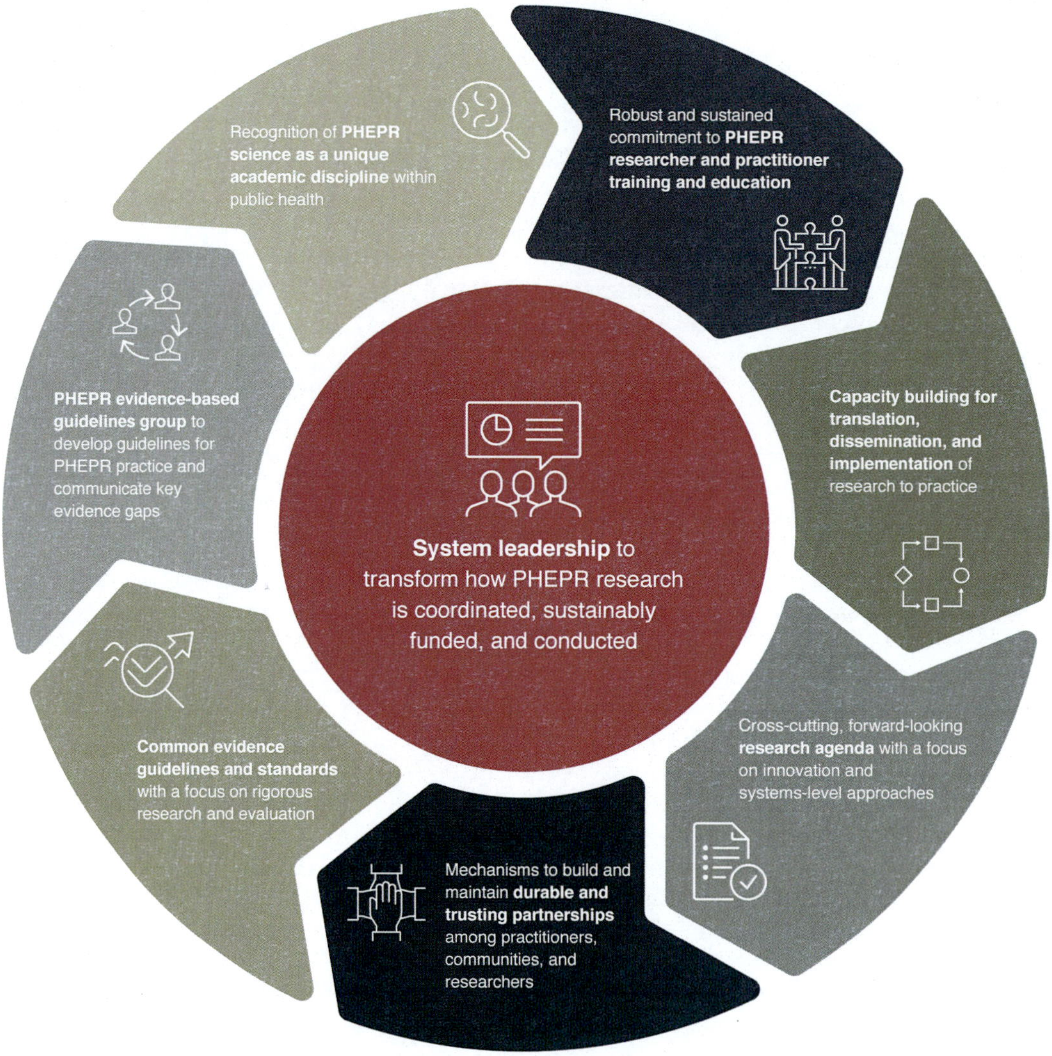
Recognition of PHEPR science as a unique academic discipline within public health
Robust and sustained commitment to PHEPR researcher and practitioner training and education
Capacity building for translation, dissemination, and implementation of research to practice
Cross-cutting, forward-looking research agenda with a focus on innovation and systems-level approaches
Mechanisms to build and maintain durable and trusting partnerships among practitioners, communities, and researchers
Common evidence guidelines and standards with a focus on rigorous research and evaluation
PHEPR evidence-based guidelines group to develop guidelines for PHEPR practice and communicate key evidence gaps
System leadership to transform how PHEPR research is coordinated, sustainably funded, and conducted

FIGURE S-1 Key components of a National PHEPR Science Framework.

mittee proposes steps to ensure the systematic and continuous development of knowledge in the PHEPR field and sets forth the aspirations for high-quality, rigorous PHEPR research and evaluation that can in turn guide practice.

Given the complexity of the PHEPR research landscape, strong leadership at all levels, but especially at the federal level, is central to the framework and essential to support systems-level change and mobilize relevant agencies to transform the way PHEPR research is coordinated, funded, and conducted. An interagency and multidisciplinary effort, led by CDC, will be necessary to develop and implement the proposed National PHEPR Science Framework; establish an authority and process for supporting high-quality, rigorous, and sustainable research before, during, and after public health emergencies; and ensure that adequate research funding, capacities, and infrastructure are in place. CDC is the funding agency with the primary mission responsibility in PHEPR, and it is important that the agency responsible for supporting PHEPR planning and implementation also lead efforts to increase the scientific evidence base that supports the execution of that responsibility. However, the committee acknowledges that no one agency can accomplish this transformation of the PHEPR research enterprise, and it will be necessary to leverage the strengths of different partners, including funding partners, in these efforts. A critical component of the committee's proposed framework is the development of a research agenda to galvanize the PHEPR research enterprise to meet the needs and respond to the concerns of PHEPR practitioners and society at large. The process for establishing research priorities should be both top down and bottom up and needs to recognize the transdisciplinary nature of this unique discipline. An important consideration is for the process to be inclusive of governmental, nongovernmental, private, and academic organizations, as well as broad public input from practitioners, policy makers, researchers, and communities.

RECOMMENDATION 3: Develop a National Public Health Emergency Preparedness and Response (PHEPR) Science Framework

To enhance and expand the evidence base for PHEPR practices and translation of the science to the practice community, the Centers for Disease Control and Prevention should work with other relevant funding agencies; state, local, tribal, and territorial public health agencies; academic researchers; professional associations; and other stakeholders to develop a National PHEPR Science Framework so as to ensure resourcing, coordination, monitoring, and execution of public- and private-sector PHEPR research. The National PHEPR Science Framework should do the following:

- Build on and improve coordination, integration, and alignment among existing PHEPR research efforts (e.g., the National Institute of Environmental Health Sciences Disaster Research Response Program), and ensure integration of these efforts with the activities of the PHEPR evidence-based guidelines group proposed in Recommendation 1.
- Recognize and support PHEPR science as a unique academic discipline within the broader public health field to address the substantial need for research and diverse and qualified researchers.
- Create a common, robust, and forward-looking PHEPR research agenda that supports advancement beyond traditional epidemiological research to include research in the fields of social science, implementation science, complex interventions, and quality improvement, as well as intervention, operations, systems, and cost-effectiveness research.

- Support meaningful partnerships between PHEPR practitioners and researchers, and develop strategies to better ensure that PHEPR research is relevant to practice.
- Prioritize sustainable strategies and mechanisms for the translation, dissemination, and implementation of PHEPR research.

RECOMMENDATION 4: Ensure Infrastructure and Funding to Support Public Health Emergency Preparedness and Response (PHEPR) Research
The Centers for Disease Control and Prevention (CDC), in collaboration with other relevant funding agencies, should ensure adequate and sustained oversight, coordination, and funding to support a National PHEPR Science Framework and to further develop the infrastructure necessary to support more efficient production of and better-quality PHEPR research. Such infrastructure should include

- sustained funding for practice-based and investigator-driven research that allows for the progression from exploratory to effectiveness to scale-up research and encourages researcher diversity;
- support for partnerships (e.g., with academic institutions, hospital systems, and state, local, tribal, and territorial public health agencies) to facilitate collaboration in research on the preparedness, response, and recovery phases of a public health emergency;
- development of a rapid research funding mechanism and interdisciplinary rapid response teams with applied research expertise (similar to CDC's Epidemic Intelligence Service) for deployment to conduct just-in-time studies related to the implementation of PHEPR practices at the time of events; and
- enhanced mechanisms to enable routine, standardized, efficient data collection with minimal disruption to delivery of services (including preapproved, adaptable research and institutional review board protocols and a research arm within the response structure).

Supporting Methodological Improvements to PHEPR Research and Practice Evaluation

Improving and expanding the evidence base as envisioned through the proposed National PHEPR Science Framework will require incentives for PHEPR researchers and practitioners. As discussed further in Chapter 8, other disciplines (e.g., education) have improved the quality and usefulness of the evidence base by setting priorities and standards for research and using them to guide funding decisions. Similar improvements could be achieved in the PHEPR field if the experiences of these other fields can be leveraged to implement policies and practices that can improve how PHEPR research is conducted, disseminated, and translated into practice. The goal should be to ensure that scarce evaluation dollars are used most productively to advance the evidence available to inform policy and practice. Achieving this goal will necessitate the careful balancing of several factors: the importance of the questions studied, the rigor with which those questions can and will be studied, the timeliness of the research findings, and the accessibility and usability of those findings.

Going forward, there is a need for clear guidelines for evaluation methods and study designs that will produce credible answers to various types of questions important to the PHEPR field. Though important for causal inference, experimental study designs are not the only method for exploring what works in PHEPR (and when, why, and for whom). Well-crafted guidance will incorporate the full range of research and evaluation methods, from exploratory case studies to randomized controlled trials and modeling studies. Qualitative research methodologies (e.g., ethnographic observations, interviews, and focus group discussions) can inform why and how PHEPR practices may or may not be effective, which may help explain study results or inform intervention design, and can also be useful in generating theories that can be tested empirically. As PHEPR research is transdisciplinary, design methodologies used in such fields as public health services and systems research, operations research, organizational research, and quality improvement can also provide evidence for understanding PHEPR practices. Behavioral and social science approaches may be particularly useful in elucidating contextual factors (social, political, cultural, historical, psychological) that may facilitate or constrain specific PHEPR outcomes. Simulation-based methods (e.g., exercises), systematic expert opinion methodologies (e.g., Delphi's), and systems science approaches (e.g., social network analyses, causal process diagrams, adaptive systems theories, modeling, machine learning, and big data analyses) can provide insight on systems-level outcomes and the interdependent relationships among the many components of the PHEPR system. Moreover, comprehensive guidance will include suggestions for strategically mixing methods to enhance understanding of the findings, including their breadth and limitations. The PHEPR research community would also be strengthened by the development of a unified taxonomy of research methods, accompanied by guidelines for judging the credibility of study findings intended to address various types of questions. Needed as well are guidelines for reporting the design and results of evaluations of the effectiveness of PHEPR practices to promote the transparency and reproducibility of research, as well as to facilitate implementation in practice settings. Federal funding agencies, professional associations, and journals all have important roles in the adoption of and commitment to reporting standards.

RECOMMENDATION 5: Improve the Conduct and Reporting of Public Health Emergency Preparedness and Response (PHEPR) Research
The Centers for Disease Control and Prevention, the Office of the Assistant Secretary for Preparedness and Response, the National Institutes of Health, the U.S. Department of Homeland Security, the National Science Foundation, and other relevant PHEPR research funders should use funding requirements to drive needed improvements in the conduct and reporting of research on the effectiveness and implementation of PHEPR practices. Such efforts should include

- developing guidance on and incorporating into funding decisions the use of appropriate research methods as determined by the level of research (e.g., exploratory, effectiveness, scale-up) and type of research question(s) being addressed, including but not limited to encouraging the use of concurrent comparison groups when feasible and assessment of baseline measures;
- establishing guidelines for evaluations using different designs and evidence streams and concepts from emerging evaluation approaches, such as complex intervention evaluations; and
- developing reporting guidelines, including essential reporting elements (e.g., addressing contextual factors, confounding factors, and negative results), in partnership with professional associations, journal editors, researchers, and methodologists for PHEPR intervention studies.

Public health agencies and PHEPR practitioners also need incentives to contribute to expanding the quality of the evidence base. Much of the available PHEPR evidence related to effectiveness and implementation is currently practice-based evidence that is largely descriptive and generated from evaluations in real-world contexts, such as after action reports (AARs).[4] It is vital to determine how to best use this type of evidence for informing practice in the immediate future and to improve its evidentiary value. In particular, though imperfect, AARs have the potential to offer rich information about what works, why, and how, and their use to advance the science could be greatly facilitated if the data they contain were increasingly reliable and capable of being analyzed in a systematic and rigorous manner. To help ensure that future AARs result in more useful and meaningful information for the evaluation of PHEPR practices (including the establishment of credible baselines for evaluation), it will be necessary to focus on strengthening methodological approaches, establishing mechanisms for analysis and dissemination of lessons learned from the reviews, and fostering a culture of improvement.

RECOMMENDATION 6: Pursue Efforts to Further a Process of Quality Improvement to Enhance the Quality and Utility of After Action Reports (AARs)
The Centers for Disease Control and Prevention, in collaboration with the Office of the Assistant Secretary for Preparedness and Response and the Federal Emergency Management Agency, should convene an expert panel of relevant federal agencies; state, local, tribal, and territorial public health agencies; and professional associations to advance a process for quality improvement at the local, regional, state, and national levels to enhance the quality and utility of AARs and support their use as sources of evidence for evaluating the effectiveness of public health emergency preparedness and response (PHEPR) practices. This process should foster a culture of improvement in public health emergency response and include, but not be limited to, discussions aimed at

- raising standards and expectations regarding the quality of information reported in AARs by defining the essential core elements of a PHEPR AAR;
- establishing an independent review panel with a standardized after action reporting process, with the aims of reducing bias and increasing the utility of AARs produced following public health emergency responses;
- establishing and maintaining a national repository of AARs or of reports based on analysis of AARs that is readily accessible to support the dissemination of key findings, lessons learned, and best practices for public health emergency response; and
- exploring the relevant privacy issues and the protection of information in AARs from use in legal proceedings or other punitive actions against practitioners and organizations, as has been done for "peer-review" data in other fields (medicine, aviation, and occupational health).

Training and Supporting the PHEPR Practitioner and Researcher Workforce

Expanding and improving the PHEPR evidence base will depend on developing and supporting PHEPR researchers and practitioners with the skills necessary to ensure the conduct of quality PHEPR research and program evaluation, respectively, and on strengthening

[4] AARs are documents created by public health authorities and other response organizations following an emergency or exercise, primarily for the purposes of quality improvement. They contain narrative descriptions of what was done, but may also contain "lessons learned" (i.e., what was perceived to work well and not well) and recommendations for future responses.

the implementation capacity of SLTT public health agencies. PHEPR practitioners often lack opportunities to develop and maintain research and evaluation skills. Moreover, not everyone is equally suited or professionally able to be both a practitioner and a researcher. It is therefore necessary to develop stronger systems, infrastructure, and norms around the notion of an integrated PHEPR research and practice system that includes both those focused on advancing the science and those applying this knowledge. Such enhancements of workforce capacity, which have the potential to bridge the traditional divide between practice and research, could be achieved through a combination of training, technical assistance, peer networking, and sustainable practitioner–researcher partnerships. On the research side, there has been virtually no investment in the development of a researcher pipeline, a gap that also reflects the relative dearth of funding opportunities for PHEPR research. Ensuring a diverse, adequately trained, and sufficiently available interdisciplinary cadre of disaster researchers will require investment in improved researcher training programs and grants (e.g., career development awards), particularly those aimed at increasing PHEPR research capacity to evaluate complex interventions and present findings in a succinct and accessible manner.

RECOMMENDATION 7: Support Workforce Capacity Development and Technical Assistance Programs for Public Health Emergency Preparedness and Response (PHEPR) Researchers and Practitioners

The Centers for Disease Control and Prevention (CDC) and the Office of the Assistant Secretary for Preparedness and Response should work with professional and academic organizations that represent multiple disciplines to guide and support the creation of the workforce capacity development and technical assistance programs necessary to ensure the conduct of quality PHEPR research and evaluation and improve the implementation capacity of state, local, tribal, and territorial public health agencies. Such efforts should include

- developing a research training infrastructure and career development grants—institutional and individual predoctoral, postdoctoral, loan repayment, and career awards—to develop and support researchers in PHEPR in order to address research gaps in the field;
- providing training grants so that PHEPR researcher and practitioner teams can learn how to develop PHEPR practices that are grounded in science and theory and to evaluate the effectiveness and implementation of PHEPR practices using rigorous and appropriate designs;
- providing ongoing technical assistance and peer networking for both PHEPR researchers and practitioners; and
- creating a training and certification program for CDC project officers and state preparedness directors to ensure their familiarity with evidence-based practices and promote consistent creation and evaluation of real-world evidence as captured in after action reports.

DEVELOPING AN EVIDENCE-BASED PROCESS TO INFORM PHEPR DECISION MAKING

The research and other evidence generated by the proposed National PHEPR Science Framework will be useful to PHEPR practitioners only if it can be synthesized and translated into evidence-based practices. Systems for evaluating the evidence supporting given practices and interventions are a valued resource for practitioners, policy makers, and others who seek to use the best available evidence for decision making, but who lack the time, resources, or expertise needed to review and interpret a large and potentially inconsistent body of evidence. In response to its charge and to support PHEPR practitioners' decision making, the committee developed a transparent process for systematically reviewing and evaluating PHEPR evidence and for understanding the balance of benefits and harms of PHEPR practices.

Developing and Applying an Evidence Review and Evaluation Methodology

In developing its methodology, the committee considered ways to address a number of challenges that characterize the PHEPR evidence base. The PHEPR system is an inherently complex one that encompasses policies, organizations, and programs. Its complexity also stems in part from the nature of public health emergencies, which are often unpredictable, may evolve rapidly, and are highly heterogeneous in terms of setting and type (e.g., weather events, disease outbreaks, terrorist events). "Setting" in this context is not limited to geographic location, but also encompasses the sociocultural and demographic environment and the characteristics of the communities and the responding agencies (e.g., organizational structure, managerial experience, capabilities, and resources). PHEPR practices themselves may also be complex, featuring multiple interacting components that target multiple levels (e.g., individual, population, system), and implementation is often tailored to local conditions. Consequently, a considerable challenge when reviewing evidence to determine the effectiveness of PHEPR practices and implementation strategies relates to the often convoluted and uncertain links between practices and important health outcomes (morbidity and mortality), as well as other potential outcomes of interest (e.g., organizational, economic, or social).

Because of these characteristics and based on a review of the literature and discussions with experts,[5] the committee concluded that none of the evidence evaluation frameworks it reviewed were sufficiently flexible, by themselves, to be universally applicable to all of the questions of interest to PHEPR practitioners and researchers without adaptation. Nor would existing methods be ideally suited to the context-sensitive nature of PHEPR practices and the diversity of evidence types and outcomes of interest, many of which are at the level of organizations or systems and thus often difficult to measure. Therefore, the committee developed a fit-for-purpose, mixed-method review methodology, drawing on—and in some cases adapting—elements of existing frameworks and approaches that were deemed most applicable to PHEPR, including those of the Community Preventive Services Task Force and Grading of Recommendations Assessment, Development and Evaluation (GRADE), as well as GRADE-Confidence in the Evidence from Reviews of Qualitative Research (CERQual) for qualitative evidence. This approach enabled the committee to use the appropriate methodology to answer different types of questions of interest to PHEPR stakeholders.

The committee's approach also was informed by more recently developed and evolving methods for the review and evaluation of interventions that are complex or implemented within complex systems, methods that focus on the integration of diverse and heterogeneous types of evidence. The PHEPR system draws on a broad evidence base, ranging from randomized controlled trials to surveys, modeling studies, and AARs, and the committee's methodology needed to accommodate that diversity. In addition to both quantitative and qualitative research-based evidence, the approach makes use of experiential evidence from

[5] The committee held a 1-day public workshop on evidence evaluation frameworks used in health and nonhealth fields, which is documented separately in a Proceedings of a Workshop—in Brief (see Appendix E).

past response scenarios. This feature of the committee's approach offers the potential for validation of research findings in practice settings, as well as improved understanding of context effects, trade-offs, and the range of implementation approaches or components for a given practice. In applying this approach, nonempiric evidence was mapped onto research findings from quantitative and qualitative syntheses to consider the coherence of evidence from across methodological streams (including evidence from quantitative impact studies, cross-sectional surveys, modeling studies, qualitative studies, case reports, and AARs, as well as parallel and mechanistic evidence[6]), and thereby to assess the certainty of the evidence (COE) of effectiveness for a practice (refer to the left side of Figure S-2) and develop summary findings for each element of the committee's Evidence to Decision (EtD) framework (refer to the right side of Figure S-2). The EtD framework enabled the committee to take into account systematically the balance of benefits and harms of a practice, the acceptability of the practice and stakeholder preferences, feasibility and PHEPR system considerations, resource and economic considerations, equity, and ethical issues in decisions regarding practice recommendations.

A key element of the committee's task was to develop and apply criteria for the selection of PHEPR practices to include in the systematic reviews. Rather than using a sequential approach involving the development of the evidence review and evaluation methodology in the abstract and then applying this methodology to the PHEPR practices selected for review, the committee selected the practices with the intent of using them to simultaneously develop and test the methodology through a highly iterative process, the steps of which are described in detail in Chapter 3. The practice selection criteria, therefore, were developed with the aim of yielding a set of PHEPR practices that would be diverse with respect to both the research and evaluation methodologies used to generate the evidence base for them and their characteristics, such as the type and scope of event in which a practice is implemented, the practice setting, whether the practice is complex or simple, whether it is within the direct purview of public health agencies, and whether it is preparedness or response oriented. This process was intended to result in a methodology that would be applicable across the full range of PHEPR practices. The committee also engaged with stakeholders (PHEPR practitioners and policy makers)[7] and referred to published literature identifying practitioners' research needs to inform the selection of practices to review. This selection process, which is depicted in Figure 3-1, yielded the following four practices[8] as the focus of the committee's review and this report:

- engaging with and training community-based partners to improve the outcomes of at-risk populations[9] after public health emergencies (falls under Capability 1, Community Preparedness);

[6] For the purposes of this report, the committee defined mechanistic evidence as evidence that denotes relationships for which causality has been established—generally within other scientific fields, such as chemistry, biology, economics, and physics—and that can reasonably be applied to the PHEPR context through mechanistic reasoning, defined as "the inference from mechanisms to claims that an intervention produced" an outcome.

[7] Stakeholder engagement occurred through the committee's public meetings and through discussions with SLTT PHEPR practitioner consultants appointed to advise the committee on the systematic literature review process. The Delphi-like practitioner engagement activity described in Appendix A was conducted after the committee's four evidence review topics had been selected and therefore did not inform the selection process. The activity was intended to inform priorities for future PHEPR evidence reviews.

[8] The review topics were selected prior to the COVID-19 pandemic.

[9] For the purposes of this report, the committee defined at-risk populations as comprising individuals with social and/or structural vulnerabilities whose access and functional needs may not be fully met by traditional service providers or who feel they cannot comfortably or safely use the standard resources offered during preparedness, response, and recovery efforts. A more comprehensive description of at-risk populations is provided in Box 4-1 in Chapter 4.

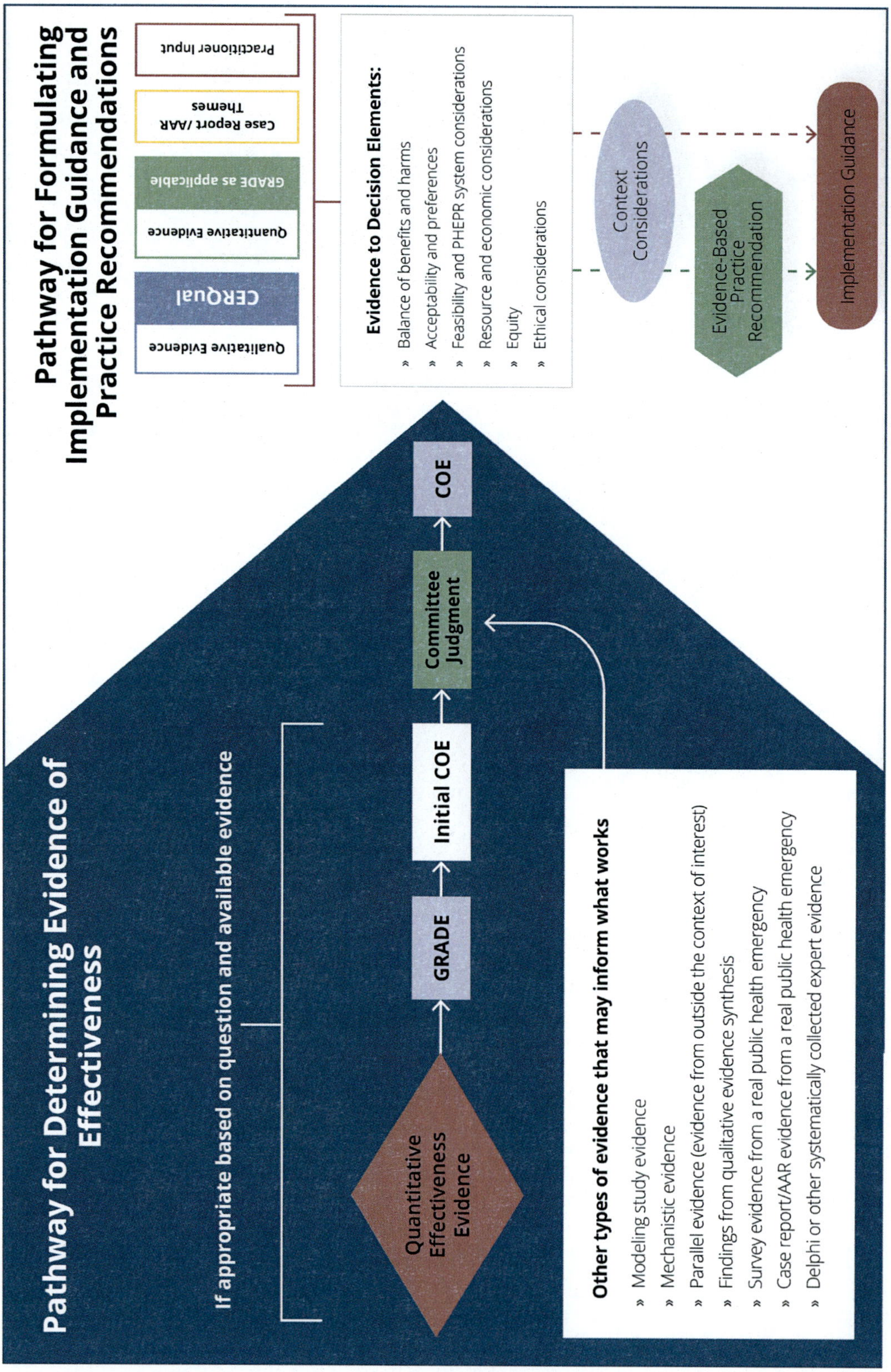
Pathway for Determining Evidence of Effectiveness
If appropriate based on question and available evidence
Quantitative Effectiveness Evidence
GRADE
Initial COE
Committee Judgment
COE
Other types of evidence that may inform what works
» Modeling study evidence
» Mechanistic evidence
» Parallel evidence (evidence from outside the context of interest)
» Findings from qualitative evidence synthesis
» Survey evidence from a real public health emergency
» Case report/AAR evidence from a real public health emergency
» Delphi or other systematically collected expert evidence
Pathway for Formulating Implementation Guidance and Practice Recommendations
Qualitative Evidence
CERQual
Quantitative Evidence
GRADE as applicable
Case Report /AAR Themes
Practitioner Input
Evidence to Decision Elements:
» Balance of benefits and harms
» Acceptability and preferences
» Feasibility and PHEPR system considerations
» Resource and economic considerations
» Equity
» Ethical considerations
Context Considerations
Evidence-Based Practice Recommendation
Implementation Guidance

FIGURE S-2 Framework for integrating evidence to inform recommendation and guidance development for PHEPR practices.

NOTES: This framework is intended for those interested in the details of the committee's methodology for evaluating evidence for PHEPR practices. Depicted are two interconnected pathways. The lefthand panel (blue) shows the committee's process for integrating evidence from quantitative impact studies with other evidence that may inform what works to determine the certainty of the evidence (COE) of effectiveness for a given outcome. The COE (for all relevant outcomes) feeds into the righthand panel (white), which shows the pathways for integrating diverse evidence for various elements (evidence to decision elements) that, along with context considerations, may inform the formulation of evidence-based practice recommendations and implementation guidance. In cases in which the review is focused on implementation and not on determining the effectiveness of a practice, it is possible to follow the pathway depicted in the righthand panel without assessing the COE as shown in the lefthand panel. Other types of evidence that may inform what works may be used to examine coherence with direct quantitative effectiveness evidence or may be used to inform committee judgment in the absence of direct quantitative evidence. AAR = after action report; CERQual = Confidence in the Evidence from Reviews of Qualitative Research; COE = certainty of the evidence; GRADE = Grading of Recommendations Assessment, Development and Evaluation; PHEPR = public health emergency preparedness and response.

- activating a public health emergency operations center (Capability 3, Emergency Operations Coordination [EOC]);
- communicating public health alerts and guidance with technical audiences during a public health emergency (Capability 6, Information Sharing); and
- implementing quarantine to reduce or stop the spread of a contagious disease (Capability 11, Non-Pharmaceutical Interventions).

Key findings and practice recommendations for each of these four review topics are presented in Table S-1. A summary of the review findings supporting the practice recommendations and/or implementation guidance for each of these four practices are presented in Chapters 4–7, respectively. The four chapters each begin with a two-page action sheet summarizing key review findings, recommendations, and guidance for practitioners; detailed descriptions of the evidence are provided in Appendixes B1–B4. Despite the limitations of the evidence base—which was often sparse and characterized by a predominance of descriptive reports and studies with notable shortcomings in their design or conduct—and challenges in the application of GRADE to practices that are dependent on context and implementation fidelity, the committee's mixed-method, layering approach enabled the development of practice recommendations for three of the four review topics. For the fourth topic (activating a public health emergency operations center), the committee was able to draw on qualitative and experiential evidence to identify specific considerations to guide decision making regarding EOC activation, thus demonstrating the utility of the methodology for answering operational questions of interest to PHEPR practitioners concerning implementation even in the absence of evidence of effect.

TABLE S-1 Key Findings and Practice Recommendations from the Committee's Evidence Review and Evaluation Process

Review Topic	Key Review Findings	Recommendation
Engaging with and training community-based partners to improve the outcomes of at-risk populations after public health emergencies	Culturally tailored preparedness training programs for community-based partners (CBPs) and at-risk populations they serve improve the public health emergency preparedness and response (PHEPR) knowledge (moderate certainty of the evidence [COE]) and preparedness behaviors (moderate COE) of trained at-risk populations. CBPs appear to support and value engagement and training, particularly when implemented using a participatory approach, but capacity limitations for both CBPs and public health organizations should be considered when selecting specific strategies.	Practice Recommendation: Engaging and training CBPs serving at-risk populations is recommended as part of state, local, tribal, and territorial (SLTT) public health agencies' community preparedness efforts so that those CBPs are better able to assist at-risk populations they serve in preparing for and recovering from public health emergencies. Recommended CBP training strategies include • the use of materials, curricula, and training formats targeted and/or tailored to the individual CBPs and the at-risk populations they serve; and • train-the-trainer approaches that utilize peer or other trusted trainers to train at-risk populations. CBP engagement and training should be accompanied by targeted monitoring and outcome evaluation or conducted in the context of research when feasible so as to improve the evidence base for engagement and training strategies.

TABLE S-1 Continued

Review Topic	Key Review Findings	Recommendation
Activating a public health emergency operations center (PHEOC)	Partly because of its long tenure as a common and standard practice, direct research evidence does not focus on whether a PHEOC should be utilized, but rather on how it should be implemented. Experiential evidence from a synthesis of case reports and after action reports (from within and outside of PHEPR) suggests that PHEOCs are probably effective at improving response and may have few undesirable effects in the short term, and speaks to the confidence in the PHEOC model among experienced practitioners across diverse situations. PHEPR practitioners consider activating public health emergency operations to be an acceptable and justifiable practice. The feasibility of this practice is variable, and the evidence highlights several feasibility issues to consider before public health emergency operations are activated.	Activating a PHEOC is a common and standard practice, supported by national and international guidance and based on earlier social science around disaster response. Despite widespread use and minimal apparent harms, there is insufficient evidence to determine the effectiveness of activating a PHEOC or of specific PHEOC components at improving response. This does not mean that the practice does not work or should not be implemented, but that more research and monitoring and evaluation around how and in what circumstances a PHEOC should be implemented are warranted before an evidence-based practice recommendation can be made.
Communicating public health alerts and guidance with technical audiences during a public health emergency	Electronic messaging systems, such as email, fax, and text messaging, are effective communication channels for increasing technical audiences' awareness of public health alerts and guidance during a public health emergency (moderate COE). Technologies employed as electronic messaging systems for communicating public health alerts and guidance to technical audiences during a public health emergency to increase awareness and appropriate guidance use have differing impacts. However, the available data are insufficient to support a conclusion as to what technology is best for which audiences in which scenarios. Reported harms are not related to the particular medium, but to how communication strategies are implemented (e.g., alert fatigue/information overload, leaving people out of the messaging loop, guidance not aligning with what is feasible).	Practice Recommendation: Inclusion of electronic messaging channels (e.g., email) is recommended as part of SLTT public health agencies' multipronged approach for communicating public health alerts and guidance to technical audiences in preparation for and in response to public health emergencies. The practice should be accompanied by targeted monitoring and evaluation or conducted in the context of research when feasible so as to improve the evidence base for strategies used to communicate public health alerts and guidance to technical audiences.
Implementing quarantine to reduce or stop the spread of a contagious disease	Quarantine can be effective at reducing overall contagious disease transmission in the community in certain circumstances (high COE), but can be associated with harms, including • increased risk of infection among those in a shared setting (high COE); • psychological harms, the risk of which increases with the longer duration of quarantine (moderate COE); and • individual financial hardship (high COE). Concerns about undesirable effects and harms may make this practice unacceptable to some communities. Implementing quarantine effectively, especially at a large scale, is very challenging and resource intensive, and the evidence highlights several feasibility issues with respect to implementation.	Practice Recommendation: Implementation of quarantine by SLTT public health agencies is recommended to reduce disease transmission and associated morbidity and mortality during an outbreak only after consideration of the best available science regarding the characteristics of the disease, the expected balance of benefits and harms, and the feasibility of implementation.

Enduring Support for Ongoing PHEPR Evidence Reviews

In developing the systematic review and evidence evaluation methodology described above, the committee aimed for a process with sufficient flexibility not only to accommodate the diversity of evidence for the four selected PHEPR practices but also to be applied and adapted as needed to support future PHEPR evidence reviews. While the committee acknowledges that tools other than systematic review methods may be useful in addressing the evidentiary needs of PHEPR practitioners and policy makers, there remains a clear need for an ongoing process that can be used to generate evidence-based PHEPR recommendations and guidelines. Given the time and resource requirements associated with conducting systematic reviews, the committee was limited to reviewing only the small selection of PHEPR practices described in Table S-1 as proof of concept. Hundreds of such reviews could be conducted to guide practitioners in operationalizing the CDC PHEPR Capabilities. Moreover, the evidence base for PHEPR practices is continually evolving with the field. As new studies and reports are published, it will be essential to have a sustained mechanism for capturing and analyzing new evidence over time and for updating prior reviews as needed. In addition to guiding PHEPR practice and decision making, such a mechanism has the potential to drive improvements in the evidence base over time and guide the research agenda through the identification of evidence gaps.

Given the complexity of the committee's review methodology, the implications for the multidisciplinary group of experts who will need to be involved in future reviews, and the importance of practice guidelines being issued by an authoritative source with the trust of the PHEPR community and the ability to disseminate this guidance widely, the committee concludes that a centralized approach supported by CDC is the best model for a process for ongoing evidence reviews of PHEPR practices. A sustainable evidence-based review process for PHEPR practices will require organizational support and leadership; multifaceted capabilities; adequate funding; and a functional, coordinated system. The committee believes CDC should create an independent task force that would oversee methods development, topic selection, and evidence reviews; ensure appropriate external input; and generate recommendations. Importantly, as reviewers gain more experience with the evaluation of PHEPR evidence and as review methodologies continue to evolve, it will be important to assess and refine the committee's proposed methodology to ensure that it is consistent with current review and guideline development practice and is meeting the needs of PHEPR stakeholders.

RECOMMENDATION 1: Appoint a Public Health Emergency Preparedness and Response (PHEPR) Evidence-Based Guidelines Group
The Centers for Disease Control and Prevention (CDC) should appoint and support an independent group to develop methodologically rigorous and transparent evidence-based guidelines for PHEPR practices on an ongoing basis. This group should take the methodology developed by the committee as a starting point, but should also be charged with its continued development based on the full range of available evidence, incorporating advances in the synthesis of quantitative, qualitative, and experiential evidence. The group should also identify and communicate key PHEPR evidence gaps in annual reports to CDC and Congress to guide future research on the effectiveness of PHEPR practices.

RECOMMENDATION 2: Establish Infrastructure to Support Ongoing Public Health Emergency Preparedness and Response (PHEPR) Evidence Reviews
The Centers for Disease Control and Prevention should establish the infrastructure, policies, and procedures needed to ensure a sustained process for conducting and updating

evidence reviews and generating evidence-based practice guidelines, in collaboration with other relevant federal agencies. The infrastructure should include an open-access repository for evidence-based PHEPR practices.

BRIDGING THE GAP BETWEEN PHEPR RESEARCH AND PRACTICE

While there is a clear need to strengthen the evidence base for PHEPR practices through improvements in research and evaluation, an equally pressing challenge is the translation, dissemination, and implementation of the evidence to practice. It is essential for evidence-based practices to reach the hands of the policy makers and practitioners who need them most, in the most timely manner. Impediments to the uptake of evidence-based practices begin with the disconnect between PHEPR practitioners and researchers, who operate within distinct disciplines in a system that poses numerous barriers to collaboration and integration. Additional barriers include varying awareness of the existing evidence base among practitioners and a lack of guidance on how to implement evidence-based practices successfully, inadequate capacity and incentives to implement proven practices, and the failure of most studies to engage practitioners early and often. The complex nature of public health emergencies often makes it difficult to identify core practice components that are applicable across the range of such events, and additional research to identify the core components of PHEPR practices could therefore enable researchers and practitioners to better operationalize interventions in various settings. The often daunting gap between research and practice can be narrowed through such sustainable strategies and mechanisms as ensuring that research is demand-driven and training specialists in translation and implementation science, particularly for the PHEPR field. Creating a shared agenda for research and implementation is vitally important to the development and implementation of evidence-based PHEPR practices. Changes to federal programs and policy—such as asking Public Health Emergency Preparedness Cooperative Agreement grantees to use evidence-based practices when available and if not, to justify why, and leveraging such accreditation processes as that of the Public Health Accreditation Board—could facilitate the use of evidence-based practices by public health agencies.

RECOMMENDATION 8: Ensure the Translation, Dissemination, and Implementation of Public Health Emergency Preparedness and Response (PHEPR) Research to Practice
The Centers for Disease Control and Prevention (CDC) should use a coordinated implementation science approach to ensure that the evidence-based practice recommendations resulting from the PHEPR evidence-based guidelines group proposed in Recommendation 1 achieve broad reach and become the standard of practice of the target audience. Strategies to this end include

- incorporating evidence-based practices into the *Public Health Emergency Preparedness and Response Capabilities: National Standards for State, Local, Tribal, and Territorial Public Health* guidance document;
- building evidence-based practices into the design of and funding decisions for the Public Health Emergency Preparedness Cooperative Agreement program;
- incentivizing and requiring state, local, tribal, and territorial public health agencies to test and evaluate new or adapted practices and embed program evaluations into routine operations to help better understand whether evidence-based practices worked, under what conditions, with what impacts and consequences, and at what cost;

- publishing evidence-based practices in CDC communication platforms (e.g., *Morbidity and Mortality Weekly Report,* blogs) and partnering with public health professional organizations, such as the Association of State and Territorial Health Officials and the National Association of County & City Health Officials (NACCHO), to disseminate evidence-based practices;
- incorporating the requirement of utilizing evidence-based PHEPR practices into such processes as the Public Health Accreditation Board accreditation and such recognition programs as NACCHO's Project Public Health Ready; and
- incorporating implementation science principles, such as the conduct of research to understand core components required for intervention effectiveness, into PHEPR research.

CONCLUDING REMARKS

It is essential for research and continuous learning to become the expectation, not the exception, for the PHEPR field such that individuals are resourced and incentivized to conduct and participate in research, and engagement and partnerships among practitioners, communities, and researchers are promoted and maintained to build insight and trust. In short, research needs to be embedded within the PHEPR system, conducted for the PHEPR system, and applied by the PHEPR system. Grounding PHEPR practice in evidence will require transformation of both the research and practice fields. Practitioners will have to turn routinely to PHEPR research when making important decisions or implementing practices, and PHEPR researchers will have to produce research that is relevant to practitioners.

The committee is aware that the PHEPR field is relatively young and has been evolving rapidly over the past two decades. During this time, changes in policy and practice have been driven by and shaped in reaction to unexpected and often traumatic events, and rarely have been influenced by research or evidence. However, the evidence examined by the committee for this study shows a field that is maturing and will no longer be deterred by the oft-cited refrain that the relative rarity of public health emergencies prohibits the development of an evidence base for PHEPR. The nation is increasingly facing public health emergencies that present opportunities to observe and learn and conduct real-time research in order to develop a strong empirical and analytical evidence base. Most recently, the emergence of COVID-19 has highlighted critical evidence gaps and lost opportunities to expand the PHEPR evidence base. As discussed in the "Note on COVID-19" included in the Preface to this report, the COVID-19 pandemic reinforces the critical, ongoing need to have processes and programs in place to perform research and evaluation, even in real time, to better inform future decisions. Without such efforts, practitioners will continue to implement ineffective or inappropriate practices that risk wasting valuable resources and failing to protect the public's health, and the ultimate result will be the needless loss of lives during this and future public health emergencies. As this report demonstrates, it is clear that, while challenging, strategies exist for remedying the lack of an established scientific evidence base in the PHEPR field. As the PHEPR research field continues to evolve and mature, it is the committee's assertion that such an evidence base represents the essential foundation of future policy and practice changes.

1

Advancing Public Health Emergency Preparedness and Response System Capabilities to Respond to Increasing Threats

Communities across the nation are increasingly facing complex public health emergencies. State, local, tribal, and territorial (SLTT) public health agencies play a vital role in protecting and securing the nation's health. These agencies routinely make difficult decisions on the front lines of emergency response and recovery and must be prepared to respond effectively to diverse public health threats, including infectious diseases, natural disasters, and human-made events. Yet, little concerted effort has been made to establish a scientific evidence base to guide and inform the actions of SLTT public health agencies, and public health emergency preparedness and response (PHEPR) practitioners in particular. The PHEPR field consequently has been based largely on long-standing rather than evidence-based practice.

PHEPR practitioners require knowledge of evidence-based practices to make effective decisions regarding strategies to mitigate the impact of public health emergencies on the public's health and to save lives. As the nation approaches two decades since September 11, 2001, this is an opportune time to take stock of the state of the evidence on PHEPR practices and the improvements necessary to move the field forward and to strengthen the PHEPR system. Without efforts to synthesize and evaluate PHEPR research in a coherent, transparent, and rigorous manner, practitioners will continue to implement ineffective or inappropriate practices that waste valuable resources and fail to protect the public's health, researchers will continue to face difficulty in identifying critical research gaps, and funders will continue to be challenged by deciding where to focus their resources. The PHEPR field needs to be informed by and grounded in robust evidence for what works, where, why, and for whom. This report documents the results of a study undertaken to examine the actions, opportunities, and resources necessary to achieve this vision.

This chapter presents the study charge, the study committee's conceptual framework for a complex PHEPR system, and the underlying reasons for the current state of the PHEPR evidence base, and explains the importance of a process for the development of evidence-based PHEPR guidelines. It concludes with an overview of the report.

STUDY CHARGE

Recognizing that the research in the PHEPR field has not been synthesized and evaluated in a coherent manner and seeking to ensure the development of an evidence-based culture within the PHEPR field, the Centers for Disease Control and Prevention (CDC) charged the National Academies of Sciences, Engineering, and Medicine with developing the methodology for and subsequently conducting a systematic review and evaluation[1] of the evidence for PHEPR practices. The committee was also charged with providing recommendations for future research needed to address critical gaps in evidence-based PHEPR practices, as well as processes needed to improve the overall quality of evidence within the field. The full charge to the committee is presented in Box 1-1. To respond to this charge, the National Academies convened a 20-member ad hoc committee comprised of experts in the fields of PHEPR practice, PHEPR research, quantitative and qualitative evidence review methodology, operations and systems research, and ethics. Biographies of the committee members are presented in Appendix F.

[1] Although the term "comprehensive review" was used in the committee's Statement of Task (see Box 1-1), the committee uses the field-accepted term "systematic review" throughout this report. The committee applied a mixed-method approach to its systematic review.

BOX 1-1 STATEMENT OF TASK

The National Academies of Sciences, Engineering, and Medicine will appoint an ad hoc committee to conduct a comprehensive review and grading of existing evidence for public health emergency preparedness and response (PHEPR) practices generated since September 11, 2001. The committee will use published literature, gray literature including publicly available reports, public input and information-gathering sessions, and the committee's original analysis and reasoning to determine which of the 15 Capabilities ("PHEPR Capabilities") defined in the Centers for Disease Control and Prevention's *Public Health Emergency Preparedness and Response Capabilities: National Standards for State, Local, Tribal, and Territorial Public Health* to prioritize for inclusion in the comprehensive review, with an emphasis given to those capabilities determined by the committee to be most critical to preparedness and response. In identifying preparedness and response practices to evaluate for each of the prioritized PHEPR capabilities and functions, the committee will focus on practices applicable to state, territorial, local, and tribal public health preparedness and response practitioners. Specifically, the committee will

1. Develop the methodology for conducting a comprehensive review of the evidence base for public health preparedness and response practices, including the criteria by which to assess the strength of evidence for specific practices and a tiered grading scheme (e.g., best, promising; A-level, B-level, etc.) to be applied in the development of recommendations for evidence-based practices. In doing so, the committee should draw from accepted scientific approaches for comprehensive literature review and existing models for assessing and grading strength of evidence (e.g., the evidence strength assessment model used for The Guide to Community Preventive Services);
2. Develop and apply criteria to determine which PHEPR Capabilities and sub-functions should be prioritized for inclusion in the comprehensive review, along with other topics that have emerged as important across multiple capabilities but which are not adequately represented within the current set (e.g., mental health, environmental health, administrative preparedness, etc.);

BOX 1-1 CONTINUED

3. Identify research regarding preparedness and response practices within the prioritized PHEPR Capabilities and functions, and apply the committee's evidence review methodology to assess the quality of and summarize the body of evidence regarding effectiveness of these practices;
4. Develop recommendations for preparedness and response practices within the prioritized areas that communities and state, territorial, local, and/or tribal agencies should or should not adopt, based on evidence demonstrating the effectiveness or ineffectiveness of those practices; and
5. Provide recommendations for future research needed to address critical gaps in evidence-based preparedness and response practices, including, as appropriate, additional research on promising but not yet proven practices within the prioritized PHEPR Capabilities and functions, as well as processes needed to improve the overall quality of evidence within the field.

Literature regarding preparedness practices will be included for evaluation only to the extent that there is a measurable and explicit connection to response practices, as determined by the committee. Literature regarding recovery practices is not within the scope of this study, except in the event where initial recovery practices are unable to be distinguished from response practices. Literature regarding practices specific to the Hospital Preparedness Program will also be excluded from this study; however, areas where public health and health care delivery functions intersect may be included as appropriate.

CONCEPTUALIZING THE COMPLEX PHEPR SYSTEM

The Building Blocks of the PHEPR System

The PHEPR system, with its multifaceted mission to prevent, protect against, quickly respond to, and recover from public health emergencies, is inherently complex, encompassing policies, organizations, and programs (Nelson et al., 2007b). To guide the committee's approach to its task and ground the committee's thinking about the PHEPR system as a whole, the committee developed a conceptual framework to explore the complexity and various interdependencies of the current PHEPR system (see Figure 1-1).

Since 2011, 15 foundational capabilities set forth by CDC have guided public health agencies in assessing, building, and sustaining PHEPR capacity (CDC, 2018). Before 2011, there were no standards to guide the PHEPR work of public health agencies. These 15 capabilities, updated in 2018, are defined in the agency's *Public Health Emergency Preparedness and Response Capabilities: National Standards for State, Local, Tribal, and Territorial Public Health* (PHEPR Capabilities) (CDC, 2018; Martinez et al., 2019) (see Box 1-2). While the committee was charged with reviewing the evidence for practices specifically encompassed within the PHEPR Capabilities, this report is designed to be useful to those who have roles in PHEPR but are guided by different doctrines, such as first responders, health care stakeholders, and emergency management professionals.

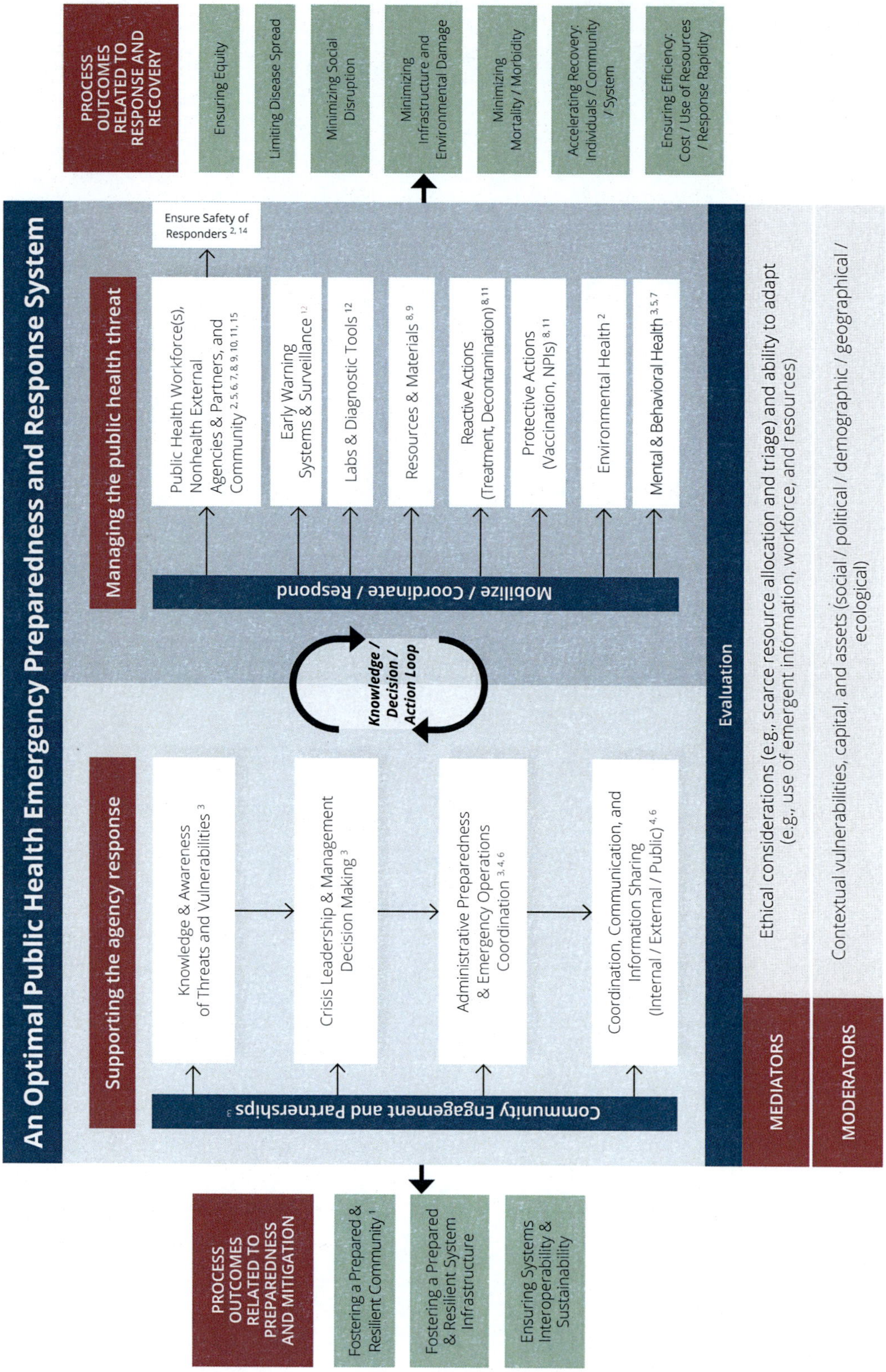
An Optimal Public Health Emergency Preparedness and Response System
Supporting the agency response
Community Engagement and Partnerships 3
Knowledge & Awareness of Threats and Vulnerabilities 3
Crisis Leadership & Management Decision Making 3
Administrative Preparedness & Emergency Operations Coordination 3,4,6
Coordination, Communication, and Information Sharing (Internal / External / Public) 4,6
Knowledge / Decision / Action Loop
Managing the public health threat
Mobilize / Coordinate / Respond
Public Health Workforce(s), Nonhealth External Agencies & Partners, and Community 2,5,6,7,8,9,10,11,15
Ensure Safety of Responders 2,14
Early Warning Systems & Surveillance 12
Labs & Diagnostic Tools 12
Resources & Materials 8,9
Reactive Actions (Treatment, Decontamination) 8,11
Protective Actions (Vaccination, NPIs) 8,11
Environmental Health 2
Mental & Behavioral Health 3,5,7
Evaluation
MEDIATORS
Ethical considerations (e.g., scarce resource allocation and triage) and ability to adapt (e.g., use of emergent information, workforce, and resources)
MODERATORS
Contextual vulnerabilities, capital, and assets (social / political / demographic / geographical / ecological)
PROCESS OUTCOMES RELATED TO RESPONSE AND RECOVERY
Ensuring Equity
Limiting Disease Spread
Minimizing Social Disruption
Minimizing Infrastructure and Environmental Damage
Minimizing Mortality / Morbidity
Accelerating Recovery: Individuals / Community / System
Ensuring Efficiency: Cost / Use of Resources / Response Rapidity
PROCESS OUTCOMES RELATED TO PREPAREDNESS AND MITIGATION
Fostering a Prepared & Resilient Community 1
Fostering a Prepared & Resilient System Infrastructure
Ensuring Systems Interoperability & Sustainability

FIGURE 1-1 Conceptual framework for an optimal PHEPR system.
NOTE: The numbers shown on the figure denote the pertinent PHEPR Capabilities:

1. Community Preparedness
2. Community Recovery
3. Emergency Operations Coordination
4. Emergency Public Information and Warning
5. Fatality Management
6. Information Sharing
7. Mass Care
8. Medical Countermeasure Dispensing and Administration
9. Medical Materiel Management and Distribution
10. Medical Surge
11. Non-Pharmaceutical Interventions (NPIs)
12. Public Health Laboratory Testing
13. Public Health Surveillance and Epidemiological Investigation
14. Responder Safety and Health
15. Volunteer Management

BOX 1-2 ***PUBLIC HEALTH EMERGENCY PREPAREDNESS AND RESPONSE CAPABILITIES: NATIONAL STANDARDS FOR STATE, LOCAL, TRIBAL, AND TERRITORIAL PUBLIC HEALTH***

The public health emergency preparedness and response (PHEPR) Capabilities are a set of 15 distinct yet interrelated capability standards designed to advance the emergency preparedness and response capacity of state and local public health systems. The PHEPR Capabilities are organized into six domains and two tiers. Tier 1 capability standards form the foundation of PHEPR, and Tier 2 capability standards are cross-cutting. Each capability standard is comprised of functions, and each function encompasses specific tasks that are supported by resource elements.

Community Resilience
- Capability 1 – Community Preparedness (Tier 1)
- Capability 2 – Community Recovery (Tier 2)

Incident Management
- Capability 3 – Emergency Operations Coordination (Tier 1)

Information Management
- Capability 4 – Emergency Public Information and Warning (Tier 1)
- Capability 6 – Information Sharing (Tier 1)

Countermeasures and Mitigation
- Capability 8 – Medical Countermeasure Dispensing and Administration (Tier 1)
- Capability 9 – Medical Materiel Management and Distribution (Tier 1)
- Capability 11 – Non-Pharmaceutical Interventions (Tier 2)
- Capability 15 – Responder Safety and Health (Tier 1)

Surge Management
- Capability 5 – Fatality Management (Tier 2)
- Capability 7 – Mass Care (Tier 2)
- Capability 10 – Medical Surge (Tier 2)
- Capability 14 – Volunteer Management (Tier 2)

Biosurveillance
- Capability 12 – Public Health Laboratory Testing (Tier 1)
- Capability 13 – Public Health Surveillance and Epidemiological Investigation (Tier 1)

SOURCE: Excerpted from CDC, 2018.

The PHEPR Capabilities alone do not constitute the PHEPR system; rather, the system comprises the interactions among the Capabilities and the context in which they are operationalized. To develop a deeper understanding of how the PHEPR Capabilities relate to each other and to various contextual factors and interact within the complex PHEPR system, the committee conducted a search for a framework that would help visualize these relationships and interactions. Previous logic models have been developed to depict various aspects of PHEPR (CDC, 2019b; Gibson et al., 2012; Stoto et al., 2017), but these models were inadequate to capture the interconnectedness and complexity of the PHEPR system. More recently, Khan and colleagues (2018) took a complex adaptive systems approach in developing a framework to represent the essential elements and interactions between these elements for a resilient public health system. While overlap exists between some of the structural elements identified in the Khan and colleagues framework and the PHEPR Capabilities (e.g., surveillance and monitoring), the committee was interested in a framework that could encompass structure, function, context, and outcomes simultaneously. To address this gap, the committee developed the framework depicted in Figure 1-1.[2]

The committee's framework is intended to depict an adaptable and scalable PHEPR system. The framework illustrates how the PHEPR Capabilities (denoted throughout the system) fit into a larger system of governmental and nongovernmental actors. The inner rectangle of the framework represents the formal PHEPR system, and is divided into two domains: "supporting the agency response," which captures the organizational features that ought to be present among responding entities; and "managing the public health threat," which identifies the practices that may be employed to respond to an event. Each domain influences the other, as indicated by the knowledge, decision, and action loop between them. The framework reinforces that leadership, management, and critical decision making are essential to the optimal operation of a PHEPR system. To the extent possible, strategic and tactical decisions should be governed by evidence and thoughtfulness and built on a robust evidence base.

Each side of the framework yields important preparedness and response outcomes for the PHEPR system. Underlying the framework are system mediators and moderators that account for the various contextual factors that may influence the execution of PHEPR practices. Thus, the committee's conceptual framework highlights how the components of the PHEPR system are intertwined. Understanding these linkages among actors, actions, and the PHEPR Capabilities is critical to informing how certain practices may interact and affect other practices and outcomes. A PHEPR research enterprise would consider how the system as a whole achieves its desired outcomes, such as equitable response, rapid recovery, and minimized harms, in addition to considering the extent to which each Capability contributes to that outcome. In addition, in viewing the committee's conceptual framework, it is important to understand the more general and fundamental characteristics that influence how systems work (see Box 1-3).

The PHEPR system consists of a multiplicity of actors from SLTT and federal response systems and organizations, including those responsible for public health, emergency management, public safety, and health care delivery, as well as other governmental and nongovernmental organizations (IOM, 2008). The committee views the PHEPR system (and this framework) as a system nested within many integrated, larger systems. Although different sectors will frequently work in isolation, their interconnectivity is often amplified during a public health emergency. Linkov and colleagues (2014) describe how management strategies for one network (e.g., telecommunications, water, gas, transportation) may be dependent on the functionality of another. Understanding in advance of an event how these different systems will affect one another can save time and effort during the response and recovery phases, and enables researchers and practitioners to consider the trade-offs inherent in operational decisions made in the midst of an event and under conditions of uncertainty.

[2] The committee developed the conceptual framework for an optimal PHEPR system through a consensus process and based on the expert opinion of the committee members. It was intended as a heuristic device to help the committee conceptualize the systemic (interdependent) nature of the PHEPR system, and to consider the pathways through which PHEPR Capabilities may be associated with system-level outcomes. Fundamentally, it is a framing device.

BOX 1-3 COMMON SYSTEM CHARACTERISTICS

- **Self-organizing**—system dynamics arise spontaneously from internal structure
- **Constantly changing**—systems adjust and readjust at many interactive timescales
- **Tightly linked**—the high degree of connectivity means that change in one sub-system affects the others
- **Governed by feedback**—a positive or negative response that may alter the intervention or expected effects
- **Nonlinear**—relationships within a system cannot be arranged along a simple input–output line
- **History dependent**—short-term effects of intervening may differ from long-term effects
- **Counterintuitive**—cause and effect are often distant in time and space, defying solutions that pit causes close to the effects they seek to address
- **Resistant to change**—seemingly obvious solutions may fail or worsen the situation

SOURCE: Excerpted from WHO, 2009.

Defining a PHEPR Practice

In PHEPR, there is seldom a discrete "intervention" as there is in clinical medicine; therefore, **the committee defined a PHEPR practice broadly as a type of process, structure, or intervention whose implementation is intended to mitigate the adverse effects of a public health emergency on the population as a whole or a particular sub-group within the population.** Given the heterogeneity, complexity, and multicomponent nature of many PHEPR practices, the committee categorized PHEPR practices based on whether they target the individual and community, organizational, or systems level (see Figure 1-2). In addition to targeting multiple levels, PHEPR practices can be strategic (e.g., long-term planning), tactical (e.g., workflow planning), or operational (e.g., real-time intervention) and be implemented by different public health agencies (federal, SLTT).

- PHEPR practices may be aimed at **individuals** through emergency risk communication efforts, dispensing and administering of medical countermeasures, preparedness education and training initiatives, and mental health interventions during emergencies.
- PHEPR practices may be aimed at the **organizational level** through information and data sharing and situational awareness practices, administrative preparedness practices, emergency operations coordination, modules and programs for training and exercising staff, and strategies to ensure a fully staffed response.
- PHEPR practices may be aimed at the **systems level** through the conduct of jurisdictional risk assessments; mapping of the locations of at-risk populations; surveillance systems; and policies related to funding, staffing, and resources.

Consistent with the charge shown in Box 1-1, the committee took as its starting point for identifying PHEPR practices the 15 PHEPR Capabilities (see Box 1-2). CDC's *Public Health Emergency Preparedness and Response Capabilities: National Standards for State, Local, Tribal, and Territorial Public Health* does not define PHEPR practices per se. Instead, each

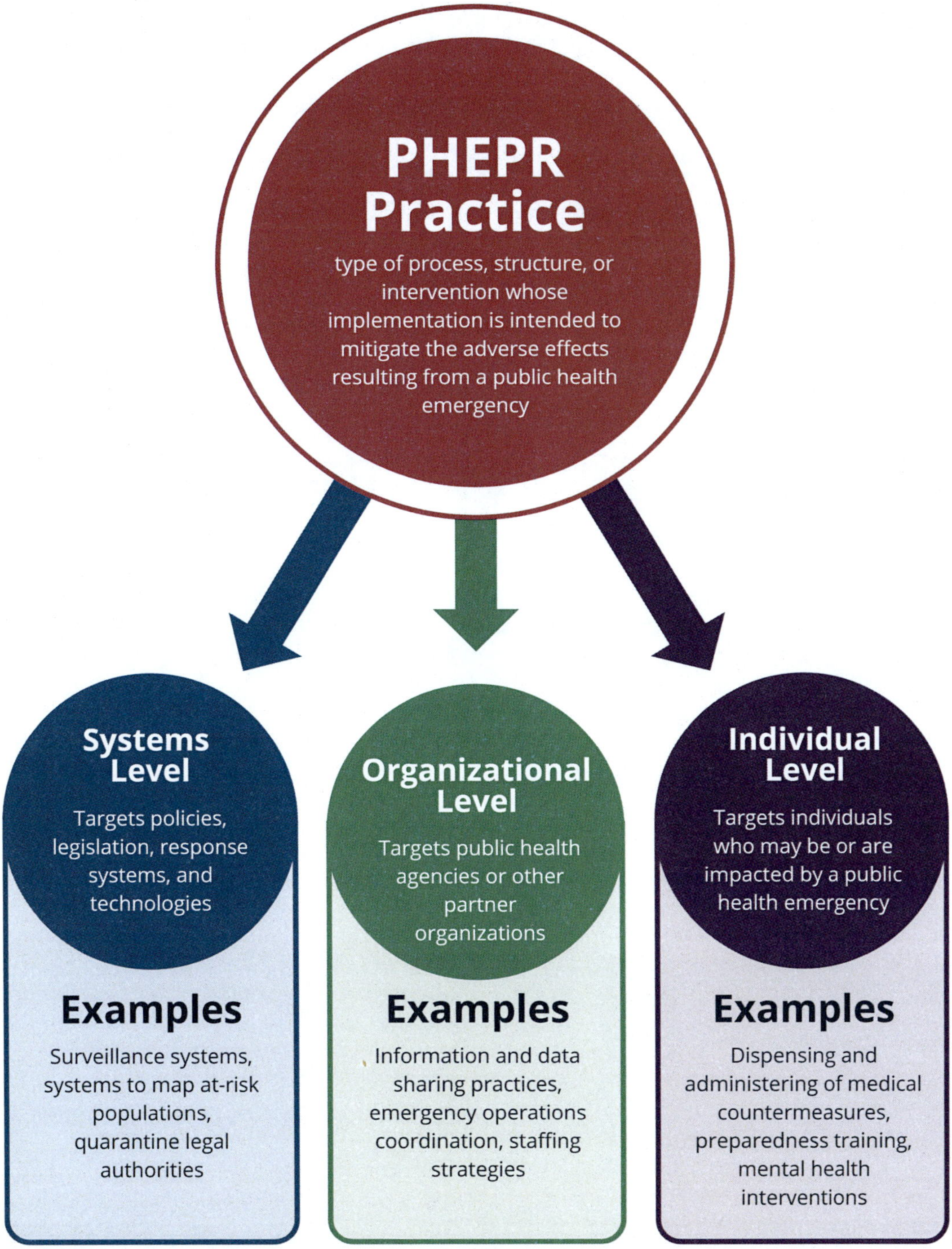

FIGURE 1-2 Levels of PHEPR practices.

Capability standard comprises Capability "functions" that must occur to achieve the standard. Specific "tasks" (or action steps) are identified for each function. The committee considered whether the Capability functions and/or tasks translated well to the concept of a PHEPR practice with the level of specificity for which an evidence review could be conducted. In many (but not all) cases, the Capability functions were too broad and the tasks too tactical to be appropriate for such a review. For example, a function within the Non-Pharmaceutical Interventions (NPIs) Capability is "Implement nonpharmaceutical interventions," and a task is "Implement NPIs in designated locations" (CDC, 2018). As the effectiveness of different NPIs is likely to differ, a specific NPI would need to be identified as the PHEPR practice to be reviewed. Ultimately, the committee developed a comprehensive list of potential PHEPR practices that was generated by breaking down the functions and tasks within the PHEPR Capabilities into topics at a level of resolution for which conclusions about effectiveness could potentially be drawn.[3]

UNDERLYING REASONS FOR THE CURRENT STATE OF THE PHEPR EVIDENCE BASE

Since the events of September 11, 2001, and the subsequent anthrax events, PHEPR practitioners have responded to countless emergencies, and the United States has invested billions of dollars and immense amounts of human capital to develop and enhance PHEPR infrastructure, systems, and science (Watson et al., 2017). These research investments, however, have been skewed toward more traditional biomedical research, such as the research and development of medical countermeasures for chemical, biological, radiological, and nuclear emergencies. For example, the National Institute of Allergy and Infectious Diseases provides $1.6 to $1.8 billion per year in funding for basic and applied research to support the development of medical countermeasures (Watson et al., 2017). However, there has been no equivalent investment in research to examine how to improve the epidemiology of biological incidents, communicate the risks, manage the distribution of medical countermeasures, or mitigate long-term consequences. Total 10-year research funding levels (2008–2017) for the Medical Countermeasure Dispensing and Administration Capability was estimated at just over $100,000 (Keim et al., 2019). This imbalance creates significant challenges for effective response by PHEPR practitioners.

The modern PHEPR research enterprise can be traced back to the CDC-funded Preparedness and Emergency Response Research Centers (PERRCs) and the Preparedness and Emergency Response Learning Centers (PERLCs). The PERRCs and the PERLCs represented the first and only major federal investment in public health systems research aimed at addressing PHEPR knowledge gaps (Savoia et al., 2018). In 2006, the Pandemic and All Hazards Preparedness Act (PAHPA)[4] articulated the need to define the existing knowledge base and establish a research agenda for PHEPR. Therefore, at the request of CDC, the Institute of Medicine (IOM) published a letter report in 2008 identifying four near-term priority research areas for PHEPR: (1) enhancing the usefulness of training, (2) improving timely emergency communications, (3) creating and maintaining sustainable response systems, and (4) generating effectiveness criteria and metrics (IOM, 2008). Guided by PAHPA and the 2008 IOM letter report on PHEPR research priorities, CDC invested $57 million in research grants through

[3] The comprehensive list of potential PHEPR practices is included in the commissioned paper documenting the scoping review, titled "Review and Evidence Mapping of Scholarly Publications Within CDC's 15 Public Health Emergency Preparedness and Response Capabilities," by Testa and colleagues (see Appendix D).

[4] Pandemic and All Hazards Preparedness Act. Public Law 116-22, 116th Cong. (January 3, 2019).

the PERRCs and $34 million in grants for workforce preparedness development through the PERLCs (Maddock et al., 2018; Qari et al., 2018). In addition to CDC, many other federal research programs made investments in PHEPR research in the years following September 11, 2001. The evolution of the PHEPR research field is discussed further in Chapter 2.

Despite past investments in PHEPR research, however, it has repeatedly been observed that the PHEPR evidence base is not proportionate to the considerable human and financial investments made in better preparing the nation for public health emergencies, and furthermore, that it is overly reliant on anecdotal and descriptive reports or studies with limited validity and generalizability (Carbone and Thomas, 2018; Khan et al., 2015; Nelson et al., 2008; Siegfried et al., 2017). Acosta and colleagues (2009) note a lack of cumulative knowledge across the field because very few studies have developed and tested clear hypotheses based on existing evidence. Several aspects of the current PHEPR field, detailed below, help explain why the development of a robust evidence base for PHEPR practices has been challenging:

- a rapidly evolving PHEPR system,
- the increasing complexity of public health emergencies and the PHEPR system,
- methodological challenges for PHEPR research,
- a poorly organized approach to PHEPR research and implications for the PHEPR researcher pipeline, and
- a well-documented gap between PHEPR research and practice.

A Rapidly Evolving PHEPR System

PHEPR is a relatively young field that has evolved rapidly over the past two decades. Immediately following the 2001 anthrax events, Congress and the executive branch rapidly and collaboratively developed legislation, Presidential Directives, and appropriations that shaped the modern PHEPR system (see Figure 1-3). The trajectory of funding sources and mechanisms has had a dramatic effect on both the scope of and infrastructure for PHEPR (Horney et al., 2019). During this time, changes in policy and practice have been driven more by reactions to public health emergencies (such as the 2001 anthrax attacks and the 2003 outbreak of severe acute respiratory syndrome [SARS]) than by systematic primary research.

Although Congress has passed several forms of supporting legislation, the largest health-focused program since 2002 is CDC's Public Health Emergency Preparedness (PHEP) Cooperative Agreement, which allocates federal funds to each state, the four largest U.S. cities, and eight U.S. territories and freely associated states for a total of 62 awardees nationwide (CDC, 2020). The 15 PHEPR Capabilities provide the framework for all PHEP program recipients, and PHEP recipients are required to build or sustain the elements identified in *Public Health Emergency Preparedness and Response Capabilities: National Standards for State, Local, Tribal, and Territorial Public Health* (CDC, 2019b). Similarly, the Office of the Assistant Secretary for Preparedness and Response (ASPR) within the U.S. Department of Health and Human Services oversees the Hospital Preparedness Program (HPP), which supports regional health care system preparedness and provides funding for health care coalitions (ASPR, 2019). The HPP is also guided by a set of specific capabilities (ASPR, 2016). While the PHEP Cooperative Agreement and HPP have been instrumental in the development of preparedness and response capacity for many jurisdictions, the past two decades have seen the emergence of additional initiatives and agencies that also have influenced the PHEPR system, including the following:

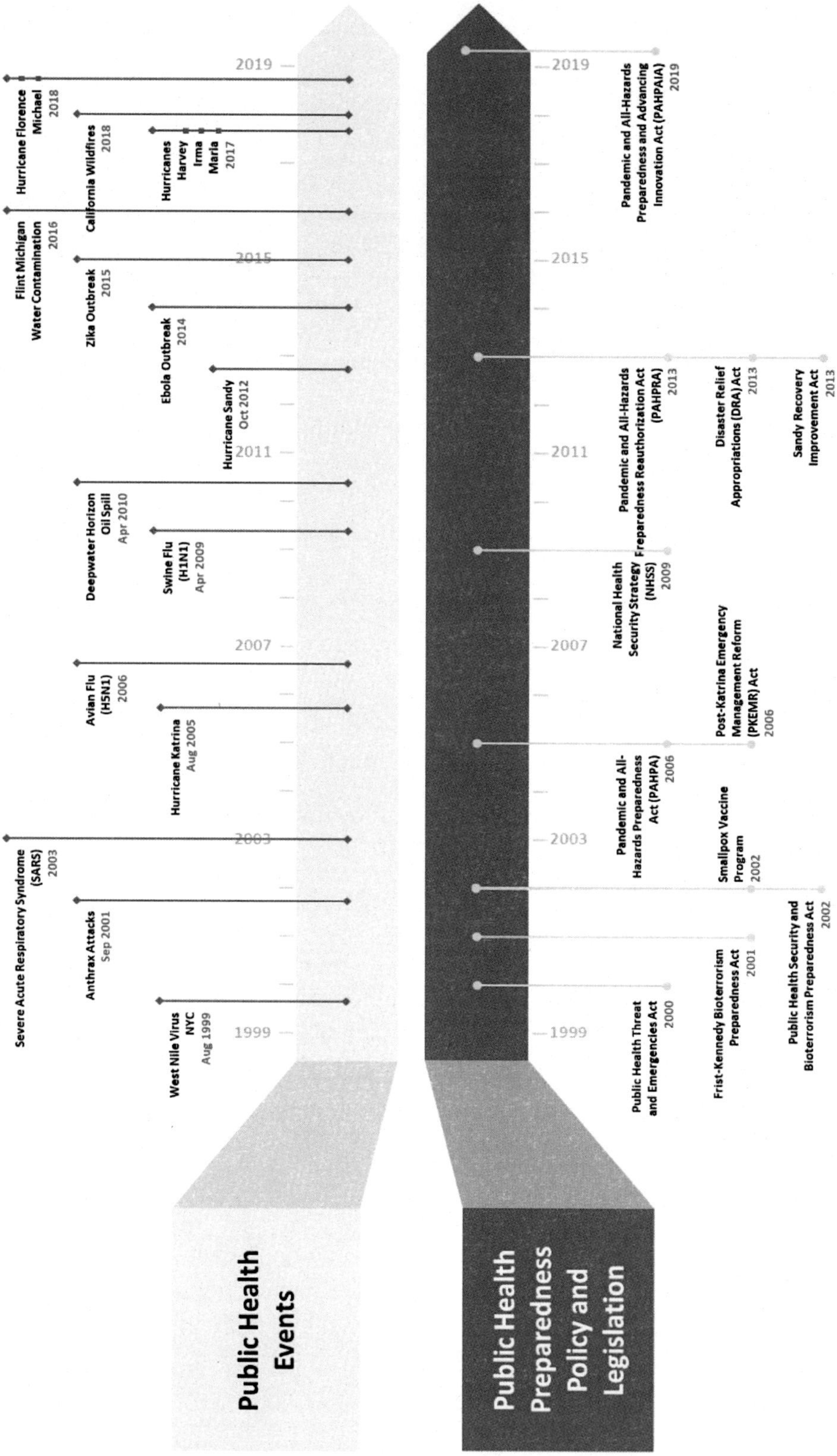

FIGURE 1-3 PHEPR system timeline: Events, policy, and legislation, 1999–2019.
SOURCE: Horney, 2019.

- CDC's Cities Readiness Initiative (CRI)—a federally funded program designed to enhance preparedness in the nation's largest population centers. State and large metropolitan public health departments use CRI funding to develop, test, and maintain plans for quickly receiving medical countermeasures from the Strategic National Stockpile (SNS) (see below) and distribute them to local communities (CDC, 2019a).
- ASPR's Biomedical Advanced Research and Development Authority—established to support the transition of medical countermeasures (e.g., vaccines, drugs, diagnostics) from research through advanced development toward consideration for approval by the U.S. Food and Drug Administration and incorporation into the SNS (HHS, 2020).
- The SNS—established to hold the nation's supply of pharmaceuticals and medical supplies for use in a public health emergency when local supplies are exhausted and SLTT responders request federal assistance to support their response efforts (HHS, 2019b).
- The Federal Emergency Management Agency's (FEMA's) Homeland Security Grant Program (HSGP)—established to support the building, sustainment, and delivery of core capabilities essential to achieving the National Preparedness Goal of a secure and resilient nation. HSGP comprises three programs—the State Homeland Security Program, the Urban Areas Security Initiative (UASI), and Operation Stonegarden (FEMA, 2020).

Initially, planning in PHEPR followed a pattern whereby SLTT public health agencies received overall guidance and direction from CDC to develop disease-specific plans. These plans included wide-area anthrax release response plans (2001), followed by smallpox plans (2002), SARS plans (2003), pandemic influenza plans (2004), Ebola response plans (2013). The PHEPR system was also heavily influenced by principles and practices from other disciplines, such as emergency management and public safety (Rose et al., 2017). Adding to the challenge was expansion of the roles and expectations of public health workers to include emergency response (VanDevanter et al., 2010). In an effort to introduce some standardization and fundamental expectations, CDC developed the PHEPR Capabilities in 2011 (updated in 2018) to help guide SLTT preparedness and response planning. Even as the PHEPR system has matured, however, determining how to implement the practices that fall within these overarching Capabilities effectively continues to be an iterative and challenging process.

The structure of funding for the PHEPR system and the funding reductions that have occurred over the years have created challenges for SLTT public health agencies in developing and maintaining the workforce and capacity to implement PHEPR practices, as well as for the monitoring and evaluation of implemented practices (Watson et al., 2017). Funding streams typically have been siloed with respect to their priorities or their targeted end users and focused on a singular disease or planning function, hampering collaboration across sectors and actors. Moreover, legislation and funding typically reflect or respond to the most recent past events, and this reactive prioritization has resulted in planning efforts that fit the needs of the last disaster rather than those of the underlying system.

Conclusion: A PHEPR system based on discrete, reactive funding streams will fail to meet the critical needs of advancing the development and use of evidence to optimize public health emergency response. As the PHEPR research field continues to evolve and mature, the committee asserts that a rigorous evidence base is the crucial foundation for future changes in policy and practice.

The Increasing Complexity of Public Health Emergencies and the PHEPR System

The knowledge gaps and paucity of high-quality evidence that currently characterize PHEPR reflect in part the inherent complexity of the PHEPR system (see Figure 1-1 earlier in this chapter) and the complexity of PHEPR practices themselves. PHEPR practices feature multiple interacting components that target multiple levels (e.g., individual and community, organizational, and systems), are implemented with an array of other practices (both public health oriented and non–health related), and often require tailoring to local conditions. Lastly, and perhaps most important, contextual factors are creating an increasingly intense and diverse threat environment (HHS, 2019a). Such factors as global migration, accelerating population density, increased proportions of unvaccinated individuals, and climate change are increasing the number, severity, and complexity of public health emergencies. In 2019 alone, 14 weather and climate disaster events resulting in losses of more than $1 billion each occurred across the United States (see Figure 1-4).

At the same time, the increased use of and dependence on technologies and the interconnectedness of supply chains mean that even local public health emergencies can have global consequences (Bunnell et al., 2019). Thus, the systemic complexities of PHEPR cannot be addressed in isolation, but are always affected by (and affecting) the broader global risk environment. Conducting research on the highly complex PHEPR system in the context of an increasingly complex environment, with many unknown public health threats, will require a comprehensive approach to transform how PHEPR research is coordinated, sustainably funded, and conducted.

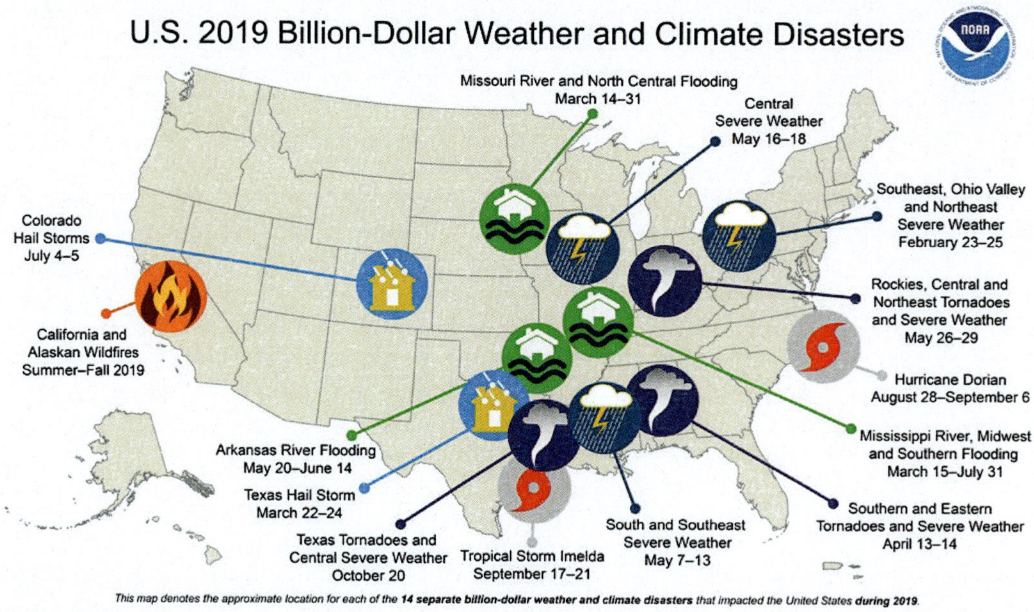

FIGURE 1-4 Billion-dollar weather and climate disasters, United States, 2019.
SOURCE: NOAA, 2020.

Methodological Challenges for PHEPR Research

The PHEPR field has generally relied on observational and quasi-experimental research designs, such as before–after studies, because more rigorous experimental designs, such as randomized controlled trials (RCTs), are often difficult and costly to develop and conduct given the unpredictability and dynamic context of public health emergencies. Because PHEPR often requires rapid decision making, such events typically allow little or no time to plan and prepare for evaluations or rapidly mobilize researchers. A number of practical issues that arise from the generally unpredictable nature of public health emergencies—such as those related to funding, ethical review, and data collection—add another layer of complexity to the conduct of research during such events. Outcomes that are more easily measurable, such as response times, are often not clearly linked to health outcomes or improved response or recovery (Nelson et al., 2007a). These challenges have impeded demonstrations of causal relationships among preparedness structures, response activities, and outcomes (Abramson et al., 2007; Asch et al., 2005; Nelson et al., 2007a).

Further differentiating PHEPR from other research fields is the inclusion of both traditional public health interventions (i.e., those aimed at improving population health outcomes) and those targeted toward improving systems and processes, such as improving the flow of information sharing, coordinating activities among response partners, or optimizing the acquisition and positioning of resources for a response. System changes often do not result in discrete outcomes but rather in adaptations within the system (Petticrew et al., 2019). While the overall aim of these system changes is to protect and improve the health of individuals and communities, their immediate effects may be shifts within the system, and it may be difficult if not impossible to attribute downstream outcomes, such as reduced mortality, to the changes with any certainty.

Past "evaluation" efforts in the PHEPR field have focused primarily on assessing the overall preparedness of the field and developing performance metrics, both of which are necessary, but differ from efforts to evaluate the effectiveness of specific PHEPR practices. For example, the National Health Security Preparedness Index was developed in an attempt to better understand the state of preparedness across SLTT agencies (RWJF, 2020). In a review of preparedness evaluation instruments, Asch and colleagues (2005) found that most of these instruments rely on subjective measures that have not been empirically validated (e.g., turn-around time for identification of pathogens in the laboratory; number of partner agencies that work together on a planning committee). Different benchmarks and performance measures have been developed and proposed over the years. For example, Khan and colleagues (2019) identified and defined a set of 67 PHEPR indicators, using a three-round modified Delphi technique, to advance performance measures for use by local and regional Canadian public health agencies in assessing readiness and measure improvement.

In the past, it has generally been held that the relative rarity of public health emergencies hinders the development of an evidence base for PHEPR. But it is becoming increasingly clear based on recent events—from hurricanes and wildfires to outbreaks of measles and the novel coronavirus responsible for the COVID-19 pandemic—that this is no longer the case. The nation now is frequently facing public health emergencies that present opportunities to observe and learn and to conduct real-time research through which to develop a strong empirical and analytical evidence base for PHEPR practices. Furthermore, there is an ever-increasing array of research and evaluation approaches for complex interventions and systems, as well as opportunities to adapt methods from complementary scientific fields, such as anthropology and operations research. The wide range of existing research and evaluation designs (discussed further in Chapter 8) has yet to be fully brought to bear on the issues facing PHEPR practitioners.

A Poorly Organized Approach to PHEPR Research and Implications for the PHEPR Researcher Pipeline

As discussed in greater detail in Chapter 2, several transformational research programs and initiatives have advanced PHEPR as a field of study and contributed to the development of a PHEPR knowledge base. However, many of these programs are no longer funded and have been discontinued. Moreover, in the absence of a formal and clearly articulated research agenda, past research funding initiatives have largely been uncoordinated and limited by event, topic, and agency. As funding for PHEPR research has repeatedly stopped and restarted since the early 2000s, many of the interventional studies produced have been one-off (i.e., lacking the repetition needed to support strong conclusions about effectiveness), and the progression of an appropriately trained research workforce has stagnated (Keim et al., 2019). Consequently, the numbers of PHEPR researchers are insufficient to address the numerous knowledge gaps in the field.

A Well-Documented Gap Between PHEPR Research and Practice

The PHEPR field is driven by a culture of response, of which research is currently not an integral component. There is a notable cultural gap between responders, who are often focused on ending an emergency quickly and mitigating its effects, and researchers, who are driven to understand the science behind these events and the proposed courses of action (McNutt, 2015). In contrast with their counterparts in other fields, PHEPR researchers are often not practitioners, which contributes to the disconnect between practice and research. Moreover, administrative or quasi-legal boundaries often preclude researchers' access to the response environment, limiting both their objective study of those environments (and hence the ability to produce useful research) and their ability to better understand the needs of practitioners through direct observation. Bridging the gap between research and practice is a daunting challenge, but PHEPR practitioners do not have decades to shift to evidence-based practices.

Furthermore, it is not clear that PHEPR practitioners have translated the evidence that does exist into their preparedness and response practices (Carbone and Thomas, 2018). Practitioners' ability to successfully implement evidence-based practices is impeded by numerous barriers, such as lack of access to research, insufficient support and time, and resource constraints. One study found that information needs and awareness of existing research-based information differed between local and state public health departments, with the former expressing a greater need for information (Siegfried et al., 2017). Thus, barriers to translating research into practice may be greater for smaller, less well-resourced local health departments. Other barriers to translation of research into practice involve gaps between the studies that researchers conduct and the information needs of PHEPR practitioners, characteristics of a practice (e.g., high resource requirements or lack of adaptability), features of a particular setting, and failure of the research design to evaluate relevant implementation information (Glasgow and Emmons, 2007). Finally, decisions to implement evidence-based practices may be influenced by the perceived generalizability or applicability of research evidence to the diverse array of PHEPR practice contexts (e.g., emergency types, settings). PHEPR practices tend to be context sensitive, meaning that although a practice may have been shown to be effective in the specific context examined in a research study, the research findings do not necessarily translate to other practice settings.

THE IMPORTANCE OF EVIDENCE-BASED PRACTICE AND GUIDELINES

This report describes a process for synthesizing evidence on PHEPR practices to improve the accessibility of research and other evidence and its utility for evidence-informed decision making. Synthesizing the evidence from research is only one aspect of evidence-informed decision making. Evidence-informed decision making is the process of distilling and disseminating the best available evidence from research and evaluation; context, systems, and environment; stakeholders' values and preferences; and practitioner experience and expert judgment and using that evidence to inform and improve practice and policy (Brownson et al., 2018) (see Figure 1-5). Figure 1-5 captures the various inputs to the evidence-informed decision-making process, and it is important to note that the nature of these inputs may be changing continuously during public health emergency response.

The direct and indirect benefits of identifying and using evidence-based practices are manifold, ranging from increasing the quality of information on which policies are based to greater workforce productivity, increased accountability, and more efficient use of resources (Brownson et al., 2009). In a recent Delphi study focused on improving the science and evidence base of disaster response, respondents agreed that the full range of review types should be used in a standardized way to synthesize evidence to inform contextually specific evidence of effectiveness in disaster response (Jillson et al., 2019).

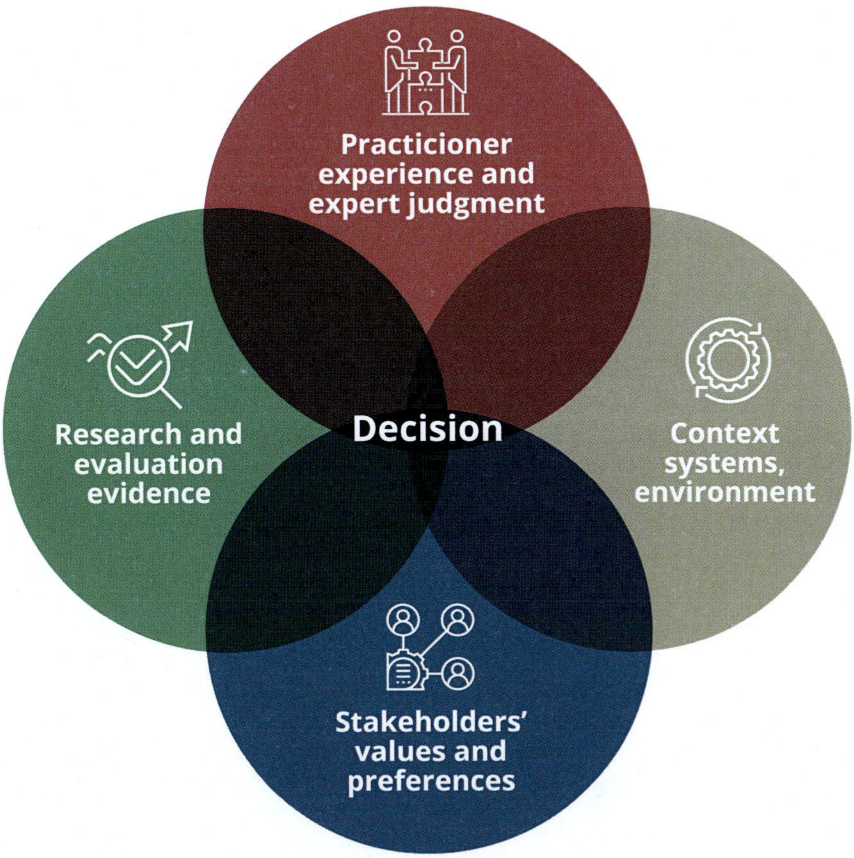

FIGURE 1-5 Evidence-informed decision making.
SOURCE: Adapted from Barends et al., 2014.

The Emergence of Evidence-Based Guidelines and Policies to Promote Evidence-Based Practice

Outside of PHEPR, research in other fields has been translated into policy and practice through the establishment of task forces and clearinghouses that evaluate evidence and make recommendations for practice. For example, the U.S. Preventive Services Task Force (USPSTF), convened by the Agency for Healthcare Research and Quality (AHRQ), which uses evidence reviews to make recommendations on clinical preventive services, has been successful in identifying both effective and ineffective practices (e.g., screenings that are both unnecessary and potentially harmful) (Guirguis-Blake et al., 2007; HHS, 2010). Similarly, The Guide to Community Preventive Services (The Community Guide) provides guidance on public health interventions and programs with the aim of promoting evidence-based practice in public health (Truman et al., 2000), using methods developed and implemented by the Community Preventive Services Task Force, convened by CDC. National and international organizations, such as Cochrane and the World Health Organization (WHO), regularly conduct robust evidence reviews that produce guidelines and recommendations (AHRQ, 2020; Cochrane, 2020; WHO, 2014). Evidence synthesis to support the uptake of evidence-based practices and policy also has spread beyond health care; other fields have adopted similar evidence review processes. Clearinghouses, such as the What Works Clearinghouse at the U.S. Department of Education and the National Institute of Justice's CrimeSolutions program, evaluate evidence and make recommendations on evidence-based practices and policies (NIJ, 2013; WWC, 2017). Historically, however, many of these guideline groups have focused more on the effectiveness of specific interventions and less on the effectiveness of systems and policies or their implementation.

The move to evidence-based practice and policy in the United States is increasingly being driven by federal policy, including the Foundations for Evidence-Based Policymaking Act of 2018.[5] That act directed federal agencies to build evidence to support policy making and programs through the development of evidence plans (to include key research questions, data needs, and planned activities), the prioritization of evaluation activities, and the development of baseline information about the resources available for evidence building. More recently, Section 201(a) of the 2019 Pandemic and All-Hazards Preparedness and Advancing Innovation Act[6] called for an evaluation of evidence-based benchmarks and objective standards in PHEPR.

Moving Beyond the Traditional Evidence Hierarchy for Evaluating the Effectiveness of PHEPR Practices

In the evaluation of interventions to improve health, the traditional hierarchy of evidence places systematic reviews of RCTs at the top (strongest evidence) and expert opinion at the bottom (weakest evidence). However, the traditional evidence hierarchy has limited applicability in such fields as PHEPR for a number of reasons. First, RCTs are likely to be unethical or infeasible for some PHEPR practices because of a lack of equipoise (genuine scientific uncertainty as to which randomization arm is best for participants) and the logistical challenges inherent in performing a randomized experiment in the context of an emergency (Durrheim and Reingold, 2010). Additionally, reductionist approaches like RCTs are not well suited to understanding the context-specific effects and interactions of systems and pro-

---

[5] Foundations for Evidence-Based Policymaking Act of 2018. Public Law 115-435, 115th Cong. (January 14, 2019).

[6] Pandemic and All-Hazards Preparedness and Advancing Innovation Act of 2019. Public Law 109-417, 116th Cong. (June 24, 2019).

cesses (Rychetnik et al., 2002), which, as discussed earlier, are inherent in much of PHEPR. Thus, evidence from such research studies may have limited relevance with respect to its application in the field (Green and Glasgow, 2006). In contrast, well-controlled observational studies may be appropriate for answering many PHEPR research questions, especially those focused on how an intervention works rather than whether it works (Petticrew, 2003). Likewise, operational research and simulation studies may have more relevance than more experimental approaches to the everyday needs of PHEPR practitioners.

As noted previously, recent years have seen the development of new research disciplines, such as implementation science, and new methodologies for evidence synthesis that consider the complexity of systems and practices and make use of diverse sources of evidence, including that derived from qualitative and process evaluation research (Dixon-Woods et al., 2016; Harden et al., 2018; Lewin et al., 2018). These methods are being adopted by international guideline bodies, including WHO, and continue to be refined (Langlois et al., 2018; Swaminathan, 2019; Wieringa et al., 2018). This report builds on these developing methods to propose an evidence review and evaluation process that is suited to the PHEPR field (see Chapter 3).

ABOUT THIS REPORT

Study Approach and Scope

In developing this report and the recommendations presented herein, the committee deliberated for more than 2 years (from January 2018 through March 2020), holding 10 in-person meetings during that period. The meetings held in January 2018, April 2018, July 2018, and January 2019 included public information-gathering sessions that allowed the committee to hear from the study sponsor (CDC) and other experts and stakeholders (all public meeting agendas can be found in Appendix D). To supplement the stakeholder input received at these public meetings, a group of PHEPR practitioners were appointed as consultants to assist in refining the committee's conceptual approach and to ensure that its recommendations would be grounded in practice.

As specified in the Statement of Task for this study (see Box 1-1), the committee was charged with selecting PHEPR practices to review from within the CDC PHEPR Capabilities (practices specific to the HPP were not within this study's scope). Recognizing the considerable challenges inherent in this study, CDC did not constrain this review to a specific number of Capabilities and did not attempt to identify the Capabilities to be included in the review a priori. The Capabilities encompass a large number of PHEPR practices and potential evidence review questions. Given time and resource constraints, the committee recognized early on that it would be able to review only a very limited number of PHEPR practices and that this report would therefore represent a proof of concept rather than a comprehensive resource for PHEPR practitioners.

This report focuses primarily on SLTT public health agencies, while recognizing that these agencies do not exist in isolation and are part of a larger preparedness and response system that includes first responders, emergency management, and health care partners, among others. The committee understands that its findings may be applicable to other disciplines and, to increase the usefulness of this report to PHEPR stakeholders, considered the evidence in the context of all hazards.

The committee began by scoping the literature in the PHEPR field (see Chapter 2) to gain a sense of the nature of the evidence base and potential challenges related to evaluating the effectiveness of PHEPR practices. The committee then explored evaluation methodologies that are used in health and other fields to synthesize and rate the strength of evidence. As discussed further in Chapter 3, there was no best-fit approach to evaluating PHEPR evidence, which does not fit easily into traditional, biomedical evidence review evaluations (Carbone and Thomas, 2018). Thus, the committee determined that a novel evidence evaluation methodology was necessary for PHEPR. The approach used to develop this proposed methodology is described in detail in Chapter 3.

Consistent with its charge, the committee applied its methodology to selected review topics to demonstrate how the methodology could accommodate different types of PHEPR practices and review questions. The committee used a careful topic selection process (described in Chapter 3 and in greater detail Appendix A) to select four review topics, which represented diverse types of practices that require a flexible approach and different kinds of evidence to evaluate. The committee solicited literature on each of the selected PHEPR practices through a call for papers (discussed in more detail in Appendix A). The four practices the committee selected for review were

- engaging with and training community-based partners to improve the outcomes of at-risk populations after public health emergencies (falls under Capability 1, Community Preparedness);
- activating a public health emergency operations center (Capability 3, Emergency Operations Coordination [EOC]);
- communicating public health alerts and guidance with technical audiences during a public health emergency (Capability 6, Information Sharing); and
- implementing quarantine to reduce or stop the spread of a contagious disease (Capability 11, Non-Pharmaceutical Interventions).

The core set of terms used throughout the report are those used routinely by policy makers, practitioners, researchers, and the public. Yet, while these terms are commonly used, their definitions are nuanced and can vary depending on the particular context and user. Box 1-4 presents the committee's definitions for these core terms. In addition to these terms, other important terms are defined throughout the report alongside the relevant discussion.

Report Audiences and Uses

In developing its evidence review methodology, the committee understood the nature of decision making required in responding to a public health emergency and the need for clear, accessible, and adaptable guidance on evidence-based practices. Throughout this report, the committee seeks to guide practitioners, policy makers, and other stakeholders in understanding and using the available evidence to inform their decision making. Accordingly, this report is intended to inform a wide range of audiences and has different potential uses for each, including the following:

- **Policy makers** can use the report to build a sustainable process with the necessary oversight and support for ongoing evaluation of the PHEPR literature to identify evidence-based practices and critical knowledge gaps that need to be addressed through future research initiatives. They can also identify other strategies for strengthening the PHEPR evidence base, for example, by incentivizing the routine evaluation of practices through quality improvement approaches, supporting the continued development of PHEPR as a unique academic discipline, and better integrating PHEPR practice and research.

BOX 1-4 CORE TERMS USED THROUGHOUT THE REPORT

Evidence-based interventions: "Public health practices and policies that have been shown to be effective based on evaluation research. Often, lists of evidence-based interventions are identified through systematic reviews, but they sometimes need adaptation to unique or varied settings, populations, or circumstances" (Brownson et al., 2018, p. 3.2).

Evidence-informed decision making: "The process of distilling and disseminating the best available evidence from research, context, and experience (political, organizational) and using that evidence to inform and improve public health practice and policy" (Brownson et al., 2018, p. 3.2).

Mixed-method evidence synthesis: An evidence synthesis approach involving the integration of quantitative, mixed-method, and qualitative evidence in a single review (Petticrew et al., 2013).

Public health emergency: For the purposes of this report, defined as a situation with health consequences whose scale, timing, or unpredictability threatens to overwhelm routine capabilities (Nelson et al., 2007b).

Public health emergency preparedness and response (PHEPR): "The capability of the public health and health care systems, communities, and individuals to prevent, protect against, quickly respond to, and recover from health emergencies, particularly those whose scale, timing, or unpredictability threatens to overwhelm routine capabilities" (Nelson et al., 2007b, p. S-9).

Public health emergency preparedness and response practice: A type of process, structure, or intervention whose implementation is intended to mitigate the adverse effects of a public health emergency on the population as a whole or a particular sub-group within the population.

Public health systems research: "A field of study that examines the organization, financing, and delivery of public health services within communities and the impact of these services on public health" (Mays et al., 2003, p. 180).

- **PHEPR researchers** can find information regarding key elements of research design and reporting that would strengthen the quality of evidence supporting PHEPR practices and improve the usefulness of their research. They can also find detailed information about critical gaps in the PHEPR evidence base that are priority areas for further exploration.
- **Methodologists** and other researchers interested in the field of evidence synthesis and guideline development can gain a deeper understanding of mixed-method approaches to evidence synthesis and the challenges associated with evaluation of complex interventions.
- **SLTT public health agencies,** and specifically **PHEPR practitioners,** can learn of strategies for engaging in the evidence review process and for implementing evidence-based practices in their own organizations, as well as ways to improve the capture of evidence from real-world practice experience. And as previously emphasized, in addition to public health agencies, this information should be useful to those who have roles in preparing for, responding to, and recovering from public health emergencies, such as first responders, health care stakeholders, and emergency management professionals.

- **Organizations that fund PHEPR research** (i.e., federal or other national agencies and nongovernmental organizations and foundations) can find information to help organize and guide their decisions about investments in PHEPR research and evaluation, as well as strategies that can be used to incentivize improvements in the quality of research.
- **Professional associations** that represent the PHEPR community, public health accreditation bodies, and journals can learn of ways to support and promote the generation, dissemination, and adoption of evidence-based PHEPR practices.

In sum, the report collectively defines a framework for a system that together practitioners, researchers, and policy makers can implement to address current gaps in PHEPR practitioners' access to information on evidence-based PHEPR practices.

Organization of the Report

This report is organized around the following two distinct aspects of the committee's Statement of Task (see Box 1-1), each of which comes with its own set of recommendations:

- developing the methodology for and subsequently conducting a systematic review and evaluation of the evidence for PHEPR practices and making recommendations on adoption of PHEPR practices based on evidence of effectiveness (bullets 1–4 in the Statement of Task); and
- providing recommendations for future research needed to address critical gaps in evidence-based PHEPR practices, as well as processes needed to improve the overall quality of evidence within the field (bullet 5 in the Statement of Task).

Review Methodology, Evidence Reviews, and Recommendations for Evidence-Based PHEPR Practices

Chapter 3 describes the committee's proposed methodology for reviewing and evaluating the evidence for PHEPR practices. So as to focus the chapter on the original aspects of the committee's methodology, details related to processes that are fairly standard in systematic reviews (i.e., the selection of review topics, the literature searches, and the data extraction and quality assessment of individual articles) are included in Appendix A. An evidence-based practice center (EPC) was commissioned to conduct the data extraction and quality assessment of individual quantitative studies. Appendix C contains a link to the EPC's report, which describes the EPC's methods and includes tables containing the extracted data and quality assessments.

As it was expected that different report audiences would be interested in different levels of detail on various topics, the committee took a layered approach to presenting the findings of its four evidence reviews (see Figure 1-6). Chapters 4–7 are oriented toward PHEPR practitioners and, respectively, present high-level summaries of the evidence for the four PHEPR practices selected for review (as detailed earlier) in a user-friendly format. Each of these chapters provides the following:

- a two-page action sheet at the front of the chapter that presents PHEPR practitioners and other users with the key takeaways from the review;
- background information on the practice, including a definition, an analytic framework with the hypothesized links between the practice and the outcomes of interest, and a description of the scope of the problem addressed by the practice;

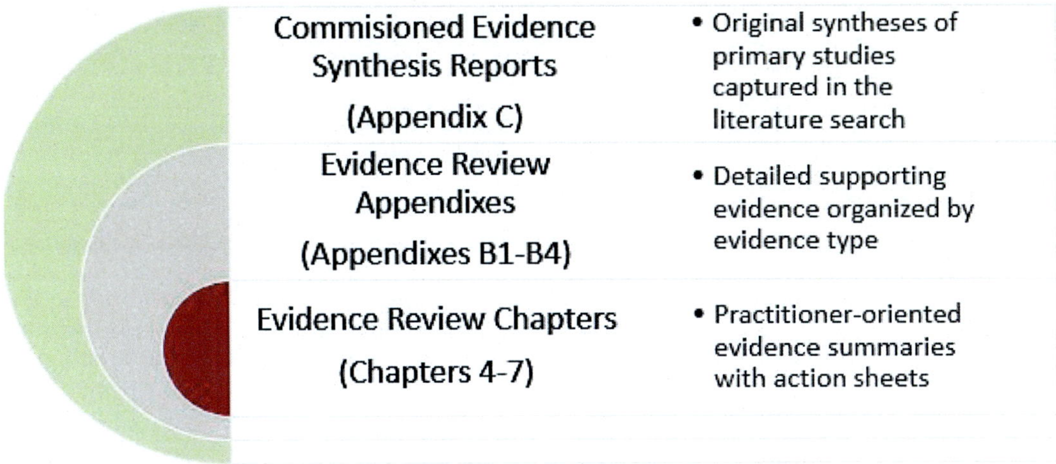

FIGURE 1-6 Layered approach to the presentation of evidence from the PHEPR practice reviews. The level of detail increases as one moves from the innermost to the outermost layer.

- an overview of the evidence base, including evidence of effectiveness, benefits and harms, acceptability and preferences, feasibility and PHEPR system considerations, resources and economic considerations, equity, and ethical considerations;
- the practice recommendation (when supported by sufficient evidence), along with a justification and specific implementation guidance; and
- priorities for future research to improve the evidence base for the practice.

For those audiences seeking additional, more detailed information, each review chapter has an associated appendix (see Appendixes B1–B4) containing a comprehensive description of the evidence base for the respective PHEPR practice. To facilitate the linkage between the evidence summaries in Chapters 4–7 and the body of studies from which the findings were generated, summaries in the evidence review chapters reference specific numbered sections in the appendixes.

Of note, external experts were commissioned to carry out some components of the committee's evidence reviews: the syntheses of the bodies of qualitative evidence, the syntheses of the experiential-based evidence from case reports and after action reports, and the synthesis of a selection of modeling studies for one of the evidence reviews. The main findings from these commissioned reports were incorporated in the detailed evidence reviews presented in Appendixes B1–B4, but for those audiences who would like to review the commissioned authors' descriptions and findings, Appendix C includes links to each of the commissioned reports.

Processes Needed to Improve the Overall Quality of Evidence Within the Field

The remaining two chapters of the report focus on the second main aspect of the committee's task—identifying and recommending processes needed to improve the overall quality of evidence within the field. Chapter 2 begins with a high-level overview of the state of PHEPR research based on the results of a commissioned scoping review for the 15 PHEPR Capabilities and associated evidence maps identifying key gaps and limitations in the PHEPR evidence base (Appendix D contains an excerpt from the commissioned authors' report and the evidence maps). The chapter then examines the evolution of the PHEPR research enterprise and the underlying reasons for the current state of the evidence. Finally, Chapter 8 presents the committee's overarching recommendations for improving the quality of PHEPR research, including the role that funders, researchers, and practitioners can play in advancing the evidence base.

Other Appendixes

Appendix E provides the agendas for the committee's public meetings and links to the committee's Workshop Proceedings—in Brief, which summarizes a public workshop on evidence evaluation methodologies and is available online through the National Academies Press. Appendix F presents biographical sketches of the committee members.

REFERENCES

Abramson, D. M., S. S. Morse, A. L. Garrett, and I. Redlener. 2007. Public health disaster research: Surveying the field, defining its future. *Disaster Medicine and Public Health Preparedness* 1(1):57–62.

Acosta, J. D., C. Nelson, E. B. Beckjord, S. R. Shelton, E. Murphy, K. L. Leuschner, and J. Wasserman. 2009. A national agenda for public health systems research on emergency preparedness. Santa Monica, CA: RAND Health.

AHRQ (Agency for Healthcare Research and Quality). 2020. *Research findings.* https://www.ahrq.gov/research/findings/index.html (accessed February 19, 2020).

Asch, S. M., M. Stoto, M. Mendes, R. B. Valdez, M. E. Gallagher, P. Halverson, and N. Lurie. 2005. A review of instruments assessing public health preparedness. *Public Health Reports* 120(5):532–542.

ASPR (Office of the Assistant Secretary for Preparedness and Response). 2016. *2017–2022 health care preparedness and response capabilities.* https://www.phe.gov/Preparedness/planning/hpp/reports/Documents/2017-2022-healthcare-pr-capablities.pdf (accessed May 14, 2020).

ASPR. 2019. *Hospital preparedness program.* https://www.phe.gov/Preparedness/planning/hpp/Pages/default.aspx (accessed March 27, 2020).

Barends, E., D. M. Rousseau, and R. B. Briner. 2014. *Evidence-based management: The basic principles.* Amsterdam, The Netherlands: Center for Evidence-Based Management. https://www.cebma.org/wp-content/uploads/Evidence-Based-Practice-The-Basic-Principles.pdf (accessed March 2, 2020).

Brownson, R. C., J. E. Fielding, and C. M. Maylahn. 2009. Evidence-based public health: A fundamental concept for public health practice. *Annual Review of Public Health* 30:175–201.

Brownson, R. C., J. E. Fielding, and L. W. Green. 2018. Building capacity for evidence-based public health: Reconciling the pulls of practice and the push of research. *Annual Review of Public Health* 39(1).

Bunnell, R. E., Z. Ahmed, M. Ramsden, K. Rapposelli, M. Walter-Garcia, E. Sharmin, and N. Knight. 2019. Global health security: Protecting the United States in an interconnected world. *Public Health Reports* 134(1):3–10.

Carbone, E. G., and E. V. Thomas. 2018. Science as the basis of public health emergency preparedness and response practice: The slow but crucial evolution. *American Journal of Public Health* 108(S5):S383–S386.

CDC (Centers for Disease Control and Prevention). 2018. *Public health emergency preparedness and response capabilities: National standards for state, local, tribal, and territorial public health.* Atlanta, GA: Centers for Disease Control and Prevention. https://www.cdc.gov/cpr/readiness/capabilities.htm (accessed February 19, 2020).

CDC. 2019a. *Cities readiness initiative.* https://www.cdc.gov/cpr/readiness/mcm/cri.html (accessed February 19, 2020).

CDC. 2019b. *Public health emergency preparedness (PHEP) cooperative agreement: CDC-RFA-TP19-1901.* https://www.grants.gov/web/grants/view-opportunity.html?oppId=310318 (accessed May 14, 2020).

CDC. 2020. *Public health emergency preparedness (PHEP) cooperative agreement.* https://www.cdc.gov/cpr/readiness/phep.htm (accessed March 3, 2020).

Cochrane. 2020. *About us.* https://www.cochrane.org/about-us (accessed February 19, 2020).

Dixon-Woods, M., S. Bonas, A. Booth, D. R. Jones, T. Miller, A. J. Sutton, R. L. Shaw, J. A. Smith, and B. Young. 2016. How can systematic reviews incorporate qualitative research? A critical perspective. *Qualitative Research* 6(1):27–44.

Durrheim, D. N., and A. Reingold. 2010. Modifying the grade framework could benefit public health. *Journal of Epidemiology and Community Health* 64(5):387.

FEMA (Federal Emergency Management Agency). 2020. *Homeland security grant program.* https://www.fema.gov/homeland-security-grant-program (accessed February 19, 2020).

Gibson, P. J., F. Theadore, and J. B. Jellison. 2012. The common ground preparedness framework: A comprehensive description of public health emergency preparedness. *American Journal of Public Health* 102(4):633–642.

Glasgow, R. E., and K. M. Emmons. 2007. How can we increase translation of research into practice? Types of evidence needed. *Annual Review of Public Health* 28(1):413–433.

Green, L. W., and R. E. Glasgow. 2006. Evaluating the relevance, generalization, and applicability of research: Issues in external validation and translation methodology. *Evaluation and the Health Professions* 29(1):126–153.

Guirguis-Blake, J., N. Calonge, T. Miller, A. Siu, S. Teutsch, E. Whitlock, and the U.S. Preventive Services Task Force. 2007. Current processes of the U.S. Preventive Services Task Force: Refining evidence-based recommendation development. *Annals of Internal Medicine* 147(2):117–122.

Harden, A., J. Thomas, M. Cargo, J. Harris, T. Pantoja, K. Flemming, A. Booth, R. Garside, K. Hannes, and J. Noyes. 2018. Cochrane qualitative and implementation methods group guidance series-paper 5: Methods for integrating qualitative and implementation evidence within intervention effectiveness reviews. *Journal of Clinical Epidemiology* 97:70–78.

HHS (U.S. Department of Health and Human Services). 2010. *Evidence-based clinical and public health: Generating and applying the evidence: Secretary's advisory committee on national health promotion and disease prevention objectives for 2020.* https://www.healthypeople.gov/sites/default/files/EvidenceBasedClinicalPH2010.pdf (accessed March 2, 2020).

HHS. 2019a. *National health security strategy 2019–2022.* https://www.phe.gov/Preparedness/planning/authority/nhss/Documents/NHSS-Strategy-508.pdf (accessed March 2, 2020).

HHS. 2019b. *Strategic national stockpile.* https://www.phe.gov/about/sns/Pages/default.aspx (accessed February 19, 2020).

HHS. 2020. *Biomedical advanced research and development authority.* https://www.phe.gov/about/barda/Pages/default.aspx (accessed February 19, 2020).

Horney, J. 2019 (unpublished). *The public health emergency preparedness and response system: A comprehensive review.* Paper commissioned by the Committee on Evidence-Based Practices for Public Health Emergency Preparedness and Response.

Horney, J., E. G. Carbone, M. Lynch, C. J. Shuang, and T. Jones. 2019. How public health agencies use the public health emergency preparedness capabilities. *Disaster Medicine and Public Health Preparedness.* https://doi.org/10.1017/dmp.2019.133.

IOM (Institute of Medicine). 2008. *Research priorities in emergency preparedness and response for public health systems: A letter report.* Washington, DC: The National Academies Press.

Jillson, I. A., M. Clarke, C. Allen, S. Waller, T. Koehlmoos, W. Mumford, J. Jansen, K. McKay, and A. Trant. 2019. Improving the science and evidence base of disaster response: A policy research study. *BMC Health Services Research* 19(1):274.

Keim, M., T. D. Kirsch, and A. Lovallo. 2019. A comparison of us federal government spending for research and development related to public health preparedness capabilities, 2008–2017. *Disaster Medicine and Public Health Preparedness* 1–8.

Khan, Y., G. Fazli, B. Henry, E. de Villa, C. Tsamis, M. Grant, and B. Schwartz. 2015. The evidence base of primary research in public health emergency preparedness: A scoping review and stakeholder consultation. *BMC Public Health* 15(432).

Khan, Y., T. O'Sullivan, A. Brown, S. Tracey, J. Gibson, M. Généreux, B. Henry, and B. Schwartz. 2018. Public health emergency preparedness: A framework to promote resilience. *BMC Public Health* 18(1344).

Khan, Y., A. D. Brown, A. R. Gagliardi, T. O'Sullivan, S. Lacarte, B. Henry, and B. Schwartz. 2019. Are we prepared? The development of performance indicators for public health emergency preparedness using a modified Delphi approach. *PLOS ONE* 14(12).

Langlois, E. V., K. Daniels, and E. A. Akl. 2018. Evidence synthesis for health policy and systems: A methods guide. World Health Organization. https://www.who.int/alliance-hpsr/resources/publications/Alliance-evidence-synthesis-MethodsGuide.pdf?ua=1 (accessed March 3, 2020).

Lewin, S., A. Booth, C. Glenton, H. Munthe-Kaas, A. Rashidian, M. Wainwright, M. A. Bohren, Ö. Tunçalp, C. J. Colvin, R. Garside, B. Carlsen, E. V. Langlois, and J. Noyes. 2018. Applying GRADE-CERQual to qualitative evidence synthesis findings: Introduction to the series. *Implementation Science* 13(1):2.

Linkov, I., T. Bridges, F. Creutzig, J. Decker, C. Fox-Lent, W. Kroger, J. H. Lambert, A. Levermann, B. Montreuil, J. Nathwani, R. Nyer, O. Renn, B. Scharte, A. Scheffler, M. Schreurs, and T. Thiel-Clemen. 2014. Changing the resilience paradigm. *Nature Climate Change* 4:407–409.

Maddock, J. E., S. A. Payne, S. Jett, and M. Kellman. 2018. Translation, dissemination, and implementation of public health preparedness research and training: Introduction and contents of the volume. 108(S5):S349–S350.

Martinez, D., T. Talbert, S. Romero-Steiner, C. Kosmos, and S. Redd. 2019. Evolution of the public health preparedness and response capability standards to support public health emergency management practices and processes. *Health Security* 17(6):430–438.

Mays, G. P., P. Halverson, and F. D. Scutchfield. 2003. Behind the curve? What we know and need to learn from public health systems research. *Journal of Public Health Management Practice* 9(3):179–182.

McNutt, M. 2015. A community for disaster science. *Science* 348(6230):11.

Nelson, C., N. Lurie, and J. Wasserman. 2007a. Assessing public health emergency preparedness: Concepts, tools, and challenges. *Annual Review of Public Health* 28(1):1–18.

Nelson, C., N. Lurie, J. Wasserman, and S. Zakowski. 2007b. Conceptualizing and defining public health emergency preparedness. *American Journal of Public Health* 97(S1):S9–S11.

Nelson, C. D., E. B. Beckjord, D. J. Dausey, E. Chan, D. Lotstein, and N. Lurie. 2008. How can we strengthen the evidence base in public health preparedness? *Disaster Medicine and Public Health Preparedness* 2(4):247–250.

NIJ (National Institute of Justice). 2013. *Crimesolutions.gov practices scoring instrument.* https://www.crimesolutions.gov/pdfs/PracticeScoringInstrument.pdf (accessed March 3, 2020).

NOAA (National Oceanic and Atmospheric Administration). 2020. *Billion-dollar weather and climate disasters: Overview.* https://www.ncdc.noaa.gov/billions (accessed Febuary 12, 2020).

Petticrew, M. 2003. Evidence, hierarchies, and typologies: Horses for courses. *Journal of Epidemiology & Community Health* 57(7):527–529.

Petticrew, M., E. Rehfuess, J. Noyes, J. P. T. Higgins, A. Mayhew, T. Pantoja, I. Shemilt, and A. Sowden. 2013. Synthesizing evidence on complex interventions: How meta-analytical, qualitative, and mixed-method approaches can contribute. *Journal of Clinical Epidemiology* 66(11):1230–1243.

Petticrew, M., C. Knai, J. Thomas, E. A. Rehfuess, J. Noyes, A. Gerhardus, J. M. Grimshaw, H. Rutter, and E. McGill. 2019. Implications of a complexity perspective for systematic reviews and guideline development in health decision making. *BMJ Global Health* 4:e000899. doi: 10.1136/bmjgh-2018-000899.

Qari, S. H., M. R. Leinhos, T. N. Thomas, and E. G. Carbone. 2018. Overview of the translation, dissemination, and implementation of public health preparedness and response research and training initiative. *American Journal of Public Health* 108(S5):S355–S362.

Rose, D. A., S. Murthy, J. Brooks, and J. Bryant. 2017. The evolution of public health emergency management as a field of practice. *American Journal of Public Health* 107(S2):S126–S133.

RWJF (Robert Wood Johnson Foundation). 2020. *National health security preparedness index.* https://nhspi.org (accessed May 20, 2020).

Rychetnik, L., M. Frommer, P. Hawe, and A. Shiell. 2002. Criteria for evaluating evidence on public health interventions. *Journal of Epidemiology and Community Health* 56(2):119–127.

Savoia, E., S. Guicciardi, D. P. Bernard, N. Harriman, M. Leinhos, and M. Testa. 2018. Preparedness emergency response research centers (PERRCs): Addressing public health preparedness knowledge gaps using a public health systems perspective. *American Journal of Public Health* 108(S5):S363–S365.

Siegfried, A. L., E. G. Carbone, M. B. Meit, M. J. Kennedy, H. Yusuf, and E. B. Kahn. 2017. Identifying and prioritizing information needs and research priorities of public health emergency preparedness and response practitioners. *Disaster Medicine and Public Health Preparedness* 11(5):552–561.

Stoto, M. A., C. Nelson, E. Savoia, I. Ljungqvist, and M. Ciotti. 2017. A public health preparedness logic model: Assessing preparedness for cross-border threats in the European region. *Health Security* 15(5):473–482.

Swaminathan, S. 2019. How to shape research to advance global health. *Nature* 569(7754):7.

Truman, B. I., C. K. Smith-Akin, A. R. Hinman, K. M. Gebbie, R. C. Brownson, L. F. Novick, R. Lawrence, M. Pappaioanou, J. E. Fielding, C. Evans, F. A. Guerra, M. Vogel-Taylor, C. Mahan, M. Fullilove, S. Zaza, and The Task Force on Community Preventive Services. 2000. Developing the guide to community preventive services: Overview and rationale. *American Journal of Preventive Medicine* 18:18–26.

VanDevanter, N., P. Leviss, D. Abramson, J. M. Howard, and P. A. Honoré. 2010. Emergency response and public health in Hurricane Katrina: What does it mean to be a public health emergency responder? *Journal of Public Health Management and Practice* 16(6):E16–E25.

Watson, C. R., M. Watson, and T. K. Sell. 2017. Public health preparedness funding: Key programs and trends from 2001 to 2017. *American Journal of Public Health* 107(S2):S165–S167.

WHO (World Health Organization). 2009. *Systems thinking for health systems strengthening.* https://apps.who.int/iris/bitstream/handle/10665/44204/9789241563895_eng.pdf;jsessionid=F75F0B4C38F0CA8AD59F8B7446D8B916?sequence=1 (accessed March 3, 2020).

WHO. 2014. *WHO handbook for guideline development, 2nd ed.* https://apps.who.int/iris/handle/10665/145714 (accessed February 19, 2020).

Wieringa, S., D. Dreesens, F. Forland, C. Hulshof, S. Lukersmith, F. Macbeth, B. Shaw, A. van Vliet, T. Zuiderent-Jerak, and AID Knowledge Working Group of the Guidelines International Network. 2018. Different knowledge, different styles of reasoning: A challenge for guideline development. *BMJ Evidence-Based Medicine* 23(3):87–91.

WWC (What Works Clearinghouse). 2017. *What Works Clearinghouse standards handbook, version 4.0.* Washington, DC: Institute of Education Sciences.

2

The Landscape and Evolution of Public Health Emergency Preparedness and Response Research in the United States

The complexities of the public health emergency preparedness and response (PHEPR) system and the unique challenges of conducting research on PHEPR practices,[1] as discussed in Chapter 1, have impeded efforts to build a cumulative evidence base for the field. This chapter examines how these challenges have been compounded by funding issues and unclear prioritization of research topics. The chapter begins with a description of the state of the evidence in the PHEPR research field, informed by a scoping review and series of evidence maps commissioned by the committee. This discussion is followed by an examination of the evolution of the PHEPR research field. The chapter concludes with an explanation of how the current approach to coordinating, funding, and conducting PHEPR research is inadequate for improving the quality of evidence in the field.

CHARACTERIZING THE RESEARCH ON PHEPR: A MAP OF THE EVIDENCE

An increasing number of PHEPR research studies have been produced over the past two decades, but these studies are often dispersed across topics and sources, and as a result, it is not clear which specific areas need further research. Several scoping reviews of the PHEPR research literature have identified important knowledge gaps and research priorities (Abramson et al., 2007; Acosta et al., 2009; Birnbaum et al., 2017; Challen et al., 2012; Khan et al., 2015; Savoia et al., 2017; Smith et al., 2018; Yeager et al., 2010). In general, these scoping reviews have found that the PHEPR evidence base was increasing with respect to the number of articles published but was overwhelmingly descriptive, lacking in objective evaluations and quantitative analyses and unbalanced in focus across the emergency cycle, with a majority of articles being focused on the preparedness and response phases.

[1] The committee defined PHEPR practices broadly as a type of process, structure, or intervention whose implementation is intended to mitigate the adverse effects of a public health emergency on the population as a whole or a particular sub-group within the population.

PHEPR research tends to be reactive and opportunistic—following a disaster, numerous event-specific research articles appear in the literature—and not always coordinated, timely, or focused on answering the most important questions (Elsevier, 2017). This situation does, however, appear to be changing. A review conducted by Savoia and colleagues (2017) found that PHEPR research has evolved over the past two decades, from generic inquiry to a more critical analysis of specific interventions and with an increase in empirical studies.

While all of these scoping reviews have added value in identifying common themes across the evidence base and noting particular knowledge gaps, none of them has focused purposefully on the 15 PHEPR Capabilities, which are fundamental in guiding state, local, tribal, and territorial public health agencies in assessing, building, and sustaining PHEPR capacity. To address this gap, the committee sought to understand the extent, range, and nature of PHEPR research across the 15 PHEPR Capabilities, with a specific focus on studies that evaluate the impact of PHEPR practices, and commissioned an expert group to visualize these findings using high-level evidence maps (see Appendix D). Evidence maps are a relatively new form of evidence synthesis whose purpose is to identify research gaps and future research needs (Miake-Lye et al., 2016). An understanding of where evidence exists and where little to no evidence exists across the 15 PHEPR Capabilities can help stakeholders interpret the state of the evidence and inform policy decision making and priorities for future research.

Overall Distribution of Articles Within the 15 PHEPR Capabilities

A total of 1,692 articles (published 2001–2019)—consisting of quantitative (comparative and noncomparative) impact, quantitative nonimpact, qualitative, and modeling studies; literature reviews; after action reports (AARs) and case reports; and commentaries—were initially included in the commissioned scoping review.[2] Ultimately, the committee was most interested in those studies that could potentially provide evidence regarding the 15 PHEPR Capabilities. Therefore, after this initial classification of all study designs, commentaries and literature reviews were excluded from subsequent analyses, resulting in a total of 1,106 articles for final inclusion.

Figure 2-1 displays the distribution of articles across the 15 PHEPR Capabilities. The highest percentage of articles mapped to the Community Preparedness Capability (20 percent of the 1,106 articles), followed by the Emergency Operations Coordination, Medical Countermeasure Dispensing and Administration, and Non-Pharmaceutical Interventions Capabilities, each at 10 percent. It is not surprising that the greatest proportion of research addresses the Community Preparedness Capability because it is the broadest of the Capabilities, covering topics from at-risk populations and community partnership building to strengthening of personal preparedness and training and education (CDC, 2018). Furthermore, research on the Capabilities is conducted primarily in nonemergency times. The Capabilities with the lowest percentage of articles include Fatality Management and Public Health Laboratory

[2] The scoping review's methodology, including search strategy, inclusion and exclusion criteria, and limitations, is described in the commissioned paper documenting the review titled "Review and Evidence Mapping of Scholarly Publications Within CDC's 15 Public Health Emergency Preparedness and Response Capabilities," by Testa and colleagues (see Appendix D). The task of finding and classifying the body of research underlying all of the 15 PHEPR Capabilities was challenging because of the broad scope, complexity, and nature of the research topics. The evidence maps that resulted from the review certainly do not contain every published study examining PHEPR practices since 2001. The scoping review did not attempt to capture after action reports not published in journals and searchable in bibliographic databases. Future efforts could focus on conducting detailed scoping reviews on specific Capabilities or practices.

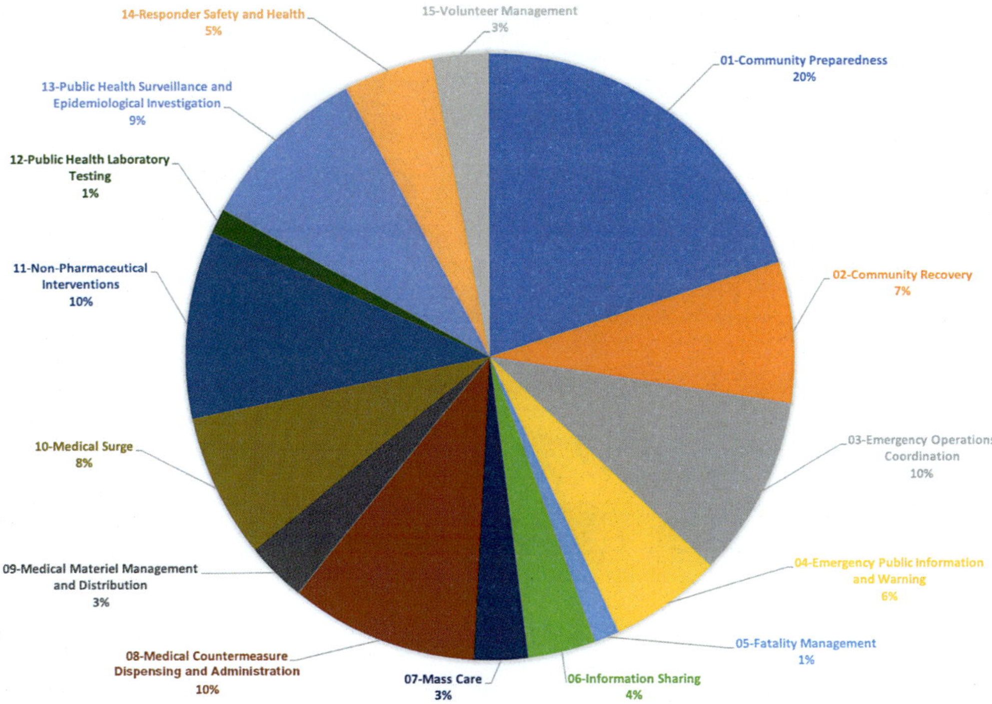

FIGURE 2-1 Distribution of evidentiary articles by PHEPR Capability (N = 1,106).

Testing, both at 1 percent. Notably, for both of these Capabilities, most of the supporting research would be expected to have occurred outside of the PHEPR field, which may help explain the low numbers of studies. Public Health Laboratory Testing is foundational public health practice, and for Fatality Management, public health agencies often play supporting roles and coordinate with partner organizations and agencies to provide services.

Figure 2-2 shows that overall, the numbers of studies are relatively evenly split across types of outcomes, with the exception of cost outcomes (1 percent of all studies). Individual health outcomes[3] are examined in 30 percent of the studies. Capabilities with individual health outcomes as their most common outcome type include Community Recovery, Fatality Management, Mass Care, Non-Pharmaceutical Interventions, Public Health Surveillance and Epidemiological Investigation, and Responder Safety and Health. These Capabilities are fundamentally different from those with process outcomes, namely Emergency Public Information and Warning, Information Sharing, Medical Countermeasure Dispensing and Administration, Medical Surge, and Public Health Laboratory Testing. The former set of Capabilities focuses on practices that more directly impact human health and well-being, while the latter set focuses on processes of the PHEPR system (e.g., information dissemination, dispensing, and testing). Individual nonhealth outcomes align most strongly with the Community Preparedness and Volunteer Management Capabilities, which likely reflects the emphasis on planning and training for those two Capabilities. Research that maps to the Emergency Operations Coordination and Medical Materiel Management and Distribution Capabilities most often assesses system-level outcomes.

[3] Individual health outcomes include morbidity-, mortality-, clinical/surgical-, and psychological-related outcomes.

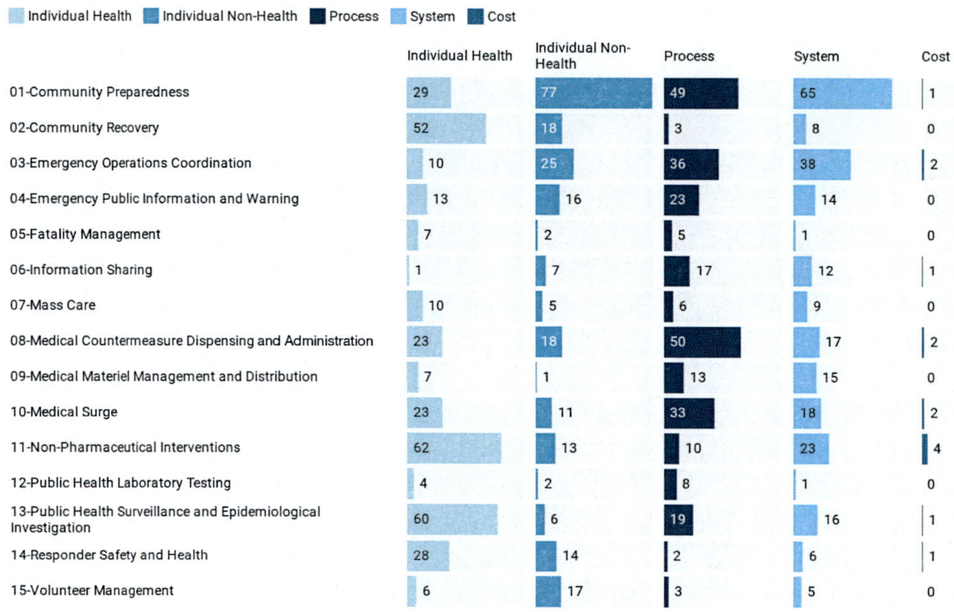

FIGURE 2-2 Type of outcome by PHEPR Capability (N = 1,106).

Quantitative Impact Studies Within the 15 PHEPR Capabilities

Among the 1,106 evidentiary studies, only 95 (8.5 percent) are categorized as quantitative impact studies—meaning they evaluated specific PHEPR practices.[4] Of these 95 studies, 22 are noncomparative and 73 comparative. The majority (72 of 95) are based in the United States. Figure 2-3 illustrates the 72 quantitative impact studies conducted in the United States by outcome (an evidence map for the non-U.S. quantitative impact studies can be found in Appendix D).

It is important to note that the distribution of U.S. quantitative impact studies across the 15 PHEPR Capabilities largely reflects the overall distribution of studies, with the exception of the Emergency Operations Coordination Capability (see Figure 2-1). Emergency Operations Coordination is examined in 10 percent of all studies, equal to the proportions for Medical Countermeasure Dispensing and Administration and Non-Pharmaceutical Interventions, but has only 3 quantitative impact studies, while the other Capabilities have 11 and 7, respectively. Given that Emergency Operations Coordination comprises largely organizational, behavioral, and management practices, which are likely to be highly context-specific, this Capability, in contrast to Medical Countermeasure Dispensing and Administration and Non-Pharmaceutical Interventions, may be better suited to quality improvement

[4] Three types of evidence are defined in evidence-based public health: Type 1 is research that describes risk–disease relations and identifies the magnitude, severity, and preventability of public health problems; Type 2 is research that identifies the relative effectiveness of specific interventions aimed at addressing a problem; and Type 3 is research on the design and implementation of an intervention, the contextual circumstances in which the intervention was implemented, and how the intervention was received. Quantitative nonimpact studies encompass Type 1 evidence, and quantitative impact studies encompass Types 2 and 3 (Rychetnik et al., 2004). All three evidence types result from "evidentiary studies," which are characterized by some form of systematic data collection and analysis that could provide evidence regarding the PHEPR Capabilities. Nonevidentiary studies include opinion pieces, concept papers, and commentaries, as well as literature reviews.

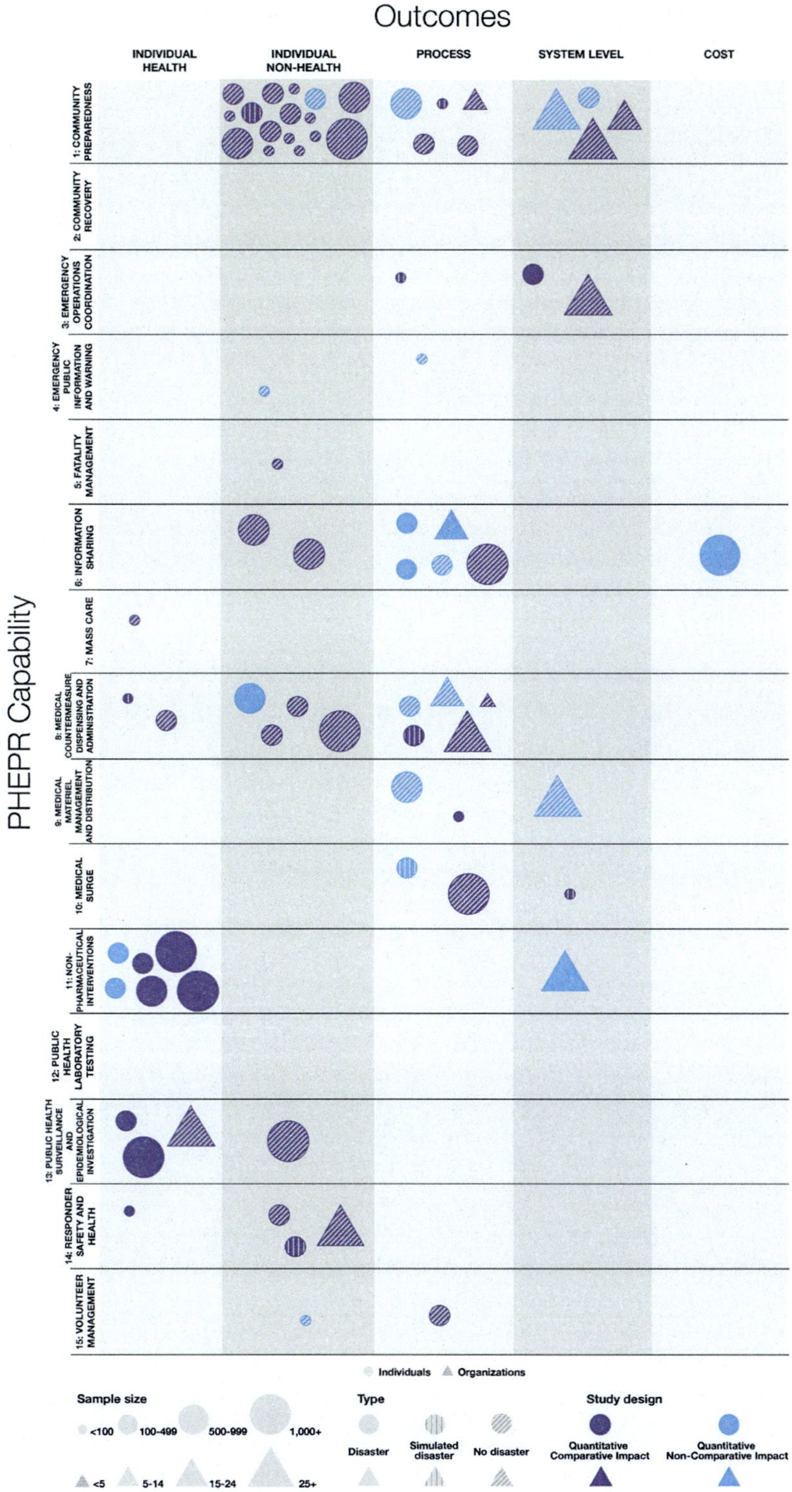

FIGURE 2-3 Evidence map: Characteristics of U.S. quantitative impact studies across the PHEPR Capabilities (N = 72).

evaluations relative to research studies aimed at generating generalizable knowledge. This notion is supported by the observation that the three Emergency Operations Coordination quantitative impact studies examine response trainings and processes.

It is unsurprising that there are only one to two quantitative impact studies each for the Capabilities of Fatality Management, Mass Care, and Volunteer Management, and none examining Public Health Laboratory Testing, as only 1 to 3 percent of all included studies fall within these Capabilities. Consistent with the overall distribution of U.S. studies, a majority of the quantitative impact studies map to Community Preparedness, and many of these comparative impact studies are pre-post test studies of trainings and educational programs. No quantitative impact studies examining Community Recovery were identified. A majority of Community Recovery studies are quantitative nonimpact designs, which is not surprising given that a large share of the focus and efforts after public health emergencies consists of assessing, monitoring, and surveilling health, disease, and injury among the impacted community to identify adverse health effects. However, this preponderance of nonimpact designs does demonstrate the significant gap in studies evaluating the impact of PHEPR programs and practices. The paucity of studies for Emergency Public Information and Warning (just two) probably reflects the fact that practices would be expected to be grounded in the risk communication literature more broadly; thus, it is likely that some impact research has occurred outside of the PHEPR field and was not captured in this scoping review.

Given the dearth of research examining cost-related outcomes across all 1,160 studies, it is not surprising that there is only one quantitative impact study (for the Information Sharing Capability) examining cost. Process and systems-level outcomes, combined, are the most predominant outcomes examined in all 1,106 studies; however, it appears that individual-level health (e.g., morbidity and mortality) and nonhealth (e.g., knowledge and behavior) outcomes are more predominant among the quantitative impact studies. As noted, the vast majority of studies examining most of the 15 PHEPR Capabilities were not conducted during a real disaster, the exception being those examining Non-Pharmaceutical Interventions.

Studies Within Specific Practice Areas of the 15 PHEPR Capabilities

The committee was interested in examining the distribution of studies not only across the 15 PHEPR Capabilities but also across specific PHEPR practice areas within individual Capabilities.[5] Evidence maps for each of the 15 PHEPR Capabilities can be found in Appendix D; one is discussed here as an illustrative example. As a whole, however, the maps in Appendix D show that the distribution of quantitative impact studies is uneven, with few (and in some cases no) such studies for the majority of PHEPR practices.

Figure 2-4 shows the characteristics of the 110 studies addressing PHEPR practice areas within the Medical Countermeasure Dispensing and Administration Capability. Notably, there are gaps in the practice areas of communication and coordination for effective dispensing and monitoring of adverse events. The monitoring of adverse events following dispensing of medical countermeasures has previously been highlighted as a gap in the field (NASEM, 2017a). The majority of the studies cluster within the practice area of initiating and managing dispensing systems, such as points of distribution and other modalities for dispensing. This Capability includes the most AARs and case reports among all 15 PHEPR Capabilities (tied with Community Preparedness) and accounts for 87 percent of U.S.-based studies. The predominant

[5] The committee developed a broad list of potential PHEPR practices by breaking the functions and tasks within the PHEPR Capabilities down into topics at a level of resolution for which conclusions about effectiveness could potentially be drawn.

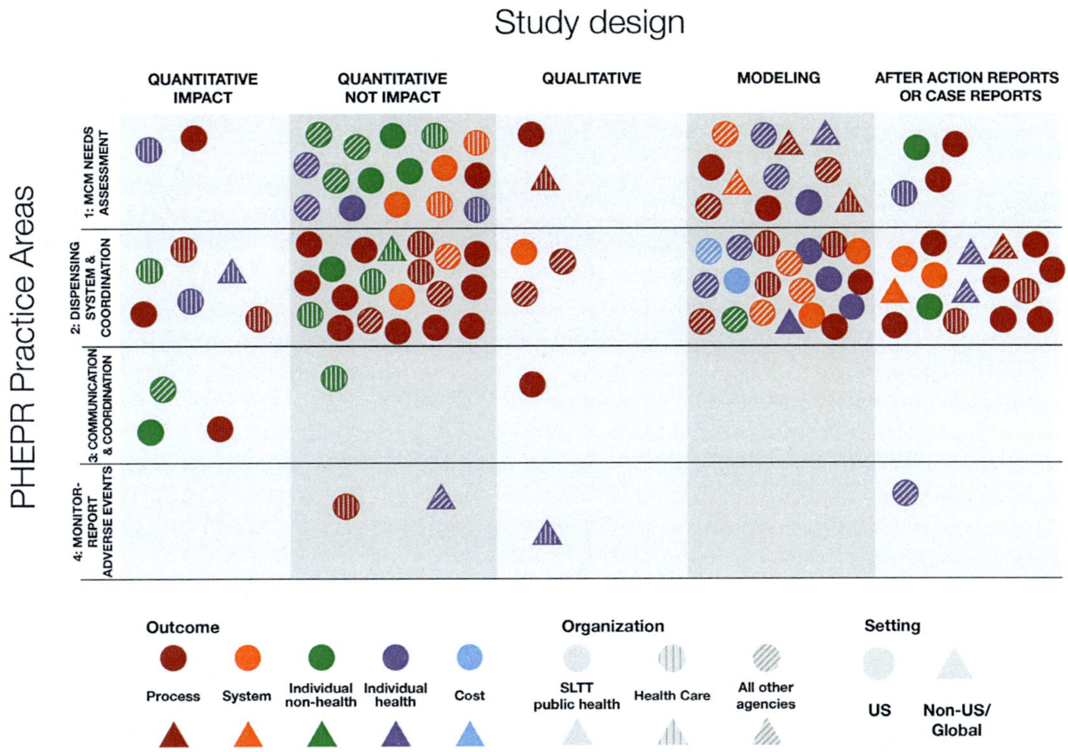

FIGURE 2-4 Evidence map: Characteristics of studies for Medical Countermeasure Dispensing and Administration (N = 110).

practice area and the numbers of U.S. studies and AARs and case reports are not surprising given that past U.S. preparedness efforts have often focused on enhancing this practice area.

Implications for Future Research and Evidence Reviews

The information gleaned from this scoping review and the series of evidence maps it produced may be useful to policy makers and PHEPR researchers as an important first step for two distinct efforts: (1) clarifying where sufficient evidence may be available for future efforts to synthesize the evidence on the effectiveness of PHEPR practices, and (2) identifying gaps that can inform priorities for future research.

Those practice areas in which quantitative impact studies tend to cluster may be good starting points for considering topics for future evidence reviews, particularly if they can be linked to important knowledge gaps identified by practitioners or policy makers. In a prioritization activity conducted by the committee with 10 PHEPR practitioners, for example, at least 66 percent of the panel indicated that reviews of several topics in Community Preparedness, Emergency Public Information and Warning, and Responder Safety and Health were of highest or high priority (see Appendix A for the full results from this activity). The map of U.S. quantitative impact studies (see Figure 2-3) shows that there is some impact evidence available for each of these three Capabilities. Capability-specific evidence maps provided in Appendix D could help further scope these reviews. For example, the PHEPR practitioner panel rated effective message formats for information sharing with at-risk populations as a high-priority practice area.

Figure 2-5 illustrates the characteristics of the 66 studies for PHEPR practice areas within the Emergency Public Information and Warning Capability. The map shows no quantitative impact studies for the at-risk population practice area, which may indicate that a review on this topic would yield little in the way of findings on effective practices and suggests that the topic is an important research gap. However, it is important to reiterate that Emergency Public Information and Warning is a broad field, and it is likely that some impact research has occurred outside of PHEPR. Evidence on risk communication practices in other contexts could, for example, be reviewed and synthesized as described in Chapter 3 as "parallel evidence" (i.e., evidence from similar practices used in other fields that could inform determinations of effectiveness).

In terms of research gaps, the evidence maps can aid in determining which areas of research are weakest and strongest. Prioritizing of which areas with little information are most deserving of further research and funding would be most useful if dependent not only on the magnitude of the evidence gaps observed, but also on the type of disaster or emergency and the resources, workforce personnel, and other components of the public health system available to public health agencies.

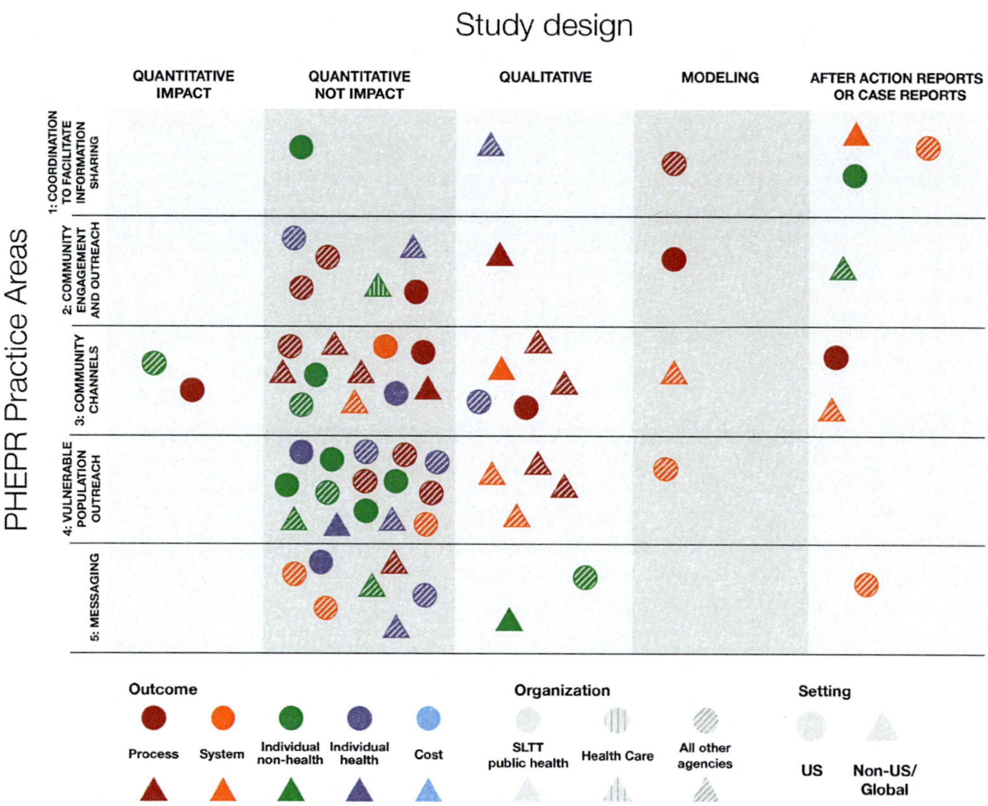

FIGURE 2-5 Evidence map: Characteristics of studies for Emergency Public Information and Warning (N = 66).

A LOOK BACK AT PHEPR RESEARCH PROGRAMS

The commissioned scoping review provides a broad overview of the research for the 15 PHEPR Capabilities and specific practice areas within these Capabilities. This section summarizes several of the transformational research programs and initiatives that contributed to the development of this PHEPR knowledge base and advanced PHEPR as a field of study. As a result of these research programs, PHEPR research has evolved in essentially two decades from focusing on program assessment and evaluation, to examining systems and health services, to being conducted during public health emergencies (Carbone and Thomas, 2018). Unfortunately, many of these programs are no longer funded and have been discontinued. As in all areas of public health, ongoing research and evaluation are essential to improving practice in the PHEPR field.

Centers for Disease Control and Prevention–Funded Academic PHEPR Workforce Development and Research Centers

Centers for Public Health Preparedness

In the PHEPR field, the Centers for Disease Control and Prevention (CDC) has long supported academic and practice linkages, particularly with schools of public health (Thielen et al., 2005; Turnock et al., 2010). In 2000, CDC funded four Centers for Public Health Preparedness (CPHPs) within schools of public health. The CPHPs were developed to be practice oriented, and to work closely with public health agencies to assess training needs and deliver competency-based training, education, and technical assistance and provide a nexus for applied research related to workforce development. From 2004 to 2010, CDC expanded the program and provided $134 million to 27 CPHPs to continue enhancing training and education for public health agencies (Baker et al., 2010; Richmond et al., 2010). The CPHPs were instrumental in strengthening academic and practice relationships related to workforce competencies (Wright et al., 2010). Furthermore, the CPHPs set the stage for some of the earliest attempts at developing evidence-based practices for workforce development by evaluating the impact of exercises and trainings and utilizing pre- and posttests to assess knowledge (Alexander et al., 2010; Hoeppner et al., 2010; Kohn et al., 2010; Potter et al., 2010).

Preparedness and Response Research Centers and Learning Centers

It was not until 2006 that provisions in the Pandemic and All-Hazards Preparedness Act (PAHPA)[6] established the need for a research agenda. A 2008 Institute of Medicine (IOM) letter report commissioned by CDC in response to PAHPA drove a focus on four topic areas: enhancing the usefulness of training, improving timely emergency communications, creating and maintaining sustainable response systems, and generating effective criteria and metrics for systems (IOM, 2008). To support the goals of PAHPA, and guided by the 2008 IOM letter report, CDC redirected resources from the CPHP program toward research and established nine Preparedness and Emergency Response Research Centers (PERRCs) at accredited schools of public health (Turnock et al., 2010). Workforce development activities were continued through 14 Preparedness and Emergency Response Learning Centers (PERLCs).

[6] Pandemic and All-Hazards Preparedness Act. Public Law 116-22, 116th Cong. (January 3, 2019).

Preparedness and Emergency Response Research Centers One of the objectives of the PERRCs was to initiate a PHEPR research enterprise in the form of multidisciplinary centers to conduct research that would enhance PHEPR planning, practices, and policies at the federal, state, local, and tribal levels (Eisenstein et al., 2014; Leinhos et al., 2014). The PERRC program, which was funded from 2008 to 2014, was the first and only U.S. Department of Health and Human Services (HHS) program to use a public health systems research approach to investigate and improve the PHEPR system (Qari et al., 2014). Over the 6 years it was funded, $57 million was provided across the PERRC program. The PERRCs supported more than 30 projects, contributed to the development of a group of future public health systems researchers through training for about 200 junior research personnel and more than 30 new investigators (Leinhos et al., 2014), and generated approximately 171 peer-reviewed publications[7] (Qari et al., 2019). The observations of Savoia and colleagues (2018) suggest that the PERRCs played a substantial role in the PHEPR research field and that without them, at least half of the existing knowledge base would not have been generated (Savoia et al., 2018).

Many of the PERRCs worked closely with public health agencies and developed their research agendas based on requests from and needs of these agencies, guided by an advisory committee comprising representatives of multiple sectors (Leinhos et al., 2014). The PERRCs engaged an estimated 500 research partners (Savoia et al., 2018). In addition to traditional collaborations within schools of public health, the PERRCs collaborated with nontraditional partners, including academic researchers in schools of engineering, law, and public policy (Eisenstein et al., 2014). For example, systems engineers at the University of North Carolina PERRC applied computer simulation tools to large-scale public health emergencies to demonstrate how modeling can improve public health emergency planning, resource allocation, and decision making (Yaylali et al., 2014).

Preparedness and Emergency Response Learning Centers The PERLC program, which was funded from 2009 to 2015, also within schools of public health, was built on a decade of activities carried out by its predecessor program, the CPHPs, and carried on the mission of strengthening linkages between academic public health programs and public health practice to improve curriculum development for both workforce development and graduate education for public health students (Richmond et al., 2014). The reduction in the total number of centers (from 27 to 14) and total funding (from $134 million to $34 million) for the PERLCs relative to the CPHPs mirrored reductions in federal funding for state and local health departments for public health preparedness (Qari et al., 2018). The PERLCs were expected to both inform and utilize the work of the PERRCs, and there were several schools where both a PERRC and a PERLC were situated. Similar to the CPHPs, the PERLCs emphasized the evaluation of trainings (Hites et al., 2014). Contributions of the PERLCs to the field include innovative methods for workforce preparedness training (Everly et al., 2014; Griffith et al., 2014; Horney and Wilfert, 2014; McCormick et al., 2014; Olson et al., 2014; Renger and Granillo, 2014; Testa et al., 2014; Uden-Holman et al., 2014; Walkner et al., 2014) and training and preparedness efforts in the community for community coalitions and at-risk populations, including Latino, limited-English-speaking, and tribal populations (D'Ambrosio et al., 2014; Frahm et al., 2014; Levin et al., 2014; Riley-Jacome et al., 2014; Tall Chief et al., 2014; Wiebel et al., 2014). The PERLCs developed more than 800 learning products intended to improve PHEPR workforce readiness and competency (Qari et al., 2018).

---

[7] A repository of PERRC publications can be accessed at https://www.cdc.gov/cpr/science/updates.htm (accessed June 23, 2020).

Translation, Dissemination, and Implementation of Public Health Preparedness and Response Research and Training Initiative

To accelerate the translation, dissemination, and implementation (TDI) of promising research findings, tools, and trainings developed by the PERRCs and the PERLCs, CDC provided through the TDI Initiative approximately $9 million in funding for nine awards at schools of public health that previously had hosted the PERRCs or the PERLCs (Qari et al., 2018). As a part of this initiative, awardees developed virtual learning communities, experiential learning approaches, and mechanisms to support the implementation of emergency and response communication tools in public health agencies and of a program to increase use of evidence-based programs in public health agencies (Arora et al., 2018; Baseman et al., 2018; Blake et al., 2018; Documet et al., 2018; Eisenman et al., 2018; Revere et al., 2018; Testa et al., 2018; Van Nostrand et al., 2018). The TDI Initiative revealed several challenges to the translation of research to practice (e.g., understanding of the product and its relevance to practice) and researchers' efforts to overcome these barriers (NORC at the University of Chicago, 2017). The initiative also demonstrated the need to evaluate the relevance and effectiveness of products developed by the PERRCs and the PERLCs for wider implementation.

Additional CDC Efforts

In addition to the CPHPs, the PERRCs, the PERLCs, and the TDI Initiative, CDC has funded other research awards related to PHEPR. In 2007, CDC's Office of Public Health Research funded Mentored Research Scientist Development Awards (K01) to provide support for intensive research career development under the guidance of a mentor in areas addressing bioterrorism, other infectious disease outbreaks, and other public health threats and emergencies, among other areas (CDC, 2007). The expectation was that awardees would launch research careers and become competitive for research project grant (R01) funding. Currently, CDC's Center for Preparedness and Response issues Broad Agency Announcements for Public Health Emergency Preparedness and Response Applied Research to solicit proposals for research funding in several topic areas of interest (CDC, 2018).

Other Federal Disaster Research Programs

Numerous other agencies and departments in the federal government have sponsored disaster research more broadly, some of which relates to PHEPR. In the absence of any single overarching research agenda across these federal efforts, each agency independently identified issues of concern and knowledge gaps to be addressed. In the early 2000s, for example, the Agency for Healthcare Research and Quality (AHRQ), which focuses on evidence-based health care, funded PHEPR research related to bioterrorism, vaccine distribution, health care system preparedness and surge capacity, and pediatric disaster preparedness (AHRQ, 2011). This program was discontinued in 2011. Following the *Deepwater Horizon* oil spill in 2010, the National Institute of Environmental Health Sciences (NIEHS) funded 4 universities and 45 community partners to conduct research related to the disaster's impacts (Guidry, 2016) on maternal and child health (Peres et al., 2016), mental health (Rung et al., 2016), and community resilience (Mayer et al., 2015). Other sources of federal disaster-related research funding include the U.S. Department of Homeland Security (DHS), the National Science Foundation, and the U.S. Department of Defense (DoD). Along the same lines, the National Center for Disaster Medicine and Public Health, housed within the Uniformed Services University, was founded as a collaboration by five federal agencies—HHS, DoD, DHS, the U.S. Department of Transportation, and the U.S. Department of Veterans Affairs—to conduct health education and research efforts related to domestic and international disasters (NCDMPH, 2020). As Table 2-1 demonstrates, the system for funding disaster research is highly fragmented and complicated, with each federal stakeholder supporting different aspects of issues related to PHEPR. Furthermore, the diversity and breadth of the federal stakeholders who conduct or support disaster research can make it challenging to coordinate efforts, especially when many of these stakeholders do not have public health as their primary mission.

Specific Efforts to Enhance the Conduct of Research During Public Health Emergencies

Recent years have seen increased recognition of critical opportunities to conduct research during response and recovery that could lead to improved assistance to those affected by the event and inform future PHEPR policy, planning, and practice (Carbone and Wright, 2016). Specific efforts to strengthen the conduct of research during public health emergencies have

TABLE 2-1 Key Federal Stakeholders in Conducting or Supporting Disaster Research

Federal Stakeholder	Role in Conducting or Supporting Disaster Research
Federal Emergency Management Agency (FEMA)	Whole-community preparedness, personal disaster preparedness, protective actions
Health Resources and Services Administration (HRSA)	Access to health care; enhancing health systems for geographically, economically, and medically vulnerable populations
National Institute for Occupational Safety and Health (NIOSH)	Responder safety and health
National Institute of Standards and Technology (NIST)	Built environment, infrastructure, communities, hazards, standards
National Institutes of Health (NIH)	Environmental health, natural disasters, biodefense
National Oceanic and Atmospheric Administration (NOAA)	Natural disasters
National Science Foundation (NSF)	Social sciences, engineering, natural hazards, built environment
Office of the Assistant Secretary for Preparedness and Response (ASPR)	Regional disaster health response, health security, medical countermeasure enterprise, science preparedness
U.S. Department of Agriculture (USDA)	Food and agriculture safety, antimicrobial resistance, climate change
U.S. Department of Defense (DoD)	Epidemiology, medical countermeasure development, biodefense
U.S. Department of Homeland Security (DHS)	Counterterrorism, homeland security, critical infrastructure, preparedness, and resilience
U.S. Department of Housing and Urban Development (HUD)	Community resilience, housing and community development
U.S. Department of the Interior (DOI)	Natural disasters
U.S. Department of Transportation (DOT)	Emergency medical services safety, innovation, and infrastructure
U.S. Department of Veterans Affairs (VA)	VA facilities and veterans' health affected by disasters
U.S. Food and Drug Administration (FDA)	Medical countermeasure law and science
U.S. Geological Survey (USGS)	Natural hazards, emergency management, environmental health

been spearheaded largely by CDC, the Assistant Secretary for Preparedness and Response (ASPR), and NIEHS (Carbone and Wright, 2016; Lurie et al., 2013; Miller et al., 2016).

In 2011, the National Biodefense Science Board (NBSB), at the behest of ASPR, issued a call to action to include scientific investigations as an integral component of disaster planning and response (NBSB, 2011). NBSB provided recommendations to establish a research office under ASPR, a separate Emergency Support Function for research, and a disaster institutional review board (see Box 2-1). In 2012, ASPR convened a workshop, "Scientific Preparedness and Response for Public Health," to discuss efforts to build the infrastructure necessary to rapidly mobilize relevant research expertise and technology in the context of a public health emergency. Continued progress toward many of these recommendations, which are still critical and relevant today, has been lacking (ASPR, 2012).

BOX 2-1 NATIONAL BIODEFENSE SCIENCE BOARD'S RECOMMENDATIONS TO MOUNT A COMPREHENSIVE AND RAPID MOBILIZATION OF SCIENTIFIC RESOURCES IN THE INVESTIGATIVE RESPONSE TO DISASTERS THAT THREATEN PUBLIC HEALTH

- Immediately convene Strategic Science Planning Panels, made up of leading expert government and civilian scientists, to identify research questions and knowledge gaps likely to arise during a variety of incident types, including those foreseen in Federal Emergency Management Agency (FEMA) National Planning Scenarios.
- Add a "Scientific Response Support Annex" to the National Response Framework, and amend the National Oil and Hazardous Substances Pollution Contingency Plan to include a scientific response.
- Establish with leadership and staff from the Office of the Assistant Secretary for Preparedness and Response an Interdepartmental Center for Scientific Investigations During Disaster Response (the Center); the Center will have a dedicated staff, and its primary mission will be to anticipate, plan for, coordinate, facilitate, and evaluate scientific investigations conducted before, during, and after disasters.
- Develop the concepts, doctrine, infrastructure, and personnel needed to begin scientific investigation and data collection rapidly in various types of incidents.
- Integrate the Public Health Emergency Research Review Board into standard operating procedures for review of research before, during, and after a disaster response.
- Appoint a liaison within the Center to the Office of Management and Budget's Office of Information and Regulatory Affairs to facilitate review of scientific protocols required by the Paperwork Reduction Act (PRA). There should also be an independent review of the benefit versus the net loss of the effect of the PRA on a timely, emergent, scientific response with consideration of possible approaches for remediation.
- Establish funding mechanisms to support a rapid and robust scientific response to disasters.
- Integrate individuals and communities affected by a disaster as full partners in scientific investigations related to the disaster.
- Standardize approaches to data collection and sharing by federal, state, and local response organizations (and encourage the same among private and volunteer organizations), giving special attention to collection of baseline data.
- Identify, acquire or develop, deploy, and maintain new information technology for collecting data in the field.

SOURCE: Excerpted from NBSB, 2011.

Following Hurricane Sandy, HHS secured funding for grants from the Disaster Relief Appropriations Act of 2013[8] to conduct research on factors related to individual and community resilience, health care system function, and adverse mental health outcomes (Carbone and Wright, 2016). Around the same time, NIEHS, the National Library of Medicine (NLM), CDC, and ASPR, in collaboration with the National Academies' Forum on Medical and Public Health Preparedness for Disasters and Emergencies, hosted a public workshop to examine strategies and diversified partnerships for enabling methodologically and ethically sound public health and medical research during future emergencies (IOM, 2015). This group also rapidly convened experts during the 2014 Ebola and 2016 Zika outbreaks to develop research priorities (IOM and NRC, 2014; NASEM, 2016). During a 2017 workshop focused on a preliminary examination of the key research findings from the Hurricane Sandy grants, it became apparent that more opportunities were needed to discuss how PHEPR research could best be conducted, interpreted, and implemented (NASEM, 2017b).

Currently, efforts to advance the conduct of research during response and recovery are sustained primarily under the Disaster Response Research (DR2) program, a partnership between NIEHS and NLM (with an interagency working group) (Miller et al., 2016). The DR2 program provides tools, protocols, researcher networks, and training exercises to support the conduct of research in response to public health emergencies as an approach to building capacity in preparedness and response.

LIMITATIONS OF PHEPR RESEARCH PROGRAMS

As previously noted, the research programs and findings that developed to inform the field over the past two decades have contributed to enhancing the PHEPR knowledge base. Unfortunately, however, the establishment of these programs did not provide a comprehensive solution to the dearth of evidence-based practices for preparing and responding to public health emergencies. This short-lived, uncoordinated approach to funding PHEPR research had several implications for the PHEPR field, discussed below, and left a number of challenges to the conduct of such research unaddressed (see Figure 2-6).

Misaligned and Unclear Research Priorities

The PERRC and the PERLC funding awards were announced before the 2011 publication of the CDC PHEPR Capabilities, which created a misalignment between research and practice. Although the research findings that emerged from the PERRCs and the PERLCs appeared retrospectively to align with the Capabilities, a formal focused and dedicated research agenda with clear goals and measurable objectives aimed at building the evidence base to support the Capabilities was never articulated (Leinhos et al., 2014; Turnock et al., 2010). Furthermore, because a formal research agenda was lacking, researchers often duplicated or recycled similar content (e.g., repeated incident command system trainings), and did not always use appropriate study designs for the research questions being asked. Moreover, the focus on research topics has been uneven, with more than half of the CDC PHEPR Capabilities receiving little to no funding (Keim et al., 2019).

In addition, much of the funding for academic programs (e.g., the CPHPs and the PERLCs) was directed at workforce development, specifically with a charge to develop, deliver, and evaluate trainings instead of conducting research (Kelliher, 2018; Richmond et

[8] Disaster Relief Appropriations Act of 2013. Public Law 113-2, 113th Cong. (January 29, 2013).

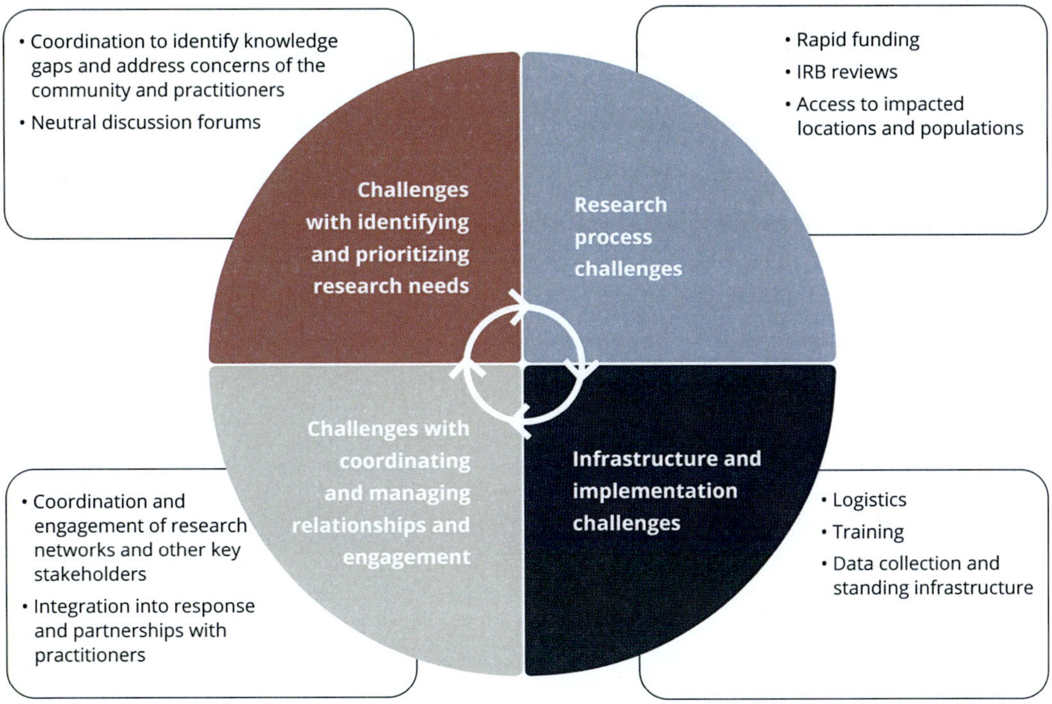

FIGURE 2-6 Major categories of challenges to the conduct of PHEPR research and how they can be addressed.
NOTE: IRB = institutional review board.
SOURCE: Adapted from Miller et al., 2016.

al., 2014). It was acknowledged that an improved evidence base likely would not emerge from these practice-oriented collaborations (Turnock et al., 2010).

Lack of Infrastructure to Support the Conduct of Quality PHEPR Research

While attempts have been made to advance the conduct of research before, during, and after public health emergencies, continued and sustained progress toward building a research infrastructure to support this approach is lacking. Inadequate infrastructure and supporting mechanisms for the conduct of PHEPR research still encompass a lack of coordination and the inability to prioritize research needs before and during response, varying institutional review board restrictions, Office of Management and Budget issues related to the Paperwork Reduction Act for surveys and user research, lack of a sustainable and rapid funding platform for this type of work, challenges with data collection and rapid mobilization of researchers, and barriers to accessing impacted locations and populations (IOM, 2015; Miller et al., 2016).

Furthermore, the response community remains hesitant to accept researchers within public health emergency settings because of cultural differences between the practice and research fields, and research is not standard practice within the given operational response structure. In a public health emergency, the first priority for a public health agency is to respond and ensure that individuals are removed from harm and continue to receive public health services (IOM, 2015). Monitoring or assisting in research can strain the resources of a public health agency and its ability to respond. The staff of public health agencies frequently lack the infrastructure or training needed to conduct such research; may lack the time, resources, incentives, or support to collect the necessary data; and may not be authorized to take part in some types of PHEPR research.

Lack of Coordination Across Funders and Shortcomings of Research Funding

The array of federal and nonfederal organizations supporting PHEPR research is highly diverse and complicated, and changes according to the phase of the disaster management cycle on which the research is focused (e.g., preparedness, response, recovery, or mitigation), as well as the type of disaster or hazard (Kirsch and Keim, 2019). This fragmentation further exacerbates the siloed nature of the topics, interests, and goals of PHEPR research, especially in the absence of an overarching national strategy or framework; at the same time, by contrast, PHEPR practice has become a more integrated system after years of collaboration across sectors through diverse responses. Most PHEPR research funding is directed or circumscribed by mission agencies, such as CDC and ASPR, and there are often barriers to using supplemental or programmatic funding for research from such agencies. This situation contributes to discontinuities in funding to support ongoing, sustainable research in the field. Furthermore, the CPHPs, the PERRCs, the PERLCs, and the TDI Initiative were collaborations limited to accredited schools of public health. Although the centers funded by these programs partnered with other disciplines, this approach potentially limited the opportunities for contributions to the evidence base by other relevant disciplines.

Research follows clear funding streams, and the more durable and long-lasting such funding is, the more focused and extensive is the research. Funding for PHEPR research has historically been short lived, repeatedly stopping and restarting, and has often been reactionary and overly focused on an immediate threat (Keim et al., 2019). The result has been an evidence base comprising one-off interventional studies (i.e., lacking the repetition needed to support strong conclusions about effectiveness). Little funding has been provided for academic PHEPR programs since the end of the PERRCs in 2015, the exception being the Broad Area Announcement for Public Health Emergency Preparedness and Response Applied Research of CDC's Center for Preparedness and Response. Substantial time and resources were invested in the PERRCs and the PERLCs to advance relationship building and research project development between academia and practitioners. Ultimately, much of that investment was lost when funding cycles were discontinued. Overall, funding for PHEPR research has declined substantially since 2009 (see Figure 2-7). Keim and colleagues (2019) determined that annual funding for research and development for the CDC PHEPR Capabilities from 2008 to 2017 averaged \$2.8 million.

Another aspect of PHEPR funding is related to rapid and sustained funding mechanisms for research during public health emergencies (IOM, 2015). Some rapid funding mechanisms are in place (as discussed earlier in this chapter in the section on other federal disaster research programs), but barriers remain, including the narrow focus of research on infrastructure or environmental health, the time required to disburse the funding to researchers, the size of the awards, and the timeframe to complete the research.

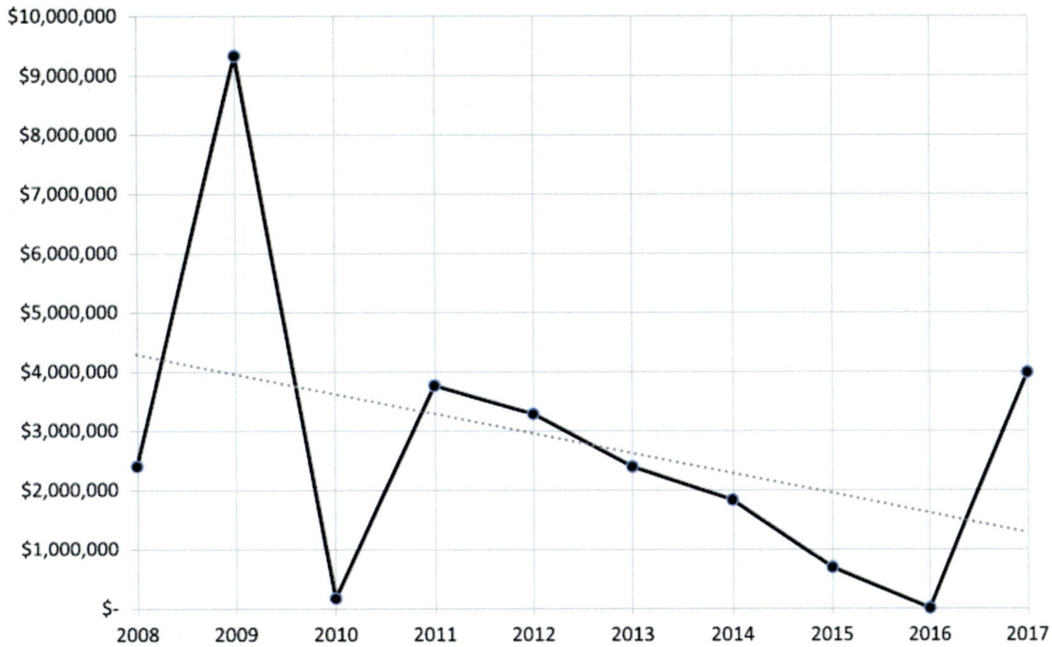

FIGURE 2-7 Total annual U.S. government funding for disaster-related research relevant to the 15 Centers for Disease Control and Prevention PHEPR Capabilities, 2008–2017.
SOURCE: Reprinted with permission from Keim et al., 2019.

CONCLUDING REMARKS

To advance the use of evidence-based practices in PHEPR, those agencies responsible for supporting PHEPR planning and implementation will have to take steps to advance the scientific evidence base for these practices. The absence of an overarching framework has contributed to a shortage of coordinated and centralized funding and infrastructure for PHEPR research and a dearth of appropriately trained researchers. Existing PHEPR research funding mechanisms do not align with how a research enterprise is normally coordinated and funded, and there are few incentives to engage in PHEPR research and many barriers to entry into the field, including limited funding opportunities. Should the field continue to be inadequately structured and supported, the PHEPR research enterprise will struggle to improve the quality of research and to address those knowledge gaps depicted in the evidence maps presented earlier in this chapter.

Research needs to become the expectation, not the exception, in the PHEPR field such that individuals are resourced and incentivized to conduct and participate in this research. As new threats emerge and response contexts evolve and become increasingly complex, it is imperative that the PHEPR system be flexible, responsive, and based on evidence to improve practice and save lives in future public health emergencies. Recommendations for ways to improve and expand the evidence base for PHEPR are presented and discussed in Chapter 8.

Conclusion: Funding for and prioritization of research before, during, and following public health emergencies are currently fragmented and disorganized, spread across multiple funding agencies, inconsistent, and do not encourage the progression of quality research or the sustainable development of research expertise. This situation has contributed to a field based on long-standing rather than evidence-based practice.

Conclusion: With the increasing complexity of both public health emergencies and the PHEPR system, policy makers and practitioners have a crucial need for access to guidance based on robust evidence to support their decisions on practices, policies, and programs for saving lives during future public health emergencies. Therefore, a coordinated and comprehensive approach to prioritizing and aligning research efforts and ensuring that research is relevant and consistently connected to practice, along with investments in research infrastructure, is necessary to strengthen the PHEPR evidence base, thereby ensuring that PHEPR practitioners have the scientific evidence they need to guide and inform their actions. At the same time, PHEPR practitioners will require incentives to base their practices, policies, and programs on evidence.

REFERENCES

Abramson, D. M., S. S. Morse, A. L. Garrett, and I. Redlener. 2007. Public health disaster research: Surveying the field, defining its future. *Disaster Medicine and Public Health Preparedness* 1(1):57–62.

Acosta, J. D., C. Nelson, E. B. Beckjord, S. R. Shelton, E. Murphy, K. L. Leuschner, and J. Wasserman. 2009. *A national agenda for public health systems research on emergency preparedness.* Santa Monica, CA: RAND Health.

AHRQ (Agency for Healthcare Research and Quality). 2011. *Public health emergency preparedness archive.* https://archive.ahrq.gov/prep (accessed February 13, 2020).

Alexander, L. K., J. A. Horney, M. Markiewicz, and P. D. M. MacDonald. 2010. Ten guiding principles of a comprehensive internet-based public health preparedness training and education program. *Public Health Reports* 125(Suppl 5):51–60.

Arora, M., B. Granillo, T. K. Zepeda, and J. L. Burgess. 2018. Experiential adult learning: A pathway to enhancing medical countermeasures capabilities. *American Journal of Public Health* 108(S5):S378–S380.

ASPR (Assistant Secretary for Preparedness and Response). 2012. *ASPR workshop: Scientific preparedness and response for public health emergencies.* https://www.phe.gov/Preparedness/legal/Documents/scientific-prep-report.pdf (accessed March 3, 2020).

Baker, E. L., M. Y. Lichtveld, and P. D. M. MacDonald. 2010. The Centers for Public Health Preparedness program: From vision to reality. *Public Health Reports* 125(Suppl 5):4–7.

Baseman, J., D. Revere, H. Karasz, and S. Allan. 2018. Implementing innovations in public health agency preparedness and response programs. *American Journal of Public Health* 108(S5):S369–S371.

Birnbaum, M. L., S. Adibhatla, O. Dudek, and J. Ramsel-Miller. 2017. Categorization and analysis of disaster health publications: An inventory. *Prehospital and Disaster Medicine* 32(5):473–482.

Blake, S. C., J. N. Hawley, A. G. Henkel, and D. H. Howard. 2018. Implementation of Florida long term care emergency preparedness portal web site, 2015–2017. *American Journal of Public Health* 108(S5):S399–S401.

Carbone, E. G., and E. V. Thomas. 2018. Science as the basis of public health emergency preparedness and response practice: The slow but crucial evolution. *American Journal of Public Health* 108(S5):S383–S386.

Carbone, E. G., and M. M. Wright. 2016. Hurricane Sandy recovery science: A model for disaster research. *Disaster Medicine and Public Health Preparedness* 10(3):304–305.

CDC (Centers for Disease Control and Prevention). 2007. *CDC Mentored Public Health Research Scientist Development award (K01).* https://grants.nih.gov/grants/guide/rfa-files/RFA-CD-07-003.html#PartII (accessed February 13, 2020).

CDC. 2018. *Research funding opportunity for 2018.* https://www.cdc.gov/cpr/research/fundingopportunity.htm (accessed February 13, 2020).

Challen, K., A. C. Lee, A. Booth, P. Gardois, H. B. Woods, and S. W. Goodacre. 2012. Where is the evidence for emergency planning? A scoping review. *BMC Public Health* 12(542).

D'Ambrosio, L., C. E. Huang, and T. Sheng Kwan-Gett. 2014. Evidence-based communications strategies: NWPERLC response to training on effectively reaching limited English-speaking (LEP) populations in emergencies. *Journal of Public Health Management and Practice* 20:S101–S106.

Documet, P. I., B. L. McDonough, and E. V. Nostrand. 2018. Engaging stakeholders at every opportunity: The experience of the emergency law inventory. *American Journal of Public Health* 108(S5):S394–S395.

Eisenman, D. P., R. M. Adams, C. M. Lang, M. Prelip, A. Dorian, J. Acosta, D. Glik, and M. Chinman. 2018. A program for local health departments to adapt and implement evidence-based emergency preparedness programs. *American Journal of Public Health* 108(S5):S396–S398.

Eisenstein, R., J. R. Finnegan, Jr., and J. W. Curran. 2014. Contributions of academia to public health preparedness research. *Public Health Reports* 129(Suppl 4):5–7.

Elsevier. 2017. *A global outlook on disaster science.* https://www.elsevier.com/__data/assets/pdf_file/0008/538091/ElsevierDisasterScienceReport-PDF.pdf (accessed March 3, 2020).

Everly, G. S. J., O. Lee McCabe, N. L. Semon, C. B. Thompson, and J. M. Links. 2014. The development of a model of psychological first aid for non–mental health trained public health personnel: The Johns Hopkins RAPID-PFA. *Journal of Public Health Management and Practice* 20:S24–S29.

Frahm, K. A., P. J. Gardner, L. M. Brown, D. P. Rogoff, and A. Troutman. 2014. Community-based disaster coalition training. *Journal of Public Health Management and Practice* 20:S111–S117.

Griffith, J. M., S. Kay Carpender, J. A. Crouch, and B. J. Quiram. 2014. A public health hazard mitigation planning process. *Journal of Public Health Management and Practice* 20:S69–S75.

Guidry, V. 2016. Deepwater Horizon *research consortia wrap up projects.* https://factor.niehs.nih.gov/2016/4/community-impact/deepwater/index.htm (accessed March 5, 2020).

Hites, L. S., M. M. Sass, L. D'Ambrosio, L. M. Brown, A. M. Wendelboe, K. E. Peters, and R. K. Sobelson. 2014. The preparedness and emergency response learning centers: Advancing standardized evaluation of public health preparedness and response trainings. *Journal of Public Health Management and Practice* 20:S17–S23.

Hoeppner, M. M., D. K. Olson, and S. C. Larson. 2010. A longitudinal study of the impact of an emergency preparedness curriculum. *Public Health Reports* 125(Suppl 5):24–32.

Horney, J. A., and R. A. Wilfert. 2014. Accelerating preparedness: Leveraging the UNC PERLC to improve other projects related to public health surveillance, assessment, and regionalization. *Journal of Public Health Management and Practice* 20:S76–S78.

IOM (Institute of Medicine). 2008. *Research priorities in emergency preparedness and response for public health systems: A letter report.* Washington, DC: The National Academies Press.

IOM. 2015. *Enabling rapid and sustainable public health research during disasters: Summary of a joint workshop by the Institute of Medicine and the U.S. Department of Health and Human Services.* Washington, DC: The National Academies Press.

IOM and NRC (National Research Council). 2014. *Research priorities to inform public health and medical practice for Ebola virus disease: Workshop in brief.* Washington, DC: The National Academies Press.

Keim, M., T. D. Kirsch, and A. Lovallo. 2019. A comparison of U.S. federal government spending for research and development related to public health preparedness capabilities, 2008–2017. *Disaster Medicine and Public Health Preparedness* 1–8.

Kelliher, R. 2018. Academic and practice partnerships: Building an effective public health system focusing on public health preparedness and response. *American Journal of Public Health* 108(S5):S353–S354.

Khan, Y., G. Fazli, B. Henry, E. de Villa, C. Tsamis, M. Grant, and B. Schwartz. 2015. The evidence base of primary research in public health emergency preparedness: A scoping review and stakeholder consultation. *BMC Public Health* 15(432).

Kirsch, T. D., and M. Keim. 2019. US governmental spending for disaster-related research, 2011–2016: Characterizing the state of science funding across 5 professional disciplines. *Disaster Medicine and Public Health Preparedness* 13(5–6):912–919.

Kohn, S., D. J. Barnett, C. Galastri, N. L. Semon, and J. M. Links. 2010. Public health-specific national incident management system trainings: Building a system for preparedness. *Public Health Reports* 125(5 Suppl):43–50.

Leinhos, M., S. H. Qari, and M. Williams-Johnson. 2014. Preparedness and emergency response research centers: Using a public health systems approach to improve all-hazards preparedness and response. *Public Health Reports* 129(Suppl 4):8–18.

Levin, K. L., M. Berliner, and A. Merdjanoff. 2014. Disaster planning for vulnerable populations: Leveraging community human service organizations direct service delivery personnel. *Journal of Public Health Management and Practice* 20:S79–S82.

Lurie, N., T. Manolio, A. P. Patterson, F. Collins, and T. Frieden. 2013. Research as a part of public health emergency response. *New England Journal of Medicine* 368(13):1251–1255.

Mayer, B., K. Running, and K. Bergstrand. 2015. Compensation and community corrosion: Perceived inequalities, social comparisons, and competition following the *Deepwater Horizon* oil spill. *Sociological Forum* 30(2):369–390.

McCormick, L. C., L. Hites, J. F. Wakelee, A. C. Rucks, and P. M. Ginter. 2014. Planning and executing complex large-scale exercises. *Journal of Public Health Management and Practice* 20:S37–S43.

Miake-Lye, I. M., S. Hempel, R. Shanman, and P. G. Shekelle. 2016. What is an evidence map? A systematic review of published evidence maps and their definitions, methods, and products. *Systematic Reviews* 5(1):28.

Miller, A., K. Yeskey, S. Garantziotis, S. Arnesen, A. Bennett, L. O'Fallon, C. Thompson, L. Reinlib, S. Masten, J. Remington, C. Love, S. Ramsey, R. Rosselli, B. Galluzzo, J. Lee, R. Kwok, and J. Hughes. 2016. Integrating health research into disaster response: The new NIH disaster research response program. *International Journal of Environmental Research and Public Health* 13(7). http://creativecommons.org/licenses/by/4.0 (accessed June 17, 2020).

NASEM (National Academies of Sciences, Engineering, and Medicine). 2016. *Potential research priorities to inform public health and medical practice for domestic Zika virus: Workshop in brief.* Washington, DC: The National Academies Press.

NASEM. 2017a. *Building a national capability to monitor and assess medical countermeasure use during a public health emergency: Going beyond the last mile: Proceedings of a workshop.* Washington, DC: The National Academies Press.

NASEM. 2017b. *Exploring the translation of the results of Hurricane Sandy research grants into policy and operations: Proceedings of a workshop—in brief.* Washington, DC: The National Academies Press.

NBSB (National Biodefense Science Board). 2011. *Call to action: Include scientific investigations as an integral component of disaster planning and response.* https://www.phe.gov/Preparedness/legal/boards/nbsb/Documents/nbsbrec14.pdf (accessed March 3, 2020).

NCDMPH (National Center for Disaster Medicine and Public Health). 2020. National Center for Disaster Medicine and Public Health. https://www.usuhs.edu/ncdmph (accessed February 23, 2020).

NORC at the University of Chicago. 2017. *Evaluation of the translation, dissemination, and implementation of public health preparedness response research and training project.* https://s3.amazonaws.com/ASPPH_Media_Files/Docs/CDC_Preparedness_Evaluation_Report (accessed March 3, 2020).

Olson, D. K., A. Scheller, and A. Wey. 2014. Using gaming simulation to evaluate bioterrorism and emergency readiness training. *Public Health Reports* 20:S52–S60.

Peres, L. C., E. Trapido, A. L. Rung, D. J. Harrington, E. Oral, Z. Fang, E. Fontham, and E. S. Peters. 2016. The *Deepwater Horizon* oil spill and physical health among adult women in southern Louisiana: The Women and Their Children's Health (WaTCH) study. *Environmental Health Perspectives* 124(8):1208–1213.

Potter, M. A., K. R. Miner, D. J. Barnett, R. Cadigan, L. Lloyd, D. K. Olson, C. Parker, E. Savoia, and K. Shoaf. 2010. The evidence base for effectiveness of preparedness training: A retrospective analysis. *Public Health Reports* 125(Suppl 5):15–23.

Qari, S., D. M. Abramson, J. A. Kushma, and P. Halverson. 2014. Preparedness and Emergency Response Research Centers: Early returns on investment in evidence-based public health systems research. *Public Health Reports* 129(Suppl 4):1–4.

Qari, S. H., M. R. Leinhos, T. N. Thomas, and E. G. Carbone. 2018. Overview of the Translation, Dissemination, and Implementation of Public Health Preparedness and Response Research and Training Initiative. *American Journal of Public Health* 108(S5):S355–S362.

Qari, S. H., H. R. Yusuf, S. L. Groseclose, M. R. Leinhos, and E. G. Carbone. 2019. Public health emergency preparedness system evaluation criteria and performance metrics: A review of contributions of the CDC-funded Preparedness and Emergency Response Research Centers. *Disaster Medicine and Public Health Preparedness* 13(3):626–638.

Renger, R., and B. Granillo. 2014. Lessons learned in testing the feasibility of evaluating transfer of training to an operations setting. *Journal of Public Health Management and Practice* 20:S30–S36.

Revere, D., S. Allan, H. Karasz, and J. Baseman. 2018. Expanding methodologies to identify high-priority emergency preparedness tools for implementation in public health agencies. *American Journal of Public Health* 108(S5):S372–S374.

Richmond, A., L. Hostler, G. Leeman, and W. King. 2010. A brief history and overview of CDC's centers for Public Health Preparedness Cooperative Agreement program. *Public Health Reports* 125(5 Suppl):8–14.

Richmond, A. L., R. K. Sobelson, and J. P. Cioffi. 2014. Preparedness and emergency response learning centers: Supporting the workforce for national health security. *Journal of Public Health Management and Practice* 20:S7–S16.

Riley-Jacome, M., B. A. G. Parker, and E. C. Waltz. 2014. Weaving Latino cultural concepts into preparedness core competency training. *Journal of Public Health Management and Practice* 20:S89–S100.

Rung, A. L., S. Gaston, E. Oral, W. T. Robinson, E. Fontham, D. J. Harrington, E. Trapido, and E. S. Peters. 2016. Depression, mental distress, and domestic conflict among Louisiana women exposed to the *Deepwater Horizon* oil spill in the WaTCH study. *Environmental Health Perspectives* 124(9):1429–1435.

Rychetnik, L., P. Hawe, E. Waters, A. Barratt, and M. Fommer. 2004. A glossary for evidence based public health. *Journal of Epidemiology and Community Health* 58:538–545.

Savoia, E., L. Lin, D. Bernard, N. Klein, L. P. James, and S. Guicciardi. 2017. Public health system research in public health emergency preparedness in the United States (2009–2015): Actionable knowledge base. *American Journal of Public Health* 107(S2):e1–e6.

Savoia, E., S. Guicciardi, D. P. Bernard, N. Harriman, M. Leinhos, and M. Testa. 2018. Preparedness Emergency Response Research Centers (PERRCs): Addressing public health preparedness knowledge gaps using a public health systems perspective. *American Journal of Public Health* 108(S5):S363–S365.

Smith, E. C., F. M. Burkle, P. Aitken, and P. Leggatt. 2018. Seven decades of disasters: A systematic review of the literature. *Prehospital and Disaster Medicine* 33(4):418–423.

Tall Chief, V., T. P. Burton, J. Campbell, D. T. Boatright, and A. Wendelboe. 2014. The Southwest Preparedness and Emergency Response Learning Center and the Oklahoma Intertribal Emergency Management Coalition: A unique partnership. *Journal of Public Health Management and Practice* 20:S107–S110.

Testa, M. A., M. L. Pettigrew, and E. Savoia. 2014. Measurement, geospatial, and mechanistic models of public health hazard vulnerability and jurisdictional risk. *Journal of Public Health Management and Practice* 20:S61–S68.

Testa, M. A., E. Savoia, M. Su, and P. D. Biddinger. 2018. Social media learning collaborative for public health preparedness. *American Journal of Public Health* 108(S5):S375–S377.

Thielen, L., C. S. Mahan, A. R. Vickery, and L. A. Biesiadecki. 2005. Academic centers for public health preparedness: A giant step for practice in schools of public health. *Public Health Reports* 120(Suppl 1):4–8.

Turnock, B. J., J. Thompson, and E. L. Baker. 2010. Opportunity knocks but twice for public health preparedness centers. *Public Health Reports* 125(5 Suppl):1–3.

Uden-Holman, T., J. Bedet, L. Walkner, and N. H. Abd-Hamid. 2014. Adaptive scenarios: A training model for today's public health workforce. *Journal of Public Health Management and Practice* 20:S44–S48.

Van Nostrand, E., N. Pillai, and A. Ware. 2018. Interjurisdictional variance in U.S. workers' benefits for emergency response volunteers. *American Journal of Public Health* 108(S5):S387–S393.

Walkner, L., D. Fife, J. Bedet, and M. DeMartino. 2014. Using a digital story format: A contemporary approach to meeting the workforce needs of public health laboratories. *Journal of Public Health Management and Practice* 20:S49–S51.

Wiebel, V., C. Welter, G. S. Aglipay, and J. Rothstein. 2014. Maximizing resources with mini-grants: Enhancing preparedness capabilities and capacity in public health organizations. *Journal of Public Health Management and Practice* 20:S83–S88.

Wright, K. S., M. W. Thomas, D. P. Durham, Jr., L. M. Jackson, L. L. Porth, and M. Buxton. 2010. A public health academic-practice partnership to develop capacity for exercise evaluation and improvement planning. *Public Health Reports* 125(Suppl 5):107–116.

Yaylali, E., J. S. Ivy, and J. Taheri. 2014. Systems engineering methods for enhancing the value stream in public health preparedness: The role of Markov models, simulation, and optimization. *Public Health Reports* 129(Suppl 4):145–153.

Yeager, V. A., N. Menachemi, L. C. McCormick, and P. M. Ginter. 2010. The nature of the public health emergnecy preparedness literature 2000–2008: A quantitative analysis. *Journal of Public Health Management and Practice* 16(5):441–449.

3 An Evidence Review and Evaluation Process to Inform Public Health Emergency Preparedness and Response Decision Making

The committee was charged with developing a methodology for and subsequently conducting a systematic review and evaluation of the evidence base for public health emergency preparedness and response (PHEPR) practices.[1] Specifically, the committee was asked to establish a tiered grading scheme to be applied in assessing the strength or certainty of the evidence (COE)[2] for specific PHEPR practices and in developing recommendations for evidence-based practices. This chapter describes the committee's approach to developing a transparent process for making judgments about the evidence for cause-and-effect relationships and understanding the balance of benefits and harms of PHEPR practices.

The chapter begins with a discussion of the evolving philosophies regarding the identification of evidence-based practices, the challenges of evaluating interventions that are complex or implemented in complex systems, and the developing methodologies to address those complexity issues. It then describes the established evidence evaluation frameworks that informed the committee's methodology. Next, the chapter details the key elements and approaches of the methodology developed and applied by the committee for reviewing and evaluating PHEPR evidence to inform decision making. Finally, the chapter concludes with lessons learned from the development and application of the committee's methodology and recommendations for supporting ongoing efforts to build a cumulative evidence base for PHEPR.

[1] The committee defined PHEPR practices as a type of process, structure, or intervention whose implementation is intended to mitigate the adverse effects (e.g., morbidity and mortality, economic impacts) of a public health emergency.

[2] "Strength of evidence" and "certainty of the evidence" are often used interchangeably. While the committee's charge used "strength of evidence," the committee uses the phrase "certainty of the evidence" throughout this report (except when referring to the grading of qualitative evidence, for which the field-accepted term "confidence" is used). "Certainty of the evidence" can be defined in different ways, depending on the context in which the term will be used. For the purposes of making recommendations, it represents the extent of confidence that the estimates of an effect are adequate to support a particular recommendation or decision. When it is not possible or helpful to generate an estimate of effect size, the certainty of the evidence may reflect the confidence that there is a non-null effect (i.e., the intervention is effective) (Hultcrantz et al., 2017).

EVOLVING PHILOSOPHIES FOR EVALUATING EVIDENCE TO INFORM EVIDENCE-BASED PRACTICE: IMPLICATIONS FOR PHEPR

Systems for evaluating the evidence supporting given practices and interventions are a valued resource for practitioners, policy makers, and others who seek to use the best available evidence for decision making, but who lack the time, resources, or expertise needed to review and interpret a large and potentially inconsistent body of evidence. Moreover, the conduct of such reviews by reputable expert groups can increase the efficiency and consistency of the process. As discussed in Chapter 1, knowledge regarding evidence-based practice is critically needed in PHEPR given the mandate of the PHEPR system to mitigate the health, financial, and other impacts of public health emergencies. To date, however, there has been little effort to develop a rigorous and transparent process for identifying evidence-based PHEPR practices. The development of such a process requires an understanding of the methodological foundation for evidence-based practice, which continues to evolve to meet the evidentiary needs of more complex problems. The following sections describe this evolution and the implications for PHEPR given the complex nature of the PHEPR system, the kinds of questions that are of interest to PHEPR practitioners, and the volume and types of evidence that exist to answer those questions.

Limitations of the Traditional Evidence Hierarchy

Issues concerning how to reach conclusions about cause-and-effect relationships have long been deliberated in the fields of science and health. The foundation for the primacy of the experimental clinical trial in a hierarchy that ranks sources of evidence of effect, generally based on experimental design, and underpins the rise of evidence-based medicine (EBM) dates back nearly 100 years (Fisher, 1925). This foundation has served the stakeholders in clinical care very well, as a plethora of advances in medicine have been shown to be beneficial in clinical trials (e.g., use of beta blockers following myocardial infarction, colorectal cancer screening in older adults), while other, once-popular interventions have been shown to be ineffective and hence discarded (e.g., extracranial–intracranial bypass to prevent stroke, Lorenzo's oil to treat cancer). Following on the successes of the EBM model, the evidence hierarchy was subsequently applied in other fields (e.g., public health, education) to support evidence-based practice and policy (Boruch and Rui, 2008; Briss et al., 2000, 2004). In its broader application, however—and increasingly within clinical medicine as well—limitations of the traditional evidence hierarchy were recognized (Durrheim and Reingold, 2010). What works well when the intervention is an immunization or a medication may not work as well when evaluating a multicomponent quality improvement intervention or a systemic organizational change (Walshe, 2007). Notably, the application of EBM methods to research and reviews of public health practice has been challenging because, in addition to variation in effects across population groups and settings, the context in which an intervention is implemented can alter the intervention itself (as may be the case, for example, in organizational interventions) (Booth et al., 2019). This context sensitivity makes it difficult to draw conclusions about the relevance of findings from an intervention studied in one set of circumstances to the use of the same intervention under different circumstances. The early application of evaluation methods in medicine focused primarily on achieving impact estimates with high internal validity—a goal that is better suited to well-controlled clinical settings and relatively homogenous physiological systems than to public health (Green et al., 2017). Demonstrating effectiveness in a controlled setting is important, but so, too, is knowing the likelihood that the findings from a study or set of studies conducted in particular contexts would apply to other settings (Leviton, 2017).

Moreover, not all interventions and practices can be studied in the context of a randomized controlled trial (RCT), for practical and/or ethical reasons (WHO, 2015). For example, communities cannot be randomized and assigned to experience a public health emergency, and in many instances, best practices for emergency response have been developed over time and cannot ethically be replaced with a placebo or no response. Nor is it always necessary to conduct an RCT to evaluate whether a cause-and-effect relationship exists. Thus, it is useful to consider any evidence that provides credible estimates of a causal impact (or lack thereof) between an intervention and the outcome of interest.

In 1965, Sir Austin Bradford Hill proposed a set of factors to apply when assessing whether an observed epidemiologic association is likely to be causal in nature. These factors draw on evidence from multiple sources and include (1) the strength of an association; (2) the consistency of the association (i.e., replicability across different studies, settings, and populations); (3) the specificity of the association; (4) the temporality of the association (i.e., whether the hypothesized cause precedes the effect); (5) the existence of a biological gradient (i.e., observation of a dose–response relationship); (6) the plausibility of the causal mechanism; (7) the coherence of the data with other evidence; (8) the availability of supporting evidence from experiments; and (9) the analogy or similarity of the observed associations with any other associations (Hill, 1965). Together these factors make up one of the earliest frameworks for evaluating evidence to reach conclusions about causal effects, and it is still widely applied for the purposes of causal inference. Hill's criteria, however, were proposed in the context of simple exposure–disease relationships and may be less directly applicable to the evaluation of cause-and-effect relationships for complex or system-level interventions.

Since Hill's time, the concept of frameworks for evaluating evidence has received increasing attention, and numerous such frameworks have been developed. Importantly, however, some authorities, including Hill himself, have argued that a rigid application of evidence criteria cannot and should not replace a global assessment of the evidence by someone with skills and training in the subject matter and methods used (Hill, 1965; Phillips and Goodman, 2004).

Evolving Methods for Evaluating Complex Health Interventions in Complex Systems

As policy makers and practitioners have increasingly recognized the importance of having an evidence base to tackle complex challenges, there has been a growing movement among those who conduct systematic reviews and develop guidelines to embrace methods that take a complexity perspective and use multiple sources and types of evidence. Early efforts to overcome methodologic challenges related to evaluating evidence for complex, multicomponent, and community-level public health interventions were undertaken during the development of The Guide to Community Preventive Services (The Community Guide) (Truman et al., 2000). More recently, three seminal report series were published that address these complexity issues and informed the committee's work: the Cochrane series on *Considering Complexity in Systematic Reviews of Interventions,* the Agency for Healthcare Research and Quality's (AHRQ's) series on *Complex Intervention Systematic Reviews,* and the World Health Organization's (WHO's) series on *Complex Health Interventions in Complex Sys-*

tems: Concepts and Methods for Evidence-Informed Health Decisions.[3] It should be noted, however, that methods for evaluating complex interventions and systems represent an active area of ongoing development.

The complexity perspective reflects a shift away from a focus on simple, linear cause-and-effect models and has been used increasingly in the health sector, particularly in public health, to "explore the ways in which interactions between components of an intervention or system give rise to dynamic and emergent behaviors" (Petticrew et al., 2019, p. 1). Multiple dimensions of intervention complexity may be considered in the evaluation of evidence, including

- **intervention complexity**—for interventions with multiple, often interacting, components;
- **pathway complexity**—for interventions characterized by complicated and nonlinear causal pathways that may feature feedback loops, synergistic effects and multiple mediators, and/or moderators of effect;
- **population complexity**—for interventions that target multiple participants, groups, or organizational levels;
- **contextual complexity**—for interventions that are context-dependent and need to be tailored to local environments; and
- **implementation complexity**—for interventions that require multifaceted adoption, uptake, or integration strategies (Guise et al., 2017).

A complex intervention perspective is different from a complex system perspective, and the choice of which to adopt when conducting a review is appropriately determined by the needs of the policy makers and practitioners. A complex system perspective is appropriate when the focus is on the system and how it changes over time and interacts with and adapts in response to an intervention (Petticrew et al., 2019). In such cases, the objective of the review may shift from determining "what works" to understanding "what happens" and to formulating theories on how those effects are produced (Petticrew, 2015).

Addressing the issues of the complexity of an intervention, the details of the implementation process, and the context in which the intervention is implemented requires the adaptation of existing or the development of new frameworks for assessing evidence. Reviewers and guideline developers have been developing and testing novel quantitative, qualitative, and mixed methods for systematic reviews and evidence synthesis and grading to better capture complexity (Briss et al., 2000; Guise et al., 2017; Noyes et al., 2019; Petticrew et al., 2013a; Waters et al., 2011). The starting point for complex reviews is commonly to develop a logic model as the analytic framework that represents an intervention and how it works in the complex system in which it is implemented as the theoretical basis for subsequent reviews (Anderson et al., 2011; Rohwer et al., 2017). In addition to quantitative reviews of intervention effects using novel methods (Higgins et al., 2019), standalone qualitative evidence syntheses are particularly useful for gaining an understanding of intervention complexity, and of how various aspects of complexity affect the acceptability, feasibility, and implementation of interventions and the way they work in specific contexts with specific populations (Flemming et al., 2019). There exist approximately 20 different

[3] In 2013, the series *Considering Complexity in Systematic Reviews of Interventions* was published by the Cochrane Review in the *Journal of Clinical Epidemiology*. The series *Complex Intervention Systematic Reviews*, which was published in 2017 in the *Journal of Clinical Epidemiology*, resulted from an expert meeting convened by AHRQ. In 2019, WHO released the series *Complex Health Interventions in Complex Systems: Concepts and Methods for Evidence-Informed Health Decisions*, which was published in *BMJ Global Health*.

qualitative synthesis methods, some of which enable theory development. Given this wide choice of methods, the European Union recently published guidance on criteria to consider when choosing a qualitative evidence synthesis method for use in health technology assessments of complex interventions (Booth et al., 2016).

Additionally, review methods for complex interventions and systems have focused on the integration of diverse and heterogeneous types of evidence. Qualitative[4] and quantitative evidence may both contribute to understanding an intervention or practice and ultimately what works, necessitating synthesis approaches that combine these different types of evidence (Noyes et al., 2019; Thomas and Harden, 2008). In some instances, guideline groups have synthesized across diverse evidence streams by mapping qualitative to quantitative findings or vice versa, so as to better understand the phenomenon of interest (Glenton et al., 2013; Harden et al., 2018; WHO, 2018). For example, to better understand how lay health worker programs work, and particularly how context affects implementation, Glenton and colleagues (2013) mapped findings on barriers and facilitators (mediators and moderators) from a qualitative evidence synthesis onto a causal model derived from a previously conducted quantitative effectiveness review. The authors suggest that this integrative synthesis approach may help decision makers better understand the elements that may promote program success. Realist review methods (a mixed-method approach) are also gaining traction as an alternative to the traditional positivist approach[5] (Gordon, 2016), focused on explaining the interactions among context, mechanisms, and outcomes (Wong et al., 2013). Realist review methods yield an evidence-informed theory of how an intervention works. By helping to understand the intervention mechanisms and the contexts in which those mechanisms function, realist reviews can assist decision makers in judging whether an intervention is likely to be useful in their own context(s), considering context-specific tailoring, and determining whether an intervention is likely to scale (Berg and Nanavati, 2016; Greenhalgh et al., 2011; Pawson et al., 2005).

Implications for Evaluating Evidence in the PHEPR System

The evolving methods described above for the review and evaluation of interventions that are complex or implemented in complex systems are of particular relevance to the PHEPR context. As discussed in Chapter 2, the PHEPR system, with its multifaceted mission to prevent, protect against, quickly respond to, and recover from public health emergencies (Nelson et al., 2007b), is inherently complex and encompasses policies, organizations, and programs. This complexity also stems in part from the nature of public health emergencies, which are often unpredictable, may evolve rapidly, and are highly heterogeneous with respect to setting and type (e.g., weather events, disease outbreaks, terrorist events) (Hunter et al., 2013). Setting is not limited to geographic location, but also encompasses the sociocultural and demographic environment, as well as the characteristics of the communities and the responding entities (e.g., organizational structure, managerial experience, staff capabili-

---

[4] While there is general understanding of quantitative evidence as numerical data derived from quantitative measurements, misconceptions regarding what constitutes qualitative research and qualitative evidence are common. Qualitative research uses "qualitative methods of data collection and analysis to produce a narrative understanding of the phenomena of interest. Qualitative methods of data collection may include, for example, interviews, focus groups, observations and analysis of documents" (Noyes et al., 2019, p. 2). Qualitative evidence can also be extracted, for example, from free-text boxes in questionnaires, but this type of qualitative data tends to be less useful as it is thin and lacks context. A questionnaire survey would not, however, be considered a qualitative research study.

[5] A positivist approach is anchored in a paradigm that assumes there is an objective truth that can be discovered through empirical evidence derived from quantitative enquiry (Ward et al., 2015).

ties, social trust, and other resources). PHEPR practices themselves may also be complex, featuring multiple interacting components that target multiple levels (e.g., individual, population, system), and with implementation that is often tailored to local conditions (Carbone and Thomas, 2018).

The questions prioritized by PHEPR stakeholders are not limited to the effectiveness of policies and practices as measured by their effects on health and system outcomes. PHEPR practitioners have identified important knowledge gaps related to implementation, such as understanding the barriers to using information-sharing systems to share data between and among states and localities (Siegfried et al., 2017) and knowing when an emergency operations center (EOC) should be activated. Addressing this wide range of operations-related questions requires assessing evidence beyond that generated through RCTs and other quantitative impact studies: evidence from qualitative studies and other sources is needed to supplement that from quantitative studies to illuminate the "hows" and "whys" in complex systems (Bate et al., 2008; Greenhalgh et al., 2004; Hohmann and Shear, 2002; Petticrew, 2015).

A considerable challenge when reviewing evidence to determine the effectiveness of PHEPR practices and implementation strategies relates to the often indirect links between the practices and primary health outcomes (e.g., morbidity and mortality) (Nelson et al., 2007a). Simple one-to-one linear cause-and-effect relationships between PHEPR practices and outcomes are the exception rather than the rule. In most circumstances, multiple pathways link practices to outcomes. Intermediate outcomes that reflect the array of potential harms and benefits may be organizational or operational, and the balance of benefits and harms is influenced by the various stakeholders' values and perceptions regarding feasibility and acceptability. Moreover, multiple interacting interventions are often implemented simultaneously, making it difficult to assess the effect of each in isolation and their additive effects, and to distinguish those that are necessary from those that are sufficient, or at least contributory, for any given event (Nelson et al., 2007a). For example, a suite of non-pharmaceutical interventions, including isolation of sick patients, quarantine of contacts, and school closures, may be implemented simultaneously during an epidemic to reduce transmission and morbidity, making the effect of any one intervention difficult to measure. Moreover, for some PHEPR practices, it may be that there is no true effect that is replicable, as effects may be inextricable from the contexts in which a practice is implemented (Walshe, 2007). This way of thinking is a departure from most EBM, which assumes there is an underlying true effect of measurable size. In such cases, traditional evidence evaluation frameworks based on a positivist approach may not be well suited to addressing the review question(s) at hand. Questions about when and in what circumstances such practices as activating public health emergency operations is effective, for example, may be better assessed using the realist approach described above.

The PHEPR system draws on a wide range of evidence types, from RCTs to after action reports (AARs),[6] and the approach to evaluating the evidence needs to reflect that diversity. In addition to research-based evidence, both quantitative and qualitative, it is important for the approach to make use of experiential evidence from past response scenarios, which offers the potential for validation of research findings in practice settings, as well as improved understanding of context effects, trade-offs, and the range of implementation approaches or components for a given practice.

---

[6] AARs are documents created by public health authorities and other response organizations following an emergency or exercise, primarily for the purposes of quality improvement (Savoia et al., 2012). They contain narrative descriptions of what was done, but may also contain "lessons learned" (i.e., what was perceived to work well and not well) and recommendations for future responses.

Finally, public health interventions often lie at the intersection of science, policy, and politics, which means that decision-making processes around implementation need to reflect not only scientific evidence but also information related to social and legal norms, ethical values, and variable individual and community preferences. Accordingly, any systematic review of the evidence necessary to make informed decisions related to PHEPR needs also to include an explicit assessment of underlying ethical, legal, and social considerations.

To inform its methodology, the committee began by reviewing existing frameworks for evaluating different sources and types of evidence, both in health care and in other areas in which experimental clinical trials may be impossible or impractical (such as aviation safety), to determine their potential to accommodate the diverse PHEPR evidence base and questions of interest to PHEPR stakeholders. These existing frameworks are described below.

HOW DO DIFFERENT FIELDS EVALUATE EVIDENCE?: A REVIEW OF EXISTING FRAMEWORKS

The charge to the committee specified that in developing its methodology, the committee should draw on accepted scientific approaches and existing models for synthesizing and assessing the strength of evidence. Thus, the committee reviewed the published literature and held a 1-day public workshop on evidence evaluation frameworks used in health and nonhealth fields. (This workshop is reported separately in a Proceedings of a Workshop—in Brief [see Appendix E].[7]) During the public workshop, the committee also heard from experts on how evidence is assessed in other areas of policy, such as transportation safety and aerospace medicine, where making decisions about cause and effect is crucial for safety but conducting randomized trials, or even concurrently controlled experimental studies, is in most cases impractical. The models for evidence evaluation reviewed and considered by the committee are summarized in Table 3-1.[8]

For each approach, the committee identified some aspects relevant to a framework for PHEPR evidence evaluation. For example, the framework used by the What Works Clearinghouse (WWC) practice guides includes a mechanism for drawing on the real-world experience of experts to inform recommendations while making clear the limitations of such evidence (WWC, 2020), which the committee thought would be applicable to evaluating evidence from AARs and integrating PHEPR practitioner input. Additionally, the user-oriented presentation of information in the WWC practice guides and the inclusion of implementation guidance was of interest given practitioners' emphasis on the importance of translation and implementation issues in PHEPR. For these reasons, the committee also carefully considered the Clearinghouse for Labor Evaluation and Research (CLEAR) approach to evaluating implementation studies.

The committee considered the causal chain of evidence approach, which employs analytic frameworks and is used by several groups, including the U.S. Preventive Services Task Force (USPSTF), the Community Preventive Services Task Force (CPSTF), and the Evaluation of Genomic Applications in Practice and Prevention (EGAPP), to be particularly relevant to PHEPR, as it was expected that there would be few, if any, studies that would provide direct evidence demonstrating the effect of a PHEPR practice on morbidity or mortality following a public health emergency. Instead, in most cases, evidence from across a chain

[7] Available at https://www.nap.edu/catalog/25510 (accessed November 7, 2019).

[8] This table is not intended to serve as an exhaustive list of all existing evidence evaluation frameworks. The committee's objective was not to review every published framework but to understand the breadth of approaches in use across diverse fields and their potential application to PHEPR.

TABLE 3-1 Examples of Evidence Evaluation Frameworks Reviewed by the Committee

Field	Evaluation Framework or Approach	Brief Description
Education	What Works Clearinghouse (WWC)	The Institute of Education Sciences founded the WWC to provide consistent methods for evaluating interventions, policies, and programs in education. The WWC has published standards, which vary by experimental design, for studies used to determine the strength of evidence.* The WWC publishes two kinds of products: intervention reports, which evaluate the effectiveness of an intervention based on studies that meet the WWC standards, and practice guides. The latter, which draw on expert input in addition to published evidence, are designed to serve as user-friendly guides for educators and provide recommendations on effective education practices, as well as implementation guidance (WWC, 2017a,b).
Labor	Clearinghouse for Labor Evaluation and Research (CLEAR)	The U.S. Department of Labor's clearinghouse adopted and adapted the WWC's methods to summarize research on topics relevant to labor, such as apprenticeships, workplace discrimination prevention, and employment strategies for low-income adults. Findings from the evidence reviews are made accessible through the agency's clearinghouse to inform decision making. Individual studies are reviewed and assigned a rating for the strength of causal evidence. Synthesis reports evaluate the body of evidence from only those studies within a given topic area that achieved high or moderate causal evidence ratings and do not make recommendations (CLEAR, 2014, 2015).
Transportation	*Countermeasures That Work*	The National Highway Traffic Safety Administration publishes *Countermeasures That Work* periodically to inform state highway safety officials and help them select evidence-based countermeasures for traffic safety problems, such as interventions to reduce alcohol-impaired driving. The guide, which does not use a transparent evidence evaluation framework, reports on effectiveness, cost, how widely a countermeasure has been adopted, and how long it takes to implement (Richard et al., 2018).
	National Transportation Safety Board (NTSB) Accident Reports	NTSB investigates aviation and other transportation accidents, reaching conclusions about causes and making safety recommendations, which are detailed in its accident reports (NTSB, 2020). Investigators identify probable causes and make recommendations based on mechanistic reasoning (e.g., theories of action based on knowledge regarding physics or chemical properties of materials), modeling, logic, expert opinion, and after action reporting from those involved in an incident.
Aerospace Medicine	National Aeronautics and Space Administration (NASA) Integrated Medical Model	NASA needs to predict and prepare for health issues that arise in space, but conducting experimental studies in this area is often infeasible for a number of logistical and ethical reasons. To overcome that barrier, empirical evidence from past experiences with space travel is integrated with a variety of other evidence sources, including longitudinal studies of astronaut health, evidence from analogous contexts (e.g., submarines), and expert opinion, in a complex simulation model that informs decision making. Each parameter in the model may be adjusted, which allows for analysis of a wide range of decisions (Minard et al., 2011).

TABLE 3-1 Continued

Field	Evaluation Framework or Approach	Brief Description
Health Care and Public Health	U.S. Preventive Services Task Force (USPSTF)	The Agency for Healthcare Research and Quality convenes USPSTF to review evidence and make recommendations on evidence-based practices for clinical preventive services (e.g., screening tests, preventive medications). USPSTF draws on evidence summaries from systematic reviews, which are conducted by evidence-based practice centers, to determine the effectiveness of a service based on the balance of potential benefits and harms. Graded recommendations are made based on the certainty of net benefit (USPSTF, 2015).
	Community Preventive Services Task Force (CPSTF)	CPSTF is a Centers for Disease Control and Prevention (CDC)-supported task force that reviews the evidence base for community preventive services and programs aimed at improving population health. Its findings and recommendations are published in The Guide to Community Preventive Services (The Community Guide). CPSTF developed its own methodology for evaluating and assessing the quality of individual studies and bodies of evidence. Because randomized controlled trials (RCTs) are often difficult to conduct for public health interventions, The Community Guide does not automatically downgrade the strength of evidence from non-RCT designs, but considers the suitability of the study design and the quality of execution for each study included in the body of evidence. CPSTF also considers the applicability of the evidence (e.g., to different populations and settings) in developing its recommendations (Briss et al., 2000; Zaza et al., 2000b).
	Grading of Recommendations Assessment, Development and Evaluation (GRADE) and GRADE-Confidence in the Evidence from Reviews of Qualitative Research (GRADE-CERQual)	GRADE is a method used to evaluate bodies of evidence to assess the certainty of the evidence (COE), up- and/or downgrading COE based on eight defined domains. In contrast to most other frameworks, GRADE does not set explicit quality standards for study inclusion, but instead adjusts the COE based on the quality and risk of bias of studies included in the analysis. GRADE also utilizes an Evidence to Decision framework for making transparent, evidence-based recommendations in the form of guidelines, considering evidence beyond that related to effect (e.g., feasibility, acceptability). Many international review and guideline groups use GRADE, and the methods are continually updated. Recently, GRADE was adapted for the assessment of qualitative evidence (GRADE-CERQual) (Guyatt et al., 2011a; Lewin et al., 2015).
	Evaluation of Genomic Applications in Practice and Prevention (EGAPP)	EGAPP, a CDC initiative, published guidelines on evidence-based processes for genetic testing and implementation in clinical practice. To generate an overall strength-of-evidence rating for a body of evidence, the EGAPP methods use different hierarchies of data sources and study designs for three distinct components of the evaluation (analytic validity, clinical validity, and clinical utility), thereby explicitly linking different evidence types to questions they are well suited to answering. EGAPP methods also consider the ethical, legal, and social implications of the genetic tests (Teutsch et al., 2009).

* While the committee uses the term "certainty of the evidence" throughout the report, some frameworks report on "strength of evidence." The summaries in this table reflect the specific terminology used in each framework.

of intermediate outcomes would need to be linked together to reach health and other downstream outcomes. Analytic frameworks (examples of which can be found in Chapters 4–7) depict the hypothesized links between an intervention/practice and intermediate and health or other final outcomes. They also provide a conceptual approach for evaluating interventions, guiding the search and analysis of evidence (Briss et al., 2000).

The committee considered the framework developed and continually updated by the Grading of Recommendations Assessment, Development and Evaluation (GRADE) group to be most applicable to those kinds of PHEPR practices for which a biomedical focus is most relevant. Examples of such practices include quarantine or the use of potassium iodide for radiological incidents. The committee's approach was also informed by a 2018 WHO report containing guidelines for emergency risk communication, which provided a timely example of how GRADE might be adapted and used in conjunction with GRADE-Confidence in the Evidence from Reviews of Qualitative Research (GRADE-CERQual) to evaluate evidence and develop recommendations on a wider range of PHEPR practices (WHO, 2018). The 2018 WHO report presents a model for synthesizing and grading evidence from quantitative and qualitative research studies, and includes guidance on inclusion of such other evidence streams as case reports and gray literature reports with similarity to AARs (e.g., governmental and nongovernmental reports containing lessons learned and improvement plans).

Although the National Transportation Safety Board (NTSB) does not rely on explicit evidence evaluation frameworks, the committee believed that organization's use of mechanistic evidence to determine the cause of an aviation disaster was relevant to the evaluation of evidence to support decision making in PHEPR. NTSB's investigation into the cause of the midair explosion of TWA Flight 800 illustrates that process. For example, an examination of the direction in which metal from the fuselage was bent and knowledge of the physics of explosions contributed to a conclusion that the explosion happened within the plane (rather than originating outside the plane, as in the case of a missile) (Marcus, 2018). This conclusion did not depend on a hypothesis-testing study with statistical tests for differences between what was observed and an alternative. This same kind of reasoning has been used to explain why one can have confidence that parachutes are better than uninhibited free fall when jumping out of a plane: it is known from physics that the rate of descent of an object dropped from the sky is slowed by the drag resistance of air, and that a parachute increases that drag such that with a big enough parachute, the descent of a 200-pound man can be slowed sufficiently for him to survive the fall.

For the purposes of this report, the committee defined mechanistic evidence as evidence that denotes relationships for which causality has been established—generally within other scientific fields, such as chemistry, biology, economics, and physics (e.g., the accelerating effect of the gravitational attraction of Earth and the slowing effect of air resistance)—and that can reasonably be applied to the PHEPR context through mechanistic reasoning, defined in turn as "the inference from mechanisms to claims that an intervention produced" an outcome (Howick et al., 2010, p. 434). For some interventions, such as the placement of auxiliary power units in hospitals at heights above expected water levels in the event of flooding, mechanistic evidence may be a significant contributor to decision making. Such evidence has not traditionally been incorporated into evidence evaluation frameworks, although processes for integrating biological mechanisms with more traditional evidence sources (e.g., data from clinical trials or epidemiological studies) have been developed (Goodman and Gerson, 2013; Rooney et al., 2014) and applied, for example, in systematic reviews of the toxicological effects of exposures (NASEM, 2017). The use of mechanistic evidence, however, can be seen as incorporating principles of a realist approach to evidence synthesis (discussed earlier in this chapter), for which it is established practice to develop theories of how an intervention works and to use diverse types of evidence to explore interactions among context, mechanisms, and outcomes to better understand causal pathways.

Also of interest to the committee was the National Aeronautics and Space Administration's (NASA's) use of modeling to understand the trade-offs among different decisions constrained by the weight and volume limitations of a space capsule. Decision models such as the Integrated Medical Model used by NASA may have utility for considering practices, such as quarantine, for which the consequences of trade-offs can be modeled in advance of having to make decisions during emergencies. Although the development of such models was beyond the scope of this study, methods for integrating evidence from existing model-based analyses with empirical evidence were examined. It should be noted, however, that this is a nascent area of methodological development (CDC, 2018a; USPSTF, 2016).

From its review of the literature and discussions with experts, the committee concluded that none of the evidence evaluation frameworks it reviewed were sufficiently flexible, by themselves, to be universally applicable to all the questions of interest to PHEPR practitioners and researchers without adaptation. Furthermore, no one framework was ideally suited to the context-sensitive nature of PHEPR practices and the diversity of evidence types and outcomes of interest, many of which are at the organizational or systems level and thus often difficult to measure. Therefore, the committee developed a mixed-method synthesis methodology[9] that draws on (and in some cases adapts) those elements of existing frameworks and approaches that the committee concluded were most applicable to PHEPR. As a starting point, the committee adopted the analytic frameworks from CPSTF and USPSTF and the GRADE evidence evaluation and Evidence to Decision (EtD) frameworks (see Box 3-1), while allowing sufficient flexibility to bring in other evidence types (e.g., mechanistic, experience-based, and qualitative) that are not accommodated by the traditional GRADE approach to the assessment of certainty in quantitative evidence. This approach allowed the committee to use the appropriate methodology to answer different types of questions of interest to PHEPR stakeholders. The development of this methodology and its application to the evaluation of evidence for four exemplar PHEPR review topics were undertaken in parallel using a highly iterative process, the steps of which are described in the sections below.

APPLYING A METHODOLOGY TO REVIEW, SYNTHESIZE, AND ASSESS THE COE FOR PHEPR PRACTICES

This section outlines the key elements and approaches of the methodology developed and applied by the committee for reviewing and evaluating PHEPR evidence to inform decision making (summarized in Box 3-2). This description is intended to inform future PHEPR evidence reviews and to serve as a foundation for future improvements and modifications to the PHEPR review methodology needed to promote its long-term sustainability.

The sections below briefly describe the committee's approach to

- formulating the scope of the review and searching the literature,
- synthesizing and assessing the certainty of the evidence, and
- formulating the practice recommendations and implementation guidance.

To allow for a more comprehensive description of the committee's processes for synthesizing the evidence, grading the evidence, and developing recommendations in this chapter,

[9] A mixed-method synthesis approach involves the integration of quantitative, mixed-method, and qualitative evidence in a single review (Petticrew et al., 2013b).

BOX 3-1 GRADING OF RECOMMENDATIONS ASSESSMENT, DEVELOPMENT AND EVALUATION EVIDENCE EVALUATION DOMAINS AND EVIDENCE TO DECISION FRAMEWORK CRITERIA

Grading of Recommendations Assessment, Development and Evaluation (GRADE) Domains for Assessing Certainty of the Evidence

Downgrading domains:

- *Risk of bias*—the potential for limitations in the study design and execution to influence estimates of the intervention effect. The overall rating for this domain is derived from the risk-of-bias assessments for all individual studies included in the body of evidence.
- *Indirectness*—considers whether the available evidence differs from the target of interest, including differences in population, interventions, outcome measures (e.g., use of surrogate outcomes removed in the putative causal pathway from important endpoints), and comparison groups.
- *Imprecision*—when study results include relatively few participants or events and thus have a wide confidence interval around the estimate of effect.
- *Inconsistency*—unexplained heterogeneity of results across studies.
- *Publication bias*—systematic underestimation or overestimation of the underlying beneficial or harmful effect due to the selective publication of studies.

Upgrading domains:

- *Large effect*—considers whether an effect is large enough that it cannot have occurred solely as a result of bias from potential confounding factors.
- *Dose–response gradient*—refers to an observation of progressively larger effect with greater exposure to the intervention.
- *Plausible residual confounding*—if confounding is likely to work counter to what the evidence demonstrates (would decrease an apparent intervention effect, or would create a spurious effect when results suggest no effect), it may confer greater confidence in the evidence.

GRADE Evidence to Decision Criteria

- *Priority of the problem*—can be determined by looking at the number of people impacted by the intervention and how substantial the desirable and undesirable anticipated effects are.
- *Certainty of the evidence*—assessed using the GRADE domains described above.
- *Balance of benefits and harms*—based on an assessment of the magnitude of desirable and undesirable effects to determine whether one significantly outweighs the other.
- *Acceptability*—considers the views of those who benefit (or are harmed) and when the benefits, adverse effects, and costs occur.
- *Values/preferences/outcome importance*—considers how important the health outcomes are to those affected, how variable they are, and whether there is uncertainty about this.
- *Equity*—can be evaluated by treating equity as a desirable outcome, assessing outcomes that are relevant to equity, assessing differences in the magnitude of effects on advantaged and disadvantaged populations, assessing the differences in the baseline risk for disadvantaged populations, and determining relevance to disadvantaged populations and settings.
- *Resource use*—identifies issues of resource use that are potentially important to stakeholders, considers the magnitude of the resource requirements and any differences in resource use between options being compared, and rates the certainty of the evidence of resource requirements and the cost-effectiveness of the intervention.
- *Feasibility*—considers the sustainability of the intervention, important barriers that limit implementation or require consideration, and capacity to meet demand.

SOURCES: Brunetti et al., 2013; Guyatt et al., 2011b; Moberg et al., 2018; Schünemann et al., 2013; Welch et al., 2017.

BOX 3-2 STEPS IN THE COMMITTEE'S PHEPR EVIDENCE REVIEW AND EVALUATION METHODOLOGY

1. Select the review topic, considering published literature on gaps and priorities and stakeholder input.
2. Develop the analytic framework and key review questions.
3. Conduct a search of the peer-reviewed and gray literature and solicit papers from stakeholders.
4. Apply inclusion and exclusion criteria.
5. Separate evidence into methodological streams (quantitative studies, including comparative, noncomparative, and modeling studies and descriptive surveys; qualitative studies; after action reports; and case reports) and extract data.
6. Apply and adapt as needed existing tools for quality assessment of individual studies based on study design.
7. Synthesize the body of evidence within methodological streams and apply an appropriate grading framework (Grading of Recommendations Assessment, Development and Evaluation [GRADE] for the body of quantitative research studies and GRADE-Confidence in the Evidence from Reviews of Qualitative Research for the body of qualitative studies to assess the certainty of the evidence [COE] and confidence in the findings, respectively).
8. Consider evidence of effect from other streams (e.g., modeling, mechanistic, qualitative evidence) and support for or discordance with findings from quantitative research studies to determine the final COE.
9. Integrate evidence from across methodological streams to populate the PHEPR Evidence to Decision framework and to identify implementation considerations.
10. Develop practice recommendations and/or implementation guidance.

the relatively standard steps of the systematic review process (formulating the scope of the reviews, searching the literature, inclusion and exclusion, and quality assessment) are only briefly mentioned herein but are described in more detail in Appendix A.

Formulating the Scope of the Reviews and Searching the Literature

The committee was charged with developing and applying criteria for the selection of PHEPR practices on which it could apply its systematic review methodology to assess the evidence of effectiveness. Rather than a sequential approach that would involve developing the evidence review and evaluation methodology in the abstract and then applying it to the PHEPR practices selected for review, the committee judged that it would be more fruitful to develop the methodology and test it on the selected PHEPR topics simultaneously. This approach was intended to result in a methodology that would be applicable across a range of different practices for which the evidence base would be expected to differ in nature. As a first step, the committee needed to select a set of review topics that would be illustrative of the diversity of PHEPR practices.

Consistent with its charge, the committee started its topic selection process with a list of the Centers for Disease Control and Prevention's (CDC's) 15 PHEPR Capabilities (CDC, 2018b) and developed criteria for prioritizing the Capabilities to select specific PHEPR practices. In considering its selection criteria, the committee sought to select test cases that would capture the expected diversity of the evidence base for various PHEPR practices resulting from different research and evaluation methodologies, as well as variability in practice characteristics. Such characteristics were defined as classification dimensions and included, for example, the type and scope of event in which a practice is implemented, the practice setting, whether the practice is complex or simple, whether it is under the direct purview of public health agencies, and whether it is preparedness or response oriented. The committee applied the classification dimensions to each PHEPR Capability to identify a set of Capabilities that were diverse with respect to those variables (see Figure 3-1). In addition to such diversity, the committee considered as criteria for selection of review topics the current needs for evidence-based guidance among key stakeholders, the potential of the review to change practice, and the relevance of a topic to national health security.[10] The committee engaged with stakeholders (PHEPR practitioners and policy makers) to inform topic selection and referred to published literature that identifies practitioners' research needs. Applying this approach, the committee, in consultation with PHEPR practitioners, selected the following four practices as topics for review:

- engaging with and training community-based partners to improve the outcomes of at-risk populations after public health emergencies (falls under Capability 1, Community Preparedness);
- activating a public health emergency operations center (Capability 3, Emergency Operations Coordination [EOC]);
- communicating public health alerts and guidance with technical audiences during a public health emergency (Capability 6, Information Sharing); and
- implementing quarantine to reduce or stop the spread of a contagious disease (Capability 11, Non-Pharmaceutical Interventions).

This chapter describes the application of the committee's evidence review and evaluation methodology to these four review topics; the details of the review findings for each topic are presented in Chapters 4–7.

The next steps, standard practice for most systematic reviews and described in more detail in Appendix A, included the development of analytic frameworks and the identification of key questions[11] for each topic area to further define the scope of the reviews; the development and execution of a comprehensive search of the peer-reviewed and gray literature; and the screening of titles, abstracts, and full-text articles by two reviewers to identify articles meeting the committee's inclusion criteria. Of note, determining the eligibility of studies required iterative discussions as the review methods, the scope of the four topics, and the outcomes used to assess effectiveness were refined over time. The analytic frameworks and the key questions were reviewed and informed by a panel of PHEPR practitioners serving as consultants to the committee (the processes for appointing the panel of PHEPR practitioner consultants and for developing the analytic frameworks and key questions are described in Appendix A).

---

[10] As noted earlier in this report, the review topics were selected prior to the COVID-19 pandemic.

[11] Key questions define the objective of an evidence review. In some guideline development processes (e.g., that of USPSTF), each linkage depicted on the analytic framework (between intervention and outcome or between two outcomes) is represented with a separate key question. The committee did not develop separate key questions for linkage in the analytic frameworks, but instead defined an overarching review question that guided the review process and sub-questions of interest generally related to benefits and harms, as well as barriers and facilitators.

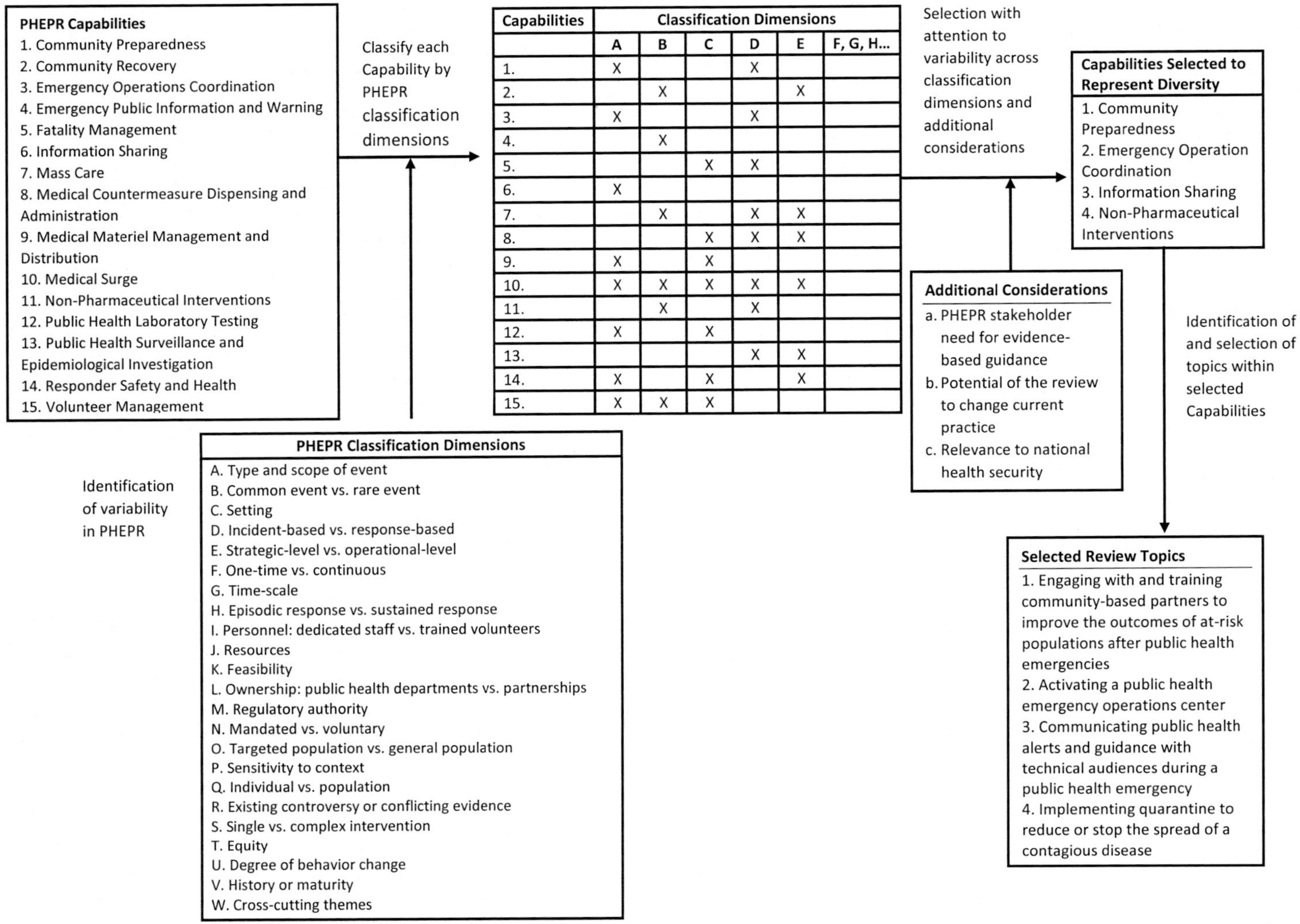

Capabilities	Classification Dimensions					
	A	B	C	D	E	F, G, H...
1.	X			X		
2.		X			X	
3.	X			X		
4.		X				
5.			X	X		
6.	X					
7.		X		X	X	
8.			X	X	X	
9.	X		X			
10.	X	X	X	X	X	
11.		X		X		
12.	X		X			
13.				X	X	
14.	X		X		X	
15.	X	X	X			

FIGURE 3-1 Selection process for the committee's review topics.

Synthesizing and Assessing the COE

To maximize the efficiency of the evidence review and evaluation process for each review topic, different component steps, described in the sections that follow, were commissioned to outside groups and individuals with the appropriate expertise. The initial classification of studies and the data abstraction and quality assessment for quantitative studies (except modeling studies) were performed by the Center for Evidence Synthesis in Health, an AHRQ-funded evidence-based practice center (EPC) at Brown University. The quality assessment and synthesis of qualitative studies were conducted by a commissioned team at Wayne State University. The evaluation and synthesis of selected modeling studies were performed by a modeling expert at Stanford University, and the evaluation and synthesis of AARs and case reports were conducted by a PHEPR expert in evaluation at Columbia University.

Classification of Studies into Methodological Streams

An overview of the evidence classification process is presented in Figure 3-2, from the point where the studies for inclusion had been identified. The evidence for the four PHEPR test cases was classified into the following categories: quantitative studies, qualitative studies, mixed-method studies, and case reports and AARs. These categories were defined by the methods employed rather than the subject of investigation, and thus encompassed the full range of evaluative studies (e.g., systems research and quality improvement studies in addition to more traditional impact studies). Mixed-method studies could be used in both quantitative and qualitative evidence syntheses, as depicted in Figure 3-2. The committee determined that no single method could be applied across these different types of evidence, and therefore describes later in this chapter separate processes for evaluating the quality and strength of each type.

Quantitative studies Quantitative studies included articles and reports with quantitative results from the evaluation of a PHEPR practice. This included quantitative comparative studies, for which there was an explicit comparison of two or more groups (or one group at two or more time points) to assess whether they were similar or different, usually with a statistical test, as well as quantitative noncomparative studies (i.e., studies that provided only postintervention results, such as posttraining knowledge scores). Modeling studies were treated as a subset of quantitative studies, as were surveys, which were further classified on the basis of the method and questions asked. Surveys that did not include an evaluation of a practice during or following a public health emergency were categorized as descriptive surveys and were not used in the evaluation of effectiveness (but could be used, for example, to populate the EtD framework or to inform implementation considerations). Modeling studies were identified only for the evidence review on quarantine. Given the diversity of purposes of the modeling studies captured in the review, the committee opted to perform an in-depth assessment of a selected group of models judged to be highly relevant. Twelve modeling studies were selected for detailed analysis based on an assessment of their modeling techniques, data sources, relevance to key review questions, potential implications for public health practice, and disease condition studied. Following a review and assessment of the selected models (described below), a commissioned modeling expert conducted a narrative synthesis of the findings of the models, with attention to common results and themes related to the circumstances in which quarantine was effective. Many other modeling studies have been conducted and may have important findings relevant to the use of quarantine; however, a detailed analysis of a representative subset was pursued based on the resources available for the study.

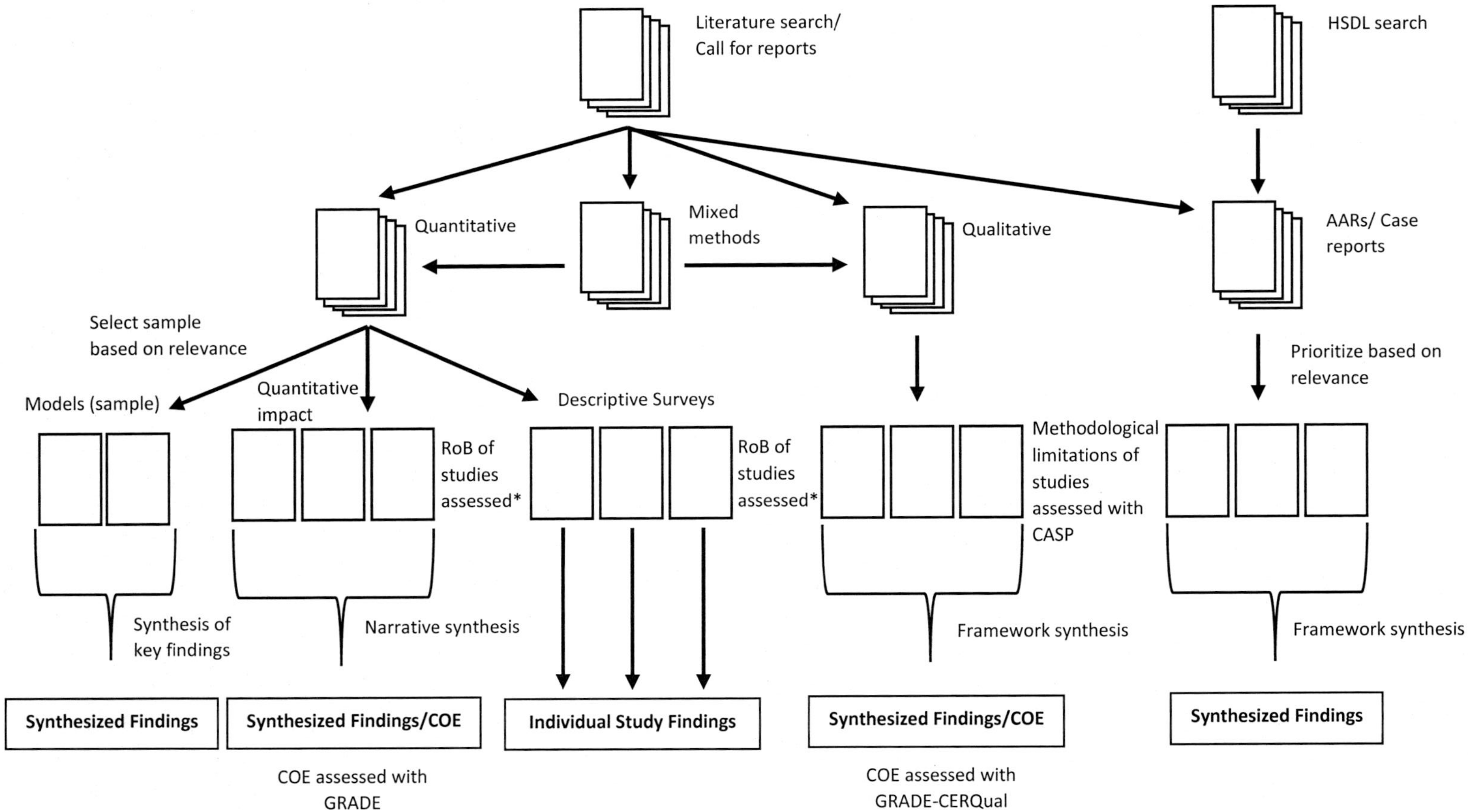

FIGURE 3-2 Classification and consolidation of studies into methodological streams.
NOTE: AAR = after action report; CASP = Critical Appraisal Skills Programme; COE = certainty of the evidence; GRADE = Grading of Recommendations Assessment, Development and Evaluation; HSDL = Homeland Security Digital Library; RoB = risk of bias.
* Risk of bias assessment tools were developed by adapting existing tools and/or published methods.

Qualitative studies Studies were classified as qualitative if they explicitly described the use of qualitative research methods, such as interviews, focus groups, or ethnographic research, and used an accepted method for qualitative analysis (Miles et al., 2014). If studies did not report the application of qualitative research methods but nonetheless collected some qualitative data, they were generally classified as case reports or AARs, depending on the context in which the data were collected (described below). In the classification process, studies were identified that contained a qualitative analysis of free-text responses to a survey. Such studies were not classified as qualitative research studies, but their findings were extracted and considered separately in the qualitative evidence synthesis to affirm or question the findings of the more complete qualitative studies.

AARs and case reports The committee sought to include a synthesis of AARs for two of its reviews (the EOC and Information Sharing Capability test cases) as an exercise in gauging the potential value of this evidence source to reviews of PHEPR practices. Case reports,[12] which included program evaluations and other narrative reports describing the design and/or implementation of a practice or program (generally in practice settings), usually with lessons learned, were grouped with AARs because of similarity of methods and intent. A synthesis of case reports was conducted and included in the evidence reviews for all four test cases. Of note, commentaries and editorials were not included as case reports; such articles were excluded in the committee's bibliographic database search and during the screening process (see Appendix A). Some case reports and AARs reported quantitative (e.g., from surveys) and/or qualitative (e.g., from interviews or focus groups) data, but such data were not collected in the context of research, and there generally was little to no description of the methods by which the data were collected. While the distinction from quantitative and qualitative studies was considered necessary for the committee's reviews given the current limitations of these two sources, should their methods and reporting be strengthened, they could conceivably be combined with quantitative or qualitative studies in the future.

Data Extraction and Quality Assessment for Individual Studies

After the included studies[13] had been sorted into one of the categories described above, individual studies were extracted and assessed for their risk of bias and/or other aspects of study quality, as described below. The full list of data extraction elements is included in Appendix A. For most studies of PHEPR practices, details about the practice itself, the context, and the implementation are necessary, and thus the committee selected for extraction some elements from the Template for Intervention Description and Replication checklist (Hoffman et al., 2014).

The quality assessment approach was determined based on study design. Many standardized tools for assessing quality or risk of bias are available, each with its own merits and shortcomings, and new tools continue to be developed. Described here is the approach taken by the committee and the groups commissioned to assess study quality and risk of bias; however, different tools and methods could reasonably be applied in future PHEPR evidence reviews. Studies were not excluded based on an assessment of the risk of bias or

[12] The synthesis of case reports, as described later in this chapter, is distinct from case study research, which is an established qualitative form of inquiry by which an issue or phenomenon is analyzed within its context so as to gain a better understanding of the issue from the perspective of participants (Harrison et al., 2017).

[13] The term "study" is used broadly here to include research studies and reports that may be descriptive in nature (e.g., AARs, case reports, program evaluations).

of methodological limitations, but this information instead was considered in the assessment of certainty for the body of evidence.

For quantitative impact studies, the Brown University EPC developed an assessment tool by drawing selected risk-of-bias domains from existing tools, including the Cochrane Risk of Bias version 2.0 tool (Sterne et al., 2019), Cochrane's suggested risk-of-bias criteria for Effective Practice and Organisation of Care reviews (Cochrane, 2017), and the Cochrane Risk of Bias in Non-Randomized Studies of Interventions (ROBINS-I) tool (Sterne et al., 2016). The Brown University EPC developed and applied a separate tool for the assessment of descriptive surveys, drawing on published methods (Bennett et al., 2010; Davids and Roman, 2014). For qualitative studies, methodological limitations were assessed using the Critical Appraisal Skills Programme qualitative tool (CASP, 2018). Additional detail on these tools and their use in quality assessment of individual quantitative and qualitative research studies is provided in Appendix A.

An expert in modeling methodology assessed the selected group of quarantine modeling studies in detail, including the specific model structures/equations and how the interventions were instantiated within these structures/equations. This assessment was intended to determine whether assumptions encoded in such structures/equations could plausibly have had a strong impact on the results reported in the studies. Likewise, a careful reading of the methods section of each paper was focused on extracting explicitly documented assumptions, as well as other implicit assumptions based on methodological decisions (e.g., no change in mixing rates as the epidemic grows because of such processes as social distancing, perfect versus imperfect case finding to be eligible for quarantine, asymptomatic transmission).

Descriptive case reports do not fit any specific analytic study design and generally report few details concerning methods, and thus are not amenable to quality assessment using tools designed for research studies. Case reports and AARs were categorized as "high" or "low" priority using the significance criterion of the AACODS (authority, accuracy, coverage, objectivity, data, significance) checklist (Tyndall, 2010), an evaluation tool used in the critical appraisal of gray literature sources. This process mirrored the general principles of the approach outlined by Cochrane for selecting qualitative studies for syntheses when a large pool of sources needs to be reduced to a manageable sample amenable to synthesis that is most likely to address the review questions (Noyes et al., 2018). Rigor was not required as a sorting criterion because the primary purpose was to synthesize experiential data to add weight to findings from research studies, provide a different perspective from that of research studies, or provide the only available perspective concerning the specific phenomena of interest. An appraisal tool for evaluating the methodological rigor of AARs published in 2019 (ECDC, 2018) was applied by the commissioned PHEPR expert to the AARs included in the committee's analyses (the tool's criteria are described in Appendix A). While the results of this analysis informed the committee's recommendations on improving the future evidentiary value of AARs (see Chapter 8), the appraisal tool was not useful in selecting reports to include in the synthesis of AARs and case reports because of the generally low scores for the majority of reports captured in the search. With improvements in the methodological rigor of AARs, however, such tools could be helpful in selecting high-quality AARs for inclusion in future evidence reviews.

Assessment of the Certainty and Confidence in Synthesized Quantitative and Qualitative Findings

After individual studies had been assessed for their quality and risk of bias, the next step was synthesizing and assessing the COE (or confidence in the case of qualitative evidence) across the body of evidence, specific to each key question, outcome, or phenomenon of interest identified in the analytic framework.

Initially, certainty of the evidence (for synthesized quantitative impact findings) and confidence in the synthesized findings from qualitative bodies of evidence were assessed separately using the GRADE and GRADE-CERQual frameworks, respectively, as discussed below. Subsequently, the coherence of evidence from across methodological streams (including evidence from cross-sectional surveys that evaluated practices,[14] modeling studies, mechanistic evidence,[15] qualitative studies, case reports, and AARs) was considered in developing summary findings for each key question. The committee employed two similar but distinct processes to integrate evidence from across methodological streams—one for assessing evidence of effectiveness, and the other for populating the EtD framework and developing implementation guidance. For evaluating evidence of effectiveness, the coherence of evidence from other streams was considered in rating the COE for each outcome.

Quantitative evidence synthesis and grading For each of the test cases, the committee first assessed the body of quantitative impact studies using the GRADE approach (see Box 3-2 earlier in this chapter for a description of the GRADE assessment domains). The committee determined that a quantitative meta-analysis was neither feasible nor warranted based on the expected context sensitivity of the PHEPR practices. Thus, the committee undertook a synthesis without meta-analysis (Campbell et al., 2020) to draw conclusions regarding effect direction. These conclusions represented global judgments based on the number, size, and methodologic strengths of the individual studies, as well as the consistency of the results. If study authors performed statistical testing of a hypothesis, the committee considered the results of such testing when drawing its conclusions about the directionality of effect. However, statistical testing was neither a necessary nor a sufficient condition for drawing these conclusions. The committee did not prespecify a minimum meaningful effect size, as it was generally unclear what would be considered meaningful for the diverse set of outcomes examined by the committee. This poses a challenge for interpreting the importance of an intervention and represents an area for future development.

Existing guidance on the application of GRADE to a narrative synthesis (Murad et al., 2017) was followed to evaluate the certainty that a practice was effective for a given outcome. Consistent with the GRADE methodology, bodies of evidence that included RCTs started at high COE, which was downgraded as appropriate based on the committee's judgment regarding risk of bias, indirectness, inconsistency, imprecision, and publication bias. Bodies of evidence that comprised only nonrandomized studies started at low COE and could be further downgraded or upgraded.[16] Modeling studies were not included in the bodies of evidence assessed with the GRADE domains, but were considered in the COE determination as discussed later in this chapter.

---

[14] There was no synthesis of noncomparative, descriptive surveys.

[15] As discussed earlier in this chapter, the committee defined mechanistic evidence as evidence that denotes relationships for which causality has been established—generally within other scientific fields, such as chemistry, biology, economics, and physics—and that can reasonably be applied to the PHEPR context through mechanistic reasoning, defined in turn as "the inference from mechanisms to claims that an intervention produced" an outcome (Howick et al., 2010, p. 434).

[16] According to GRADE, bodies of evidence comprising nonrandomized studies that were assessed with ROBINS-I (Sterne et al., 2016) could start as high COE, but would then generally be rated down by default by two levels because of risk of bias unless there was a clear reason for not downgrading (Schünemann et al., 2018). However, because ROBINS-I was not used for the quality assessment of nonrandomized studies per se (although domains from the ROBINS-I tool were considered by the Brown EPC in developing its quality assessment tool), the committee started bodies of evidence that comprised only nonrandomized studies at low COE.

TABLE 3-2 Definitions for the Four Levels of Certainty of the Evidence

COE Level	Definition
High	We are very confident that, in some contexts, there are important effects (benefits or harms). Further research is very unlikely to change our conclusion.
Moderate	We are moderately confident that, in some contexts, there are important effects, but there is a possibility that there is no effect. Further research is likely to have an important impact on our confidence and could alter the conclusion.
Low	Our confidence that there are important effects is limited. Further research is very likely to have an important impact on our confidence and is likely to change the conclusion.
Very Low	We do not know whether the intervention has an important effect.

Table 3-2 defines the four levels of the COE used in the committee's evidence reviews. Of note, the differences among the levels are not quantitative, and there is no algorithm or set of rules for determining the COE (e.g., based on the number and quality of included studies). As with other systematic review and guideline development processes, the assessment of the COE is based on the judgment of the evaluators. In some cases, a single high-quality study may provide a high COE, while in others, having multiple RCTs with consistent effects could yield a lower COE (e.g., because of indirectness). Transparency is key so that the rationale for up- and/or downgrading decisions and the ultimate COE rating are clear. While this judgment-based approach allows the evaluators flexibility in the COE determination process, a potential limitation is poor interrater reliability (i.e., others could arrive at different judgments given the same set of evidence).

Two operational decisions made by the committee regarding the GRADE process warrant additional explanation. First, for those key questions and outcomes for which the only serious limitation was in the imprecision domain and the evidence came from a single, nonrandomized study of modest size, the committee considered the upgrading domains, in particular the domain for large effect size. The second decision relates to upgrading for nonrandomized studies based on large effect size.[17] The quantitative evidence was rated for risk of bias by the Brown University EPC, and based on these ratings, an overall assessment of quality was made using a "good/moderate/poor" set of categories. Studies rated as good quality were considered to have no serious limitations for the risk-of-bias domain in GRADE, whereas those rated as poor quality were considered to have serious or very serious limitations for this domain. For studies that were rated by the EPC as having "moderate" risk of bias and had a large effect size, the committee asked the EPC to assess whether the factors contributing to the "moderate" risk-of-bias rating were likely or unlikely to be responsible for the large effect size. For those cases in which the EPC judged this to be likely, the committee did not upgrade the COE based on the large effect size. For those cases in which the EPC judged this to be unlikely, the committee considered whether to upgrade the COE based on the large effect size.

Qualitative evidence synthesis and grading For the qualitative evidence synthesis, the primary studies were uploaded into Atlas.ti (Version 8.1, Atlas.ti Scientific Software Development GmbH, Berlin, Germany), and the key findings and supporting information from

[17] Consistent with GRADE guidelines on rating the COE (Guyatt et al., 2011b), the committee upgraded for large effect when nonrandomized studies showed at least a two-fold increase or decrease in relative risk (or other measure of effect size) associated with implementation of a PHEPR practice.

each study were extracted in the form of key phrases, sentences, and direct quotations. This approach allowed researchers to identify and note evidence that mapped onto the phenomena of interest. The specific phenomena of interest were prespecified as questions around what happened when the practice was implemented, what was perceived to work, and what was perceived not to work. The EtD domains (e.g., acceptability, feasibility, equity) were also phenomena of interest for the qualitative evidence synthesis.

The Wayne State University team conducted the extraction and used the pragmatic framework synthesis method (Barnett-Page and Thomas, 2009; Pope et al., 2000), which employs an iterative deductive and inductive process to analyze and synthesize the findings. Framework synthesis is a matrix-based method that involves the a priori construction of index codes and thematic categories into which data can be coded. The method allows

- themes identified a priori to be specified as coding categories from the start,
- application of an a priori theoretical framework or logic model to inform the development of index codes and themes,
- incorporation of researcher experience and background literature and expert opinion, and
- combining with other themes emerging de novo by subjecting the data to inductive analysis.

A five-step process was used for the synthesis: (1) familiarization to create a priori descriptive codes and codebook development, (2) first-level in vivo coding[18] using descriptive codes, (3) second-level coding into descriptive themes (families of descriptive codes), (4) analytic theming (interpretive grouping of descriptive themes), and (5) charting/mapping and interpretation (the authors' more detailed description of each of these steps is provided in Box 3-3). A lead author from the two-person Wayne State University team was assigned for each review topic and was responsible for the synthesis of findings, which were developed through ongoing discussions with the other Wayne State team member and the committee.

GRADE-CERQual was used to assess the confidence in synthesized qualitative findings (analytic and some descriptive themes). CERQual provides a systematic and transparent framework for assessing confidence in individual review findings, based on consideration of four components:

- methodological limitations—the extent to which there are concerns about the design or conduct of the primary studies that contributed evidence to an individual review finding;
- coherence—an assessment of how clear and compelling the fit is between the data from the primary studies and a review finding that synthesizes those data;
- adequacy of data—an overall determination of the degree of richness and quantity of data supporting a review finding; and
- relevance—the extent to which the body of evidence from the primary studies supporting a review finding is applicable to the context (perspective or population, phenomenon of interest, setting) specified in the review question (Lewin et al., 2018).

---

[18] During in vivo coding, a label is assigned to a section of qualitative data, such as an interview transcript, using an exact word or short phrase taken from that section of the data (Tracy, 2018).

BOX 3-3 STEPS FOR THE SYNTHESIS OF FINDINGS FROM QUALITATIVE STUDIES

Step 1: The familiarization process involved an initial close reading of the project documents and the selected articles to create descriptive codes. The familiarization with the project documents unpacked the key questions, sub-key questions, evidence to decision issues, aims and objectives of the project, and analytic frameworks so that key phrases and words that meaningfully addressed the phenomenon of interest could be identified. The familiarization with the articles similarly identified key phrases and words that described various aspects of the phenomenon of interest. Both sets of key phrases and words were converted to descriptive codes, which captured the essence of the extractions and replaced the in vivo original words with ones that translated across studies, creating a common yet representative nomenclature. A codebook was developed to compile the codes with corresponding definitions, thereby forming a set of a priori descriptive codes.

Step 2: First-level in vivo coding involved multiple close readings of the articles in their entirety, with attention to findings wherever they appeared (particularly in the abstracts, results, discussions, and conclusions). The in vivo findings (consisting of verbatim key phrases, sentences, and paragraphs) related to the key questions, sub-key questions, context questions, or evidence to decision issues were highlighted and assigned a descriptive code. When there were no a priori codes that matched the essence of in vivo extractions, this was considered an emergent code. The emergent code was translated to a new descriptive code, and the code with a corresponding definition was incorporated in the codebook. During this process, attention was paid to all meaningful extractions, whether they appeared to confirm or counter previously coded extractions. For mixed-method studies that had both qualitative and quantitative portions, only the qualitative findings were coded.

Step 3: Second-level coding involved a synthesis process of creating descriptive themes, where a theme was a family of descriptive codes in which codes that formed a cohesive set were grouped together. The themes represented a nuanced description, rather than just a generalized description, of the phenomenon of interest.

Step 4: This step involved a synthesis process of creating analytic themes. This analytic theming relied on a robust interpretation of the descriptive themes and how they intersected relationally with one another. The descriptive themes were grouped together in a nuanced manner to create the analytic themes.

Step 5: Charting/mapping involved explaining how the analytic themes specifically addressed the phenomenon of interest. Additionally, evidence to decision issues were addressed in this step by looking at how the analytic themes were grounded in descriptive themes, codes, and in vivo extractions.

Based on these ratings, each synthesized finding was then assigned an overall assessment as follows:

- High confidence—It is highly likely that the finding is a representation of the phenomenon.
- Moderate confidence—It is likely that the finding is a representation of the phenomenon.
- Low confidence—It is possible that the finding is a representation of the phenomenon.
- Very low confidence—It was not clear whether the finding is a representation of the phenomenon.

Confidence in the synthesized findings was assessed by the lead author for that review topic. The second author reviewed the assessments, queried the lead author for additional information, and offered suggestions. The discussion culminated in the final assessment of confidence.

Synthesis of evidence from case reports and AARs For the framework synthesis of findings from case reports and AARs, report characteristics (e.g., type of event, type of report, location) were extracted from the reports, which were then coded using a codebook developed based on the key areas of interest and adapted from the codebook used for the qualitative evidence synthesis (see Box 3-3) to facilitate alignment between the two evidence streams when feasible. Although case reports and AARs were analyzed jointly, findings were considered by report type to assess for any differences. No assessment of the confidence in the findings from the synthesis of case reports and AARs was conducted.

Integration of Effectiveness Evidence from Across Methodological Streams

As noted earlier in this chapter and depicted in Figure 3-3, the committee took a pragmatic, layering approach to synthesizing and grading the full body of evidence to determine the COE for the effectiveness of a given PHEPR practice and to inform practice recommendations. After evaluating the body of evidence from quantitative impact studies using the GRADE domains to determine the initial COE for each outcome of interest, the committee reviewed and considered the coherence of evidence from other methodological streams, including findings from the qualitative evidence syntheses (generally related to harms) with associated CERQual confidence assessments; findings from the modeling study analysis; quantitative data from individual cross-sectional surveys, case reports, and AARs regarding practice effectiveness in a real public health emergency; mechanistic evidence (defined earlier in this chapter); and parallel evidence. Although the committee did not undertake to do so, findings from a Delphi-type activity or other systematically collected expert evidence (Schünemann et al., 2019) could be brought to bear in grading the overall body of evidence.

"Parallel evidence," as the committee uses the term in this report, is evidence on the effectiveness of similar practices from outside the PHEPR context. The consideration of supporting evidence from analogy (e.g., similar interventions or analogous contexts) was proposed by Sir Austin Bradford Hill (Hill, 1965) and has been resurrected in more recent discussions on evidence grading (Howick et al., 2009). As PHEPR is a transdisciplinary field, foundational research may have been undertaken by other disciplines (within and outside of public health) for many PHEPR practices. Consequently, it is important to consider for all PHEPR evidence reviews (at the start of the process) whether there is likely an existing body of parallel evidence that should be captured in the review process. For the committee's review on engaging community-based partners to improve outcomes for at-risk populations, for example, the committee recognized that there would be a much broader but relevant evidence base related to community engagement from outside the PHEPR context. Also important to consider are factors that might contribute to different outcomes when an intervention is applied in the PHEPR context as compared with the context from which the parallel evidence was derived. For example, educational programs aimed at reducing a known health risk (e.g., cardiovascular disease) may be more effective at motivating behavior change relative to similar programs addressing the lower-probability risk of a disaster. Such factors should influence the weight given to parallel evidence in the evidence grading process. Rather than searching for and synthesizing primary studies, it may be more expedient to conduct targeted searches of the literature for existing systematic reviews on the effectiveness of similar interventions from other contexts that could be considered in determining the COE.

Of note, the consideration of parallel evidence is also consistent with the GRADE concept of applying indirect evidence when there is a paucity of direct evidence to inform a recommendation, and including parallel evidence in the body of evidence assessed with GRADE is an alternative approach that could be taken by future PHEPR review groups. However, the COE is downgraded for indirectness in GRADE, which conflicts conceptually with the committee's view—and that of others who have undertaken similar reviews (Bruce et al., 2014; Movsisyan et al., 2016)—of parallel evidence as a construct that may in some circumstances increase certainty in the effectiveness of an intervention.

Each additional source of evidence was judged to be supportive, very supportive, inconclusive (no conclusion can be drawn regarding coherence because either results are mixed or the data are insufficient), or unsupportive (discordant with the findings from quantitative impact research studies). The distinction between supportive and very supportive evidence was based on the magnitude of the reported effect and the directness of its application to the question and outcome of interest. Mechanistic evidence, which does not lend itself to an assessment of magnitude of effect, was determined to be supportive or very supportive based on the counterfactual (i.e., how likely it is that an alternative explanation accounts for the observed effect that has been attributed to a specified mechanism of action). For example, mechanistic reasoning is applied in the quarantine evidence review discussed in Chapter 7 and Appendix B4. While an observed reduction in disease transmission may reasonably be attributed to quarantine based on its mechanism (i.e., separating individuals at risk of becoming infectious from susceptible populations), other factors (e.g., seasonal effects related to temperature and humidity) may actually be responsible for the reduced spread. In contrast, mechanistic evidence regarding the impact of congregate quarantine was deemed very supportive as there is no good alternative explanation for why infections would increase among those quarantined in the congregate setting. Following discussion by the committee, a global judgment was made as to whether there was sufficient supportive or unsupportive evidence to warrant up- or downgrading the initial COE. Table 3-3 presents the committee's decision criteria for its four evidence reviews (discussed further in Appendixes B1–B4), but these are not intended as standards. As with the up- and downgrading process using the GRADE domains, the adjustment of the COE up or down one or more levels was not based on an algorithm but on the committee's judgment. The committee judged its approach to be reasonable because it was not estimating an effect size but drawing conclusions regarding whether an intervention had an important (beneficial or harmful) effect. The results of the evidence grading process, including the committee's ratings for each of the GRADE domains, the corresponding assessment of COE, and the rationale for further up- or downgrading the COE, were captured in evidence profile tables (see Appendixes B1–B4).

Formulating the Practice Recommendations and Implementation Guidance

An Evidence to Decision Framework for Formulation of PHEPR Practice Recommendations

The committee reviewed and adapted as necessary the criteria from the Developing and Evaluating Communication Strategies to Support Informed Decisions and Practice Based on Evidence (DECIDE) project (Alonso-Coello et al., 2016) and recently published WHO INTEGRATE (Rehfuess et al., 2019) EtD frameworks to develop a novel EtD framework for the committee's use in formulating recommendations on evidence-based PHEPR practices. The PHEPR EtD framework comprised the following criteria:

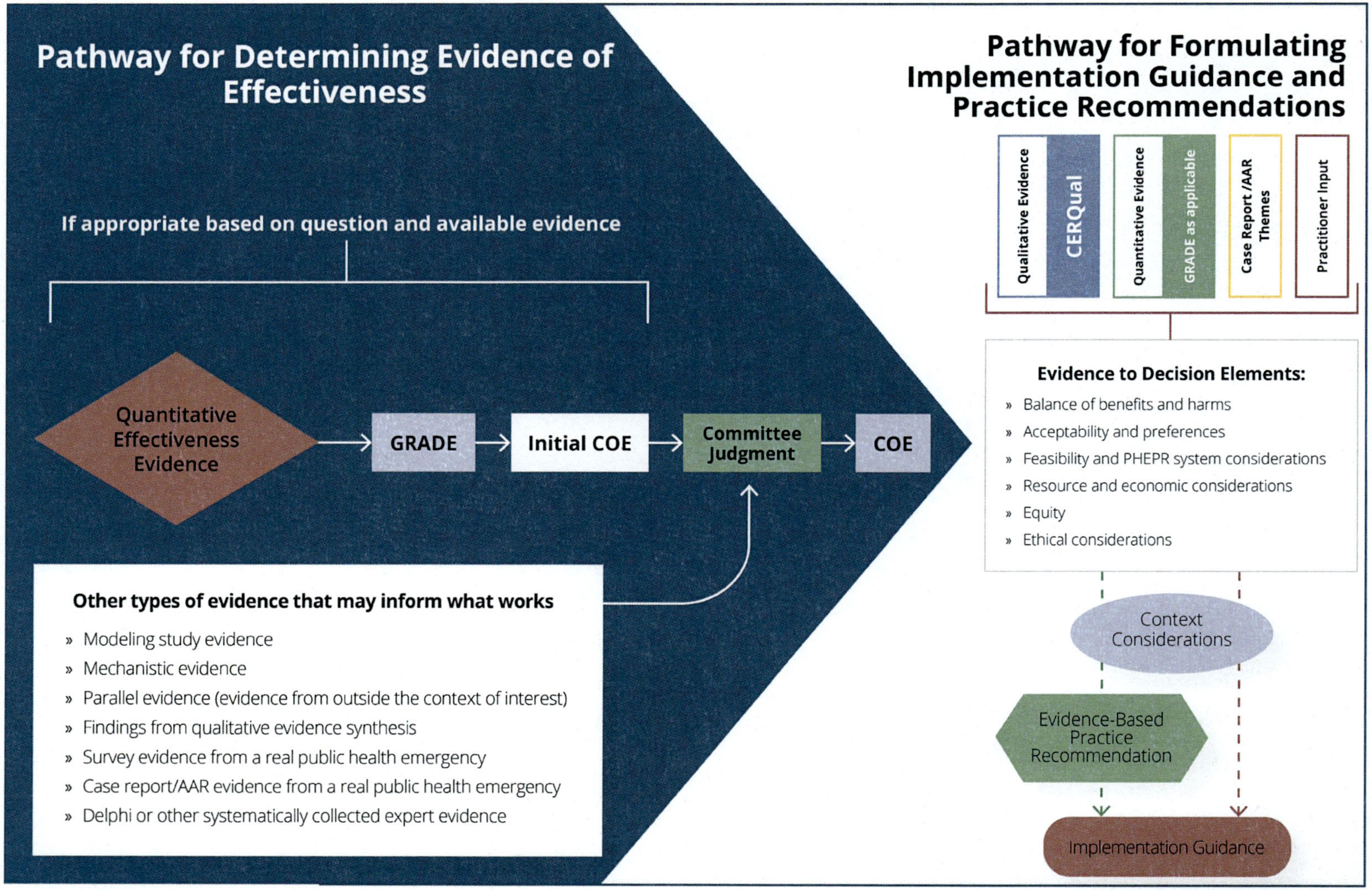
Pathway for Determining Evidence of Effectiveness
If appropriate based on question and available evidence
Quantitative Effectiveness Evidence
GRADE
Initial COE
Committee Judgment
COE
Other types of evidence that may inform what works
» Modeling study evidence
» Mechanistic evidence
» Parallel evidence (evidence from outside the context of interest)
» Findings from qualitative evidence synthesis
» Survey evidence from a real public health emergency
» Case report/AAR evidence from a real public health emergency
» Delphi or other systematically collected expert evidence
Pathway for Formulating Implementation Guidance and Practice Recommendations
Qualitative Evidence
CERQual
Quantitative Evidence
GRADE as applicable
Case Report /AAR Themes
Practitioner Input
Evidence to Decision Elements:
» Balance of benefits and harms
» Acceptability and preferences
» Feasibility and PHEPR system considerations
» Resource and economic considerations
» Equity
» Ethical considerations
Context Considerations
Evidence-Based Practice Recommendation
Implementation Guidance

FIGURE 3-3 Framework for integrating evidence to inform recommendation and guidance development for PHEPR practices.

NOTES: The framework depicts two interconnected pathways for evaluating evidence for PHEPR practices. The lefthand panel (blue) shows the committee's process for integrating evidence from quantitative impact studies with other evidence that may inform what works to determine the certainty of the evidence (COE) of effectiveness for a given outcome. The COE (for all relevant outcomes) feeds into the righthand panel (white), which shows the pathways for integrating diverse evidence for various elements (evidence to decision elements) that, along with context considerations, may inform the formulation of evidence-based practice recommendations and implementation guidance. In cases in which the review is focused on implementation and not on determining the effectiveness of a practice, it is possible to follow the pathway depicted in the righthand panel without assessing the COE as shown in the lefthand panel. Other types of evidence that may inform what works may be used to examine coherence with direct quantitative effectiveness evidence or may be used to inform committee judgment in the absence of direct quantitative evidence. AAR = after action report; CERQual = Confidence in the Evidence from Reviews of Qualitative Research; COE = certainty of the evidence; GRADE = Grading of Recommendations Assessment, Development and Evaluation; PHEPR = public health emergency preparedness and response.

TABLE 3-3 Matrix with the Generalized Approach by Which the Committee Determined the Certainty of the Evidence

Certainty of the Evidence (COE) Decision	Committee Criteria
No change in COE	Did not upgrade based solely on evidence from case reports, surveys, supportive evidence from modeling evidence, or low-confidence findings from qualitative evidence synthesis. Did not upgrade for supportive parallel evidence when direct evidence (from the PHEPR context) was available that resulted in low or moderate initial COE (see, for example, Table B1-2 in Appendix B1). Did not upgrade if evidence raised concerns about potential harmful or undesirable effects.
Upgraded COE one level	Required very supportive mechanistic or modeling evidence or high-confidence findings from qualitative evidence synthesis.
Upgraded COE two levels	Required a combination of supportive (or very supportive) findings from mechanistic, modeling, or qualitative evidence (see, for example, Table B4-2 in Appendix B4).
Downgraded COE	Although the committee did not encounter this scenario, evidence of harmful or undesirable effects could warrant downgrading the initial COE.

- balance of benefits and harms,
- acceptability and preferences,
- feasibility and PHEPR system considerations,
- resource and economic considerations,
- equity, and
- ethical considerations.

The PHEPR EtD framework enabled diverse types of evidence (e.g., from quantitative and qualitative studies, surveys, case reports, and AARs) concerning the same phenomenon of interest to be brought together in a single place. To populate this EtD framework, the committee adapted the methods described in the WHO guideline on emergency risk communication (WHO, 2018). For each EtD criterion, findings from within a methodological stream were compared and contrasted with findings from the other methodological streams (while findings were generally synthesized findings from a body of evidence, survey evidence was not synthesized and was incorporated as findings from individual studies). Whenever findings supported each other, they were combined into higher-order findings that represented syntheses across the methodological streams. These points of alignment were noted in EtD evidence summaries. Evidence from research studies was given greater weight than evidence from other sources, which was used to add weight to findings from research studies, provide a different perspective from that of research studies, or provide the only perspective concerning specific phenomena of interest in the absence of research-derived evidence. COE and confidence ratings for the within-stream findings were kept in mind during the evidence integration process, but no attempt was made to generate an overarching (across-stream) COE for the findings related to the EtD elements.

Finally, while each of the above EtD elements can be viewed through an ethics lens (i.e., harms and benefits generally map to the ethical principle of harm reduction/benefit promotion, equity to the principle of justice, and feasibility and resource considerations to the principle of stewardship, and acceptability and preferences will often include consideration of other ethical values), the committee's description of ethical considerations was not developed from the same body of studies as that from which the other EtD criteria were developed. Though some of these studies include reflections on ethical, legal, and social factors related to implementation, information about ethical considerations also often comes from essays and reflection pieces that were not explicitly encompassed by the committee's review process. Rather, the inclusion of ethical considerations as a separate category reflects the committee's discussion around general ethical principles that can help guide PHEPR practice (see Box 3-4), along with the pragmatic recognition that decision making in PHEPR is often a necessarily political matter as well as a matter of science. As such, explicit consideration of ethical, legal, and social factors has an important role in any discussion of implementation considerations and guideline development processes for PHEPR. Although the committee did not undertake to do so, analyses of regulatory and policy texts, as well as findings from a Delphi activity or other systematically collected expert evidence regarding ethical, legal, and social considerations, could be incorporated into future review processes.

Context Considerations

In addition to the EtD criteria, the committee considered the contexts in which the practices had been evaluated and whether any serious evidence gaps with regard to context (i.e., applicability concerns) should influence a recommendation. Contextual factors that were considered and may be relevant to future PHEPR reviews include

- settings (e.g., location, population density, emergency type and scale, public health system governance structure);
- populations (e.g., target study population or affected population, demographics such as race/ethnicity, age, and socioeconomic status); and
- PHEPR practice features (e.g., organization implementing the practice).

Key contextual information reported in the studies themselves should be extracted with other important data elements, but it may be necessary to supplement the literature search to identify other contextual details (Booth et al., 2019). For example, media reports may yield valuable information regarding potential political environment influences on the effectiveness and acceptability of a practice.

Practice Recommendations

For those practices for which there was sufficient evidence demonstrating a beneficial effect, the committee developed a practice recommendation. Although the committee did not encounter circumstances that warranted doing so, a recommendation against a practice could be made if there was sufficient evidence of harm or absence of effect. Other evidence review and guideline groups use multiple recommendation levels (e.g., strong and conditional recommendations), and future groups conducting reviews of PHEPR practices may determine that modifications of the committee's methodology are needed to accommodate recommendations of different strengths.

Importantly, the committee did not believe there should be a minimum required COE to make a recommendation (although recommendations when the COE for important outcomes is very low are expected to be rare). In fact, recommendations may be most useful to guide practitioners' decision making when there is a paucity of evidence but some action must be taken, such as in the response to a public health emergency. This is a notable difference from the field of preventive medicine, in which interventions are being applied to otherwise healthy (or at least asymptomatic) individuals who are unlikely to be harmed by inaction. The certainty about the benefits of a practice necessary to make a recommendation is expected to differ depending on the nature of the practice and the expected severity of any potential

BOX 3-4 GENERAL ETHICAL PRINCIPLES TO GUIDE PHEPR

Ethical approaches to PHEPR are typically informed by some combination of utilitarian (i.e., actions are right or wrong based on their consequences), deontological (i.e., actions are right or wrong based on rules and obligations), social justice, human rights, and other philosophical approaches. This complex blend is reflected in the principles below. This set of principles is not comprehensive, but can provide a set of checkpoints for ensuring that key ethical issues are considered.

Substantive Principles

Justice: An overarching ethical goal in PHEPR is that it be recognized as just, or fair, by all affected parties; this often includes considerations of fair distribution of resources, as well as fair and reciprocal obligations among stakeholders.

Harm reduction/benefit promotion: A primary duty of public health organizations and practitioners in preparation for and during public health emergencies is to promote benefits and reduce harms to people and communities in need.

Stewardship: Public health organizations and practitioners have a responsibility to be good stewards of the communal resources over which they have control, seeking to use limited resources efficiently.

Respect for persons and communities: Planning and response activities should seek to promote human rights and freedoms, including through protecting privacy, valuing autonomy, and supporting the dignity of every individual and community.

Note: Various factors in public health emergencies can generate or exacerbate tensions within and among the principles of justice, harm reduction/benefit promotion, stewardship, and respect for persons and communities. It is therefore critical to use ethical processes for making decisions in which trade-offs between these substantive principles are required.

Process Principles

Transparency: Ethically sound preparedness and response decisions reflect more than technical expertise; they reflect values, trade-offs, and often the establishment of reciprocal obligations among multiple stakeholders. Hence, broad awareness of preparedness and response decisions is important, and leaders must provide clear and honest communication about decisions, as well as opportunities for broad input into decisions when possible.

Equity: Treating like groups alike and avoiding invidious discrimination is an important way to promote fairness and foster public trust in the planning and response process.

Proportionality: Burdens imposed on individuals or groups, such as limitations on services provided or restrictions on personal liberties, should be necessary and commensurate with the scale of the public health emergency. As the situation evolves, it is also important to reassess regularly to ensure the continued optimal use of available resources.

Accountability: All decision makers should be accountable for a reasonable level of situational awareness and for incorporating evidence into decision making, including revising decisions as new data emerge.

SOURCES: Hick et al., 2020; IOM, 2009; Jennings and Arras, 2008; Jennings et al., 2016; Mastroianni et al., 2019.

undesirable effects. For example, the threshold for organizational practices, such as EOC activation, may be lower than that for practices that pose greater risks to an individual's health and well-being, such as quarantine. For interventions in the preparedness phase, a higher evidentiary threshold may be warranted given the absence of pressure to act.

When there is sufficient evidence to make a recommendation but there are notable gaps in the evidence base, a practice recommendation may also include statements regarding the need for monitoring and evaluation or rigorous research. In other cases, the body of evidence may not provide enough information about the effectiveness of a practice to serve as the basis for a recommendation. In such cases, a finding of insufficient evidence may be appropriate. Insufficient evidence does not mean that the intervention does not work, but that a determination of whether or not it works cannot be made, indicating a need for additional research into the effectiveness of the intervention or the circumstances under which it might be more or less effective or even harmful. Similarly, the absence of a practice recommendation does not indicate that the practice should not be implemented, particularly in cases in which a practice is a common or standard practice.

Implementation Guidance

The committee developed implementation guidance to accompany its practice recommendations. If a practice is in widespread use, available evidence may not address whether the practice should be conducted, but rather how it should be implemented. In such cases, implementation guidance may still be of value to practitioners in the absence of a practice recommendation. In future reviews, it is conceivable that the review question itself may focus solely on implementation, in which case this guidance may be the only product of the evidence review process. As depicted in the two panels in Figure 3-3, the committee intended its evidence review and grading methodology to allow for a focus on both effectiveness and implementation questions.

The committee included in its key review questions for each of the evidence reviews a question related to the factors that created barriers to and facilitators of implementation of the PHEPR practice, which informed its implementation guidance. To address those review questions, evidence was synthesized using much the same process as that described above for the EtD framework. Findings on barriers or facilitators that aligned across evidence streams were combined into higher-order findings that were featured most prominently in the guidance on facilitating implementation and/or other operational considerations (noting any associated confidence assessments from the qualitative evidence synthesis). Where information useful to practitioners was identified only in a single evidence stream, it was still captured in the guidance, but the absence of support from other evidence sources was noted for transparency. The lack of coherence across evidence streams may result because some types of evidence are more likely to be generated by certain study types or because a finding is novel and has not yet been explored using a multitude of methods. In some cases, implementation guidance may also be drawn from the evidence synthesis used to populate the EtD framework or other evidence sources. In the case of the committee's quarantine review, for example, implementation guidance was also informed by the modeling study analysis.

LIMITATIONS, LESSONS LEARNED, AND RECOMMENDATIONS FOR THE FUTURE

The committee undertook to develop an evidence review and evaluation methodology with sufficient flexibility such that it not only could accommodate the diversity of evidence for the four exemplar PHEPR practices but also could be applied and adapted as needed to support future PHEPR evidence reviews. In this section, the committee reflects on the limitations of its methodology, its experience in developing and applying the methodology, and the implications for future reviews of PHEPR practices. The chapter concludes with the committee's recommendations for the development of a sustainable process for conducting reviews and generating evidence-based PHEPR guidelines on an ongoing basis and the infrastructure necessary to support that process.

Limitations of the Committee's Evidence Review and Evaluation Methodology

The evidence review and evaluation methodology described in this chapter and applied to the four PHEPR practices discussed in the following chapters represents the culmination of 2 years of methodological development and consensus building through committee discussion. The strengths of that development process include the diverse expertise of the committee members, who represent methodologists (both U.S. and international), PHEPR practitioners, and PHEPR researchers; consultation with outside experts in systematic review methods and guideline development (during both public and closed session discussions); and iterative testing of the methodology on a small but diverse selection of PHEPR practices. A combination of existing and adapted methods and tools was used to synthesize and assess the quality of method-specific streams of evidence that were subsequently, in a process original to this committee, brought together in a single integrated mixed-method synthesis using a logic model as the analytical framework for integration.

At the same time, there are limitations to the process by which the methods and tools were used, adapted, or developed. Although the four practices to which the committee's methodology was applied were deliberately chosen to represent a spectrum of the types of questions and evidence relevant to PHEPR, new situations are likely to be identified in which additions to or adaptations of these methods are warranted when the methodology is applied to additional practices. Ongoing methodological refinement through iterative testing on additional PHEPR practices is therefore an important next step. Another critical component of the refinement process that is employed by other groups developing methods and tools involves the use of strategies, such as surveys, Delphi processes, and small-group feedback sessions, to gather input from a much broader group of experts (e.g., methodologists, researchers, end users) and organizations in the field (Lewin et al., 2018). The committee's time constraints and the National Academies' confidentiality requirements limited the opportunities for extensive solicitation of feedback from the field. However, such solicitation is often conducted in phases when new methods and tools are developed, and the committee's work should therefore be viewed as the first phase of the development process. The committee anticipates that additional phases of expert review and feedback on its methodology will follow the release of this report. As with any first-time application, the committee expects that with the methodology's increased use, opportunities to improve it will be identified.

Another limitation relates to the current state of methodological science with regard to the integration of different types of evidence. Mixed-method syntheses like the process adopted by the committee are relatively uncommon in guideline development, and methods for synthesizing evidence from highly diverse study designs (e.g., quantitative, qualitative, case reports, modeling) are still being developed and tested (Noyes et al., 2019). There are accepted methods for assessing the quality of individual quantitative and qualitative studies and for grading the respective bodies of evidence, but methods and tools have not yet been developed for grading findings developed from the integration of quantitative and qualitative evidence. An added challenge for the committee was the lack of existing quality assessment and grading methods for bodies of descriptive surveys and case reports and AARs. Consequently, some of the evidence streams used by the committee were synthesized and graded, while others were not. Other groups have adapted the GRADE and GRADE-CERQual methods for these evidence types (WHO, 2018), but in the absence of methods for integrating the assessments to generate a composite rating, the committee chose not to grade bodies of descriptive surveys and case reports and AARs. Given these gaps in evidence review methods, the committee took a pragmatic approach to integrating the diverse evidence types that were captured in its reviews, as described above. However, as the methodological science behind mixed-method synthesis continues to evolve, it will be important to update the methods. Thus, the methods presented here should not be viewed as the final word in how PHEPR topics should be systematically assessed, but rather the starting point to be built on in future efforts.

Reflections and Lessons Learned from the Mixed-Method Reviews

The committee recognized from the inception of this study that its evidence review and evaluation methodology needed to be aligned with the questions of interest to PHEPR stakeholders and the nature of the PHEPR evidence base. At the outset, however, the committee had an incomplete picture of what that evidence base looked like. Thus, it was unclear how well existing evidence evaluation frameworks would work, even allowing for adaptation. Accordingly, the committee undertook its work with the mindset of a learning process, allowing flexibility to adapt methods and tools as they were being applied, but also capturing the strengths and limitations of the approach and acknowledging alternatives that may be considered in the future. The committee found it was important when adapting and applying the methods and tools to its specific review questions to have input from those familiar with the subject area and the types of studies and other information available.

The committee's methodology accommodated a wide range of evidence types, including evidence from RCTs, nonrandomized experimental studies, case reports, modeling studies, and descriptive surveys, as well as mechanistic evidence and parallel evidence from other fields. Although it is common for evidence review groups to exclude studies based on study design or methodological limitations in execution, the committee chose not to set such criteria for inclusion of studies in its review. Instead, it considered the appropriateness of the study design and the quality of execution as they related to the ability to address a specific review question. For example, qualitative research methods were considered superior to quantitative methods for certain tasks, such as describing the lived experiences of people placed under quarantine, or exploring the ways in which multiple factors coalesce or conflict in the minds of decision makers choosing whether to implement an emergency operations center. Because much learning about what works and considerations for implementation accumulates through experience, it was important for the committee's mixed-method synthesis approach to accommodate experiential evidence, such as case reports and AARs, so as to corroborate research findings in the COE determination and help to explain differences in outcomes in practice settings (e.g., by illustrating differences in feasibility or acceptability across settings). However, integrating evidence from AARs and case reports presented its own challenges as these types of reports rarely include clear outcome measures or clearly elucidated cause-and-effect relationships. Moreover, such evidence, even when derived in accordance with high methodological standards, is subject to higher risk of bias compared with evidence from RCTs. The committee attempted to mitigate these risks by ensuring that the methods used to assess the quality of evidence were suited not just to the type of evidence being reviewed but also to the purpose to which that evidence was to be put, rather than holding every study to the same set of evaluative criteria. For example, the quality threshold for applying evidence to an assessment of *acceptability* differed from that for assessing *effectiveness.*

The four review topics selected by the committee as test cases represented complex practices for which diverse types of PHEPR evidence were captured. Each raised different methodological challenges, thus providing an opportunity to test and iteratively expand the range of the committee's methodology.

The EOC test case, for example, yielded a situation in which no quantitative evidence of effect was found, but other types of evidence provided information that would be useful to practitioners in considering when and in what circumstances to activate public health emergency operations. Recognizing that PHEPR practitioners must make decisions in the face of a public health emergency with the best information available, the committee sought to develop a process that, even in the absence of quantitative evidence of effectiveness, could present such useful information without an accompanying practice recommendation.

The community preparedness test case provided an opportunity to consider parallel evidence in the review process. As discussed earlier, the applicability of evidence from other fields will be important in reviews of PHEPR practices given that foundational knowledge for some practices may have been generated outside the PHEPR context. Other fields that may be relevant to PHEPR include behavioral economics, psychology, and sociology.

The information sharing test case highlighted the challenges of conducting systematic reviews on technology-based interventions that are evolving rapidly, thus raising concerns regarding the relevance of the findings and recommendations to contemporary practice. These challenges are not specific to PHEPR; the suitability of slow and often infrequently updated evidence reviews for research areas that are changing rapidly has been noted more broadly, giving rise to the concept of living systematic reviews (Elliott et al., 2017) and guidelines (Akl et al., 2017) that are continuously updated as new evidence is published.

The non-pharmaceutical intervention (quarantine) test case raised the issue of how effectiveness is defined (which outcomes matter). It also necessitated the incorporation of mechanistic evidence and evidence from modeling studies. The scoping review discussed in Chapter 2 found that modeling studies make up a substantial proportion of the evidence base for the Non-Pharmaceutical Interventions Capability (as well as the Medical Countermeasure Dispensing and Administration and Medical Materiel Management and Distribution Capabilities), emphasizing the importance of integrating modeling evidence into PHEPR evidence reviews. Although models have been incorporated into past evidence reviews, such as The Community Guide review of school closure to reduce transmission of pandemic influenza (The Community Guide, 2012), this remains an active area of methodological development and is also an intensive process. Consequently, the committee undertook only a limited analysis. As methods for review and integration of modeling evidence are refined, the methodology applied by the committee will need to be updated. The use of mechanistic evidence in evidence syntheses is uncommon, although evidence of biological mechanisms of action is increasingly being incorporated into reviews, for example, on pharmacological and toxicological topics. This is another area requiring further methodological development, one that would benefit from the efforts of a future guidelines development group (see Recommendation 1) to further develop and refine the definition and test the mechanistic upgrading assumptions.

Despite these challenges, the committee was able to use its evidence review and evaluation methodology to answer not only traditional questions about the effectiveness of a practice but also more operational questions of interest to PHEPR practitioners regarding implementation. The committee hopes this may encourage future reviewers to embrace unconventional questions to address important knowledge gaps in the PHEPR field.

In assessing the COE for the PHEPR practices, the committee experienced challenges applying some of the GRADE domains. GRADE is most suitable for discrete interventions as is typical in clinical trials, but less so for more complex areas where context and the effect of multiple interventions are prominent study characteristics. As discussed earlier in this chapter, for most PHEPR practices, the committee judged that it would not be conceptually appropriate to assume that an effect size existed independent of context and implementation fidelity. As others have done (Movsisyan et al., 2016; Rehfuess and Akl, 2013), the committee also considered whether all bodies of evidence comprising largely nonrandomized studies should start the GRADE process at low COE, but ultimately determined that there was value in adhering to the GRADE approach to the extent possible while acknowledging that this is an ongoing point of discussion in the field (Montgomery et al., 2019). Further consideration of potential modifications to GRADE or of alternative rating schemes that provide more emphasis on non-RCT methods is warranted.[19]

The committee refined its methodology as a clearer picture of the evidence base emerged. The ultimate result was a process that could be used to develop practice recommendations for three of the four exemplar review topics. It is important to note, however, that other review approaches could have been employed (e.g., the realist approach [Greenhalgh et al., 2011] described earlier in this chapter) for questions about circumstances in which a particular intervention should be implemented. Furthermore, the committee's focus on methods for systematic literature review and evidence grading reflects its charge, but does not imply that this is the best approach to inform decision making for all PHEPR practices, particularly given the substantial investment of time (see Figure 3-4) and resources required for such reviews. It may be that for some questions, other methods, such as Delphi studies to elicit expert opinion, decision analysis, or simulation modeling, would yield sufficient and perhaps even more useful information to guide decision making, in some cases in real time. It is worth noting, especially in the current context (i.e., the coronavirus outbreak that was declared a public health emergency in January 2020), that while the time required to conduct these evidence reviews is not an issue unique to PHEPR, scenarios are more likely to arise in PHEPR that would necessitate the rapid development of guidelines (Garritty et al., 2017; Schünemann et al., 2007). Standard methods for rapid guideline development and revision are actively being pursued (Garritty et al., 2016; Kowalski et al., 2018) and may inform adaptations of the committee's methodology to facilitate rapid review. Relatedly, it is conceivable that a public health emergency would warrant the expedited completion and/or early release of information from an in-progress review, and processes need to be established for such a contingency.

Need for Ongoing PHEPR Evidence Reviews

There have been repeated calls for measures and approaches for evaluation in the PHEPR field (Acosta et al., 2009; IOM, 2008). However, there has been no concerted effort to change the methodologies used in evaluating PHEPR practice or evidence. While the committee acknowledges that methods other than systematic review may be useful in addressing the evidentiary needs of PHEPR practitioners and policy makers, there remains a clear need for an evidence review process to generate evidence-based PHEPR recom-

[19] As noted earlier in this chapter, had individual nonrandomized studies been assessed for risk of bias using ROBINS-I, the starting COE for bodies of such studies could have been set at high according to GRADE guidance (Schünemann et al., 2018), but would immediately have been downgraded two levels because of risk of bias from lack of randomization, ending up at low.

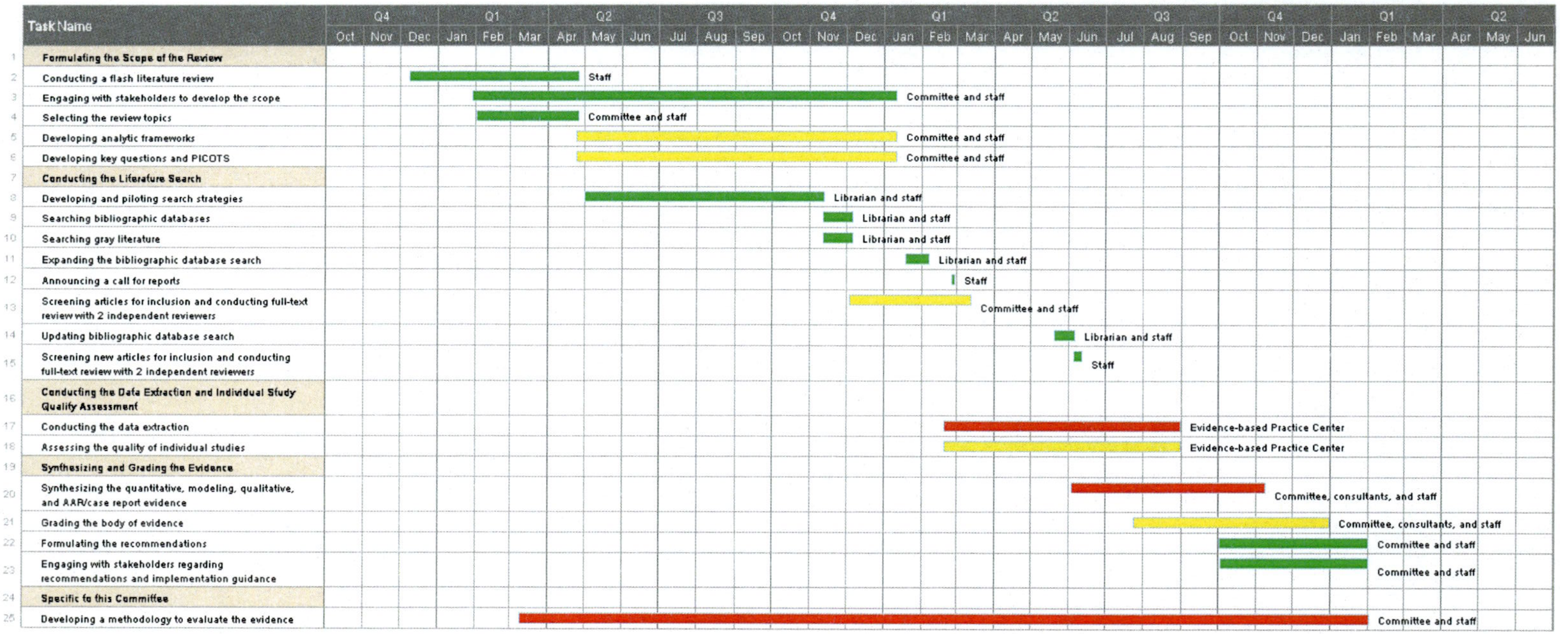

FIGURE 3-4 Burden (time and intensity) of the committee's methodology development and mixed-method review process.
NOTES: Green = lowest-intensity tasks; yellow = moderate-intensity tasks; red = highest-intensity tasks. AAR = after action report; PICOTS = population, intervention, comparator, outcome, timing, setting.

mendations and guidelines. Given the time and resources required to conduct systematic reviews, the committee was limited to reviewing only a small selection of PHEPR practices as proof of concept. Hundreds of such reviews could be conducted on PHEPR practices to guide practitioners in operationalizing the 15 PHEPR Capabilities. Scoping reviews such as those discussed in Chapter 2 can help guide the selection of review topics for which a systematic review is likely to be worthwhile, as can structured priority-setting activities (Zaza et al., 2000a), including such Delphi-type processes as the practitioner engagement activity the committee undertook to inform future potential PHEPR review topics (described in Box 3-5).[20] Moreover, the evidence base for PHEPR practices is continually evolving with the field. As new studies and reports are published, a sustained mechanism will be needed for capturing and analyzing new evidence over time and for updating prior reviews as needed.

In addition to guiding PHEPR practice and decision making, systems that support ongoing evidence reviews have the potential to drive improvements in the evidence base over time and guide the research agenda through the identification of evidence gaps (as discussed further in Chapter 8). As limitations in study design and execution are systematically catalogued, standards and guidance to researchers can be developed to improve the evidentiary value of future studies.

Evidence review and evaluation methods are continuing to evolve, and particularly relevant to PHEPR are the emerging methods for complex interventions and complex systems. In the interest of sustainability, the committee adopted as the foundation for its layered grading approach the widely adopted GRADE framework for evaluating quantitative evidence of effectiveness, its EtD criteria, and the GRADE-CERQual method for assessing synthesized qualitative findings, although the integrated COE assessment described in this chapter went beyond the GRADE approach. The GRADE methodology is continually refined through the work of the GRADE working groups, one of which is actively developing methods for assessing the certainty of the body of evidence for complex health and social interventions (Norris et al., 2019; Rehfuess and Akl, 2013). Moreover, training courses and workshops are provided to assist users with applying the GRADE methods, and such events are noted on the GRADE Working Group's website.[21] Consequently, the use of GRADE and GRADE-CERQual gives reviewers access to widely used evidence evaluation tools that are regularly updated. Over time, and as reviewers gain more experience with PHEPR evidence reviews, it will be important to assess and refine the review methods to ensure that they are consistent with current review and guideline development practice and are meeting the needs of PHEPR stakeholders.

An Infrastructure to Sustain PHEPR Evidence Reviews

There are two distinct approaches for ongoing guideline development—centralized and decentralized or "franchised." In the centralized approach, guidelines are developed by a single organization, whereas in the decentralized model, any group (often professional organizations and academic groups) can apply a standard methodology to produce a guideline (Grol, 1993; IOM, 1992). Although a decentralized approach allows for greater capacity to conduct reviews and may stimulate wider interest in evidence-based methods, the resulting products exhibit significant variability, and concerns have been raised regard-

[20] The Delphi-like practitioner engagement activity described in Box 3-5 and in Appendix A was conducted after the committee's four evidence review topics had been selected and therefore did not inform the selection process. The activity was intended to inform priorities for future PHEPR evidence reviews.

[21] See https://www.gradeworkinggroup.org (accessed February 22, 2020).

BOX 3-5 PRIORITY TOPICS FOR FUTURE PHEPR EVIDENCE REVIEWS

The committee engaged with a panel of state, local, tribal, and territorial practitioners to assess the relative priority (from the practitioner perspective) of potential future evidence review topics encompassed within the 15 Centers for Disease Control and Prevention PHEPR Capabilities (see Appendix A for additional details regarding this activity). Building on the work by Siegfried and colleagues (2017), the committee employed a modified Delphi-like process that yielded the following list of topics rated by at least 66 percent of the panel as "highest-priority" or "high-priority" after two rounds of voting:

- Engaging, educating, training, and motivating communities to prepare for, withstand, and recover from emergencies
- Strategies for engaging at-risk populations in community preparedness activities and in protective actions during and immediately after an emergency
- Strategies to integrate preparedness activities into routine public health practice
- Effective message formats for information sharing with at-risk populations (e.g., populations that rely on oral traditions, populations with limited English proficiency, and individuals without Internet access or smartphones)
- Information management strategies for public risk perception during an emergency
- Monitoring and tracking health issues (physical safety and mental and behavioral health) of responders prior to, during, and following response

ing the potential to use the process to promote special interests. Centralized approaches, in contrast, are characterized by lower throughput and may be threatened by budget cuts when dependent on federal support, but ensure greater consistency in the application of the methods and the quality of the reports (although it should be noted that a centralized approach can mitigate but does not entirely obviate the possibility of conflicts of interest or other biases on the part of the agency or individuals charged with carrying out the reviews).

The complexity of the review methods developed by the committee has clear implications for the expertise required in the multidisciplinary group that will need to be involved in future reviews of PHEPR practices. The group's composition will need to include PHEPR practitioners; PHEPR researchers; and experts with deep knowledge of review methodologies, including methods for synthesizing and grading both quantitative and qualitative evidence. A review group will also benefit from including legal, ethical, and social science expertise, especially when addressing issues affecting implementation. Considering the requisite diversity of expertise and the need for guidelines to issue from an authoritative source with the trust of the PHEPR community and the ability to disseminate the guidelines widely, the committee concluded that a centralized approach supported by CDC is the best model for a system for ongoing evidence reviews of PHEPR practices. Importantly, CDC has extensive experience in overseeing evidence-based review processes, with notable examples including the CPSTF; the Advisory Committee on Immunization Practices (Lee et al., 2018); the Healthcare Infection Control Practices Advisory Committee, which notably incorporates GRADE into its guideline process (CDC, 2019; Umscheid et al., 2010); and, formerly, EGAPP.

There are a number of ways to operationalize a centralized evidence review model, each with its advantages and limitations. The evidence review system can be internal to a federal agency, or centralized reviews can be conducted by independent, external groups that are convened by and work closely with a federal sponsor. Durable exemplars of these two models are CPSTF and USPSTF (USPSTF, 2015; Zaza et al., 2000b). The 35-year-old USPSTF is an independent task force that is convened and funded by AHRQ and makes recommendations on clinical preventive services. It selects topics and oversees the evidence reviews, which are conducted by the separately funded EPCs. The task force reviews the evidence and makes recommendation statements, which are published separately from the EPC reports. CPSTF is convened and overseen by CDC, and in contrast to the USPSTF process, CDC staff have a central role in topic selection and conduct of the evidence reviews, although the recommendations that result are those of the task force.

For a complex task such as PHEPR evidence reviews, an independent, external review group could help avoid conflict of interest while ensuring the broad range of inputs and skills necessary to produce credible, rigorous recommendations. An additional advantage is that its recommendations would not need to be vetted through a government approval process. CDC could still play different roles in these processes, including funding the evidence review system, convening a task force, suggesting topics, overseeing contractors that perform the reviews, soliciting public input, and disseminating recommendations.

A sustainable evidence-based review process for PHEPR will require organizational support and leadership; multifaceted capabilities; adequate funding; and a functional, coordinated system. An initial investment in infrastructure will need to include a curated catalog/guide for the evidence reviews that is made widely available and supported by outreach, education, and implementation resources. In addition to the initial costs for standup of the evidence review group and process, annual funding will be needed to support the group's ongoing activities. This funding can be roughly estimated, based on the USPSTF annual budget,[22] at approximately $10 million annually. This annual cost is not insignificant, but pales in the context of annual spending by the National Institutes of Health (NIH) on research project grants (approximately $6 billion in 2019).[23] Because of the vagaries of year-to-year priorities and changing personnel, there are significant advantages to establishing the funding and structure in legislation, although care would be necessary to ensure that the language of such legislation is not so prescriptive that those responsible for implementation lack the necessary flexibility. In addition to providing some measure of stability (i.e., protection against agency budget cuts), legislation can facilitate needed oversight. For example, both CPSTF and USPSTF send annual reports to Congress highlighting high-priority research gaps, which could also help secure funding for critical PHEPR research.

RECOMMENDATION 1: Appoint a Public Health Emergency Preparedness and Response (PHEPR) Evidence-Based Guidelines Group

The Centers for Disease Control and Prevention (CDC) should appoint and support an independent group to develop methodologically rigorous and transparent evidence-based guidelines for PHEPR practices on an ongoing basis. This group should take the methodology developed by the committee as a starting point, but should also be charged with its continued development based on the full range of available evidence, incorporating advances in the synthesis of quantitative, qualitative, and experiential evidence. The group should also identify and communicate key PHEPR evidence gaps in annual reports to CDC and Congress to guide future research on the effectiveness of PHEPR practices.

---

[22] In 2019, the AHRQ budget for USPSTF was $11.6 million according to AHRQ's 2020 operating plan, available at https://www.ahrq.gov/sites/default/files/wysiwyg/cpi/about/mission/operating-plan/operating-plan-2020.pdf (accessed February 21, 2020).

[23] Data on NIH research project grant funding are available at https://report.nih.gov/nihdatabook/category/6 (accessed February 21, 2020).

RECOMMENDATION 2: Establish Infrastructure to Support Ongoing Public Health Emergency Preparedness and Response (PHEPR) Evidence Reviews
The Centers for Disease Control and Prevention should establish the infrastructure, policies, and procedures needed to ensure a sustained process for conducting and updating evidence reviews and generating evidence-based practice guidelines, in collaboration with other relevant federal agencies. The infrastructure should include an open-access repository for evidence-based PHEPR practices.

REFERENCES

Acosta, J. D., C. Nelson, E. B. Beckjord, S. R. Shelton, E. Murphy, K. L. Leuschner, and J. Wasserman. 2009. *A national agenda for public health systems research on emergency preparedness.* Santa Monica, CA: RAND Health.

Akl, E. A., J. J. Meerpohl, J. Elliott, L. A. Kahale, H. J. Schünemann, T. Agoritsas, J. Hilton, C. Perron, E. Akl, R. Hodder, et al. 2017. Living systematic reviews: Living guideline recommendations. *Journal of Clinical Epidemiology* 91:47–53.

Alonso-Coello, P., H. J. Schünemann, J. Moberg, R. Brignardello-Petersen, E. A. Akl, M. Davoli, S. Treweek, R. A. Mustafa, G. Rada, S. Rosenbaum, A. Morelli, G. H. Guyatt, and A. D. Oxman. 2016. GRADE evidence to decision (ETD) frameworks: A systematic and transparent approach to making well informed healthcare choices: Introduction. *BMJ* 2016:353. https://doi.org/10.1136/bmj.i2016.

Anderson, L. M., M. Petticrew, E. Rehfuess, R. Armstrong, E. Ueffing, P. Baker, D. Francis, and P. Tugwell. 2011. Using logic models to capture complexity in systematic reviews. *Research Synthesis Methods* 2(1):33–42.

Barnett-Page, E., and J. Thomas. 2009. Methods for the synthesis of qualitative research: A critical review. *BMC Medical Research Methodology* 9(1):59.

Bate, P., P. Mendel, and G. Robert. 2008. *Organizing for quality: The improvement journeys of leading hospitals in Europe and the United States.* New York: Radcliffe Publishing.

Bennett, C., S. Khangura, J. C. Brehaut, I. D. Graham, D. Moher, B. K. Potter, and J. M. Grimshaw. 2010. Reporting guidelines for survey research: An analysis of published guidance and reporting practices. *PLOS Medicine* 8(8):e1001069.

Berg, R. C., and J. Nanavati. 2016. Realist review: Current practice and future prospects. *Journal of Practice Research* 12(1).

Booth, A., J. Noyes, K. Flemming, A. Gerhardus, P. Wahlster, G. J. Wilt, K. Mozygemba, P. Refolo, D. Sacchini, M. Tummers, and E. Rehfuess. 2016. *Guidance on choosing qualitative evidence synthesis methods for use in health technology assessments of complex interventions.* https://www.integrate-hta.eu/wp-content/uploads/2016/02/Guidance-on-choosing-qualitative-evidence-synthesis-methods-for-use-in-HTA-of-complex-interventions.pdf (accessed March 4, 2020).

Booth, A., G. Moore, K. Flemming, R. Garside, N. Rollins, Ö. Tunçalp, and J. Noyes. 2019. Taking account of context in systematic reviews and guidelines considering a complexity perspective. *BMJ Global Health* 4(Suppl 1).

Boruch, R., and N. Rui. 2008. From randomized controlled trials to evidence grading schemes: Current state of evidence-based practice in social sciences. *Journal of Evidence-Based Medicine* 1(1):41–49.

Briss, P. A., S. Zaza, M. Pappaioanou, J. Fielding, L. K. Wright-De Aguero, B. I. Truman, D. P. Hopkins, P. Dolan Mullen, R. S. Thompson, S. H. Woolf, V. G. Carande-Kulis, L. Andersin, A. R. Hinman, D. V. McQueen, S. M. Teutsch, J. R. Harris, and The Task Force on Community Preventive Services. 2000. Developing an evidence-based guide to community preventive services—methods. *American Journal of Preventive Medicine* 18(1S):35–43.

Briss, P. A., R. C. Brownson, J. E. Fielding, and S. Zaza. 2004. Developing and using the guide to community preventive services: Lessons learned about evidence-based public health. *Annual Review of Public Health* 25(1):281–302.

Bruce, N., A. Pruss-Ustun, D. Pope, H. Adair-Rohani, and E. Rehfuess. 2014. Methods used for evidence assessment. *WHO indoor air quality guidelines: Household fuel combustion.* Geneva, Switzerland: World Health Organization.

Brunetti, M., I. Shemilt, S. Pregno, L. Vale, A. D. Oxman, J. Lord, J. Sisk, F. Ruiz, S. Hill, G. H. Guyatt, R. Jaeschke, M. Helfand, R. Harbour, M. Davoli, L. Amato, A. Liberati, and H. J. Schünemann. 2013. GRADE guidelines: 10. Considering resource use and rating the quality of economic evidence. *Journal of Clinical Epidemiology* 66(2):140–150.

Campbell, M., J. E. McKenzie, A. Sowden, S. V. Katikireddi, S. E. Brennan, S. Ellis, J. Hartmann-Boyce, R. Ryan, S. Shepperd, J. Thomas, V. Welch, and H. Thomson. 2020. Synthesis without meta-analysis (SWIM) in systematic reviews: Reporting guideline. *BMJ* 368:l6890.

Carbone, E. G., and E. V. Thomas. 2018. Science as the basis of public health emergency preparedness and response practice: The slow but crucial evolution. *American Journal of Public Health* 108(S5):S383–S386.

CASP (Critical Appraisal Skills Programme). 2018. *CASP appraisal checklists.* http://casp-uk.net/casp-tools-checklists (accessed June 23, 2020).

CDC (Centers for Disease Control and Prevention). 2018a. *Introduction to prevention effectiveness.* https://www.cdc.gov/publichealth101/prevention-effectiveness.html (accessed February 15, 2020).

CDC. 2018b. *Public health emergency preparedness and response capabilities: National standards for state, local, tribal, and territorial public health.* Atlanta, GA: Centers for Disease Control and Prevention. https://www.cdc.gov/cpr/readiness/00_docs/CDC_PreparednesResponseCapabilities_October2012_Final_508.pdf (accessed March 4, 2020).

CDC. 2019. *Update to the Centers for Disease Control and Prevention and the Healthcare Infection Control Practices Advisory Committee recommendation categorization scheme for infection control and prevention guideline recommendations.* https://www.cdc.gov/hicpac/pdf/recommendation-scheme-update-H.pdf (accessed March 4, 2020).

CLEAR (Clearinghouse for Labor Evaluation and Research). 2014. *Operational guidelines for reviewing implementation studies.* https://clear.dol.gov/sites/default/files/CLEAR_Operational%20Implementation%20Study%20GuGuidelin.pdf (accessed March 4, 2020).

CLEAR. 2015. *Clear causal evidence guidelines, version 2.1.* https://clear.dol.gov/sites/default/files/CLEAR_Evidence-Guidelines_V2.1.pdf (accessed March 4, 2020).

Cochrane. 2017. *Suggested risk of bias criteria for EPOC reviews.* https://epoc.cochrane.org/sites/epoc.cochrane.org/files/public/uploads/Resources-for-authors2017/suggested_risk_of_bias_criteria_for_epoc_reviews.pdf (accessed February 15, 2020).

Davids, E. L., and N. V. Roman. 2014. A systematic review of the relationship between parenting styles and children's physical activity. *African Journal for Physical, Health Education, Recreation and Dance* 228–246.

Durrheim, D. N., and A. Reingold. 2010. Modifying the GRADE framework could benefit public health. *Journal of Epidemiology and Community Health* 64(5):387.

ECDC (European Centre for Disease Prevention and Control). 2018. *Best practice recommendations for conducting after-action reviews to enhance public health preparedness.* Stockholm, Sweden: European Centre for Disease Prevention and Control. https://www.ecdc.europa.eu/sites/default/files/documents/public-health-preparedness-best-practice-recommendations.pdf (accessed March 4, 2020).

Elliott, J., A. Synnot, T. Turner, M. Simmonds, E. Akl, S. McDonald, G. Salanti, J. Meerpohl, H. MacLehose, J. Hilton, I. Shemilt, J. Thomas, T. Agoritsas, R. Hodder, and J. Yepes-Nuñez. 2017. Living systematic review: Introduction: The why, what, when and how. *Journal of Clinical Epidemiology* 91.

Fisher, R. A. 1925. *Statistical methods for research workers.* Edinburgh, Scotland: Oliver and Boyd.

Flemming, K., A. Booth, R. Garside, Ö. Tunçalp, and J. Noyes. 2019. Qualitative evidence synthesis for complex interventions and guideline development: Clarification of the purpose, designs and relevant methods. *BMJ Global Health* 4(Suppl 1):e000882.

Garritty, C., A. Stevens, G. Gartlehner, V. King, C. Kamel, and on behalf of the Cochrane Rapid Reviews Methods Group. 2016. Cochrane Rapid Reviews Methods Group to play a leading role in guiding the production of informed high-quality, timely research evidence syntheses. *Systematic Reviews* 5(1):184.

Garritty, C. M., S. L. Norris, and D. Moher. 2017. Developing who rapid advice guidelines in the setting of a public health emergency. *Journal of Clinical Epidemiology* 82:47–60.

Glenton, C., C. J. Colvin, B. Carlsen, A. Swartz, S. Lewin, J. Noyes, and A. Rashidian. 2013. Barriers and facilitators to the implementation of lay health worker programmes to improve access to maternal and child health: Qualitative evidence synthesis. *Cochrane Database of Systematic Reviews* (10).

Goodman, S. N., and J. Gerson. 2013. *Mechanistic evidence in evidence-based medicine: A conceptual framework.* AHRQ. https://effectivehealthcare.ahrq.gov/products/mechanistic-evidence-framework/white-paper (accessed May 23, 2020).

Gordon, M. 2016. Are we talking the same paradigm? Considering methodological choices in health education systematic review. *Medical Teacher* 38(7):746–750.

Green, L. W., R. C. Brownson, and J. E. Fielding. 2017. Introduction: How is the growing concern for relevance and implementation of evidence-based interventions shaping the public health research agenda? *Annual Review of Public Health* 38:i–iii.

Greenhalgh, T., G. Robert, F. MacFarlane, P. Bate, and O. Kyriakidou. 2004. Diffusion of innovations in service organizations: Systematic review and recommendations. *The Milbank Quarterly* 82(4):581–629.

Greenhalgh, T., G. Wong, G. Westhorp, and R. Pawson. 2011. Protocol—realist and meta-narrative evidence synthesis: Evolving standards (RAMESES). *BMC Medical Research Methodology* 11(1):115.

Grol, R. 1993. Development of guidelines for general practice care. *British Journal of Medical Practice* 43:146–151.

Guise, J.-M., C. Chang, M. Butler, M. Viswanathan, and P. Tugwell. 2017. AHRQ series on complex intervention systematic reviews—paper 1: An introduction to a series of articles that provide guidance and tools for reviews of complex interventions. *Journal of Clinical Epidemiology* 90:6–10.

Guyatt, G., A. D. Oxman, E. A. Akl, R. Kunz, G. Vist, J. Brozek, S. Norris, Y. Falck-Ytter, P. Glasziou, H. Debeer, R. Jaeschke, D. Rind, J. Meerpohl, P. Dahm, and H. J. Schünemann. 2011a. GRADE guidelines: 1. Introduction—GRADE evidence profiles and summary of findings tables. *Journal of Clinical Epidemiology* 64(4):383–394.

Guyatt, G. H., A. D. Oxman, S. Sultan, P. Glasziou, E. A. Akl, P. Alonso-Coello, D. Atkins, R. Kunz, J. Brozek, V. Montori, R. Jaeschke, D. Rind, P. Dahm, J. Meerpohl, G. Vist, E. Berliner, S. Norris, Y. Falck-Ytter, M. H. Murad, H. J. Schünemann, and GRADE Working Group. 2011b. GRADE guidelines: 9. Rating up the quality of evidence. *Journal of Clinical Epidemiology* 64(12):1311–1316.

Harden, A., J. Thomas, M. Cargo, J. Harris, T. Pantoja, K. Flemming, A. Booth, R. Garside, K. Hannes, and J. Noyes. 2018. Cochrane Qualitative and Implementation Methods Group guidance series-paper 5: Methods for integrating qualitative and implementation evidence within intervention effectiveness reviews. *Journal of Clinical Epidemiology* 97:70–78.

Harrison, H., M. Birks, R. Franklin, and J. Mills. 2017. Case study research: Foundations and methodological orientations. *Forum: Qualitative Social Research* 18(1). http://www.qualitative-research.net/index.php/fqs/article/view/2655/4079 (accessed May 7, 2020).

Hick, J. L., D. Hanfling, M. K. Wynia, and A. T. Pavia. 2020. *Duty to plan: Health care, crisis standards of care, and novel coronavirus SARS-CoV-2.* National Academy of Medicine. https://nam.edu/duty-to-plan-health-care-crisis-standards-of-care-and-novel-coronavirus-sars-cov-2 (accessed May 23, 2020).

Higgins, J. P. T., J. A. Lopez-Lopez, B. J. Becker, S. R. Davies, S. Dawson, J. M. Grimshaw, L. A. McGuinness, T. H. M. Moore, E. A. Rehfuess, J. Thomas, and D. M. Caldwell. 2019. Synthesising quantitative evidence in systematic reviews of complex health interventions. *BMJ Global Health* 4(Suppl 1):e000858.

Hill, A. B. 1965. The environment and disease: Association or causation? *Proceedings of the Royal Society of Medicine* 58(5):295–300.

Hoffmann, T. C., P. P. Glasziou, I. Boutron, R. Milne, R. Perera, D. Moher, D. G. Altman, V. Barbour, H. Macdonald, M. Johnston, S. E. Lamb, M. Dixon-Woods, P. McCulloch, J. C. Wyatt, A.-W. Chan, and S. Michie. 2014. Better reporting of interventions: Template for intervention description and replication (TIDieR) checklist and guide. *BMJ* 348:g1687.

Hohmann, A. A., and M. K. Shear. 2002. Community-based intervention research: Coping with the "noise" of real life in study design. *The American Journal of Psychiatry* 159(2):201–207.

Howick, J., P. Glasziou, and J. K. Aronson. 2009. The evolution of evidence hierarchies: What can Bradford Hill's "Guidelines for Causation" contribute? *Journal of the Royal Society of Medicine* 102(5):186–194.

Howick, J., P. Glasziou, and J. K. Aronson. 2010. Evidence-based mechanistic reasoning. *Journal of the Royal Society of Medicine* 103(11):433–441.

Hultcrantz, M., D. Rind, E. A. Akl, S. Treweek, R. A. Mustafa, A. Iorio, B. S. Alper, J. J. Meerpohl, M. H. Murad, M. T. Ansari, S. V. Katikireddi, P. Ostlund, S. Tranaeus, R. Christensen, G. Gartlehner, J. Brozek, A. Izcovich, H. Schünemann, and G. Guyatt. 2017. The GRADE Working Group clarifies the construct of certainty of evidence. *Journal of Clinical Epidemiology* 87:4–13.

Hunter, J. C., J. E. Yang, A. W. Crawley, L. Biesiadecki, and T. J. Aragón. 2013. Public health response systems in-action: Learning from local health departments' experiences with acute and emergency incidents. *PLOS ONE* 8(11):e79457. https://doi.org/10.1371/journal.pone.0079457.

IOM (Institute of Medicine). 1992. Developing clincal practice guidelines. In *Guidelines for clinical practice: From development to use.* Washington, DC: National Academy Press.

IOM. 2008. *Research priorities in emergency preparedness and response for public health systems: A letter report.* Washington, DC: The National Academies Press.

IOM. 2009. *Guidance for establishing crisis standards of care for use in disaster situations: A letter report.* Washington, DC: The National Academies Press.

Jennings, B., and J. Arras. 2008. *Ethical guidance for public health emergency preparedness and response: Highlighting ethics and values in a vital public health service.* Ethics Subcommittee, Advisory Committee to the Director, Centers for Disease Control and Prevention. https://www.cdc.gov/od/science/integrity/phethics/docs/white_paper_final_for_website_2012_4_6_12_final_for_web_508_compliant.pdf (accessed March 4, 2020).

Jennings, B., J. D. Arras, D. H. Barrett, and B. A. Ellis. 2016. *Emergency ethics: Public health preparedness and response.* New York: Oxford University Press.

Kowalski, S. C., R. L. Morgan, M. Falavigna, I. D. Florez, I. Etxeandia-Ikobaltzeta, W. Wiercioch, Y. Zhang, F. Sakhia, L. Ivanova, N. Santesso, and H. J. Schünemann. 2018. Development of rapid guidelines: Systematic survey of current practices and methods. *Health Research Policy and Systems* 16(1):61.

Lee, G., W. Carr, and ACIP Evidence-Based Recommendations Work Group. 2018. Updated framework for development of evidence-based recommendations by the Advisory Committee on Immunization Practices. *Morbidity and Mortality Weekly Report* 67:1271–1272. https://www.cdc.gov/mmwr/volumes/67/wr/mm6745a4.htm?s_cid=mm6745a4_w (accessed March 4, 2020).

Leviton, L. C. 2017. Generalizing about public health interventions: A mixed-methods approach to external validity. *Annual Review of Public Health* 38:371–391.

Lewin, S., C. Glenton, H. Munthe-Kaas, B. Carlsen, C. J. Colvin, M. Gulmezoglu, J. Noyes, A. Booth, R. Garside, and A. Rashidian. 2015. Using qualitative evidence in decision making for health and social interventions: An approach to assess confidence in findings from qualitative evidence syntheses (GRADE-CERQual). *PLOS Medicine* 12(10):e1001895.

Lewin, S., A. Booth, C. Glenton, H. Munthe-Kaas, A. Rashidian, M. Wainwright, M. A. Bohren, O. Tuncalp, C. J. Colvin, R. Garside, B. Carlsen, E. V. Langlois, and J. Noyes. 2018. Applying GRADE-CERQual to qualitative evidence synthesis findings: Introduction to the series. *Implementation Science* 13(Suppl 1):2.

Marcus, J. 2018. *Additional evidence evaluation methods for assessing the effectiveness of interventions and practices: National Transportation Safety Board.* Paper presented to the Committee on Evidence-Based Practices for Public Health Emergency Preparedness and Response, July 26, Washington, DC.

Mastroianni, A. C., J. P. Kahn, and N. E. Kass, eds. 2019. *The Oxford handbook of public health ethics.* Oxford University Press. https://www.oxfordhandbooks.com/view/10.1093/oxfordhb/9780190245191.001.0001/oxfordhb-9780190245191 (accessed May 23, 2020).

Miles, M. B., M. A. Huberman, and J. Saldana. 2014. *Qualitative data analysis: A methods sourcebook.* Thousand Oaks, CA: SAGE Publications.

Minard, C. G., M. F. de Carvalho, and M. S. Iyengar. 2011. Optimizing medical resources for spaceflight using the integrated medical model. *Aviation Space and Environmental Medicine* 82(9):890–894.

Moberg, J., A. D. Oxman, S. Rosenbaum, H. J. Schünemann, G. Guyatt, S. Flottorp, C. Glenton, S. Lewin, A. Morelli, G. Rada, P. Alonso-Coello, and G. W. Group. 2018. The GRADE Evidence to Decision (ETD) framework for health system and public health decisions. *Health Research Policy and Systems* 16(1):45.

Montgomery, P., A. Movsisyan, S. P. Grant, G. Macdonald, and E. A. Rehfuess. 2019. Considerations of complexity in rating certainty of evidence in systematic reviews: A primer on using the GRADE approach in global health. *BMJ Global Health* 4(Suppl 1).

Movsisyan, A., G. J. Melendez-Torres, and P. Montgomery. 2016. Users identified challenges in applying GRADE to complex interventions and suggested an extension to GRADE. *Journal of Clinical Epidemiology* 70:191–199.

Murad, M. H., R. A. Mustafa, H. J. Schünemann, S. Sultan, and N. Santesso. 2017. Rating the certainty in evidence in the absence of a single estimate of effect. *Journal of Evidence-Based Medicine* 22(3):85–87.

NASEM (National Academies of Sciences, Engineering, and Medicine). 2017. *Application of systematic review methods in an overall strategy for evaluating low-dose toxicity from endocrine active chemicals.* Washington, DC: The National Academies Press.

Nelson, C., N. Lurie, and J. Wasserman. 2007a. Assessing public health emergency preparedness: Concepts, tools, and challenges. *Annual Review of Public Health* 28(1):1–18.

Nelson, C., N. Lurie, J. Wasserman, and S. Zakowski. 2007b. Conceptualizing and defining public health emergency preparedness. *American Journal of Public Health* 97:S9–S11.

Norris, S. L., E. A. Rehfuess, H. Smith, Ö. Tunçalp, J. M. Grimshaw, N. P. Ford, and A. Portela. 2019. Complex health interventions in complex systems: Improving the process and methods for evidence-informed health decisions. *BMJ Global Health* 4(Suppl 1).

Noyes, J., A. Booth, K. Flemming, R. Garside, A. Harden, S. Lewin, T. Pantoja, K. Hannes, M. Cargo, and J. Thomas. 2018. Cochrane Qualitative and Implementation Methods Group guidance series-paper 3: Methods for assessing methodological limitations, data extraction and synthesis, and confidence in synthesized qualitative findings. *Journal of Clinical Epidemiology* 97:49–58.

Noyes, J., A. Booth, G. Moore, K. Flemming, Ö. Tunçalp, and E. Shakibazadeh. 2019. Synthesising quantitative and qualitative evidence to inform guidelines on complex interventions: Clarifying the purposes, designs and outlining some methods. *BMJ Global Health* 4(Suppl 1).

NTSB (National Transportation Safety Board). 2020. *About the National Transportation Safety Board.* https://www.ntsb.gov/about/Pages/default.aspx (accessed May 23, 2020).

Pawson, R., T. Greenhalgh, G. Harvey, and K. Walshe. 2005. Realist review: A new method of systematic review designed for complex policy interventions. *Journal of Health Services Research and Policy* 10(Suppl 1):21–34.

Petticrew, M. 2015. Time to rethink the systematic review catechism? Moving from "what works" to "what happens." *Systematic Reviews* 4:36.

Petticrew, M., L. Anderson, R. Elder, J. Grimshaw, D. Hopkins, R. Hahn, L. Krause, E. Kristjansson, S. Mercer, T. Sipe, P. Tugwell, E. Ueffing, E. Waters, and V. Welch. 2013a. Complex interventions and their implications for systematic reviews: A pragmatic approach. *Journal of Clinical Epidemiology* 66(11):1209–1214.

Petticrew, M., E. Rehfuess, J. Noyes, J. P. T. Higgins, A. Mayhew, T. Pantoja, I. Shemilt, and A. Sowden. 2013b. Synthesizing evidence on complex interventions: How meta-analytical, qualitative, and mixed-method approaches can contribute. *Journal of Clinical Epidemiology* 66(11):1230–1243.

Petticrew, M., C. Knai, J. Thomas, E. A. Rehfuess, J. Noyes, A. Gerhardus, J. M. Grimshaw, H. Rutter, and E. McGill. 2019. Implications of a complexity perspective for systematic reviews and guideline development in health decision making. *BMJ Global Health* 4(Suppl 1).

Phillips, C. V., and K. J. Goodman. 2004. The missed lessons of Sir Austin Bradford Hill. *Epidemiologic Perspectives and Innovations* 1(1):3.

Pope, C., S. Ziebland, and N. Mays. 2000. Qualitative research in health care: Analysing qualitative data. *BMJ Clinical Research Edition* 320(7227):114–116.

Rehfuess, E. A., and E. A. Akl. 2013. Current experience with applying the GRADE approach to public health interventions: An empirical study. *BMC Public Health* 13:9.

Rehfuess, E. A., J. M. Stratil, I. B. Scheel, A. Portela, S. L. Norris, and R. Baltussen. 2019. The WHO-INTEGRATE evidence to decision framework version 1.0: Integrating WHO norms and values and a complexity perspective. *BMJ Global Health* 4(Suppl 1).

Richard, C., K. Magee, P. Bacon-Abdelmoteleb, and J. Brown. 2018. *Countermeasures that work: A highway safety countermeasure guide for state highway safety offices.* 9th ed. Washington, DC: National Highway Traffic Safety Administration.

Rohwer, A., L. Pfadenhauer, J. Burns, L. Brereton, A. Gerhardus, A. Booth, W. Oortwijn, and E. Rehfuess. 2017. Clinical epidemiology in South Africa, paper 3: Logic models help make sense of complexity in systematic reviews and health technology assessments. *Journal of Clinical Epidemiology* 83:37–47.

Rooney, A. A., A. L. Boyles, M. S. Wolfe, J. R. Bucher, and K. A. Thayer. 2014. Systematic review and evidence integration for literature-based environmental health science assessments. *Environmental Health Perspectives* 122(7):711–718.

Savoia, E., F. Agboola, and P. D. Biddinger. 2012. Use of after action reports (AARs) to promote organizational and systems learning in emergency preparedness. *International Journal of Environmental Research and Public Health* 9(8):2949–2963.

Schünemann, H. J., S. R. Hill, M. Kakad, G. E. Vist, R. Bellamy, L. Stockman, T. F. Wisloff, C. Del Mar, F. Hayden, T. M. Uyeki, J. Farrar, Y. Yazdanpanah, H. Zucker, J. Beigel, T. Chotpitayasunondh, T. T. Hien, B. Ozbay, N. Sugaya, and A. D. Oxman. 2007. Transparent development of the WHO rapid advice guidelines. *PLOS Medicine* 4(5):e119.

Schünemann, H., J. Brožek, G. Guyatt , and A. Oxman. 2013. *GRADE handbook.* GRADE Working Group. https://gdt.gradepro.org/app/handbook/handbook.html (accessed March 4, 2020).

Schünemann, H. J., C. Cuello, E. A. Akl, R. A. Mustafa, J. J. Meerpohl, K. Thayer, R. L. Morgan, G. Gartlehner, R. Kunz, S. V. Katikireddi, J. Sterne, J. P. Higgins, G. Guyatt, and GRADE Working Group. 2018. GRADE guidelines: 18. How ROBINS-I and other tools to assess risk of bias in nonrandomized studies should be used to rate the certainty of a body of evidence. *Journal of Clinical Epidemiology* 111:105–114.

Schünemann, H. J., Y. Zhang, A. D. Oxman, and Expert Evidence in Guidelines Group. 2019. Distinguishing opinion from evidence in guidelines. *BMJ* 366:l4606.

Siegfried, A. L., E. G. Carbone, M. B. Meit, M. J. Kennedy, H. Yusuf, and E. B. Kahn. 2017. Identifying and prioritizing information needs and research priorities of public health emergency preparedness and response practitioners. *Disaster Medicine and Public Health Preparedness* 11(5):552–561.

Sterne, J. A., M. A. Hernan, B. C. Reeves, J. Savovic, N. D. Berkman, M. Viswanathan, D. Henry, D. G. Altman, M. T. Ansari, I. Boutron, J. R. Carpenter, A. W. Chan, R. Churchill, J. J. Deeks, A. Hrobjartsson, J. Kirkham, P. Juni, Y. K. Loke, T. D. Pigott, C. R. Ramsay, D. Regidor, H. R. Rothstein, L. Sandhu, P. L. Santaguida, H. J. Schünemann, B. Shea, I. Shrier, P. Tugwell, L. Turner, J. C. Valentine, H. Waddington, E. Waters, G. A. Wells, P. F. Whiting, and J. P. Higgins. 2016. ROBINS-I: A tool for assessing risk of bias in non-randomised studies of interventions. *BMJ* 355:i4919.

Sterne, J. A., J. Savović, M. J. Page, R. G. Elbers, N. S. Blencowe, I. Boutron, C. J. Cates, H. Y. Cheng, M. S. Corbett, S. M. Eldridge, J. R. Emberson, M. A. Hernán, S. Hopewell, A. Hróbjartsson, D. R. Junqueira, P. Jüni, J. J. Kirkham, T. Lasserson, T. Li, A. McAleenan, B. C. Reeves, S. Shepperd, I. Shrier, L. A. Stewart, K. Tilling, I. R. White, P. F. Whiting, and J. P. Higgins. 2019. RoB 2: A revised tool for assessing risk of bias in randomised trials. *BMJ* 366:l4898.

Teutsch, S. M., L. A. Bradley, G. E. Palomaki, J. E. Haddow, M. Piper, N. Calonge, W. D. Dotson, M. P. Douglas, A. O. Berg, and EGAPP Working Group. 2009. The evaluation of genomic applications in practice and prevention (EGAPP) initiative: Methods of the EGAPP working group. *Genetics in Medicine* 11(1):3–14.

The Community Guide. 2012. *Emergency preparedness and response: School dismissals to reduce transmission of pandemic influenza: Summary evidence tables—economic review.* https://www.thecommunityguide.org/sites/default/files/assets/SET-schooldismissals-econ.pdf (accessed March 4, 2020).

Thomas, J., and A. Harden. 2008. Methods for the thematic synthesis of qualitative research in systematic reviews. *BMC Medical Research Methodology* 8:45.

Tracy, S. J. 2018. A phronetic iterative approach to data analysis in qualitative research. *Semantic Scholar* 19(2):61–76. https://pdfs.semanticscholar.org/e6b9/48c979223e21c695003636d2b73ed8a692dc.pdf?_ga=2.166166476.1259835723.1583341124-540380720.1583341124 (accessed March 4, 2020).

Truman, B. I., C. K. Smith-Akin, A. R. Hinman, K. M. Gebbie, R. C. Brownson, L. F. Novick, R. Lawrence, M. Pappaioanou, J. E. Fielding, C. Evans, F. A. Guerra, M. Vogel-Taylor, C. Mahan, M. Fullilove, S. Zaza, and The Task Force on Community Preventive Services. 2000. Developing the guide to community preventive services: Overview and rationale. *American Journal of Preventive Medicine* 18:18–26.

Tyndall, J. 2010. *AACODS checklist.* https://dspace.flinders.edu.au/xmlui/bitstream/handle/2328/3326/AACODS_Checklist.pdf (accessed March 4, 2020).

Umscheid, C. A., R. K. Agarwal, and P. J. Brennan. 2010. Updating the guideline development methodology of the healthcare infection control practices advisory committee (HICPAC). *American Journal of Infection Control* 38(4):264–273.

USPSTF (U.S. Preventive Services Task Force). 2015. *U.S. Preventive Services Task Force procedure manual.* https://www.uspreventiveservicestaskforce.org/Page/Name/procedure-manual (accessed March 4, 2020).

USPSTF. 2016. *Use of decision models in the development of evidence-based clinical preventive services recommendations.* https://www.uspreventiveservicestaskforce.org/Page/Name/use-of-decision-models-in-the-development-of-evidence-based-clinical-preventive-services-recommendations (accessed February 15, 2020).

Walshe, K. 2007. Understanding what works—and why—in quality improvement: The need for theory-driven evaluation. *International Journal for Quality in Health Care* 19(2):57–59.

Ward, K., K. J. Hoare, and M. Gott. 2015. Evolving from a positivist to constructionist epistemology while using grounded theory: Reflections of a novice researcher. *Journal of Research in Nursing* 20(6):449–462.

Waters, E., B. J. Hall, R. Armstrong, J. Doyle, T. L. Pettman, and A. de Silva-Sanigorski. 2011. Essential components of public health evidence reviews: Capturing intervention complexity, implementation, economics and equity. *Journal of Public Health* 33(3):462–465.

Welch, V. A., E. A. Akl, K. Pottie, M. T. Ansari, M. Briel, R. Christensen, A. Dans, L. Dans, J. Eslava-Schmalbach, G. Guyatt, M. Hultcrantz, J. Jull, S. V. Katikireddi, E. Lang, E. Matovinovic, J. J. Meerpohl, R. L. Morton, A. Mosdol, M. H. Murad, J. Petkovic, H. Schünemann, R. Sharaf, B. Shea, J. A. Singh, I. Solà, R. Stanev, A. Stein, L. Thabaneii, T. Tonia, M. Tristan, S. Vitols, J. Watine, and P. Tugwellan. 2017. GRADE equity guidelines 3: Considering health equity in GRADE guideline development: Rating the certainty of synthesized evidence. *Journal of Clinical Epidemiology* 90:76–83.

WHO (World Health Organization). 2015. *Ethics in epidemics, emergencies and disasters: Research, surveillance and patient care.* Geneva, Switzerland: World Health Organization.

WHO. 2018. *Communicating risk in public health emergencies: A WHO guideline for emergency risk communication (ERC) policy and practice.* Geneva, Switzerland: World Health Organization.

Wong, G., T. Greenhalgh, G. Westhorp, J. Buckingham, and R. Pawson. 2013. RAMESES publication standards: Realist syntheses. *BMC Medicine* 11:21.

WWC (What Works Clearinghouse). 2017a. *Procedures handbook: Version 4.0.* https://ies.ed.gov/ncee/wwc/Docs/referenceresources/wwc_procedures_handbook_v4.pdf (accessed March 4, 2020).

WWC. 2017b. *Standards handbook: Version 4.0.* https://ies.ed.gov/ncee/wwc/Docs/referenceresources/wwc_standards_handbook_v4.pdf (accessed March 4, 2020).

WWC. 2020. *Standards handbook: Version 4.1.* https://ies.ed.gov/ncee/wwc/Docs/referenceresources/WWC-Standards-Handbook-v4-1-508.pdf (accessed March 4, 2020).

Zaza, S., R. S. Lawrence, C. S. Mahan, M. Fullilove, D. Fleming, G. J. Isham, and M. Pappaioanou. 2000a. Scope and organization of the Guide to Community Preventive Services: The task force on community preventive services. *American Journal of Preventive Medicine* 18(1 Suppl):27–34.

Zaza, S., L. K. Wright-De Aguero, P. A. Briss, B. I. Truman, D. P. Hopkins, M. H. Hennessy, D. M. Sosin, L. Andersin, V. G. Carande-Kulis, S. M. Teutsch, M. Pappaioanou, and Task Force on Community Preventive Services. 2000b. Data collection instrument and procedure for systematic reviews in the guide to community preventive services. *American Journal of Preventive Medicine* 18(1S):44–74.

Engaging with and Training Community-Based Partners to Improve the Outcomes of At-Risk Populations

Engaging and training community-based partners (CBPs) serving at-risk populations is recommended as part of state, local, tribal, and territorial (SLTT) public health agencies' community preparedness efforts so that those CBPs are better able to assist at-risk populations they serve in preparing for and recovering from public health emergencies.

4

Finding Statements and Certainty of the Evidence

●●●● High ●●● Moderate ●● Low ● Very Low

Finding Statement	**Certainty**
Culturally tailored preparedness training programs improve public health emergency preparedness and response (PHEPR) knowledge of CBP representatives	●●
Culturally tailored preparedness training programs improve attitudes and beliefs of CBP representatives regarding their preparedness to meet needs of at-risk individuals	●
Culturally tailored preparedness training programs increase CBP disaster planning	●
Culturally tailored preparedness training programs improve the PHEPR knowledge of trained at-risk populations	●●●
Culturally tailored preparedness training programs improve attitudes and beliefs of trained at-risk populations regarding their preparedness	●●
Culturally tailored preparedness training programs improve preparedness behaviors of trained at-risk populations	●●●
CBP engagement in preparedness outreach activities improves the attitudes and beliefs of at-risk populations toward preparedness behaviors	●
CBP engagement and training in coalitions addressing public health preparedness/resilience increases the diversity of coalitions, the coordination of CBPs with other response partners, or capacity to reach and educate at-risk populations before an emergency	●

Recommended CBP training strategies include

- » the use of materials, curricula, and training formats targeted and/or tailored to the individual CBPs and the at-risk populations they serve
- » train-the-trainer approaches that utilize peer or other trusted trainers to train at-risk populations

CBP engagement and training should be accompanied by targeted monitoring and outcome evaluation or conducted in the context of research when feasible so as to improve the evidence base for engagement and training strategies.

Implementation Guidance

- ☑ Ensure that CBP engagement efforts feature a clearly articulated purpose and goals, a shared language, an acceptable power balance, and a sense of shared ownership
- ☑ Ensure that multistakeholder collaborations with CBPs are diverse and inclusive, with particular attention to those groups that are often excluded and marginalized
- ☑ Engage umbrella organizations (e.g., American Red Cross, United Way) to reach smaller, local, community-based organizations
- ☑ Consider participatory engagement strategies that allow for ongoing, bidirectional communication with CBPs to build trust and buy-in prior to an emergency
- ☑ Develop formal agreements to clarify the nature of membership roles and responsibilities in collaborations with CBPs
- ☑ Consider designating a coordinator to maintain the focus of coalitions, mitigate problems of competing priorities, and minimize perceptions of uneven power dynamics
- ☑ Identify information technology (e.g., resource databases) and existing data sources that can be used to facilitate more timely engagement of CBPs and to link at-risk populations with needed services during an emergency
- ☑ Tailor the curriculum and format of CBP preparedness training programs to the learning needs and preferences of specific audiences, and ensure that they are culturally sensitive and appropriate
- ☑ Consider soliciting stakeholder feedback in the evaluation of training program materials and content

Context Considerations

Setting

Settings reflected in this evidence review were primarily U.S. based and included a mix of rural and urban/suburban settings.

Population

At-risk populations reflected in this evidence review were multiple and included low-income minority populations, adults with disabilities, tribal populations, and rural populations.

CBPs reflected in this evidence review were multiple and included community health workers, tribal leaders, nongovernmental organizations serving adults with disabilities, faith-based organizations, and other community-based organizations.

Emergency Phase

Studies in this evidence review focused on CBP engagement and training during the preparedness phase. No studies focused on response-phase strategies.

DESCRIPTION OF THE PRACTICE

Defining the Practice

The committee examined the evidence for strategies used to engage with and train community-based partners (CBPs) to improve the outcomes of at-risk populations (defined in Box 4-1) who may be disproportionately affected by a public health emergency. The committee also examined the factors that may facilitate or act as barriers to CBP engagement and training (e.g., trust, organizational capacity). Engaging with and training CBPs to improve the outcomes of at-risk populations falls primarily under Capability 1: Community Preparedness (CP Capability) in the Centers for Disease Control and Prevention's (CDC's) *Public Health Emergency Preparedness and Response Capabilities: National Standards for State, Local, Tribal, and Territorial Public Health* (CDC PHEPR Capabilities) (CDC, 2018a). However, addressing the access and functional needs of at-risk individuals is a topic that cuts across the CDC PHEPR Capabilities (see Box 4-2).

For the purposes of this review, the committee defined CBPs to include those organizations and individuals that are representative of a community or a defined segment of a community and have established relationships with and/or serve at-risk populations. CBPs may include governmental (e.g., social services agencies) and nongovernmental (e.g., faith- and community-based organizations) entities, as well as individuals who represent or routinely work with populations that may be at increased risk of adverse outcomes during and following a public health emergency (e.g., community health workers and tribal leaders). This definition of CBPs distinguishes practices considered for this review from the broader class of community engagement practices that fall within the CP Capability and are aimed at improving community preparedness and resilience more generally. Practices aimed at directly engaging at-risk populations without the involvement of CBPs as an intermediary were outside the scope of this review.

In public health, the engagement and training of CBPs to better reach and improve outcomes for individuals with social vulnerabilities has much broader application beyond preparedness and response. For example, public health practitioners may seek to leverage relationships with trusted community-based organizations to improve childhood vaccination rates (Willis et al., 2016) or HIV management (Remien et al., 2015) in socially vulnerable groups. Although limitations of time and resources necessitated the committee's narrow focus on CBP engagement and training practices oriented specifically to public health emergency preparedness and response (PHEPR), the committee recognizes that this broader body of evidence from public health practice may have some applicability to the practices evaluated in this review.

Scope of the Problem Addressed by the Practice

The impacts of disasters and public health emergencies on health and well-being are not distributed equally across an affected population (HHS, 2011). Rather, the impacts are often felt disproportionately by groups with features that limit individuals' capability to respond or the effectiveness of such traditional response practices as evacuation or English-language messages (CDC, 2015). These at-risk populations are often those who are already the most vulnerable in a community and suffer from health and other disparities (Blumenshine et al., 2008). In the PHEPR context, social determinants of health (e.g., access to health care services, safe housing, and healthy food) can also be framed as social determinants of vulnerability (IOM, 2015). Such issues, which are often structural in nature, can be resolved only

BOX 4-1 DEFINING AT-RISK POPULATIONS

The Centers for Disease Control and Prevention's (CDC's) 2018 *Public Health Emergency Preparedness and Response Capabilities: National Standards for State, Local, Tribal, and Territorial Public Health* describes at-risk populations as "individuals with access and functional needs, such as needs related to communication, maintaining health, independence, support, safety, self-determination, and transportation (CMIST)" (CDC, 2018a, p. 3). However, the committee adopted a broader definition of at-risk populations, adapted from CDC's *Public Health Workbook to Define, Locate, and Reach Special, Vulnerable and At-Risk Populations in an Emergency,* that encompasses individuals with social and/or structural vulnerabilities whose access and functional needs may not be fully met by "traditional service providers or who feel they cannot comfortably or safely use the standard resources offered during preparedness, response, and recovery efforts" (CDC, 2018b, p. 4).

CDC has defined five broad categories that may inform the identification of at-risk populations, depending on the context of the emergency (individuals often may fall within more than one category):

- economic disadvantage,
- language and literacy,
- medical issues and disability (physical, mental, cognitive, or sensory),
- isolation (cultural, geographic, or social), and
- age.

Examples of at-risk populations include individuals who

- "Are at higher risk of severe complications from infectious diseases, such as pandemic influenza, for example, older adults, pregnant women, children, and people with pre-existing chronic medical conditions, such as diabetes or heart disease
- Have limitations that interfere with the receipt of and response to information, such as individuals who may not be able to hear, see, understand, or act on safety information
- Rely on personal care assistance to manage or maintain health
- Function independently if they have durable medical equipment or other assistive devices, service animals, or personal assistance service providers
- Find it difficult to cope in a new environment, such as those with autism, dementia, or intense anxiety
- Have transportation needs, including those who use public transit or accessible vehicles, such as lift-equipped or vehicles suitable for transporting individuals who use oxygen tanks" (CDC, 2018a, pp. 20–21).

While these categories can guide the identification of at-risk populations, the populations that will be at risk for any given public health emergency are defined in part by the nature of the hazard and environmental conditions (both physical and socioeconomic). Thus, at-risk populations may be defined by both structural and emergent properties. Moreover, one must take care when drawing conclusions about the effectiveness of practices targeting at-risk groups because not everyone in a given demographic group is equally at risk.

The term "at-risk population" is used in this review for consistency with the terminology used in CDC's 2018 *Public Health Emergency Preparedness and Response Capabilities: National Standards for State, Local, Tribal, and Territorial Public Health* (CDC, 2018a). However, a number of terms are also used by other sources, including "vulnerable," "marginalized," "underresourced," and "underserved," as alternatives to "at-risk." Given that some terms may unintentionally promote stigmatization of certain communities, consulting partners in the appropriate use of acceptable terminology is important to minimize the risk of "othering" members of the community and/or overlooking their strengths.

BOX 4-2 HOW ENGAGING WITH AND TRAINING COMMUNITY-BASED PARTNERS TO IMPROVE THE OUTCOMES OF AT-RISK POPULATIONS RELATES TO THE CENTERS FOR DISEASE CONTROL AND PREVENTION'S PHEPR CAPABILITIES

Capability 1: Community Preparedness—emphasizes the need for processes to identify at-risk populations that may be disproportionately impacted by public health emergencies and the need for collaborations with community partners to assess and plan for the access and functional needs of those populations. It also promotes training and education of community partners and stakeholders to support preparedness and recovery for at-risk populations.

Capability 2: Community Recovery—the transition between response and recovery is rarely well defined, and in both phases community-based partners (CBPs) can provide critical services to mitigate the effects of public health emergencies on at-risk populations and to assist with their recovery. Partnerships established with CBPs during the preparedness phase may be leveraged during recovery to coordinate services, identify and address gaps, and ensure that at-risk populations are integrated into community recovery planning efforts.

Capability 3: Emergency Operations Coordination—includes the ability to coordinate with emergency management, internal public health stakeholders, and external CBPs and to direct and support the response to an incident or event with public health or health care implications. Central to this Capability are identifying and sharing knowledge about public health risks, hazards, threats, and vulnerabilities. In this function, CBPs are important to understanding the needs of at-risk populations and help coordinate emergency response.

Capability 4: Emergency Public Information and Warning—includes practices to reach at-risk populations with public health messages during an emergency. There is growing recognition of the need to leverage trusted messengers when communicating risks and guidance to at-risk populations.

Capability 6: Information Sharing—refers to the effective interagency exchange of health-related information and situational awareness among different government agencies and other partners. CBPs offer vital avenues to and from at-risk populations that are necessary to conduct health-related information exchange and to gather situational awareness data.

SOURCE: CDC, 2018a.

through a substantial commitment to reducing the conditions that contribute to increased risk of adverse outcomes, so that the response of a community can be more effective when an emergency rises. Hurricane Katrina and its effects on at-risk populations served as a wake-up call for the need to prioritize and invest in preparedness for these populations and communities (Gibson and Hayunga, 2006; HHS, 2011; Turner et al., 2010; Wells et al., 2013). Failure to attend adequately to the needs of these populations before an emergency occurs risks exacerbating the underlying conditions that contribute to disparities in outcomes.

The challenges faced by at-risk populations may intersect and magnify each other. For example, ethnic communities with limited English proficiency may have difficulty receiving public health messages and may be distrustful of the government agencies disseminating them, or may have fewer resources for response actions, such as evacuation (Messias et al., 2012). This pernicious combination of factors was evident during the 2017 California wildfires, when it took several days to get appropriately translated risk messages to migrant farmworkers who continued working in the fields, often without proper respiratory protection, despite the hazardous conditions (NASEM, 2020). Moreover, the same family networks that may be supportive in one set of circumstances may make evacuation more challenging if elder members are difficult to move and strain the network's resources (Eisenman et al., 2007; Messias et al., 2012; Rowel et al., 2012). This example emphasizes the interconnectedness of populations such that when the needs of vulnerable populations are not adequately attended to, the risks to those who otherwise would not have been identified as at risk may be exacerbated. Consequently, focusing on meeting the needs of these populations before, during, and after a public health emergency has the potential to benefit the community writ large.

Integration of at-risk populations into emergency preparedness has been identified as a pressing need that requires more than recognizing that these populations will face particular challenges or including mention of them in preparedness plans; proactive planning for responses is needed (Edgington et al., 2014; Gibson and Hayunga, 2006; NCD, 2005). Hurricane Sandy demonstrated that socially, physically, and geographically vulnerable populations often have limited capacity to take protective action when facing acute adversity (Hernandez et al., 2018). Understanding and overcoming the barriers faced by such populations will necessitate their engagement in the development of response protocols. Failure to adequately meet the needs of at-risk populations following a disaster or public health emergency contributes to mistrust that may pose a barrier to their engagement and the engagement of CBPs that serve them in future events.

Historically, governmental preparedness programs, messages, and messengers have been best suited to mainstream audiences (Eisenman et al., 2009; Fothergill et al., 1999). Racially and ethnically diverse at-risk populations of low socioeconomic status may perceive government as unfair, and cultural and language factors may impede the uptake of institution-derived programs and messages (Andrulis et al., 2011; Eisenman et al., 2004, 2012). Furthermore, government entities themselves face institutional-level barriers to best serving at-risk populations, such as a lack of funds for at-risk and diversity initiatives, limited knowledge about diverse communities, and limited collaboration with communities and potential partners based therein (Bevc et al., 2014).

CBPs can be vital partners in reaching at-risk populations both before and after a public health emergency as they are often trusted agents familiar with and relied on by these populations for care and information during nonemergency situations (Eisenman et al., 2009; Gin et al., 2016). Existing networks with at-risk populations established for other purposes (e.g., focused on ensuring access to health and social services) can be useful in engaging these populations in preparedness efforts. Public health plays a key role in establishing and maintaining partnerships that promote community preparedness and response activities targeted at at-risk populations. However, little guidance is available on evidence-based strategies for developing and maintaining these partnerships or on the best approaches for related training for CBPs. PHEPR practitioners have expressed the need to better understand how best to implement partnerships and train CBPs in PHEPR (DHS, 2018).

OVERVIEW OF THE KEY REVIEW QUESTIONS AND ANALYTIC FRAMEWORK

Defining the Key Review Questions

The overarching review question that guided this review addresses the effectiveness of different strategies for engaging with and training CBPs to improve the outcomes of at-risk populations after public health emergencies. Engaging with CBPs to meet the needs of at-risk populations may take place in the preparedness, response, and recovery phases of the emergency cycle. Recovery practices were outside the committee's scope of work, but separate key review sub-questions were formulated for the preparedness and response phases. The committee also posed sub-questions related to documented benefits and harms of CBP engagement and training strategies and the factors that create barriers to and facilitators of implementation of such strategies (see Box 4-3).

Analytic Framework

For the purposes of this review, the committee developed an analytic framework to present the causal pathway and interactions between CBP engagement and training approaches and outcomes of interest (see Figure 4-1). The theory behind the practice is that when public health agencies adequately engage with and train CBPs who have established relationships with and/or serve at-risk populations to impart preparedness and response knowledge and concepts, the result is increased capacity to reach these populations before and during a public health emergency, and thus the potential to reduce disaster-associated morbidity and mortality and ameliorate health disparities.

Engaging and training CBPs may improve the outcomes of at-risk populations following a public health emergency through a number of presumed pathways. Such pathways generally focus on ensuring at-risk individuals' postdisaster access to critical services and/or resources (e.g., food, medication, information). CBP intermediaries may provide needed services and resources directly or may assist public health agencies (or other emergency responders) in reaching at-risk populations to deliver these services and resources before or after an emergency (e.g., by enabling access through their venues or by passing along information on how to access services and resources). CBPs also can be well positioned to help ensure the cultural appropriateness of preparedness and response materials, services, and training so they are functionally accessible (e.g., available in different languages for non-English-speaking individuals) and likely to be well received (Andrulis et al., 2011).

BOX 4-3 KEY REVIEW QUESTIONS

What is the effectiveness of different strategies for engaging with and training community-based partners (CBPs) to improve the outcomes of at-risk populations after public health emergencies?

- What is the effectiveness of strategies for engaging with and training CBPs before a public health emergency?
- What is the effectiveness of strategies for engaging with and leveraging existing CBPs during a public health emergency?
- What benefits and harms (desirable and/or undesirable impacts) of different strategies for engaging with and training community-based partners have been described or measured?
- What are the barriers to and facilitators of effective engagement and training of CBPs?

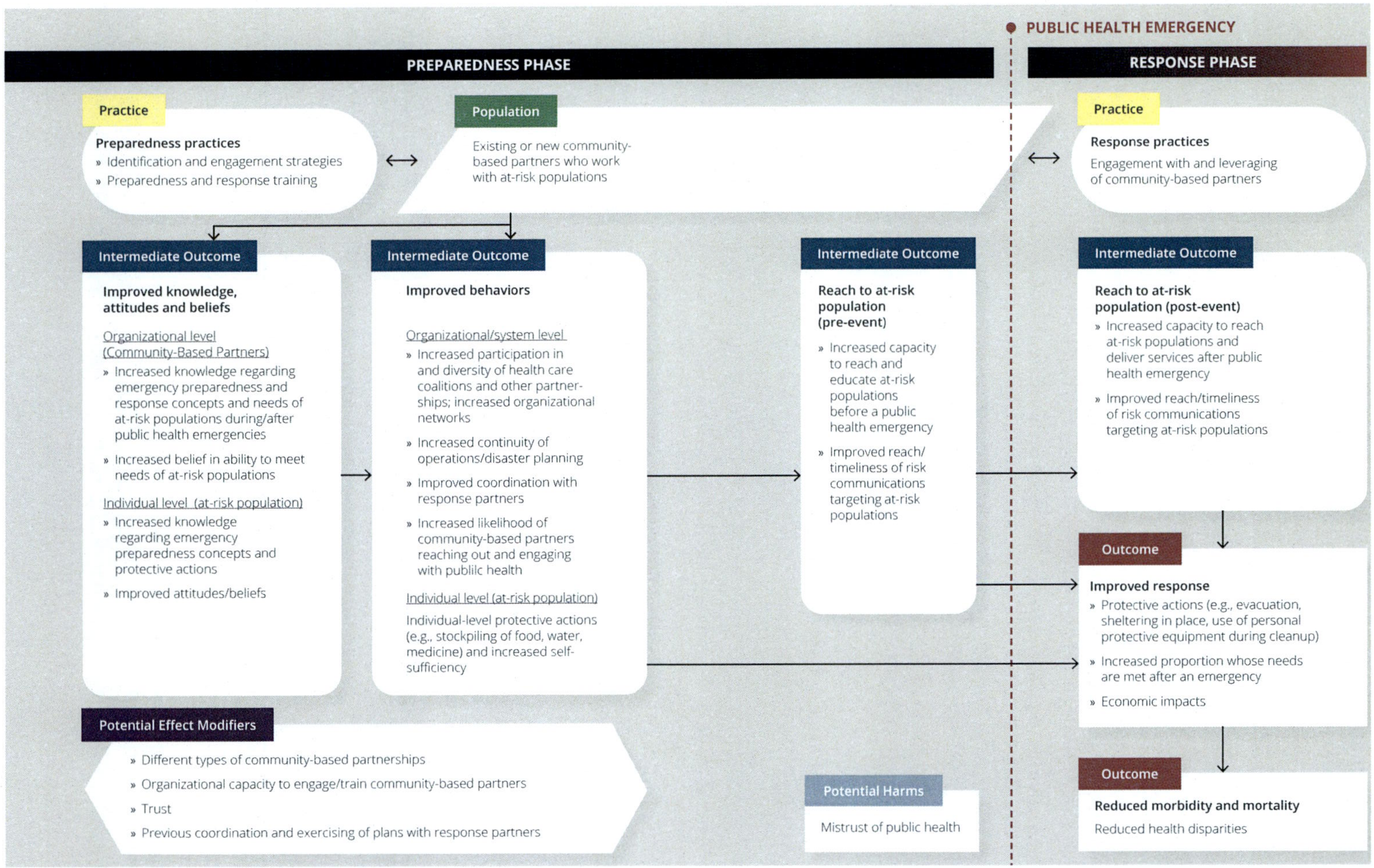

FIGURE 4-1 Analytic framework for engaging with and training community-based partners to improve the outcomes of at-risk populations.
NOTES: Arrows in the framework indicate hypothesized causal pathways between interventions and outcomes. Double-headed arrows indicate feedback loops.

Training CBPs may help better prepare them to mitigate the effects of public health emergencies on at-risk populations. The objectives of such training may include the following:

- Improving the knowledge of CBP employees and volunteers with respect to disaster risks (to themselves, their organizations, and the at-risk populations they serve) and preparedness approaches. Such training may help ensure continuity of operations and educate CBPs in providing critical services, resources, and information to at-risk populations after a public health emergency.
- Developing collaborations, engaging in constructive interactions, and coordinating efforts with governmental and other response partners in advance of public health emergencies. Preexisting relationships between CBPs and other response partners may facilitate meeting the needs of at-risk populations (e.g., access to culturally and linguistically appropriate risk messages, as well as resources and critical services).
- Educating CBPs in how to train members of at-risk populations so they are better prepared to meet their own needs during and after a public health emergency or to obtain assistance from their social networks. At-risk individuals may be more receptive to training on protective preparedness behaviors when it is delivered by trusted messengers, such as CBP representatives.

OVERVIEW OF THE EVIDENCE SUPPORTING THE PRACTICE RECOMMENDATION[1]

This section summarizes the evidence from the mixed-method review examining strategies for engaging with and training CBPs to improve the outcomes of at-risk populations. Following the summary of the evidence of effectiveness, summaries are presented for each element of the Evidence to Decision (EtD) framework (encompassing balance of benefits and harms, acceptability and preferences, feasibility and PHEPR system considerations, resource and economic considerations, equity, and ethical considerations), which the committee considered in formulating its practice recommendation. Full details on the review strategy and findings can be found in the appendixes: Appendix A provides a detailed description of the study eligibility criteria, search strategy, data extraction process, and individual study quality assessment criteria, Appendix B1 provides a full description of the evidence, including the literature search results, evidence profile tables, and EtD framework for engaging with and training CBPs to improve the outcomes of at-risk populations; and Appendix C links to all of the commissioned analyses that informed this review. Table 4-1 shows the types of evidence included in this review.

Effectiveness

Seven quantitative comparative and four quantitative noncomparative studies directly address the overarching key question regarding the effectiveness of different strategies for engaging with and training CBPs to improve the outcomes of at-risk populations after public health emergencies. (Refer to Section 1, "Determining Evidence of Effect," in Appendix B1 for additional detail.) All 11 studies describe strategies for engaging with or training CBPs *before* a public health emergency (preparedness phase); no quantitative research studies were found that address the effectiveness of strategies for engaging with and leveraging existing CBPs

[1] To enhance readability for an end user audience, this section does not include references. Citations supporting the findings in this section appear in Appendix B1.

TABLE 4-1 Evidence Types Included in the Mixed-Method Review of Strategies for Engaging with and Training Community-Based Partners to Improve the Outcomes of At-Risk Populations

Evidence Type[a]	Number of Studies (as applicable)[b]
Quantitative comparative	7
Quantitative noncomparative (postintervention measure only)[c]	4
Qualitative	23
Modeling	0
Descriptive surveys	7
Case reports	15[d]
After action reports	N/A
Mechanistic	N/A
Parallel (systematic reviews)[e]	13

[a] Evidence types are defined in Chapter 3.
[b] Note that sibling articles (different results from the same study published in separate articles) are counted as one study in this table. Mixed-method studies may be counted in more than one category.
[c] Quantitative noncomparative studies were considered separately for the purpose of evaluating evidence of effect but were included in the synthesis of case reports (or qualitative evidence in the case of mixed-method studies) to identify themes relevant to the Evidence to Decision framework.
[d] A sample of case reports was prioritized for inclusion in this review based on relevance to the key questions, as described in Chapter 3.
[e] Parallel evidence for the purposes of this review was derived from existing systematic reviews of similar practices from outside the PHEPR context.

during a public health emergency (response phase strategies). Ten of these 11 studies evaluate strategies that involve both engaging and training CBPs.

Strategies identified by the committee in the body of evidence fall into two broad categories: (1) those aimed at training and/or engaging individual CBPs with a goal of reaching particular at-risk populations (training programs may be targeted solely to CBPs or may be aimed at training both CBPs and members of the at-risk populations they serve); and (2) those aimed at engaging multiple CBPs in a coalition or other multistakeholder partnership. From these two categories, three strategies for training and/or engaging CBPs were identified and evaluated separately:

- implementation of culturally tailored[2] preparedness training programs for CBPs and at-risk populations they serve,
- engagement of CBPs in preparedness outreach activities targeting at-risk populations, and
- engagement and training of CBPs in coalitions addressing public health preparedness/resilience.

Consistent with the methods described in Chapter 3, in making its final judgment on the evidence of effectiveness for strategies for engaging with and training CBPs to improve the outcomes of at-risk populations, the committee considered other types of evidence that could inform a determination of what works for whom and in which contexts, ultimately coming to

[2] The committee uses the term "culturally tailored" to describe an intervention that is targeted and/or tailored to ensure that it meets the unique needs of the target group by incorporating its experiences and norms and values.

consensus on the certainty of the evidence (COE) for each outcome. Including other forms of evidence beyond quantitative comparative studies is particularly important when assessing evidence in settings where controlled studies are challenging to conduct and/or other forms of quantitative comparative data are difficult to obtain. Descriptive evidence from real-world implementation of practices offers the potential to corroborate research findings or explain differences in outcomes in practice settings, even if it has less value for causal inference. Moreover, qualitative studies can complement quantitative studies by providing additional useful evidence to guide real-world decision making, because well-conducted qualitative studies produce deep and rich understandings of how interventions are implemented, delivered, and experienced. Other forms of evidence considered for evaluation of effectiveness included findings from quantitative data reported in case reports that involved a real disaster or public health emergency, and parallel evidence from systematic reviews on community engagement and cultural tailoring of interventions outside the PHEPR context. The parallel evidence was considered recognizing that the engagement and training of CBPs to better reach and improve outcomes for individuals with social vulnerabilities has much broader application in public health beyond the PHEPR context, and the committee believed that this broader body of evidence may have some applicability to the PHEPR activities evaluated in this review.

Implementation of Culturally Tailored Preparedness Training Programs for CBPs and At-Risk Populations They Serve

The evidence suggests that culturally tailored preparedness training may be effective in improving outcomes for at-risk populations following a public health emergency, although there is little evidence linking preparedness phase outcomes (e.g., improved knowledge and preparedness behaviors) with health and other outcomes after an event. There is low COE based on three quantitative studies that culturally tailored preparedness training programs for CBPs and at-risk populations they serve improve the PHEPR knowledge of trained CBP representatives, and one quantitative study yielded very low COE that such training improves the attitudes and beliefs of CBP representatives regarding their preparedness to meet the needs of at-risk populations or increases their organizations' disaster planning.

When at-risk populations are trained by trained CBP representatives using a train-the-trainer model or at the same time as CBP representatives, there is moderate COE supported by four quantitative studies that culturally tailored preparedness training programs improve the PHEPR knowledge of those trained at-risk populations. Improved PHEPR knowledge may prompt trained at-risk individuals to engage in preparedness behaviors including stockpiling critical supplies and developing a family communication plan (moderate COE based on four quantitative studies). Three quantitative studies yielded low COE that culturally tailored preparedness training programs improve the preparedness attitudes and beliefs of trained at-risk populations. It should also be noted that, while these findings suggest that this training improves the preparedness of both CBPs and, in some cases, at-risk individuals, short follow-up periods were employed in these studies. Therefore, it is unclear how long these effects last and whether they translate to improved outcomes for at-risk populations following a public health emergency.

Engagement of CBPs in Preparedness Outreach Activities Targeting At-Risk Populations

The committee found limited evidence on the effects of engaging CBPs in preparedness outreach activities targeting at-risk populations. Based on a single quantitative study, there is very low COE that CBP engagement in preparedness outreach activities improves the attitudes and beliefs of at-risk populations toward preparedness behaviors. No impact data were identified for other relevant outcomes.

Engagement and Training of CBPs in Coalitions Addressing Public Health Preparedness/Resilience

The committee found limited evidence on the effects of engaging and training CBPs in coalitions addressing public health preparedness/resilience. There is very low COE based on a single quantitative study that CBP engagement and training in such coalitions increases the diversity of coalitions, the coordination of CBPs with other response partners, or capacity to reach and educate at-risk populations before an emergency.

Balance of Benefits and Harms

Engagement and training of CBPs in PHEPR can benefit communities in multiple ways, particularly when undertaken using a participatory approach and, in the context of multi-stakeholder collaborations, when inclusive of diverse membership. These benefits can be observed at the individual, organizational, and community and system levels.

At the individual level, engaging and training CBPs may increase reach to at-risk populations, many of which are traditionally underserved. This increased reach may yield opportunities to improve at-risk individuals' knowledge regarding risks from public health emergencies and potential mitigation strategies, which in turn may effect change in preparedness behaviors. Increased reach following a public health emergency may also ensure access of at-risk individuals to critical services. (Evidence source: synthesis of evidence of effect, qualitative evidence synthesis, case report evidence synthesis.)

At the organizational level, benefits of CBP engagement and training may include capacity building and enhanced CBP preparedness to meet the needs of at-risk populations following a public health emergency through increased PHEPR knowledge and integration of preparedness into CBP core services. (Evidence source: synthesis of evidence of effect, qualitative evidence synthesis, case report evidence synthesis.) In addition, public health agencies and CBPs may benefit from improved mutual awareness of existing community and organizational roles and capacities during routine times. This improved awareness provides the basis for leveraging and coordinating available services when an emergency event occurs, and also aids in identifying and developing strategies for covering gaps in needed services. (Evidence source: qualitative evidence synthesis, case report evidence synthesis.)

Benefits observed at the community and system level include new partnerships that enhance the inclusion of CBPs and promote a shared sense of ownership of community preparedness efforts. Relationship building may benefit routine operations, create opportunities for new collaborations, and facilitate coordination of partners during emergencies. Other community and system-level benefits include greater appreciation of varied community and cultural perspectives (cultural competence) and understanding of the needs and expectations of underserved populations, as well as opportunities for shared learning and enhanced trust in public health and other government agencies. (Evidence source: qualitative evidence synthesis, case report evidence synthesis.)

There are also a number of potential undesirable effects related to engagement and training of CBPs, including the potential to raise difficult and uncomfortable issues (e.g., implicit bias, marginalization), especially when trainers come from socially advantaged groups (e.g., based on race, education, or social status) and those being trained come from less advantaged groups. Additionally, people can become disenchanted with preparedness-focused collaborations when past collaborations have failed to achieve desired results or when members have had negative experiences (e.g., conflict, perceived power imbalance). Such disenchantment may impede future engagement efforts. There is also potential for disenchantment with preparedness training if there are no opportunities to apply it (in routine or emergency contexts). Finally, when collaborations cannot be sustained because of the often short-term nature of preparedness funding or shifting priorities, trust and confidence issues may be exacerbated. (Evidence source: qualitative evidence synthesis. Refer to Section 2, "Balance of Benefits and Harms," in Appendix B1 for additional detail.)

Acceptability and Preferences

CBPs generally value inclusion and shared ownership of community preparedness efforts and are willing to collaborate with public health agencies. Participatory approaches, leadership support, organizational commitment to CBP engagement and training, and transparency are likely to be important facilitators of acceptability. (Evidence source: qualitative evidence synthesis, case report evidence synthesis, evidence from descriptive surveys.)

Some public health departments may require an internal culture change to embrace and align with a community partnering approach. Reframing public health emergency preparedness activities to include a commitment to leveraging existing community health activities, along with a strong emphasis on health equity, can facilitate this organizational shift toward collaborative strategies and community preparedness. (Evidence source: case report evidence synthesis. Refer to Section 3, "Acceptability and Preferences," in Appendix B1 for additional detail.)

Feasibility and PHEPR System Considerations

Engaging and training CBPs to improve the outcomes of at-risk populations may be time and resource intensive, with intensity varying depending on the specific strategy. Capacity challenges (e.g., human and nonhuman resource limitations, policy impediments) and competing priorities, for both public health organizations and CBPs, are likely to be common barriers. Feasibility may be improved by working strategically to reduce capacity-related barriers through financial support and by leveraging opportunities to expand capacity, for example, through coordination. (Evidence source: qualitative evidence synthesis, case report evidence synthesis, evidence from descriptive surveys.)

Studies note legal issues regarding separation of church and state as a potential consideration when engaging faith-based organizations. Guidelines in accordance with the U.S. and state constitutions that include nondiscriminatory requirements, separation of public health services and religious activities, and no furthering of religious activities may be helpful in addressing this issue. (Evidence source: case report evidence synthesis. Refer to Section 4, "Feasibility and PHEPR System Considerations," in Appendix B1 for additional detail.)

Resource and Economic Considerations

Community preparedness efforts may be perceived as having to do more with no concomitant increase in resources. Framing preparedness efforts as an adaptation of existing activities rather than as additional services may reduce concerns regarding resource requirements. Many CBPs and public health agencies are already facing challenges in sustaining underfunded programs while dealing with high staff turnover, which may discourage engagement efforts and impede the ability of CBP representatives to attend trainings. Competing priorities for limited resources may necessitate prioritization of engagement and training initiatives (e.g., targeting specific at-risk groups based on local needs), but identifying opportunities to leverage existing resources and programs can help address financial constraints. Collaboration building and maintenance require a long-term investment. Such activities need to be undertaken with an understanding of the importance of longitudinal funding and appropriate outcome evaluations. Failure to sustain partnerships and lack of clear outcomes from engagement and training initiatives may contribute to disenchantment with preparedness-related engagement efforts. (Evidence source: qualitative evidence synthesis, case report evidence synthesis. Refer to Section 5, "Resource and Economic Considerations," in Appendix B1 for additional detail.)

Equity

Although none of the studies included in this review assess the potential effects on equity outcomes, engagement and training of CBPs is presumed to yield equity-related benefits by mitigating the often disproportionate effects of disasters on at-risk populations, many of which have been marginalized historically. The body of qualitative studies suggests that representation and meaningful participation in community preparedness efforts may help counteract feelings of being discounted and mitigate mistrust associated with government initiatives in some populations. In the absence of an inclusive approach to engagement and training, however, many CBPs will continue to be underrepresented, with continued marginalization of the at-risk populations with whom they work. Such models as community-based participatory research that promote two-way knowledge exchange, equal power in the development and evaluation of programs, and building of community capacity to apply findings may help promote equitable outcomes, mutual respect, and inclusive participation, but this is an important research gap. As discussed further in the section below on evidence gaps and future research priorities, equity outcomes need to be measured in future studies to better capture the opportunities to embrace a health equity framing and community asset approach to CBP engagement and preparedness training. Careful attention is needed to ensure that participants in CBP engagement and training efforts are representative of the populations intended to be served. (Evidence source: qualitative evidence synthesis, case report evidence synthesis. Refer to Section 6, "Equity," in Appendix B1 for additional detail.)

Ethical Considerations

The section above on equity notes several ways in which engaging communities, when done well, can promote the ethical principles of justice, or fairness, and equity. The earlier section on balancing benefits and harms also describes some ways in which poorly designed or implemented engagement efforts, even when intended to promote principles of transparency and accountability, can generate mistrust, frustration, or alienation. Overall, these observations suggest that engaging communities is ethically justified if it achieves harm reduction and/or benefit promotion for relevant stakeholders. Similarly, if engaging communities in preparedness activities is an efficient means of achieving better preparedness, it is supported by the principle of stewardship, which often is considered to be of special importance in public health emergencies, when resources can be very limited. Still, it is important to bear in mind that community engagement, like all human relationships, also can hold intrinsic value. That is, building open and trusting relationships is important because it reflects the value placed on respect for persons and communities. The principle of respect for persons and communities posits that one has a fundamental obligation to engage people in decisions that might affect their well-being and the well-being of those they care about, and this holds true even if doing so does not change ultimate decisions. (Evidence source: committee discussion drawing on key ethics and policy texts. Refer to Section 7, "Ethical Considerations," in Appendix B1 for additional detail.)

CONSIDERATIONS FOR IMPLEMENTATION

The following considerations for implementation are drawn from the committee's synthesis of evidence of effectiveness, the qualitative evidence synthesis, and the synthesis of case report evidence. The findings from these syntheses are presented in Appendix B1. Note that this is not an exhaustive list of considerations; additional implementation resources should be consulted before the practice recommendation is implemented.

Facilitators for CBP Engagement

The effectiveness of efforts to engage CBPs in preparedness and response to improve the outcomes of at-risk populations will likely be improved by a shared understanding and acceptance of the aims and operating aspects of the collaboration. Specifically, it is important to attend to clearly articulating a purpose and goals, adopting a shared language, bridging differences in decision-making processes, and ensuring that there are no unacceptable differentials in power. Participatory approaches are likely to enhance effectiveness by improving cultural appropriateness, building a sense of shared ownership, and enhancing CBP capacity. Additionally, multistakeholder collaborations are likely to be effective in reaching and improving the outcomes of at-risk populations when CBP membership is diverse and inclusive, with particular attention to those who are often excluded and marginalized and services that are aligned with the needs of the target audience. (Evidence source: qualitative evidence synthesis, case report evidence synthesis.)

Engaging umbrella organizations that often serve at-risk populations (e.g., American Red Cross, United Way) may serve to connect local public health agencies with smaller, local, community-based organizations to which these agencies would not otherwise have access. Attention will also be needed, however, to developing connections with populations that are not formally served by an agency or provider (e.g., by reaching out to neighborhood and grassroots groups, including faith-based organizations and limited-English-speaking communities). Strategies that allow for ongoing, bidirectional communication with CBPs may help build trust and buy-in prior to an emergency, which could then be leveraged to foster more effective engagement during an emergency. (Evidence source: case report evidence synthesis.)

Formal agreements may help clarify the nature of membership roles and responsibilities in collaborations, which in turn can aid in setting expectations and minimize conflicts over inequitable participation. It may be beneficial for such agreements to openly address how perceived barriers and harms from past experiences will be minimized. Important elements of such agreements include expectations for attendance, participation, and engagement; roles of individual members within the coalition; and organizational commitment. A designated coordinator may also help maintain the focus of a coalition, mitigate problems associated with competing priorities, and minimize perceptions of uneven power dynamics among the coalition members. Consideration is needed as well to the time commitment required for this role so as not to add responsibilities to an already overburdened employee. (Evidence source: qualitative evidence synthesis.)

One case report shows that leveraging information technology, such as a community-based resource database, may facilitate more timely engagement of CBPs and link at-risk populations with needed services during an emergency. Another suggests that data already being collected by agencies serving at-risk populations could be leveraged if stripped of any identifying or confidential information, although difficulties could be faced in achieving the necessary trust and buy-in from CBPs. (Evidence source: case report evidence synthesis. Refer to Section 8, "Facilitators for CBP Engagement," in Appendix B1 for additional detail.)

Facilitators for CBP Training

Preparedness trainings are more likely to be effective at recruiting, engaging, and educating CBPs when their curriculum and format are tailored to the learning needs and preferences of specific audiences and are culturally sensitive and appropriate. Soliciting stakeholder feedback in the development and evaluation of program materials and training content can help ensure the quality of materials and promote stakeholder buy-in. Highlighting the importance of personal preparedness and self-care during partner trainings may also help promote buy-in for their role as promoters of client preparedness and may enable providers to serve those in need more effectively. In implementing training programs for CBPs and at-risk populations they serve, the following are also important considerations:

- employing capable, credible, and trusted trainers;
- making training accessible through location (physical or virtual) and affordability;
- adjusting the length of any training session to accommodate learners' attention spans and availability of time;
- facilitating bidirectional discussion, interaction, and feedback loops in training activities; and
- evaluating training and facilitating opportunities for deliberate practice.

(Evidence source: synthesis of evidence of effectiveness, qualitative evidence synthesis, case report evidence synthesis. Refer to Section 9, "Facilitators for CBP Training," and Section 1, "Determining Evidence of Effect," in Appendix B1 for additional detail.)

PRACTICE RECOMMENDATION, JUSTIFICATION, AND IMPLEMENTATION GUIDANCE

Practice Recommendation

Engaging and training community-based partners (CBPs) serving at-risk populations is recommended as part of state, local, tribal, and territorial public health agencies' community preparedness efforts so that those CBPs are better able to assist at-risk populations they serve in preparing for and recovering from public health emergencies. Recommended CBP training strategies include

- the use of materials, curricula, and training formats targeted and/or tailored to the individual CBPs and the at-risk populations they serve; and
- train-the-trainer approaches that utilize peer or other trusted trainers to train at-risk populations.

continued

CBP engagement and training should be accompanied by targeted monitoring and outcome evaluation or conducted in the context of research when feasible so as to improve the evidence base for engagement and training strategies.

Justification for the Practice Recommendation

The practice recommendation is based on moderate certainty of the evidence (COE) that culturally tailored preparedness training programs for CBPs, when also used to train at-risk populations, improve the public health emergency preparedness and response (PHEPR) knowledge and protective preparedness behaviors of at-risk populations. There is low COE that culturally tailored preparedness training programs for CBPs and the at-risk populations they serve are effective in increasing CBP representatives' PHEPR-related knowledge and improving the attitudes and beliefs of trained at-risk populations regarding their preparedness.

The recommended training strategies were found to be beneficial in multiple different at-risk populations, strengthening the conclusion that the evidence is likely applicable to populations beyond those in which the strategies have been evaluated. However, the limited number of studies for each population indicates a need for additional research and evaluation. For example, only one study evaluates the effectiveness of strategies for engaging and training tribal community partners, and none of the studies were conducted in territorial settings.

Although there is insufficient evidence to recommend specific strategies for engaging CBPs in PHEPR outreach activities targeting at-risk populations or for engaging CBPs in community coalitions, the qualitative evidence suggests numerous benefits of CBP engagement in public health preparedness and response. CBPs appear to support and value engagement and training, particularly when implemented using a participatory approach, but capacity limitations for both CBPs and public health organizations should be considered when selecting specific strategies.

Implementation Guidance

Considerations for CBP Engagement

- Ensure that CBP engagement efforts feature a clearly articulated purpose and goals, a shared language, an acceptable power balance, and a sense of shared ownership.
- Ensure that multistakeholder collaborations with CBPs are diverse and inclusive, with particular attention to those groups that are often excluded and marginalized.
- Engage umbrella organizations (e.g., American Red Cross, United Way) to reach smaller, local, community-based organizations.
- Consider participatory engagement strategies that allow for ongoing, bidirectional communication with CBPs to build trust and buy-in prior to an emergency.
- Develop formal agreements to clarify the nature of membership roles and responsibilities in collaborations with CBPs.
- Consider designating a coordinator to maintain the focus of coalitions, mitigate problems of competing priorities, and minimize perceptions of uneven power dynamics.
- Identify information technology (e.g., resource databases) and existing data sources that can be used to facilitate more timely engagement of CBPs and to link at-risk populations with needed services during an emergency.

Considerations for CBP Training

- Tailor the curriculum and format of CBP preparedness training programs to the learning needs and preferences of specific audiences, and ensure that they are culturally sensitive and appropriate.
- Consider soliciting stakeholder feedback in the evaluation of training program materials and content.

EVIDENCE GAPS AND FUTURE RESEARCH PRIORITIES

None of the strategies for engaging with and training CBPs reviewed by the committee are supported by high COE. For strategies to engage CBPs in preparedness/resilience-focused coalitions or outreach activities targeting at-risk populations, there is very low COE regarding effectiveness, indicating a need for further research to expand the body of evidence on these CBP engagement and training strategies. The committee's commissioned qualitative evidence synthesis suggests a number of engagement and training approaches for which empirical data are limited (e.g., framing of preparedness efforts in terms of community resilience, use of virtual versus in-person training formats). Other novel strategies for leveraging CBPs to improve preparedness and postevent outcomes for at-risk populations that have not yet been rigorously evaluated through research studies include employing audience segmentation approaches (Adams et al., 2017), activating social networks, activating home health workers (Eisenman et al., 2014), working with pharmacists or the hospital discharge process to improve preparedness (e.g., with respect to medications) (Carameli et al., 2013), and using behavioral economic approaches.

The committee noted a number of limitations in the body of research it reviewed that need to be addressed in future research to advance the state of the science on CBP engagement and training strategies. The use of objective, validated measures, when feasible, and the collection of baseline data would mitigate concerns related to risk of bias and strengthen the conclusions that can be drawn regarding causal relationships between practices and outcomes. Particularly concerning is the absence of long-term outcomes from which conclusions can be drawn about the duration of the practice's effects. For example, evaluation of training effectiveness was almost always conducted immediately following the training, and it is unclear how long such knowledge is retained. Future research needs to include longer-term follow-up outcomes and, for training interventions, to evaluate the frequency of refresher training necessary to ensure that perishable knowledge is retained. As discussed earlier in this chapter, accomplishing this will require that funders acknowledge and support the need for long-term investments in research studies.

Another observed limitation of the existing body of research is the absence of evidence linking pre-event intermediate outcomes (e.g., posttraining knowledge, preparedness behaviors) to improved outcomes for at-risk populations after a public health emergency. Although this evidence gap is challenging to address through prospective research studies given uncertainty as to the location and timing of future emergencies, communities that have made investments in CBP engagement in preparedness activities and training need to consider how the effect of those investments can be rigorously evaluated in the event of a public health emergency.

While it is encouraging that engagement and training strategies have been evaluated for multiple types of CBPs (e.g., nongovernmental social services organizations, faith-based organizations, community health workers) that work with different types of at-risk populations (e.g., low-income minorities, adults with disabilities, tribal populations), the limited number of studies for each such population makes conclusions regarding the applicability of the evidence base premature. It will be important for future studies not only to replicate the findings of previous studies in the same populations, but also to consider other CBPs and at-risk populations not addressed in the current literature base.

There also are important knowledge gaps related to the implementation of CBP engagement and training strategies in real-world settings. For example, capacity limitations of CBPs are cited in the qualitative and case report literature as barriers to engagement and training. There also may be barriers to preparedness behaviors promoted in trainings targeting at-risk populations, such as insurance barriers to stockpiling extra medications (Carameli et al., 2013). Qualitative studies may inform strategies for overcoming such barriers that can then be tested and evaluated in order to translate research into practice. Simulations and tabletop exercises offer opportunities to identify gaps in partnerships with community organizations serving at-risk populations using real-world scenarios and to better prepare for real-time decision making in the midst of a public health emergency (Chandra et al., 2015; Paige et al., 2010). Simulations and exercises can also be incorporated into a larger research study as a means of evaluating improvements in partnerships and coordination over time as a result of an intervention focused on CBP engagement (Chandra et al., 2015). Pragmatic trial designs whereby whole communities can be randomized (discussed further in Chapter 8) are well suited to evaluating practices in real-world settings and are feasible to execute for preparedness phase interventions. For example, trials with a stepped-wedge design are increasingly used in the evaluation of community-level service delivery and policy interventions (Hemming et al., 2015). In this design, all clusters (e.g., communities) are initially observed in the control condition. In subsequent phases, some are randomly assigned to the intervention until finally all are observed in the intervention condition. While appropriate statistical methods are needed to adjust for the confounding effect of time, this design permits evaluation of each community under both experimental conditions, providing increased statistical power. Importantly, such trials allow for the kind of participatory approach that is valued by communities while meeting the need for robust evaluation, ideally moving the field away from weaker pre-post designs.

The COVID-19 pandemic that emerged in the course of the committee's work has provided yet another disturbing example of the disproportionate morbidity and mortality observed during and after public health emergencies in those populations that already face health disparities in everyday circumstances. While data are still being collected, early evidence suggests that ethnic and racial minority populations in particular are overrepresented in hospitalizations related to COVID-19 (CDC, 2020). While such disparities are certainly not unique to COVID-19, they underscore how the lack of evidence on equity-related outcomes observed in the committee's review represents a critical knowledge gap that future research should seek to address. Going forward, the application of critical race theory methods (Ford and Airhihenbuwa, 2010)—which are grounded in social justice—to the design and execution of research may increase understanding of racial and ethnic disparities associated with disasters and public health emergencies and opportunities to address them. The PROGRESS (place of residence, race/ethnicity/culture/language, occupation, gender/sex, religion, education, socioeconomic status, and social capital) framework is a tool that may facilitate the application of an equity lens to the conduct and reporting of research focused on improving outcomes for at-risk populations after disasters and public health emergencies (O'Neill et al., 2014). As additional research on interventions focused on improving outcomes for at-risk populations is published, it may be helpful to undertake future systematic reviews with an explicit equity focus (Welch et al., 2016).

The COVID-19 pandemic is also challenging some long-standing assumptions based on the more common geological and meteorological hazards that have been the focus of preparedness and response efforts. It has generally been held that the kinds of structural vulnerabilities that put populations at risk cannot be addressed in the midst of a public health emergency. However, a protracted emergency like the current pandemic may illuminate the conditions of vulnerability, such as lack of health insurance or inadequate job site protections, and may provide unique opportunities to address those conditions through, for example, legislation or programs targeting socioeconomic risk factors. It is conceivable that CBPs could be mediators of such efforts, and given the absence of studies identified for this review examining the effectiveness of interventions that leverage CBPs during a public health emergency, careful consideration of potential methods for measuring the impact of any such interventions that may be implemented in response to COVID-19 is warranted.

REFERENCES

References marked with an asterisk (*) are formally included in the mixed-method review. The full reference list of articles included in the mixed-method review can be found in Appendix B1.

Adams, R. M., B. Karlin, D. P. Eisenman, J. Blakley, and D. Glik. 2017. Who participates in the great shakeout? Why audience segmentation is the future of disaster preparedness campaigns. *International Journal of Environmental Research and Public Health* 14(11).

*Andrulis, D. P., N. J. Siddiqui, and J. P. Purtle. 2011. Integrating racially and ethnically diverse communities into planning for disasters: The California experience. *Disaster Medicine and Public Health Preparedness* 5(3):227–234.

*Bevc, C. A., M. C. Simon, T. A. Montoya, and J. A. Horney. 2014. Institutional facilitators and barriers to local public health preparedness planning for vulnerable and at-risk populations. *Public Health Reports* 129(Suppl 4):35–41.

Blumenshine, P., A. Reingold, S. Egerter, R. Mockenhaupt, P. Braveman, and J. Marks. 2008. Pandemic influenza planning in the United States from a health disparities perspective. *Emerging Infectious Diseases* 14(5):709–715.

Carameli, K. A., D. P. Eisenman, J. Blevins, B. d'Angona, and D. C. Glik. 2013. Planning for chronic disease medications in disaster: Perspectives from patients, physicians, pharmacists, and insurers. *Disaster Medicine and Public Health Preparedness* 7(3):257–265.

CDC (Centers for Disease Control and Prevention). 2015. *Planning for an emergency: Strategies for identifying and engaging at-risk groups: A guidance document for emergency managers.* https://www.cdc.gov/nceh/hsb/disaster/atriskguidance.pdf (accessed March 11, 2020).

CDC. 2018a. *Public health emergency preparedness and response capabilities: National standards for state, local, tribal, and territorial public health.* https://www.cdc.gov/cpr/readiness/00_docs/CDC_PreparednesResponseCapabilities_October2018_Final_508.pdf (accessed March 11, 2020).

CDC. 2018b. *Public health workbook—to define, locate, and reach special, vulnerable, and at-risk populations in an emergency.* https://emergency.cdc.gov/workbook/pdf/ph_workbookfinal.pdf (accessed March 11, 2020).

CDC. 2020. *Hospitalization rates and characteristics of patients hospitalized with laboratory-confirmed coronavirus disease 2019—COVID-NET, 14 states, March 1–30, 2020.* https://www.cdc.gov/mmwr/volumes/69/wr/mm6915e3.htm?s_cid=mm6915e3_w (accessed May 23, 2020).

Chandra, A., M. V. Williams, C. Lopez, J. Tang, D. Eisenman, and A. Magana. 2015. Developing a tabletop exercise to test community resilience: Lessons from the Los Angeles County Community Disaster Resilience Project. *Disaster Medicine and Public Health Preparedness* 9(5):484–488.

DHS (U.S. Department of Homeland Security). 2018. *Engaging faith-based and community organizations: Planning considerations for emergency managers.* https://www.fema.gov/media-library-data/1528736429875-8fa08bed9d957cdc324c2b7f6a92903b/Engaging_Faith-based_and_Community_Organizations.pdf (accessed March 11, 2020).

Edgington, S., D. Canavan, F. Ledger, and R. L. Ersing. 2014. *Integrating homeless service providers and clients in disaster preparedness, response, and recovery.* Silver Spring, MD: National Health Care for the Homeless Council.

Eisenman, D. P., C. Wold, C. Setodji, S. Hickey, B. Lee, B. D. Stein, and A. Long. 2004. Will public health's response to terrorism be fair? Racial/ethnic variations in perceived fairness during a bioterrorist event. *Biosecurity and Bioterrorism: Biodefense Strategy, Practice, and Science* 2(3).

Eisenman, D. P., K. M. Cordasco, S. Asch, J. F. Golden, and D. Glik. 2007. Disaster planning and risk communication with vulnerable communities: Lessons from Hurricane Katrina. *American Journal of Public Health* 97(Suppl 1):S109–S115.

Eisenman, D. P., D. Glik, R. Maranon, L. Gonzales, and S. Asch. 2009. Developing a disaster preparedness campaign targeting low-income Latino immigrants: Focus group results for project PREP. *Journal of Health Care for the Poor and Underserved* 20(2):330–345.

Eisenman, D. P., M. V. Williams, D. Glik, A. Long, A. L. Plough, and M. Ong. 2012. The public health disaster trust scale: Validation of a brief measure. *Journal of Public Health Management and Practice* 18(4):E11–E18.

*Eisenman, D. P., A. Bazzano, D. Koniak-Griffin, C. H. Tseng, M. A. Lewis, K. Lamb, and D. Lehrer. 2014. Peer-mentored preparedness (PM-PREP): A new disaster preparedness program for adults living independently in the community. *Intellectual and Developmental Disabilities* 52(1):49–59.

Ford, C. L., and C. O. Airhihenbuwa. 2010. Critical race theory, race equity, and public health: Toward antiracism praxis. *American Journal of Public Health* 100:S3–S35.

Fothergill, A., E. G. M. Maestas, and J. D. Darlington. 1999. Race, ethnicity and disasters in the United States: A review of the literature. *Disasters* 23(2):156–173.

Gibson, M. J., and M. Hayunga. 2006. *We can do better: Lessons learned for protecting older persons in disasters.* Washington, DC: AARP. https://assets.aarp.org/rgcenter/il/better.pdf (accessed March 11, 2020).

Gin, J. L., R. Saia, A. Dobalian, and D. Kranke. 2016. Disaster preparedness in homeless residential organizations in Los Angeles County: Identifying needs, assessing gaps. *Natural Hazards Review* 17(1).

Hemming, K., T. P. Haines, P. J. Chilton, A. J. Girling, and R. J. Lilford. 2015. The stepped wedge cluster randomised trial: Rationale, design, analysis, and reporting. *BMJ* 350:h391.

Hernandez, D., D. Chang, C. Hutchinson, E. Hill, A. Almonte, R. Burns, P. Shepard, I. Gonzalez, N. Reissig, and D. Evans. 2018. Public housing on the periphery: Vulnerable residents and depleted resilience reserves post-Hurricane Sandy. *Journal of Urban Health* 95(5):703–715.

HHS (U.S. Department of Health and Human Services). 2011. *Guidance for integrating culturally diverse communities into planning for and responding to emergencies: A toolkit: Recommendations of the national consensus panel on emergency preparedness and cultural diversity.* https://www.aha.org/system/files/content/11/OMHDiversityPreparednesToolkit.pdf (accessed March 11, 2020).

IOM (Institute of Medicine). 2015. *Healthy, resilient, and sustainable communities after disasters: Strategies, opportunities, and planning for recovery.* Washington, DC: The National Academies Press.

*Messias, D. K. H., C. Barrington, and E. Lacy. 2012. Latino social network dynamics and the Hurricane Katrina disaster. *Disasters* 36(1):101–121.

NASEM (National Academies of Sciences, Engineering, and Medicine). 2020. *Implications of the California wildfires for health, communities, and preparedness: Proceedings of a workshop.* Washington, DC: The National Academies Press.

NCD (National Council on Disability). 2005. *Saving lives: Including people with disabilites in emergency planning.* https://ncd.gov/rawmedia_repository/fd66f11a_8e9a_42e6_907f_a289e54e5f94.pdf (accessed March 11, 2020).

O'Neill, J., H. Tabish, V. Welch, M. Petticrew, K. Pottie, M. Clarke, T. Evans, J. Pardo Pardo, E. Waters, H. White, and P. Tugwell. 2014. Applying an equity lens to interventions: Using PROGRESS ensures consideration of socially stratifying factors to illuminate inequities in health. *Journal of Clinical Epidemiology* 67(1):56–64.

Paige, S., M. Jones, L. D'Ambrosio, W. Taylor, D. Bonne, M. Loehr, and A. Stergachis. 2010. Strengthening community partnerships with local public health through regional pandemic influenza exercises. *Public Health Reports* 125(3):488–493.

Remien, R. H., L. J. Bauman, J. E. Mantell, B. Tsoi, J. Lopez-Rios, R. Chhabra, A. DiCarlo, D. Watnick, A. Rivera, N. Teitelman, B. Cutler, and P. Warne. 2015. Barriers and facilitators to engagement of vulnerable populations in HIV primary care in New York City. *Journal of Acquired Immune Deficiency Syndromes* 69(Suppl 1):S16–S24.

*Rowel, R., P. Sheikhattari, T. M. Barber, and M. Evans-Holland. 2012. Introduction of a guide to enhance risk communication among low-income and minority populations: A grassroots community engagement approach. *Health Promotion Practice* 13(1):124–132.

Turner, D. S., W. A. Evans, M. Kumlachew, B. Wolshon, V. Dixit, V. P. Sisiopiku, S. Islam, and M. D. Anderson. 2010. Issues, practices, and needs for communicating evacuation information to vulnerable populations. *Transportation Research Record* 2196(1):159–167.

Welch, V., M. Petticrew, J. Petkovic, D. Moher, E. Waters, H. White, P. Tugwell and the PRISMA-Equity Bellagio group. 2016. Extending the PRISMA statement to equity-focused systematic reviews (PRISMA-E 2012): Explanation and elaboration. *Journal of Development Effectiveness* 8(2):287–324.

*Wells, K. B., B. F. Springgate, E. Lizaola, F. Jones, and A. Plough. 2013. Community engagement in disaster preparedness and recovery: A tale of two cities—Los Angeles and New Orleans. *Psychiatric Clinics of North America* 36(3):451–466.

Willis, E., S. Sabnis, C. Hamilton, F. Xiong, K. Coleman, M. Dellinger, M. Watts, R. Cox, J. Harrell, D. Smith, M. Nugent, and P. Simpson. 2016. Improving immunization rates through community-based participatory research: Community health improvement for Milwaukee's children program. *Progress in Community Health Partnerships* 10(1):19–30.

5

Activating a Public Health Emergency Operations Center

Activating a public health emergency operations center (PHEOC) is a common and standard practice, supported by national and international guidance and based on earlier social science around disaster response. Despite widespread use and minimal apparent harms, there is insufficient evidence to determine the effectiveness of activating a PHEOC or of specific PHEOC components at improving response. This does *not* mean that the practice does not work or should not be implemented, but that more research and monitoring and evaluation around how and in what circumstances a PHEOC should be implemented are warranted before an evidence-based practice recommendation can be made.

Justification for the Insufficient Evidence Statement

Partly because of its long tenure as a common and standard practice, direct research evidence does not focus on whether PHEOCs should be utilized, but rather how they should be implemented. Experiential evidence from a synthesis of case reports and after action reports (from within and outside of public health emergency preparedness and response [PHEPR]) suggests that PHEOCs are probably effective at improving response and may have few undesirable effects in the short term, and speaks to the confidence in the PHEOC model among experienced practitioners across diverse situations. PHEPR practitioners consider activating a PHEOC to be an acceptable and justifiable practice. The feasibility of this practice is variable, and the evidence highlights several feasibility issues to consider before a PHEOC is activated.

Implementation Guidance

Considerations for *when* to activate public health emergency operations

☑ **A public health emergency is large in size and complex in scope.** Such events are likely to exceed the capacity of existing resources and/or the capabilities of the agency

☑ **A novel response may require multiple new tasks or partnerships.** Err on the side of activating early to handle new tasks or partnerships that may emerge

☑ **An event occurs that requires public health support functions, large-scale information sharing, or response coordination.** Consider activating for planned events and environmental disasters with potential for public health implications

☑ **Resource, cost, technological, legal, and logistical constraints need to be overcome.** Resource needs change throughout an event and may entail moderate to large resources

☑ **An incident requires high levels of interagency partnership.** Even if a response is small, interagency coordination may require PHEOC activation

Considerations for *when to refrain* from activating public health emergency operations

☑ The cost of activating is higher than any potential resource needs for the event

☑ Leadership has minimum experience with PHEOC operations, and staff have minimum PHEOC training. Lack of prior activation experience or training could lead to interagency distrust and chain-of-command disruption

☑ Leadership prioritizes maintaining routine public health functions over response needs

Considerations for *how* to make the decision to activate public health emergency operations

☑ Respect staff knowledge, and involve staff with past emergency experience in leadership discussions

☑ Ensure strong leadership, even using leaders outside the regular hierarchy

☑ Provide support to address the social functioning of the PHEOC

☑ Resource common operating picture functions to increase shared understanding

☑ Encourage staff flexibility within the PHEOC

☑ Conduct just-in-time training to minimize disruptions caused by less-experienced staff

☑ Continuously monitor and evaluate response functions to ensure and prove utility

Context Considerations

Setting

Settings reflected in this evidence review were primarily U.S. based, at the state and local level, and included a mix of rural and urban and suburban settings.

Agency Activated

The agencies activated in this evidence review were public health, health care, or emergency management, and the activations were primarily multiagency activations. No studies examined emergency operations conducted by tribal or territorial public health agencies.

Emergency Phase

The evidence review included a mix of preparedness and response phase studies.

Emergency Type

Emergencies included a mix of real and simulated events and were diverse (all hazards, natural disasters, and infectious disease epidemic).

DESCRIPTION OF THE PRACTICE

Defining the Practice

The committee examined the evidence on the circumstances in which activating a public health emergency operations center (PHEOC) is appropriate. It also examined various aspects of public health emergency operations (e.g., how response changes following activation). For the purposes of this review, public health emergency operations is defined as the ability to coordinate, direct, and support response to an event with public health or health care implications by "establishing a standardized, scalable system of oversight, organization, and supervision that is consistent with jurisdictional standards and practices and the National Incident Management System (NIMS)" (CDC, 2018, p. 12). Public health emergency operations fall under Capability 3: Emergency Operations Coordination (EOC Capability) in the Centers for Disease Control and Prevention's (CDC's) *Public Health Emergency Preparedness and Response Capabilities: National Standards for State, Local, Tribal, and Territorial Public Health* (CDC PHEPR Capabilities). Activating a PHEOC allows for relevant public health expertise to be employed and resources to be used that would improve the efficiency and outcomes of a response relative to a response without public health involved. The EOC Capability is closely linked to other CDC PHEPR Capabilities (see Box 5-1).

BOX 5-1 HOW PUBLIC HEALTH EMERGENCY OPERATIONS RELATES TO THE CENTERS FOR DISEASE CONTROL AND PREVENTION'S PHEPR CAPABILITIES

Capability 1: Community Preparedness—successful public health emergency operations require engaging in preparedness activities, including the strengthening of community partnerships, to ensure that the access and functional needs of the whole community are met during and after an event.

Capability 3: Emergency Operations Coordination—is the ability to coordinate, direct, and support response to an event with public health or health care implications by establishing a standardized, scalable system of oversight, organization, and supervision.

Capability 6: Information Sharing—is the ability to exchange health-related information and situational awareness data among different levels of government agencies and other partners. This capability is important to establish a common operating picture, a necessary element of successful public health emergency operations.

Capability 13: Public Health Surveillance and Epidemiological Investigation—involves the ability to coordinate surveillance and epidemiological activities with jurisdictional laboratories, partners, and stakeholders who can provide data to potentially activate public health emergency operations as well as support routine and emergency responses requiring surveillance and epidemiological investigation.

Capability 15: Volunteer Management—is the ability to coordinate with partners to identify, recruit, register, verify, train, and engage volunteers to support the activities during predeployment, deployment, and postdeployment. The capacity to notify, organize, assemble, and deploy volunteers is critical to the EOC Capability.

SOURCE: CDC, 2018.

Under NIMS guidance, an emergency operations center (EOC) is the central location (physical or virtual) where responsible personnel gather to coordinate operational information and resources for emergency operations. More recently, practitioners have used the term PHEOC to define the central location for the strategic management of public health emergencies (WHO, 2015a). Public health agencies typically, but not always, use an incident command system (ICS) within a PHEOC. An ICS is a "scalable, flexible system for organizing emergency response functions and resources characterized by principles such as standardized roles, modular organization, and unity of command" (Rose et al., 2017, p. S130). Many components go into creating a PHEOC, including plans and procedures, physical infrastructure, information and communication technology, systems, and equipment. In addition to these components are PHEOC leaders and staff. This collection of expertise in close collaboration is deemed a core component of a PHEOC.

The process of activating a PHEOC may include, but is not limited to, the following actions:

- conducting a preliminary assessment to determine the need for and level of activation of public health emergency operations (e.g., whether public health will have a lead, supporting, or no role);
- activating necessary public health functions;
- supporting mutual aid according to the public health role and incident requirements;
- identifying personnel with the skills necessary to fulfill the required incident command for activation; and
- establishing primary and alternative locations for the PHEOC and notifying personnel to report either physically or virtually to the PHEOC (CDC, 2018).

Scope of the Problem Addressed by the Practice

Chaos, poor information flow, unexpected tasks, extreme resource needs—these are the factors that often characterize public health emergencies. Standardized, bureaucratic hierarchies, on the other hand, are designed to perform the same tasks repeatedly. Beyond public health, the EOC model was developed in the period after World War II, as civil defense, to address this mismatch and coordinate emergency management's response to a wide range of emergencies (Botterell and Griss, 2011).

ICS and EOC

ICSs and EOCs are often conflated in response guidance and training, but it is important to differentiate them in any search for an evidence-based approach to their use.

The ICS model—a generic set of flexible, scalable organization structures designed to facilitate integrated response based on military antecedents—was born out of the response to California wildfires in the 1960s. In 1972, an interagency group representing federal, state, and local agencies was convened to address the problem, and eventually developed the Wildfire ICS (Jensen and Waugh, 2014). In 2004, the U.S. Department of Homeland Security established NIMS to provide a consistent, nationwide response approach for all levels of government (Jensen and Waugh, 2014; Rose et al., 2017). The initial release of NIMS mandated training on the ICS model, fostering its official use across U.S. response agencies.

ICS was developed for direct incident management, and its implementation varies. In his distillation of 40 years of research in the area of incident management, social scientist Enrico Quarantelli (1997) cites a still ongoing debate around the implementation and effectiveness of the ICS model, especially as applied to public health threats (Jensen and Thompson, 2016; Jensen and Waugh, 2014; Rimstad and Braut, 2015; Rose et al., 2017). As a fundamentally hierarchical model, ICS has drawn criticism from scholars with respect to a lack of flexibility and a rigid command and control mentality (Buck et al., 2006). However, it has often been implemented, especially in recent years, with a more intense focus on collaboration and the networked aspects of incident response (Moynihan, 2009). Regardless, the key purpose of any ICS is the direct management of an emergency situation.

By contrast, NIMS is clear that EOCs are structures designed primarily for incident support, decision making, and coordination across a jurisdiction (FEMA, 2017). They may support multiple ICS structures in different geographic and functional regions; they may or may not direct tactical operations. Quarantelli's (1997) research review points to a "well-functioning EOC" as a key success factor for disaster response. As he notes:

> Organised crisis-time activity in a disaster is clearly aided if responding organizations, local and otherwise, are aware of and represented at a common place or location, such as a fully staffed and adequately equipped EOC. (pp. 51–52)

According to Quarantelli, an EOC needs to be primarily a successful *social* system (rather than a *physical* one) in order to function well. On the other hand, he does not identify a particular structure (whether ICS or otherwise) as helpful. Having the right people together, collaborating on the correct functions (e.g., evacuation, risk communication) is the key point, as opposed to any focus on organization. In fact, NIMS currently addresses three potential EOC structures without mandating any one of them: an ICS structure modifed to remove its field components, a variant support model focused on communication and resourcing, and a structure that simply mimics day-to-day relationships among government agencies (FEMA, 2017).

PHEOC

The idea of the PHEOC blurs this ICS–EOC distinction, because in a public health emergency, the PHEOC combines the tactical elements of ICS (e.g., for public health operations) with the coordination and decision making of a jurisdictional EOC. For this reason, as well as some skepticism within the medical community regarding the idea of "command and control," it took some time for public health agencies to adopt an EOC model, although they were often represented in the jurisdictional EOCs described above. For example, it was not until after the 2001 anthrax attacks that CDC developed a PHEOC model for its own public health emergency responses (CDC, 2019). Used during the 2000s in response to severe acute respiratory syndrome, H5N1 planning, and the Hurricane Katrina response, PHEOCs did not become a national focal point for public health responses until the 2009 H1N1 epidemic. Since then, CDC's PHEOC has been mobilized for more than 17 distinct incidents, from leading roles in major international disease outbreaks such as Zika and the coronavirus disease 2019 (COVID-19) pandemic (in progress as of this writing) to support for the response to such nondisease incidents as oil spills and even a mass influx of unaccompanied immigrant children. CDC has credited its PHEOC model with increasing its ability to respond flexibly, increasing the speed of its resource allocation, and improving its leadership model, among other benefits (Redd and Frieden, 2017).

After its massive Ebola response in 2014, the World Health Organization (WHO) retooled its emergency response efforts from the top down, adopting a more stringent PHEOC model and a modified version of the ICS framework for global health emergencies. Crucially, both

CDC and WHO have adopted ICS principles (e.g., scalability, defined positions, rigorous training) without the rigid organizational structures of early ICS models. Both organizations now have integrated ICS frameworks that outline the key concepts and essential requirements for maintaining public health emergency operations in an EOC (Rose et al., 2017; WHO, 2015a). At the same time, their models continue to emphasize the key role that adaptability, partnerships, and clinical expertise must play in these events in ways that the Federal Emergency Management Agency (FEMA), for example, does not. Rose and colleagues (2017, p. S130) suggest that the main purpose of an ICS in a public health context includes

> coordination between functional units or groups of expertise within and across organizations; information collection, integration, and sharing internal to the [ICS] but also external to response partners and other stakeholders; developing and disseminating public information and warning and crisis and emergency risk communication messages to target audiences and the general public; and providing access to and deployment of resources such as staff and equipment to an EOC or the field (including the management and logistical support of surge staff).

This functional model, rather than any organizational doctrine, is key to maintaining a focus on health outcomes during the urgency of an emergency.

The Decision to Activate

Today, EOCs may be established at various jurisdictional levels, ranging from local and regional to national or international (WHO, 2015b). Federal and international guidance indicates that EOCs mitigate the impact of emergencies by facilitating an effective, coordinated response. Without these common structures, agencies would need to redevelop their emergency operations procedures with each new incident. This lack of established procedures would likely place stress on the agency and staff responsible for the response. Also, EOCs enable the consolidated movement of substantial resources, which helps emergency managers address the large-scale impacts of incidents (WHO, 2015a).

At the same time, however, the decision to activate emergency operations necessitates careful deliberation, because maintaining and operating an EOC requires the substantial use of finite resources. FEMA has provided general guidance on when to activate an EOC (FEMA, 2019) (see Box 5-2).

The public health emergency response and preparedness (PHEPR) field adds several unique features to the debate about when to activate a PHEOC. These include an ongoing debate about how PHEOCs relate to jurisdictional EOCs. For example, if a jurisdictional EOC is mobilized for a natural hazard (e.g., a hurricane or snowstorm), should a PHEOC be mobilized as well? Or is it better for public health practitioners to deploy to the jurisdictional EOC? Conversely, during an epidemic when a PHEOC assumes response leadership, how should it relate to a jurisdictional EOC that is used to coordinating emergencies of other types? As abstract and bureaucratic as these questions may appear, they have real consequences for health care resourcing, coordinated decision making, and patient care. Different jurisdictions may answer these questions in different ways, but WHO makes it clear that close collaboration is necessary throughout any system of EOCs (WHO, 2015a).

In addition, many public health agencies in the United States are small, and this low-resource status may make PHEOC mobilization difficult, especially since PHEOCs are generally staffed with public health practitioners instead of drawing on multiple agencies, as with jurisdictional EOCs. Thus concerns about resource drain linked to PHEOC mobilization may be especially critical among public health entities. This concern may lead to delayed mobilization of PHEOCs, lessening their utility.

BOX 5-2 ACTIVATING AN EMERGENCY OPERATIONS CENTER

The jurisdictional policy determines emergency operations center (EOC) activation. The decision-making process for EOC activation should be outlined in a policy. Listed below are possible circumstances that would trigger an EOC activation.

- A Unified Command or Area Command is established.
- More than one jurisdiction becomes involved in a response.
- The Incident Commander indicates an incident could expand rapidly or involve cascading events.
- A similar incident in the past required EOC activation.
- The Chief Executive Officer or similar top executive directs that the EOC should be activated.
- An emergency is imminent (e.g., hurricane warnings, slow river flooding, predictions of hazardous weather, elevated threat levels, major community events).
- Threshold events described in the Emergency Operations Plan occur.

All personnel need to be aware of

- Who makes the decision to activate the EOC.
- What are the circumstances for activation.
- When activation occurs.
- How the level of activation is determined.

SOURCE: Excerpted from FEMA, 2019, p. 1.

Finally, as CDC and WHO have noted, both public health emergencies and the essential practice of public health have unique characteristics that must not be lost during an EOC mobilization (Redd and Frieden, 2017; WHO, 2015b). Clinical and technical expertise, for example, must not be subsumed by bureaucracy. Such key public health functions as prevention services and technical guidance must be represented. Most important, novel public health emergencies are characterized by high levels of uncertainty. The importance of the ability of a PHEOC to adapt both its functions and its structure as new information emerges should never be underestimated. Public health emergency operations must continually evolve, just as the emergencies that they manage do.

OVERVIEW OF THE KEY REVIEW QUESTIONS AND ANALYTIC FRAMEWORK

Defining the Key Review Questions

As described above, activating a PHEOC is a common and standard practice in response to a public health emergency. Therefore, the committee approached this review with the objective of better understanding how the PHEPR system interacts with and changes in response to the activation of a PHEOC to inform when and under what circumstances activation should occur. Adopting a systems perspective, the committee posed the following overarching question in this review: "In what circumstances is activating public health emergency operations appropriate?" To further identify evidence of interest, the committee explored several specific sub-questions related to activation, separate public health emergency operations, changes in response, benefits and harms, and the factors that create barriers and facilitators (see Box 5-3).

Analytic Framework

For the purposes of this review, the committee developed an analytic framework to present the causal pathway and interactions between public health emergency operations and its components, populations, and outcomes of interest (see Figure 5-1). The underlying theory is that activating a PHEOC facilitates the coordination of resources and information flow, thereby improving response efforts by increasing the efficiency and timeliness of response (CDC, 2019). As illustrated in the analytic framework, activating a PHEOC or involving public health in multiagency emergency operations should ultimately lead to cohesive and effective response operations and an improved ability to provide emergency services. This improved coordination and more robust service delivery should, in turn, lead to better health outcomes by reducing morbidity and mortality and improving social well-being. Unfortunately, this is a difficult causal pathway to prove.

To begin with, a preliminary assessment in coordination with response partners is required to determine the need for and level of activation, as well as whether public health should assume a lead role, a supporting role, or no role in the emergency operations (CDC, 2018). Deciding whether to activate a PHEOC requires consideration of assigned or recruited staff who may be pulled away from their primary responsibilities, legal issues, and the resources and costs of running the operation. As with many interventions in the PHEPR field, the effectiveness of a response intervention is often measured by intermediate outcomes rather than health outcomes. The committee hypothesized the following intermediate outcomes:

BOX 5-3 KEY REVIEW QUESTIONS

In what circumstances is activating public health emergency operations appropriate?

- What factors (e.g., type and scale of event, type of command, complexity, past experience, mutual aid requests, policy) are useful for determining when to activate public health emergency operations?
- In what circumstances should public health agencies activate a separate public health emergency operations center (PHEOC), lead a multiagency PHEOC, or play a supporting role in a multiagency PHEOC based on identified or potential public health consequences?
- How does the response change following the activation of public health emergency operations?
- What benefits and harms (desirable and/or undesirable impacts) of activation of public health emergency operations have been described or measured?
- What are the barriers to and facilitators of successful public health emergency operations using an incident command center?

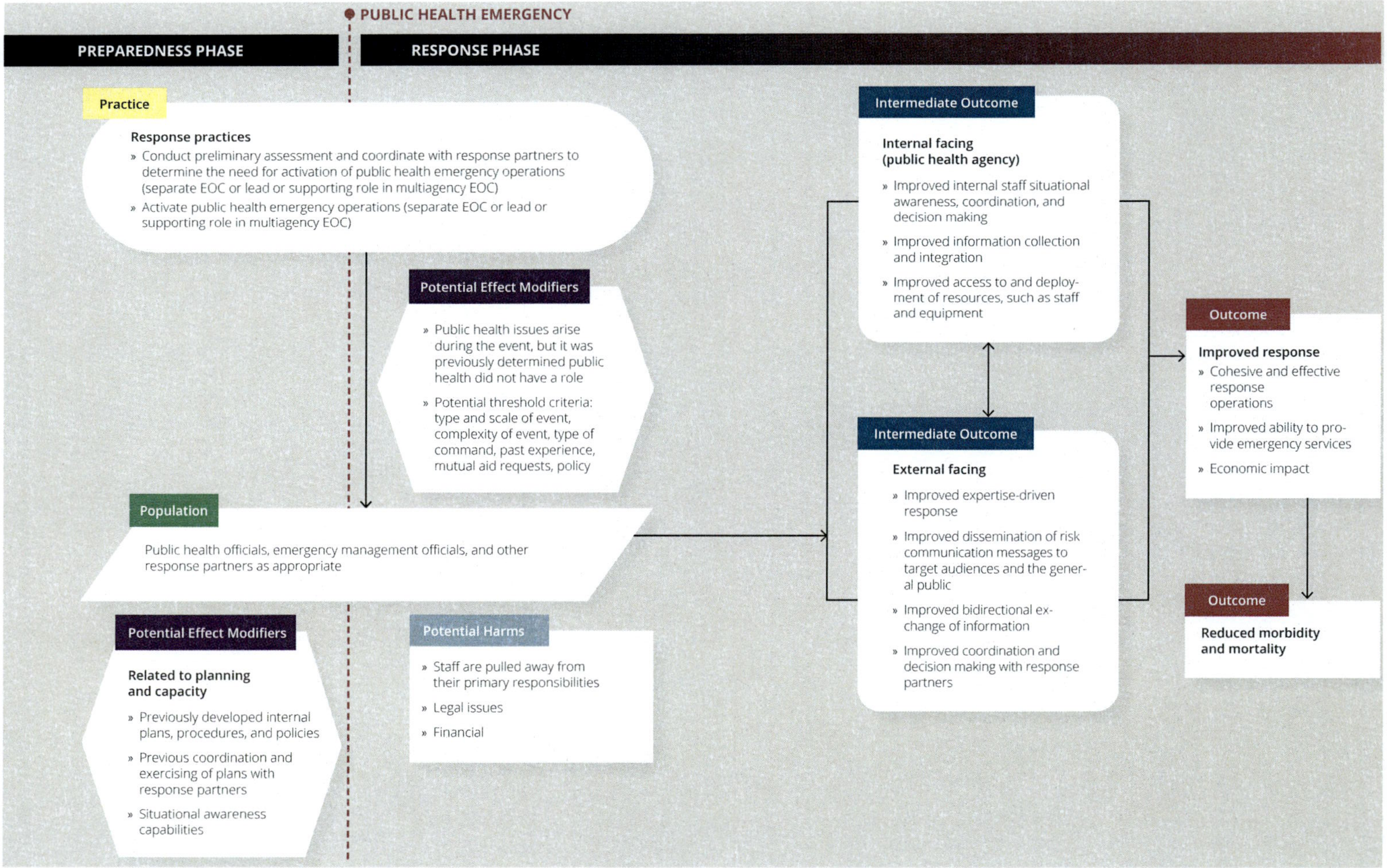

FIGURE 5-1 Analytic framework for public health emergency operations.
NOTES: Arrows in the framework indicate hypothesized causal pathways between interventions and outcomes. Double-headed arrows indicate feedback loops. EOC = emergency operations center.

- Internal-facing (i.e., public health agency) intermediate outcomes
  - Improved internal staff situational awareness, coordination, and decision making
  - Improved information collection and integration
  - Improved access to and deployment of resources, such as staff and equipment
- External-facing intermediate outcomes
  - Improved expertise-driven response
  - Improved dissemination of risk communication messages to target audiences and the general public
  - Improved bidirectional exchange of information
  - Improved coordination and decision making with response partners

OVERVIEW OF THE EVIDENCE SUPPORTING THE PRACTICE RECOMMENDATION[1]

This section summarizes the evidence from the mixed-method review examining PHEOC activation. Following the summary of the evidence of effectiveness, summaries are presented for each element of the Evidence to Decision (EtD) framework (encompassing balance of benefits and harms, acceptability and preferences, feasibility and PHEPR system considerations, resource and economic considerations, equity, and ethical considerations), which the committee considered in formulating its practice recommendation. Full details on the review strategy and findings can be found in the appendixes: Appendix A provides a detailed description of the study eligibility criteria, search strategy, data extraction process, and individual study quality assessment criteria; Appendix B2 provides a full description of the evidence, including the literature search results, evidence profile tables, and EtD framework for activating a PHEOC; and Appendix C links to all the commissioned analyses that informed this review. Table 5-1 shows the types of evidence included in this review.

Effectiveness

The review identified no quantitative comparative or noncomparative studies or modeling studies eligible for inclusion, but information gleaned from the qualitative evidence synthesis and the case report and after action report (AAR) evidence synthesis contributed to the committee's understanding of the circumstances in which activating a PHEOC is appropriate. This is a difficult evidentiary situation; the lack of quantitative studies, in particular, speaks to the committee's high-level finding that more and improved research is needed with respect to this practice. Still, the committee's overriding goal was to distill the available evidence so as to provide practitioners with the best possible guidance. Therefore, the evidence gleaned was used to construct a high-level view of what happened and what appeared to work. (Refer to Section 1, "Determining Evidence of Effect," in Appendix B2 for additional detail.)

Balance of Benefits and Harms

As stated above, no quantitative research on the effectiveness of PHEOC activation was identified. The evidence from qualitative studies and from case reports and AARs indicates that activation generally results in more efficient response operations and improved ability to

[1] To enhance readability for an end user audience, this section does not include references. Citations supporting the findings in this section appear in Appendix B2.

TABLE 5-1 Evidence Types Included in the Mixed-Method Review of Activating Public Health Emergency Operations

Evidence Type[a]	Number of Studies (as applicable)[b]
Quantitative comparative	0
Quantitative noncomparative (postintervention measure only)	0
Qualitative	21
Modeling	0
Descriptive surveys	1
Case reports	29[c]
After action reports	35[c]
Mechanistic	N/A
Parallel (systematic reviews)	N/A

[a] Evidence types are defined in Chapter 3.
[b] Note that sibling articles (different results from the same study published in separate articles) are counted as one study in this table. Mixed-method studies may be counted in more than one category.
[c] A sample of case reports and after action reports was prioritized for inclusion in this review based on relevance to the key questions, as described in Chapter 3.

respond to emergent needs with greater flexibility, and as a result may have implicit benefits in relation to improving population health during a public health emergency. The timeliness of response activities also improves because of the increased availability of resources and/or capabilities. Moreover, activation may enable greater access to subject-matter experts during responses with potential public health implications. A long-term benefit of activation is the accumulation of institutional knowledge of what does and does not work (i.e., practical experience) gained by the public health agency under urgent and/or emergent conditions.

Important factors in deciding whether activating a PHEOC will lead to any harms include the potential need for more intensive staffing due to long hours and the need to continue routine public health services, as well as the potential for adaptation-generated interorganizational distrust and chain-of-command disruption. These harms are likely to be present only during an event and not to persist postevent for any appreciable length of time. In some cases, however, such harms may become embedded in the public health system and carry over from event to event (e.g., if a negative interpersonal relationship forms that creates barriers to future successful collaboration). Simply activating a PHEOC is not a comprehensive solution; public health agencies must be ready to manage them effectively, and without that readiness, more harms may be experienced. (Evidence source: qualitative evidence synthesis and case report and AAR evidence synthesis. Refer to Section 2, "Balance of Benefits and Harms," in Appendix B2 for additional detail.)

Acceptability and Preferences

PHEPR practitioners generally find their roles in participating in emergency operations acceptable and are amenable to the resulting changes in work patterns. PHEPR practitioners prefer to use an ICS but appreciate the ability to modify the structure to better suit their operational context and jurisdiction.

Furthermore, to facilitate the implementation of public health emergency operations, practitioners must believe that implementation of the NIMS and ICS has the potential to solve real problems and is clear and specific, that incentives and sanctions are not only provided but also likely, and that capacity-building resources are being provided. Ongoing support for meaningful work is important, and PHEOCs that provide this support are therefore likely to be more successful. (Evidence source: case report and AAR evidence synthesis and descriptive survey study evidence. Refer to Section 3, "Acceptability and Preferences," in Appendix B2 for additional detail.)

Feasibility and PHEPR System Considerations

Many barriers impact the feasibility of successful PHEOC activation, and these barriers are often related to challenges involving general management practices. These challenges include interorganizational awareness, relationships, and cultural differences; differences in team members' knowledge and experience; adequate staffing to implement the activation with all of its components, structures, and processes; communication technology; rules and regulations; the volume of information; and a lack of training in NIMS and ICS, partner roles, and job-specific roles. If these interorganizational characteristics are not conducive to implementation, actual implementation behavior can be negatively impacted regardless of what jurisdictions intend. (Evidence source: qualitative evidence synthesis, case report and AAR evidence synthesis, and descriptive survey study evidence. Refer to Section 4, "Feasibility and PHEPR System Considerations," in Appendix B2 for additional detail.)

Resource and Economic Considerations

The resource, cost, and logistical constraints of activating a PHEOC are important considerations in deciding whether to activate. These considerations often change over the course of an event and may be sizable depending on the scope of the event. Salient resources include training; databases; supplies; and mechanism(s) for communicating with the public and media, among which is the creation of liaison and point-of-contact positions. These resource needs may dictate the level at which the public health emergency operations should be coordinated (e.g., local, regional, state, and/or national). Baseline PHEOC operations require an infusion of resources beyond normal operations, in general, and public health agencies need to be prepared to manage those costs, ideally with support from other levels of government. (Evidence source: qualitative evidence synthesis and case report and AAR evidence synthesis. Refer to Section 5, "Resource and Economic Considerations," in Appendix B2 for additional detail.)

Equity

Inequities in the implementation of public health emergency operations for different populations due to variability in the availability of resources, infrastructure, and funding likely exist among state, local, tribal, and territorial public health agencies (and are also related to the resource and economic considerations discussed above). Activating a PHEOC can help ensure that the needs of particular at-risk populations are addressed during the response to an event. Accomplishing this requires interagency planning based within the PHEOC that entails establishing a task force to help these population(s), creating a database to collect relevant risk information, providing targeted care in shelters, ensuring access to medications, and addressing specific medical needs caused by power outages and unique transportation requirements. Another approach involves welcoming community representatives into the PHEOC for more inclusive decision making. Additional research is needed to better understand how biases or inequities internal to a PHEOC relate to equitable response outcomes. PHEOCs likely reflect the implicit biases of their decision makers and will support equity more or less well based on the perspective of those individuals. (Evidence source: qualitative evidence synthesis and case report and AAR evidence synthesis. Refer to Section 6, "Equity," in Appendix B2 for additional detail.)

Ethical Considerations

The section on equity above addresses ethical considerations in PHEOC operations related to the principle of justice or fairness. In addition, the primary ethical principle underlying the initiation of a PHEOC is that of stewardship of limited resources. This principle, often framed as a duty to produce the greatest good for the greatest number of people as efficiently as possible, is frequently seen as particularly important during public health emergencies, because resources in emergencies are typically limited and need to be allocated with care. As a result, ethical concerns related to implementing a PHEOC are centered primarily on the pragmatic benefits and harms of doing so: namely, the possibility that implementing a PHEOC will waste resources and generate harms due to the neglect of other programs while team members are reassigned to PHEOC operations. Some of the procedural principles in play can include transparency, which is supported when a PHEOC improves communication, and proportionality (acting only in proportion to need, or using the least restrictive means to achieve a desired outcome), which is supported when having an activated PHEOC improves situational awareness and therefore averts unnecessary implementation of interventions. (Evidence source: committee discussion drawing on key ethics and policy texts. Refer to Section 7, "Ethical Considerations," in Appendix B4 for additional detail.)

CONSIDERATIONS FOR IMPLEMENTATION

The following considerations for implementation were drawn from the synthesis of qualitative research studies, the synthesis of case reports and AARs, and descriptive surveys, the findings of which are presented in Appendix B2. Note that this is not an exhaustive list of considerations; additional implementation resources need to be consulted.

Factors in Determining When to Activate a PHEOC

Establishment of Pre-Event and Ad Hoc Activation Triggers

An essential element of activation of PHEOC activation is determination of the critical point or specific threshold that elicits an activation decision. Having predefined activation triggers is useful in determining when to activate, reactivate, or deactivate response operations. These triggers can be defined in interagency protocols and memoranda of understanding before an emergency event occurs, thus facilitating rapid activation. It is important for such predefined triggers to be flexible and not necessarily rely on a state's declaration of an emergency, as response needs can still overburden resources in the absence of such a formal declaration. In certain circumstances, particularly novel diseases, new, ad hoc triggers may need to be developed. Five factors may influence the time required to activate a PHEOC:

- previous knowledge and experience;
- the degree to which an emergency event is atypical;

- the amount, speed, and quality of the situation data available;
- the integration of data into building a picture of the situation; and
- perception of the urgency of making a decision.

Triggers can help overcome the hesitation sometimes inherent in PHEOC mobilization based on resource concerns among executive leadership, especially given the finding that practitioners generally consider early PHEOC activation more useful. (Evidence source: qualitative evidence synthesis and case report and AAR evidence synthesis. Refer to Section 8, "Factors in Determining When to Activate a PHEOC," in Appendix B2 for additional detail.)

Determination of Separate, Lead, or Support Public Health Emergency Operations

Public health agencies appropriately lead a multiagency EOC in response to acute public health threats (e.g., infectious disease outbreaks) when coordination and information sharing among response agencies are critical to the achievement of response objectives. Public health agencies appropriately support a multiagency EOC during planned events or incidents with potential public health implications (e.g., environmental disasters such as oil spills or refinery fires). During such events, public health agencies can help with

- family reunification;
- surveillance and epidemiology, environmental health, and mental health and psychological support functions; and
- mass care and management and distribution of medical supplies.

It is less clear from the evidence when public health agencies should activate fully separate public health emergency operations, although many public health agencies engage in this practice for relatively small epidemics. (Evidence source: qualitative evidence synthesis and case report and AAR evidence synthesis. Refer to Section 8, "Factors in Determining When to Activate a PHEOC," in Appendix B2 for additional detail.)

Events That Are Large in Size, Complex in Scope, and Novel

It is helpful to activate a PHEOC for multijurisdictional responses to events that are large in size and complex in scope when the event poses threats to public health; it is also helpful to activate early even if the size and scope of an event are initially unknown. There is often a period of initial uncertainty about size and complexity, particularly with regard to novel diseases or events. Risk assessments and foresight can be useful in carefully weighing the potential public health impacts against the cost implications of a resource-intensive activation. In general, the larger, more rapidly developing, and more novel an incident, the more likely it is that a PHEOC structure will benefit a public health agency. (Evidence source: qualitative evidence synthesis and case report and AAR evidence synthesis. Refer to Section 8, "Factors in Determining When to Activate a PHEOC," in Appendix B2 for additional detail.)

Need for Effective Surge

Understanding the burden of operations required can assist in deciding whether to activate a PHEOC by helping to determine the necessary scope of the activation. If the needs imposed by the incident go beyond the capacity of existing resources, activating public health emergency operations can provide a means for an effective surge response. This is especially true if public health agencies use the PHEOC mobilization to involve public and private partners that can bring additional resources to bear quickly. (Evidence source: qualitative evidence synthesis and case report and AAR evidence synthesis. Refer to Section 8, "Factors in Determining When to Activate a PHEOC," in Appendix B2 for additional detail.)

Need for Coordination Among Federal, State, and Local Public Health Agencies

PHEOC activation at the local level is beneficial to support state-level response to public health threats. Activation allows local jurisdictions to keep pace with the response and improves interagency coordination if other agencies are involved. Public health agencies need to clarify the respective roles of the state and local PHEOCs. Doing so is particularly important to ensure clear chains of command and decision-making authority during a response. Regardless of the structure established, public health agencies across the federal, state, and local levels need to work to integrate their functions. In particular, cross-staffing PHEOCs with personnel from public health agencies at all three levels can aid cohesion, as can joint strategic sessions involving leadership at these levels. (Evidence source: case report and AAR evidence synthesis. Refer to Section 8, "Factors in Determining When to Activate a PHEOC," in Appendix B2 for additional detail.)

Other Implementation Considerations

The following conceptual findings inform the perspectives and approaches to be considered when implementing public health emergency operations.

Leverage Strong, Decisive Leadership

During emergencies, strong, decisive leadership is essential despite uncertainties associated with the event. Information will always be imperfect, but indecision that results in taking no action is generally undesirable, because the speed of an emergency magnifies the impact of delay. In addition, leadership needs to have the ability to receive new, sometimes unexpected information and the flexibility to revise objectives as needed. Leadership needs to promote trust by creating a shared sense of purpose and highlighting the contributions of different network members. (Evidence source: qualitative evidence synthesis and case report and AAR evidence synthesis. Refer to Section 9, "Other Implementation Considerations," in Appendix B2 for additional detail.)

Create Shared Understanding in Response

A key consideration in the activation of a PHEOC is its ability to aid in building a shared understanding of the incident at hand, as well as the organizational response structure. Flexibility will be successful only if there is a shared understanding of the nature of the response throughout the response structure. Otherwise, staff are likely to reject change, especially when it is rapid.

Cognitively, any time practitioners are involved in a preparedness exercise or an ongoing event, they are creating a shared understanding. Although the picture (or "mental model") that results from such involvement may exist fully in the mind of one leader, the understanding of the different aspects of an event more often is distributed across multiple leaders and staff. These mental models evolve, and during the chaos of an emergency, they may be quite different for different aspects of the response. Reality is strained under this kind of chaos, and the mental models of some staff may not reflect the reality of any part of the emergency at all. This is not their fault, but may be due to limited or incorrect information.

One way to think about coordination, then, is to see it as coordination of the varying mental models of staff and leaders within and across agencies. Sharing accurate mental models can lead to a shared understanding of key roles, missions, and needed outcomes, and staff in one location working toward defined objectives can more easily share understanding relative to disparate staff in different locales working under different structures. (Evidence source: qualitative evidence synthesis and case report and AAR evidence synthesis. Refer to Section 9, "Other Implementation Considerations," in Appendix B2 for additional detail.)

Ensure Simultaneous Rigidity and Flexibility in a PHEOC

Standard roles and functions likely help increase understanding; however, response decisions must be flexible based on context. This apparent contradiction is, in fact, necessary, and it is important to conceptualize public health emergency operations as command and control functions with the potential to necessitate adjustments to plans and ad hoc improvisations. The often changing, complex, and dynamic environment of an emergency creates unique demands, and preplanned command and control functions may not apply in their entirety. In these situations, it is essential to encourage new organizational structures and functions to meet new needs. Many methods have been used to reconfigure formal structures in emergencies—for example, structure elaborating (building out rapid new organizations such as call centers), role switching (switching to new leadership for new strategic direction), and authority migrating (formally reassigning large portfolios of work suddenly during emergencies). The goal is always to enhance organizational flexibility and reliability (or its perception) during a high-consequence event. At the same time, however, the basic, well-trained PHEOC (or ICS) structures that help to keep the shared understanding operational within the response must remain locked in order to maintain cohesion. (Evidence source: qualitative evidence synthesis and case report and AAR evidence synthesis. Refer to Section 9, "Other Implementation Considerations," in Appendix B2 for additional detail.)

View Public Health Emergency Operations Teams as Social Groups

To help balance these different demands, it is important to see public health emergency operations teams not just as task groups but also as social groups. Focusing on their social dynamics can help improve relationships and decision-making affinities across different aspects of the response. This social cohesion is a critical factor when a situation is moving too rapidly for the hierarchies involved in standard bureaucratic structures. During the preparedness phase, it can be improved through joint training and exercises and such collaborative activities as planning. However, PHEOCs that can address these social issues during response tend to be more successful as well. For instance, a useful strategy can entail recognizing cultural differences among staff from different organizational cultures and working to bridge those differences. So, too, can being transparent about preexisting social, economic, and political power differentials and addressing them respectfully. In addition, emotional issues, such as the personal safety concerns of staff members, tend to be overlooked during the urgency of an emergency. Encouraging staff to share concerns and then addressing those concerns when possible will improve cohesion. In short, ensuring that a PHEOC will be able to support the social group it creates is an important consideration for successful implementation. (Evidence source: qualitative evidence synthesis. Refer to Section 9, "Other Implementation Considerations," in Appendix B2 for additional detail.)

Understand How Response Changes Following PHEOC Activation

It is clear from the above discussion that activating a PHEOC will change the response to an event, potentially for both good and ill. Understanding the nature of these changes is an important implementation consideration. Metrics for gauging these changes are thus helpful in determining whether and when to activate.

The Dynes typology, drawn from the emergency management literature, offers one such set of metrics. Organized by tasks and structure, it can be used to classify emergency response into four categories: established organized response (regular task–old structural arrangements), expanding organized response (regular task–new structural arrangements), extending organized response (nonregular task–old structural arrangements), and emergent organized response (nonregular task–new structural arrangements). Building an understanding of how a public health agency's response might change following PHEOC activation can inform decision-making processes. Coupling that understanding with a tool such as the Dynes typology that delineates adaptation types will likely improve success. It is important to remember that the likelihood of adaptation is highest in the earliest phases of an event, an argument that supports early consideration of PHEOC activation. (Evidence source: qualitative evidence synthesis. Refer to Section 9, "Other Implementation Considerations," in Appendix B2 for additional detail.)

Leverage Staff with Past Response Experience

Leveraging the knowledge and experience of staff regarding prior emergencies can be a practical means of determining whether to activate in a particular situation, providing more context than can be gleaned from any written plan and facilitating positive outcomes. This experience can also be helpful during the preparedness phase in the development of effective, context-driven activation triggers. Ensuring that experienced staff participate in activation discussions, even those generally limited to higher-ranking executives, can thus help foster improved decision making. While it is helpful to leverage experienced staff and subject-matter experts early on in an event, it is also important to recognize that overreliance on a few key personnel can lead to staff fatigue. (Evidence source: case report and AAR evidence synthesis. Refer to Section 9, "Other Implementation Considerations," in Appendix B2 for additional detail.)

PRACTICE RECOMMENDATION, JUSTIFICATION, AND IMPLEMENTATION GUIDANCE

Insufficient Evidence Statement

Activating a public health emergency operations center (PHEOC) is a common and standard practice, supported by national and international guidance and based on earlier social science around disaster response. Despite widespread use and minimal apparent harms, there is insufficient evidence to determine the effectiveness of activating a PHEOC or of specific PHEOC components at improving response. This does *not* mean that the practice does not work or should not be implemented, but that more research and monitoring and evaluation around how and in what circumstances a PHEOC should be implemented are warranted before an evidence-based practice recommendation can be made.

Justification for the Insufficient Evidence Statement

Partly because of its long tenure as a common and standard practice, direct research evidence does not focus on whether PHEOCs should be utilized, but rather on how they should be implemented. Experiential evidence from a synthesis of case reports and after action reports (AARs) (from within and outside of public health emergency preparedness and response [PHEPR]) suggests that PHEOCs are probably effective at improving response and may have few undesirable effects in the short term, and speaks to the confidence in the PHEOC model among experienced practitioners across diverse situations. PHEPR practitioners consider activating a PHEOC to be an acceptable and justifiable practice. At the same time, the feasibility of this practice is variable, and the evidence highlights several feasibility issues to consider before a PHEOC is activated.

The evidence reviewed demonstrates coverage across multiple agencies and disciplines, strengthening the conclusion that the evidence is likely applicable to agencies beyond those in which PHEOC activation has been evaluated. However, it is important to note that no studies have examined PHEOCs activated by tribal or territorial public health agencies. Additionally, there is concern about the applicability of studies conducted during an exercise to real-world decision making.

Implementation Guidance

While the available evidence does not address *whether* PHEOCs should be implemented, it does address *how* PHEOCs should be implemented. The committee offers a set of implementation considerations based on the evidence from qualitative studies and experiential evidence from case reports and AARs to support planning. Based on this evidence, public health agencies should consider the following factors to make more successful decisions regarding the activation of public health emergency operations.

Considerations for *when* to activate public health emergency operations:

- **A public health emergency is large in size and complex in scope.** Such events are likely to exceed the capacity of existing resources and/or the capabilities of the agency.
- **A novel response may require multiple new tasks or partnerships.** Given high uncertainty, an agency should err on the side of activating early to handle new tasks or partnerships that may emerge. Public health emergency operations can always be scaled back.
- **An event occurs that requires public health support functions, large-scale information sharing, or response coordination.** Such events include, for example, environmental disasters with the potential for short-term and/or long-term public health impacts. In these incidents, the focus should be on providing support and leadership to the jurisdictional EOC. Activation of emergency operations should also be considered for planned events with potential for public health implications.
- **Resource, cost, technological, legal, and logistical constraints need to be overcome.** Resource needs often change throughout an event and may entail moderate to large resource requirements, depending on the size and scope of the event.
- **An incident requires high levels of interagency partnership.** Even if a response is small, interagency coordination may require PHEOC activation, especially if a partner agency has mobilized its own EOC structure. An agency should focus on ensuring that other agencies coordinate within the PHEOC to achieve the most shared understanding.

continued

Considerations for *when to refrain* from activating public health emergency operations:

- The cost of activating is higher than any potential resource needs for the emergency.
- Leadership has minimum experience with PHEOC operations, and staff have minimum PHEOC training. Lack of prior PHEOC activation experience or training could lead to interagency distrust and chain-of-command disruption, which in turn could negatively impact the success of the response.
- Leadership prioritizes maintaining routine public health functions over the needs of the emergency response. A key aspect of this consideration is leadership's willingness to allow staff to work at or with the PHEOC, possibly for long hours.

Considerations for *how* to make the decision to activate public health emergency operations:

- Respect staff knowledge, and involve staff with past emergency experience in leadership discussions.
- Ensure strong leadership, even using leaders outside the regular hierarchy if necessary, or switching out established leaders for newer leaders better suited to the flexibility in decision making needed in emergency response.
- Provide support to address the social functioning of the PHEOC.
- Resource common operating picture functions to increase shared understanding across the PHEOC.
- Create an environment that encourages staff flexibility within the PHEOC.
- Conduct just-in-time training to minimize disruptions caused by less-experienced staff.
- Continuously monitor and evaluate response functions to ensure and prove utility.

EVIDENCE GAPS AND FUTURE RESEARCH PRIORITIES

A significant limitation of the evidence for this practice was the lack of quantitative evidence on the effectiveness of activating a PHEOC, a gap that could be addressed if activation were accompanied by targeted monitoring and evaluation (M&E) when feasible. M&E for a PHEOC involves establishing a system for consistently reviewing how a PHEOC is progressing, what needs to be improved, and whether the response goals are being met. This process entails the regular and systematic collection and analysis of data (quantitative, process, or output data, as well as qualitative data) and assessment of the degree to which anticipated outcomes are met (Gossip et al., 2017; USAID, 2020; WHO, 2015a). Ongoing monitoring is critical to generate information for use in evaluations and AARs.

M&E systems, capacities, and capabilities are best created in the preparedness phase to ensure rapid activation in the event of a public health emergency. Establishing an M&E system for a PHEOC, whether within an agency (at a minimum) or at the national level, can enable standard data collection across different events and aid in conducting analyses over time. Quasi-experimental designs could make use of these data to evaluate the effectiveness of PHEOCs. To guide public health agencies (from low resourced to high resourced) in conducting rigorous M&E, future research could initially focus on identifying the key components of a formalized M&E system for a PHEOC. For example, PHEOCs manage public health emergencies via objectives meant to improve population health outcomes. Keim (2013) notes that these objectives can be standardized across responses, which makes it possible to develop objective-driven performance measures that can be adapted and implemented across jurisdictions during public health emergencies. The importance of addressing this gap was also confirmed during the committee's prioritization of review topics with 10 PHEPR practitioners, at least half of whom indicated that resources and tools are needed to capture critical information during an emergency that involves public health (see Appendix A for the full results of this prioritization activity).

The committee was unable to identify any quantitative research on the effectiveness of activating a PHEOC. Future research could take advantage of the heterogeneity inherent in the response to a public health emergency and use natural experiments to evaluate PHEOCs (e.g., examining cases in which one agency activates and another does not, or looking at different activations within the same agency). Matched comparison group studies are an example of such a methodology. Additional examples are presented in Tables 8-2 and 8-4 in Chapter 8.

Because there was no quantitative research on the effectiveness of PHEOC activation, the committee relied on other types of evidence, including evidence from qualitative studies, case reports, and AARs, to inform its work on this practice. It will be important for future efforts to focus on ways of ensuring that evaluators adhere to rigorous protocols for data collection, analysis, and interpretation for these types of evidence because they can be useful in particular for topics such as this. Such research could be strengthened through the use of more robust methods, such as qualitative comparative analyses (Baptist and Befani, 2015) and data collection (e.g., routine data captured in a future M&E system). A qualitative comparative analysis is a comparative method that allows evaluators to identify and understand what different combinations of factors are most important for a given outcome and the influence of context on that outcome.

It is important to note that one of the review findings was supported by evidence from only case reports and AARs, which could indicate an issue that has arisen in practice but has not been examined within the context of a research study. This finding was related to the interaction among different PHEOCs at the federal, state, and local levels. The case reports and AARs briefly discuss the importance of activating a PHEOC at the local level to support state-level responses and to improve coordination among the different levels and agencies. The field could benefit from research exploring what is known about the interactions and coordination among various EOCs. Large-scale implementation of PHEOCs is already under way. Therefore, greater investment in implementation science methods and approaches is needed. Implementation science is a rapidly advancing field that is used to help bridge the divide between research and practice. One focus of implementation science is the core components of an intervention. In thinking about adopting a PHEPR practice for implementation in different contexts, identifying its core components can help determine what should remain intact and what can be modified without jeopardizing outcomes. The core components of a PHEOC have not been adequately examined. The lack of a sufficient narrative describing a PHEOC in the corpus of qualitative studies, case reports, and AARs made it difficult for the committee to determine the impact of PHEOC activation. Furthermore, the lack of uniform terminology and insufficient reporting and articulation of methodology hampered consistency in searching and reviewing the literature, especially when the committee was attempting to review public health emergency operations, which involves a fairly new terminology. For example, one jurisdiction's PHEOC may be another's command center or ICS. Because public health emergency operations are complicated in that a public health agency may activate separately, lead a multiagency effort, or play a supporting role in a multiagency effort, and are context-specific depending on the jurisdiction, this level of detail and the use of common terminology are critical to future evaluations. Also related to implementation science, no studies examined PHEOCs activated by tribal or territorial public health agencies, a gap the committee believes to be significant in understanding the effectiveness of activating a PHEOC in these contexts. Future research needs to make a point of seeking out best practices in these areas.

More broadly, the committee acknowledges the limitations of its evidence review methodology in reviewing the practice of PHEOC activation. Methods used in other fields, such as the behavioral, organizational, structural, and quality improvement fields, could be employed to better understand PHEOC functioning. Decision trees, systems dynamics, systematic expert opinion methodologies such as Delphi, and other methods could be beneficial in informing those circumstances in which to activate a PHEOC. At the time of this writing, the COVID-19 pandemic was occurring, and many public health agencies had activated PHEOCs at differing times and levels to respond. The COVID-19 pandemic presents a unique opportunity to examine the timing of PHEOC activations and compare the benefits and harms of differing activation approaches. Several key gaps in current research and practice could immediately be observed: (1) the need for evidence on the impact of sustaining activation for a long period, (2) the importance of having an M&E system in place prior to an emergency to enable the collection of data on PHEOCs during an actual emergency, and (3) the need to understand the interrelationships of activation and scalability. In a true catastrophe, the question is not just mobilization of a PHEOC, but the scale at which that mobilization occurs and the PHEOC's ability to improvise new functions as needed in response to shifts in the situation. During and following the COVID-19 pandemic, it will be crucial to coordinate research efforts to ensure that priority questions related to public health emergency operations are answered with appropriate and rigorous methods (see Chapter 8 for additional detail regarding methodological improvements).

REFERENCES

Baptist, C., and B. Befani. 2015. *Qualitiative comparative analysis: A rigorous qualitative method for assessing impact.* Coffey International. https://www.betterevaluation.org/sites/default/files/Qualitative-Comparative-Analysis-June-2015%20(1).pdf (accessed March 12, 2020).

Botterell, A., and M. Griss. 2011. *Toward the next generation of emergency operations systems.* Paper read at the 8th International Information Systems for Crisis Response And Management (ISCRAM) Conference, Lisbon, Portugal.

Buck, D. A., J. E. Trainor, and B. E. Aguirre. 2006. A critical evaluation of the incident command system and NIMS. *Journal of Homeland Security and Emergency Management* 3(3).

CDC (Centers for Disease Control and Prevention). 2018. *Public health emergency preparedness and response capabilities: National standards for state, local, tribal, and territorial public health.* Atlanta, GA: Centers for Disease Control and Prevention. https://www.cdc.gov/cpr/readiness/capabilities.htm (accessed March 12, 2020).

CDC. 2019. *CDC Emergency Operations Center.* https://www.cdc.gov/cpr/eoc.htm (accessed March 22, 2020).

FEMA (Federal Emergency Management Agency). 2017. *National Incident Management System: Third edition.* https://www.fema.gov/media-library-data/1508151197225-ced8c60378c3936adb92c1a3ee6f6564/FINAL_NIMS_2017.pdf (accesed May 20, 2020).

FEMA. 2019. *Lesson 7: Activating and deactivating the EOC.* https://emilms.fema.gov/IS2200/groups/323.html (accessed April 1, 2020).

Gossip, K., H. Gouda, Y. Y. Lee, S. Firth, R. I. Bermejo, W. Zeck, and E. J. Soto. 2017. Monitoring and evaluation of disaster response efforts undertaken by local health departments: A rapid realist review. *BMC Health Services Research* 17(450).

Jensen, J., and S. Thompson. 2016. The incident command system: A literature review. *Disasters* 40(1):158–182.

Jensen, J., and W. L. Waugh. 2014. The United States' experience with the incident command system: What we think we know and what we need to know more about. *Journal of Contingencies and Crisis Management* 22(1):5–17.

Keim, M. E. 2013. An innovative approach to capability-based emergency operations planning. *Disaster Health* 1(1):54–62.

Moynihan, D. 2009. The network governance of crisis response: Case studies of incident command systems. *Journal of Public Administration Research and Theory* 19(4):895–915.

Quarantelli, E. L. 1997. Ten criteria for evaluating the management of community disasters. *Disasters* 21(1):39–56.

Redd, S. C., and T. R. Frieden. 2017. CDC's evolving approach to emergency response. *Health Security* 15(1):41–52.

Rimstad, R., and G. S. Braut. 2015. Literature review on medical incident command. *Prehospital and Disaster Medicine* 30(2):205–215.

Rose, D. A., S. Murthy, J. Brooks, and J. Bryant. 2017. The evolution of public health emergency management as a field of practice. *American Journal of Public Health* 107(S2):S126–S133.

USAID (U.S. Agency for International Development). 2020. *Unit 9: Monitoring and evaluation.* https://sbccimplementationkits.org/sbcc-in-emergencies/lessons/unit-9-monitoring-and-evaluation (accessed May 20, 2020).

WHO (World Health Organization). 2015a. *Framework for a public health emergency operations centre.* https://apps.who.int/iris/bitstream/handle/10665/196135/9789241565134_eng.pdf;jsessionid=931A229892C8BD19F6B995B37FE0325F?sequence=1 (accessed March 12, 2020).

WHO. 2015b. *Summary report of systematic reviews for public health emergency operations centres: Plans and procedures; communication technology and infrastructure; minimum datasets and standards; training and exercises.* https://apps.who.int/iris/bitstream/handle/10665/197379/9789241509787_eng.pdf?sequence=1 (accessed March 12, 2020).

6

Communicating Public Health Alerts and Guidance with Technical Audiences During a Public Health Emergency

Inclusion of electronic messaging channels (e.g., email) is recommended as part of state, local, tribal, and territorial public health agencies' multipronged approach for communicating public health alerts and guidance with technical audiences in preparation for and in response to public health emergencies.

The practice should be accompanied by targeted monitoring and evaluation or conducted in the context of research when feasible so as to improve the evidence base for strategies used to communicate public health alerts and guidance with technical audiences.

Finding Statements and Certainty of the Evidence

●●●● High ●●● Moderate ●● Low ● Very Low

Finding Statement	Certainty
Electronic messaging systems such as email, fax, and text messaging are effective communication channels for increasing technical audiences' awareness of public health alerts and guidance during a public health emergency	●●●
Electronic messaging systems are effective communication channels for increasing technical audiences' use of current public health guidance during a public health emergency	●

Implementation Guidance

- ☑ Engage technical audiences in the development of communication plans, protocols, and channels
- ☑ Consider contextual factors, such as the level of uncertainty or urgency, cultural preferences, and stakeholders' technical capabilities in the selection of communication channels
- ☑ Establish vetting processes in advance of public health emergencies and coordinate with response partners on messaging to prevent information overload, duplication of effort, and conflicting recommendations
- ☑ Reduce message volume when feasible, and highlight new information and any differences from previous or other existing guidance
- ☑ Develop distribution lists in advance of public health emergencies, and ensure that contact information is kept up to date
- ☑ Consider designating liaisons and institutional points of contact and leverage existing networks (e.g., medical societies and associations) to facilitate broad message dissemination

Context Considerations

Setting

Settings reflected in this evidence review included a mix of U.S. and non-U.S. settings.

Population

Technical audiences reflected in this evidence review were primarily health care professionals.

Emergency Phase

The evidence review included a mix of preparedness and response phase studies.

Emergency Type

Emergencies were primarily infectious disease events.

Type of Communication Channel

The type of communication channel reflected in this evidence review was primarily electronic messaging systems (e.g., fax, email, text). Social media is a notable gap area.

DESCRIPTION OF THE PRACTICE

Defining the Practice

The committee examined the evidence for different communication channels used to share public health alerts and guidance with technical audiences. It also examined the factors that may mediate the effectiveness of such communications (e.g., engagement of technical audiences in communication plans prior to an incident, frequency of messaging, designated liaisons). Communicating with technical audiences during a public health emergency falls primarily under Capability 6: Information Sharing (IS Capability) in the Centers for Disease Control and Prevention's (CDC's) *Public Health Emergency Preparedness and Response Capabilities: National Standards for State, Local, Tribal, and Territorial Public Health* (CDC PHEPR Capabilities) (CDC, 2018a). Information sharing is "the ability to conduct multijurisdictional and multidisciplinary exchange of health-related information and situational awareness data among federal, state, local, tribal and territorial levels of government and the private sector" (CDC, 2018a, p. 62). The IS Capability and the more specific practices for communicating alerts and guidance with technical audiences are closely linked to other CDC PHEPR Capabilities (see Box 6-1). In particular, the IS Capability is closely related to but distinct from the Emergency Public Information and Warning Capability, which is focused on dissemination of information, alerts, warnings, and notifications to the public. Channels and approaches for communicating with the public, while a critically important aspect of communication during response to a public health emergency, were not within the scope of this review. Elements of effective emergency risk communication with the public were the focus of a recent World Health Organization mixed-method systematic review (WHO, 2018). It should be noted that many of the broad principles of good emergency risk communication (related to, for example, time sensitivity and credibility) are applicable across different audience types and scenarios (CDC, 2018b).

Technical audiences for the purpose of this review include those response partners (governmental and nongovernmental) to whom a public health agency communicates public health alerts and guidance in preparation for and response to public health emergencies. Technical audiences may include multijurisdictional and multidisciplinary partners and stakeholders (see Table 6-1). Alerts and guidance may be disseminated by public health agencies at all levels—federal, state, local, tribal, and territorial. Public health alerts are time-sensitive communications that notify technical audiences of and provide updated status on public health threats (e.g., infectious disease outbreaks). Alerts may convey information requiring immediate action, action in the near future, or no action. Public health guidance specifies actions that should or should not be taken (or considered) in response to a public health threat (e.g., information on diagnostic testing methods, directions for submitting confirmed cases, information on use of personal protective equipment) (CDC, 2018a).

Communication channels (see Table 6-1) may allow only unidirectional reporting of information from public health agencies to technical audiences or may facilitate bidirectional exchange (e.g., dissemination of alerts and/or guidance and receipt of reports from technical audiences). The committee considered unidirectional reporting of information (disease cases or adverse events) to public health agencies to be a public health surveillance activity and did not include it in the scope of this review. However, the review did encompass communication channels that facilitate the bidirectional exchange of information if public health agencies may use the information shared by technical audiences to inform future guidance and alerts.

BOX 6-1 HOW COMMUNICATING PUBLIC HEALTH ALERTS AND GUIDANCE WITH TECHNICAL AUDIENCES DURING A PUBLIC HEALTH EMERGENCY RELATES TO THE CENTERS FOR DISEASE CONTROL AND PREVENTION'S PHEPR CAPABILITIES

Capability 1: Community Preparedness—a key aspect is the engagement of and coordination with state, local, tribal, and territorial partners and other stakeholders within communities, many of whom represent technical audiences to whom public health alerts and guidance need to be communicated. Establishing relationships and partnerships with these stakeholders in advance of a public health emergency may facilitate communication of public health information during response.

Capability 3: Emergency Operations Coordination—emergency operations centers are activated, in part, to facilitate improved coordination and information sharing across response partners, which may include the sharing of public health alerts and guidance.

Capability 4: Emergency Public Information and Warning—involves the coordinated development and dissemination of information, alerts, warnings, and notifications to the public. Alerts and guidance shared with technical audiences may in some cases be similar to public health information shared with the public. As with the Information Sharing Capability, selection of communication channels and the coordination of messaging are important issues for this capability.

Capability 6: Information Sharing—is more broadly focused, including, for example, data sharing for situational awareness, but all three of the Capability's functions are relevant to communicating alerts and guidance with technical audiences. Function 1 is focused on identifying stakeholders that should be incorporated into information flow and defining information-sharing needs, Function 2 relates to the identification and development of guidance, standards, and systems for information exchange, and Function 3 is focused on the process of sharing information during response.

Capability 13: Public Health Surveillance and Epidemiological Investigation—often involves reporting of events (e.g., disease cases, adverse treatment effects) by external partners, such as health care providers, to public health agencies. Some surveillance systems may allow bidirectional communication and the delivery of public health alerts.

SOURCE: CDC, 2018a.

TABLE 6-1 Technical Audiences and Communication Channels Used to Share Public Health Alerts and Guidance

Technical Audiences	Communication Channels
• Health care partners (e.g., hospitals, clinics, long-term care facilities, emergency departments, providers, health care coalitions, health and hospital associations, college health services, vaccine providers, community health centers) • Response agencies (emergency medical services, law enforcement, emergency management) • Other: syndromic surveillance partners, pharmacies, diagnostic laboratories, child care providers, shelter staff, veterinarians	• Health Alert Network • Electronic health record alert • Agency-run notification systems, with alert mechanisms that include email, text, phone call, pager, radio, and fax • WebEOC, teleconferences, in-person meetings, briefings • Bidirectional surveillance and messaging systems • Hotline/call center • Website, SharePoint, document libraries (e.g., Google drive), discussion threads • Webinar/webcast • Professional listservs/electronic newsletters • Social media

NOTE: These lists are not intended to be comprehensive but to capture the technical audiences and communication channels reported in the studies examined for this review.

Scope of the Problem Addressed by the Practice

Emergencies require exchanging large amounts of information at a rapid pace with multiple stakeholders, often using multiple modes of communication. The rapidly evolving nature of many emergencies and significant uncertainty are critical factors that contribute to changing information and specific challenges in communication with technical audiences (CDC, 2018b). The success of the public health emergency preparedness and response (PHEPR) system relies on the effective communication of information both horizontally across involved organizations and individuals who make up a complex network of response partners and vertically from the federal level down to the regional, state, and local levels. Challenges related to communication with response partners are commonly noted in after action reports (AARs) (Savoia et al., 2012). In an analysis of 31 AARs that addressed information sharing, Savoia and colleagues (2012) note the following themes:

- difficulty sharing information with external partners, often resulting from exclusion of key partners, such as health care and schools, from communication networks, as well as challenges with communication systems and inconsistency of messages;
- difficulty sharing information across different internal groups;
- lack of training in the use of communication technology (e.g., Health Alert Network [HAN], WebEOC, conference call or radio systems); and
- difficulty tracking information in the face of rapidly changing information, lengthy situational reports, and frequent and redundant alerts resulting in information overload.

Public health agencies are often well positioned to notify technical audiences regarding public health emergencies. Clinicians and other stakeholders also rely on public health authorities for guidance on the detection and management of infectious agents and other public health threats. During the H1N1 epidemic, for example, public health guidance informed the use of personal protective equipment, diagnostic testing, and antiviral therapies (Staes et al., 2011). In this context, public health agencies must collect and analyze information and share it with technical audiences during public health emergencies to support decision making and to mitigate health threats (e.g., disease and injury). A notable challenge, however, is ensuring that stakeholders have clear and up-to-date information, particularly in the face of public health guidance that changes as new information becomes available during response (Staes et al., 2011). Moreover, technical audiences may seek and/or receive information from different sources, and inconsistencies across sources can lead to confusion and potentially inappropriate actions by the recipients. In the absence of clear and consistent messaging from public health authorities, technical audiences may obtain and use information from the media or other unreliable sources, which may be inaccurate or out of date.

A wide variety of communication channels are commonly used to disseminate public health alerts and guidance with technical audiences (Revere et al., 2011), and more channels are becoming available as technology continues to evolve at a rapid pace, bringing both opportunities and challenges. In recent years, for example, use of social media during disasters has become both a valuable tool in information sharing and a difficult information-management challenge (Merchant et al., 2011). Facing an ever-growing menu of options for information-sharing vehicles, some of which represent significant resource investments, public health agencies have had little evidence-based guidance to support them in selecting communication channels and strategies. For example, a systematic review by Revere and colleagues (2011) identifies 25 different systems for communicating public health alerts and guidance to health care providers but notes a paucity of rigorous scientific evaluations of their effectiveness. Ongoing assessment of both traditional technologies and innovations is needed to ensure that public health authorities have the tools and knowledge they need to ensure that urgent public health information reaches target audiences and can be translated into action during public health emergencies. The review described in this chapter builds and expands on the Revere et al. (2011) systematic review.

OVERVIEW OF THE KEY REVIEW QUESTIONS AND ANALYTIC FRAMEWORK

Defining the Key Review Questions

The overarching question that guided this review addresses the effectiveness of different channels for communicating public health alerts and guidance with technical audiences during a public health emergency. To answer this question, the committee sought evidence on several sub-questions related to documented benefits and harms associated with the channels themselves, as well as the engagement of technical audiences in the development of communication plans and channels. The committee also examined the evidence on the factors that create barriers to and facilitators of effective communication with technical audiences (see Box 6-2).

Analytic Framework

For the purposes of this review, the committee developed an analytic framework to present the causal pathway and interactions between the activation of communication channels during a public health emergency and outcomes of interest (see Figure 6-1). Effective communication channels provide a conduit for the transmission of information from public health authorities to recipient technical audiences (and in some cases, allow for bidirectional exchange). The objective of such information-sharing processes is to ensure that technical audiences are aware of and understand up-to-date information about a particular public health threat. Awareness of current alerts and guidance may influence the behaviors of information recipients (e.g., changes in diagnostic testing protocols, use of personal protective

BOX 6-2 KEY REVIEW QUESTIONS

What is the effectiveness of different channels for communicating public health alerts and guidance with technical audiences during a public health emergency (e.g., Health Alert Network, conference calls, bidirectional text-based messaging/SMS, provider access line, email, website, written guidance documents)?

- What are the benefits and harms of engaging technical audiences in the development of communication plans, protocols, and channels?
- What benefits and harms (desirable and/or undesirable impacts) of different communication channels have been described or measured?
- What are the barriers to and facilitators of effective communication with technical audiences?

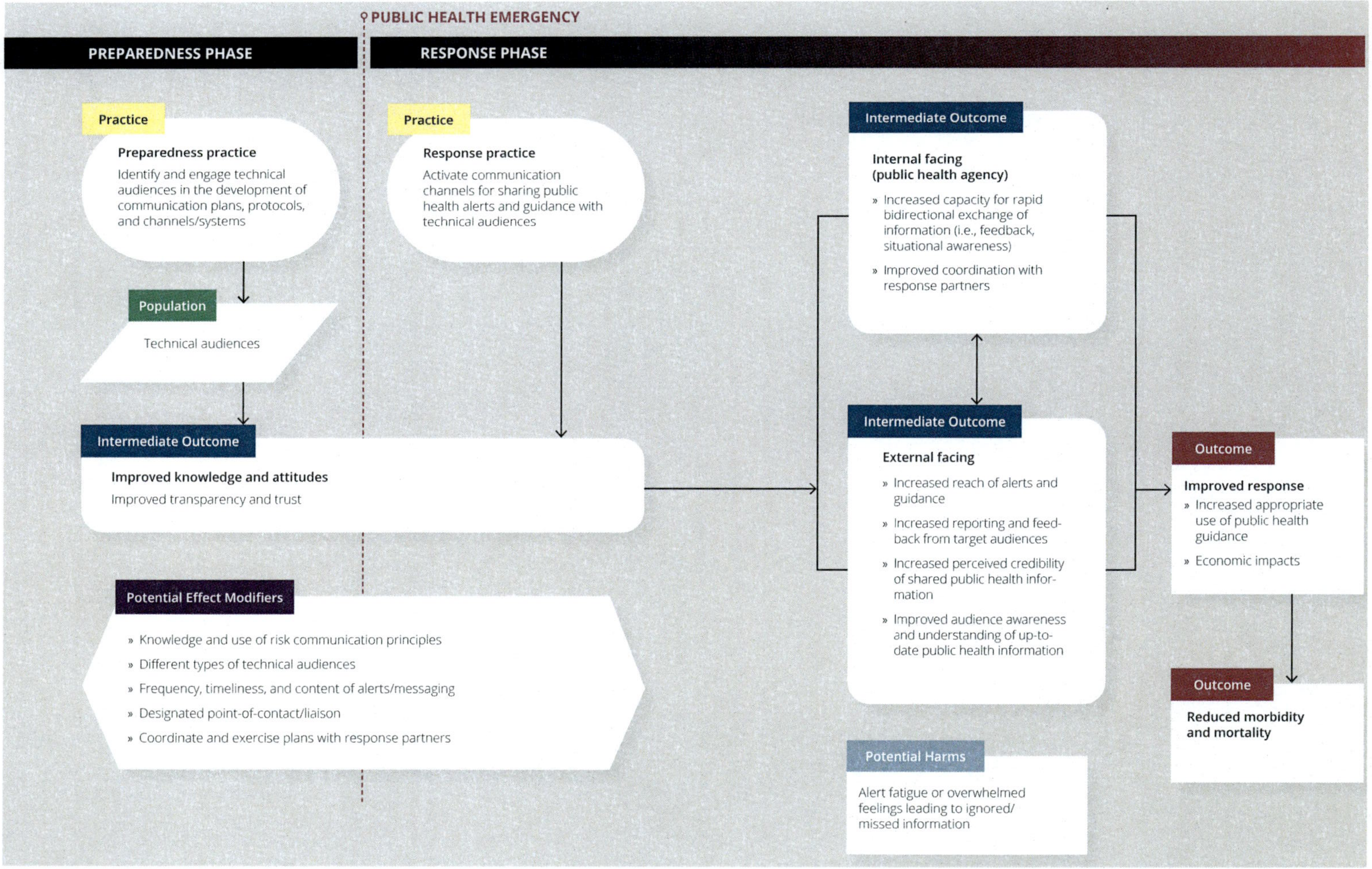

FIGURE 6-1 Analytic framework for communicating public health alerts and guidance with technical audiences during a public health emergency.
NOTES: Arrows in the framework indicate hypothesized causal pathways between interventions and outcomes. Double-headed arrows indicate feedback loops.

equipment, case reporting), which may in turn improve the response to a public health threat (e.g., through improved situational awareness and coordination of response partners) and reduce associated morbidity and mortality (e.g., by reducing or better managing infections).

Communication can be categorized as either active (push type) or passive (pull type). Active communication approaches seek to draw the attention of the target audience(s) to information being shared (e.g., emails, alerts embedded in electronic health records), whereas passive mechanisms (e.g., websites) rely on information-seeking behavior among the target audience(s). Understanding the needs and behaviors of the target audience(s) is necessary to combine active and passive approaches effectively. Defining key target audiences and a means of reaching them (e.g., contact information, alert system) in advance of a public health emergency enables more timely information dissemination.

OVERVIEW OF THE EVIDENCE SUPPORTING THE PRACTICE RECOMMENDATION[1]

This section provides a summary of the evidence from the mixed-method review examining different channels for communicating public health alerts and guidance with technical audiences during a public health emergency. Following the summary of the evidence of effectiveness, summaries are presented for each element of the Evidence to Decision (EtD) framework (encompassing balance of benefits and harms, acceptability and preferences, feasibility and PHEPR system considerations, resource and economic considerations, equity, and ethical considerations), which the committee considered in formulating its practice recommendation. Full details on the review strategy and findings can be found in the appendixes: Appendix A provides a detailed description of the study eligibility criteria, search strategy, data extraction process, and individual study quality assessment criteria; Appendix B3 provides a full description of the evidence, including the literature search results, evidence profile tables, and EtD framework for communicating public health alerts and guidance with technical audiences during a public health emergency; and Appendix C links to all the commissioned analyses that informed this review. Table 6-2 shows the types of evidence included in this review.

Effectiveness

Two quantitative comparative studies directly addressed the overarching key question regarding the effectiveness of different channels for communicating public health alerts and guidance with technical audiences during a public health emergency. Both studies evaluated types of electronic messaging systems (e.g., email, fax, text messaging) that are used to push information out to target audiences (rather than relying on target audiences to pull down information). (Refer to Section 1, "Determining Evidence of Effect," in Appendix B3 for additional detail.)

Consistent with the methods described in Chapter 3, in making its final judgment on the evidence of effectiveness for electronic messaging channels for communicating public health alerts and guidance with technical audiences during a public health emergency, the committee considered other types of evidence that could inform a determination of what works for whom and in which contexts, ultimately reaching consensus on the certainty of the evidence (COE) for each outcome. Including other forms of evidence beyond quantitative comparative studies is particularly important when assessing evidence in settings where

[1] To enhance readability for an end user audience, this section does not include references. Citations supporting the findings in this section appear in Appendix B3.

TABLE 6-2 Evidence Types Included in the Mixed-Method Review of Channels for Communicating Public Health Alerts and Guidance with Technical Audiences During a Public Health Emergency

Evidence Type[a]	Number of Studies (as applicable)[b]
Quantitative comparative	2
Quantitative noncomparative (postintervention measure only)	0
Qualitative	8[c]
Modeling	0
Descriptive surveys	8
Case reports	12[d]
After action reports	29[d]
Mechanistic	N/A
Parallel (systematic reviews)	N/A

[a] Evidence types are defined in Chapter 3.
[b] Note that sibling articles (different results from the same study published in separate articles) are counted as one study in this table. Mixed-method studies may be counted in more than one category.
[c] Two surveys containing a qualitative analysis of free-text responses were included in the qualitative evidence synthesis. The two studies were not classified as qualitative research studies and are not included in the qualitative study count for this table. As described in Chapter 3, the findings from these sources were extracted and considered separately in the qualitative evidence synthesis to affirm or question those findings from the more complete qualitative studies.
[d] A sample of case reports and after action reports was prioritized for inclusion in this review based on relevance to the key questions, as described in Chapter 3.

controlled studies are challenging to conduct and/or other forms of quantitative comparative data are difficult to obtain. Descriptive evidence from real-world implementation of practices offers the potential to corroborate research findings or explain differences in outcomes in practice settings, even if it has lesser value for causal inference. Moreover, qualitative studies can complement quantitative studies by providing additional useful evidence to guide real-world decision making, because well-conducted qualitative studies produce deep and rich understandings of how interventions are implemented, delivered, and experienced. Other forms of evidence considered for evaluation of effectiveness included findings from surveys, case reports, and AARs that involved a real disaster or public health emergency.

The evidence suggests that electronic messaging systems are effective channels for communicating public health alerts and guidance with technical audiences. There is moderate COE supported by two quantitative studies that such electronic messaging systems as email, fax, and text messaging are effective communication channels for increasing technical audiences' awareness of public health alerts and guidance during a public health emergency. However, these effects may be dampened by alert fatigue associated with excessive message volume. Additionally, awareness of alerts and guidance does not necessarily translate to behavior change. There is very low COE based on a single quantitative study that electronic messaging systems are effective for increasing technical audiences' use of current public health guidance during a public health emergency. The committee concluded that there is evidence that different technologies used as electronic messaging systems for communicating public health alerts and guidance with technical audiences during a public health emergency to increase awareness and appropriate use have differing impacts; however, data are insufficient to conclude what technology is best for which audiences in which scenarios.

Of note, some surveys, case reports, and AARs included in this review report on passive electronic messaging systems that rely on information-seeking behavior among the target audience (e.g., websites) and communication channels other than electronic messaging systems (e.g., telephone conferencing, hotlines). In the absence of comparative data from which conclusions about their effectiveness could be drawn, however, these other communication channels were not included in the committee's synthesis of quantitative evidence. While it is clear that channels other than electronic messaging systems are being used in practice to communicate public health alerts and guidance with technical audiences, the effectiveness of these channels has not yet been rigorously studied in the PHEPR context.

Balance of Benefits and Harms

Although only two quantitative comparative research studies evaluate the effectiveness or benefits of specific channels for communicating public health alerts and guidance, case reports and AARs also cite improved audience awareness and the timeliness of messaging as benefits for some communication channels, such as electronic messaging systems (e.g., fax, email, web-based alerting and surveillance systems), teleconferences, and hotlines. (Evidence source: synthesis of evidence of effect, case report and AAR evidence synthesis.)

Reported harms and undesirable impacts rarely relate to a specific communication channel but arise as a result of how communication is implemented. For example, several evidence sources note the potential for important stakeholders to be left out of the loop if excluded from the systems used to distribute messages (e.g., CDC's HAN, teleconferences) and/or if contact information is not kept up to date. Also commonly reported as undesirable impacts of public health messaging are alert fatigue and information overload (particularly when guidance is constantly changing), with potential downstream effects of loss of credibility for the public health agency and disillusionment with future preparedness and response efforts. (Evidence source: qualitative evidence synthesis, case report and AAR evidence synthesis, evidence from descriptive surveys.) Finally, one study notes that when guidance does not align with what can feasibly be carried out in practice, it may be ignored. (Evidence source: qualitative evidence synthesis. Refer to Section 2, "Balance of Benefits and Harms," in Appendix B3 for additional detail.)

Acceptability and Preferences

Email and fax have consistently been reported as preferred channels for communicating public health alerts and guidance, although published technology preferences may be outdated given the rapid pace of technology development and adoption. Recent AARs may be useful sources of more current information on preferred communication channels (e.g., webcasts, social media). Technical audiences generally prefer information from local sources (public health or health care institutional sources) or such national authorities as CDC and medical societies. Engaging technical audiences in communication strategies, providing a direct line of communication, offering opportunities for bidirectional exchange, and ensuring information reciprocity (i.e., returning results generated from information submitted by stakeholders to demonstrate the utility and value of the shared information) may improve the acceptability of and responsiveness to messaging. Tailoring guidance to specific audiences, sending just-in-time guidance, and ensuring that guidance is congruent with practice and allows sufficient flexibility in implementation may help enable the translation of information to appropriate action. (Evidence source: quantitative study evidence, qualitative evidence synthesis, case report and AAR evidence synthesis, evidence from descriptive surveys. Refer to Section 3, "Acceptability and Preferences," in Appendix B3 for additional detail.)

Feasibility and PHEPR System Considerations

Some communication channels are more feasible than others for public health agencies and technical audiences to implement. The widespread use of traditional channels (e.g., email, fax, phone calls) indicates their feasibility, but further research is needed on the acceptability and feasibility of newer channels (e.g., health information exchange–based and electronic health record–based alerting, purpose-built bidirectional surveillance and alert systems). For example, while advances in information technology may lead the public health system to examine and adopt new communication channels, the adoption of these new channels may raise concerns about adding to the burden of message volume and about the availability of needed resources, such as personal or work devices, and technical support. (Evidence source: qualitative evidence synthesis, case report and AAR evidence synthesis. Refer to Section 4, "Feasibility and PHEPR System Considerations," in Appendix B3 for additional detail.)

Resource and Economic Considerations

Resource requirements for communicating public health alerts and guidance with technical audiences include both technology costs (e.g., phones, radios, computers, servers, software platforms) and human resources. Little research has examined the cost-effectiveness of different communication channels. Many public health agencies and technical audiences already have the technology necessary for traditional communication methods, such as email and conference calls. The initial costs for some purpose-built systems may exceed tens or even hundreds of thousands of dollars, which does not include ongoing maintenance costs. However, such systems often have multiple functions of value to public health agencies, including situational awareness and surveillance. Moreover, the indirect costs of new technologies related to training and technical support need to be added to the direct costs. Designated liaisons and communication networks may help amplify messaging and build or maintain trusted relationships, but the human resource costs of these strategies need to be considered. (Evidence source: qualitative evidence synthesis, case report and AAR evidence synthesis. Refer to Section 5, "Resource and Economic Considerations," in Appendix B3 for additional detail.)

Equity

Equity issues associated with different channels for communicating public health alerts and guidance with technical audiences are rarely raised in research studies and evaluations (e.g., AARs), and represent an important evaluation gap. One such issue is access to technology, which may be a consideration with respect to rural and underserved populations. Improving relationships with technical audiences that serve disadvantaged populations could lead to more targeted and tailored information sharing during a public health emergency, which in turn could help address equity issues. (Evidence source: qualitative evidence synthesis, case report and AAR evidence synthesis. Refer to Section 6, "Equity," in Appendix B3 for additional detail.)

Ethical Considerations

In addition to the equity concerns noted above, which are often viewed as reflecting ethical values, the primary value of communication using appropriate channels is often considered to be instrumental, meaning that it is important because using appropriate channels to convey information presumably leads to better information delivery, which in turn can facilitate better decision making. In the language of ethical principles, communication using appropriate channels is important because it promotes the principle of harm reduction/benefit promotion. But problems of overcommunication (such as information overload or alert fatigue) can also occur when appropriate communication channels are used, problems that can lead to worse or delayed decisions. In addition, communication using appropriate channels has intrinsic value; that is, setting aside whether decision making is improved by better information delivery, communicating with individuals and communities in ways that are most effective for them is important to achieve transparency, which reflects the principle of respect for persons and communities. As in considering the instrumental value of using more effective channels for communication, one should remember that while communication using ineffective channels is obviously disrespectful, overloading effective communication channels is also disrespectful during crises when recipients have limited time and bandwidth. In sum, selecting appropriate communication channels is ethically important, and so is careful selection of the information to be delivered over those channels. (Evidence source: committee discussion drawing on key ethics and policy texts. Refer to Section 7, "Ethical Considerations," in Appendix B3 for additional detail.)

CONSIDERATIONS FOR IMPLEMENTATION

The following considerations for implementation are drawn from the synthesis of qualitative research studies, the synthesis of case reports and AARs, and evidence from descriptive surveys, the findings of which are presented in Appendix B3. Note that this is not an exhaustive list of considerations, and that it is important to consult additional implementation resources before implementing the practice recommendation.

Engaging Technical Audiences in the Development of Communication Plans, Protocols, and Channels

The act and process of engaging technical audiences prior to public health emergencies supports relationship building that enhances trust and facilitates understanding of institutional needs, sharing of expertise, coordination among response partners, and enhanced situational awareness. It also allows for the identification of designated points of contact that support direct lines of communication. For the development of new communication channels, a bottom-up approach to identification of system requirements may help ensure that the channel is accepted and meets stakeholder needs. Engaging technical audiences in the development of communication plans and channels also appears to help in the dissemination of public health guidance and may improve the usefulness of such guidance through advance consideration of how the guidance will be translated into actionable knowledge. Conversely, insufficient engagement of partners in planning processes may impede effective communication during emergency responses as a result of planning gaps and unclear communication channels and vetting processes, potentially raising questions about the credibility of public health information. Beyond engaging technical audiences in advance of an emergency, public health communication strategies may also be improved by soliciting real-time feedback during a public health emergency to better meet stakeholder needs. (Evidence source: qualitative evidence synthesis, case report and AAR evidence synthesis, evidence from descriptive surveys. Refer to Section 8, "Engaging Technical Audiences in the Development of Communication Plans, Protocols, and Channels," in Appendix B3 for additional detail.)

Considerations for Selection of Communication Channels

Although few studies evaluate the effectiveness of different communication channels, several provide information on considerations that might inform the selection of channels based on contextual factors, such as the level of uncertainty or urgency. Table 6-3 summarizes considerations discussed in the qualitative studies that may inform the use of different channels for communicating public health alerts and guidance with technical audiences, although it should not be considered an exhaustive list of considerations or communication channels.

Multipronged approaches featuring simultaneous or sequential use of multiple communication channels are commonly reported and may facilitate effective communication when

TABLE 6-3 Considerations for Selection of Communication Channels

Face to Face	Direct contact through in-person meetings is synchronous (i.e., allows real-time exchange of information), which allows for degrees of nuance and flexibility related to the uptake and understanding of public health guidance. In-person meetings between public health personnel and clinicians are useful, especially when there is perceived anxiety or discomfort about particular guidance.
Phone Calls	Direct contact through phone calls and teleconferences is also synchronous and is helpful for very urgent communication. Conference calls allow for collaborative, cross-agency decision making. In one example, the use of two-tiered conference calls (a triage call followed by a coordination call) expedited specific decision making for coordinated patient care decisions.
Email	Despite its limitations and regardless of situational context (emergency versus nonurgent) and message recipients (target audience[s]), email is a favored modality for receiving public health messages and has been reported as a timely way to convey information to clinicians. This is a push-type channel, generally used in the one-way delivery of alerts and guidance to target audiences. Effective email-based dissemination of alerts and guidance during a public health emergency relies on an established listserv, prepared in advance. Communication failures may result when key people are not on the list and/or the list has not been maintained with up-to-date contact information.
Fax	Fax has often been used in tandem with email. Faxes still may arrive when phone calls cannot connect.
Internet/Websites/ Social Media	Websites rely on information-seeking behavior among technical audiences (a pull-type channel). In one study, providers were as likely to seek information from Google as from the Centers for Disease Control and Prevention. Increasingly, health care providers and community-based organizations (and to some degree public health agencies) are using social media as a communication channel.
Text Messaging/ SMS	Text messaging provides rapid, in-the-field short messages, probably helpful in emergencies but not for mass communications. When information is lengthy, email appears to be better suited and preferred. Texts may also include hyperlinks to additional information to overcome the space limitation. Both public health agencies and their stakeholders note multiple values and uses as well as concerns regarding two-way public health text messaging. Use of texts may facilitate communication, for example, by readily providing "eyes on the ground" reports, short polls, and postdisaster check-in of status and availability. It also is an alternative when phone lines are out of service. Conversely, there are concerns with text messaging, including the receipt of text messages on personal phones, restrictive screen space, limited cell coverage, security, and the inability to forward messages. Texts also are not persistent and are easy to ignore. Whether mobile phones are sufficiently made available or supported by workplaces appears to be understudied.
Electronic Health Records	Use of electronic health records may enable public health guidance to arrive directly to the point of individual care. However, many issues—related to technology, resources, and compatibility with emergency guidance—would need to be considered and managed before effective implementation could occur.

adequate attention is paid to contextual dynamics (e.g., needs related to access, accuracy, coordination, reciprocity, and timeliness). The choice of a specific communication strategy needs to balance message content (emergency versus routine communications), delivery (one- versus two-way), and channel (e.g., text, email) with stakeholder preferences and technical capabilities while also mitigating the risk of message overload. The decision to use bidirectional communication strategies is complex and needs to be based on consideration of the balance of benefits (e.g., ability to receive confirmation of message receipt and information from recipients for purposes of surveillance or surge capacity awareness) and such concerns as burden; management; technology requirements; and considerations related to privacy, security, or the Health Insurance Portability and Accountability Act[2] when health-related information is transmitted to public health agencies. (Evidence source: qualitative evidence synthesis. Refer to Section 9, "Considerations for Selection of Communication Channels," in Appendix B3 for additional detail.)

Facilitating Communication with Technical Audiences During a Public Health Emergency

A recurring theme within and across different evidence sources is the challenge posed by the dynamic information environment characteristic of response scenarios. Rapidly changing conditions during response often necessitate repeated messaging to disseminate updated guidance and other public health information. Technical audiences may have difficulty tracking the most current guidance, and additional confusion and frustration may result from inconsistencies in guidance disseminated by different sources (e.g., national, state, local, institutional). Efforts to ensure clearer and more coordinated messaging can help prevent information overload, duplication of effort, and conflicting recommendations. For example, reviewing and comparing multiple guidance notifications for discrepancies is too time-consuming for technical audiences during response, so new information and differences in guidance (e.g., between that from local public health agencies and CDC or that from health care institutions and public health agencies) need to be clearly noted and explained. Including executive summaries at the beginning of informational emails and other sources may be another way to quickly highlight new, important information for technical audiences. In addition, vetting processes for the review of alerts and guidance and their distribution to appropriate target audiences need to be formally documented and shared prior to a public health emergency to minimize confusion over roles and responsibilities. Given the urgency of disseminating updated information, simplified review protocols and easily customizable alerting frameworks are essential for providing timely decision support to technical audiences.

Effective communication of alerts and guidance is dependent on access to communication platforms and contact information for target audiences. A lack of preexisting, accurate, and up-to-date distribution lists can hinder the reach and timeliness of public health guidance. Standard distribution lists with multiple types of individual contact information (e.g., cell phone, email) need to be developed and maintained for health care providers, local health departments, executive leadership, and response managers. Determining in advance which communications will need to be sent to each stakeholder based on that stakeholder's information needs and developing an automated system for delivery can ensure that targeted audiences receive the appropriate information. Maintaining these lists and systems as part of

[2] Health Insurance Portability and Accountability Act, HR 3103. Public Law 104-901, 104th Cong. (August 21, 1996).

routine preparedness activities can save valuable time during responses. Another commonly reported barrier is a lack of access to common communication platforms, such as WebEOC, across the local, state, and regional levels, and establishing these links can facilitate vertical communication. There are also cases in which communication systems fail because of either technical issues or power outages. Therefore, redundant systems are critical to ensure that technical audiences receive alerts and guidance in a timely manner.

In addition to technological systems, designated individuals and established networks can facilitate message dissemination and coordination, and in some cases may help ensure that guidance is consistent with practice. These message amplifiers might include designated public information officers (who might also be responsible for communicating information to the general public), liaisons, and institutional points of contact. These individuals may be well positioned to reach contacts in target audience institutions and to facilitate bidirectional information sharing. Although existing networks and coalitions may also enhance the dissemination of public health messages, they can be time intensive to maintain. (Evidence source: qualitative evidence synthesis, case report and AAR evidence synthesis, evidence from descriptive surveys. Refer to Section 10, "Barriers and Facilitators to Communicating Alerts and Guidance During a Public Health Emergency," in Appendix B3 for additional detail.)

A number of other strategies that may facilitate dissemination of public health information to technical audiences are discussed in individual case reports, AARs, and surveys captured in this review. The following list of these strategies, although potentially of use to public health stakeholders, should not be viewed as exhaustive, and additional evidence is needed before these strategies can be recommended as evidence-based practices:

- posting webinar highlights on relevant websites;
- sharing meeting notes after conference calls;
- leveraging media and social media to amplify message dissemination;
- routing notifications regarding public health alerts and guidance through medical societies and institutional (e.g., health care institution) communication channels; and
- disseminating talking points as an attachment to notifications so recipients can pass information along to others in their institution during in-person meetings.

PRACTICE RECOMMENDATION, JUSTIFICATION, AND IMPLEMENTATION GUIDANCE

Practice Recommendation

Inclusion of electronic messaging channels (e.g., email) is recommended as part of state, local, tribal, and territorial public health agencies' multipronged approach for communicating public health alerts and guidance with technical audiences in preparation for and in response to public health emergencies. The practice should be accompanied by targeted monitoring and evaluation or conducted in the context of research when feasible so as to improve the evidence base for strategies used to communicate public health alerts and guidance with technical audiences.

Justification for the Recommendation

The practice recommendation is based on moderate-quality evidence that electronic messaging systems are effective in increasing technical audiences' awareness of public health alerts and guidance, and substantial evidence from other sources indicating that technical audiences prefer to receive alerts and guidance through electronic messaging channels, such as email. The evidence suggests that different technologies employed as electronic messaging systems for communicating public health alerts and guidance with technical audiences during a public health emergency to increase awareness and use of appropriate guidance have differing impacts. However, the available data are insufficient to support a conclusion as to what technology is best for which audiences in which scenarios. Stakeholder preferences need to be monitored continuously as technology continues to evolve. The vast majority of the evidence relates to stakeholders from the health care field in the context of a disease epidemic, raising questions about the applicability of the evidence to other technical audiences and settings. No studies examine the communication needs or processes of tribal or territorial public health agencies. Further research and/or evaluation is needed to address these evidence gaps.

Implementation Guidance

- Engage technical audiences in the development of communication plans, protocols, and channels.
- Consider contextual factors, such as the level of uncertainty or urgency, cultural preferences, and stakeholders' technical capabilities, in the selection of communication channels.
- Establish vetting processes in advance of public health emergencies and coordinate with response partners on messaging to prevent information overload, duplication of effort, and conflicting recommendations.
- Reduce message volume when feasible, and highlight new information and any differences from previous or other existing guidance.
- Develop distribution lists in advance of public health emergencies, and ensure that contact information is kept up to date.
- Consider designating liaisons and institutional points of contact and leverage existing networks (e.g., medical societies and associations) to facilitate broad message dissemination.

EVIDENCE GAPS AND FUTURE RESEARCH PRIORITIES

Few rigorous evaluations salient to this practice have been published since Revere and colleagues (2011) conducted their systematic review. The committee identified only two quantitative studies that evaluated the effectiveness of channels for communicating public health alerts and guidance with technical audiences: one did not evaluate communication channels during a real public health emergency (Baseman et al., 2016), and the other had serious methodological limitations (van Woerden et al., 2007). Both studies evaluated a subset of electronic messaging system channels (i.e., email, fax, text). Other channels (electronic and nonelectronic) were discussed in case reports, surveys, and AARs, but no quantitative data were available from which conclusions regarding effectiveness could be drawn. More research is needed to generate evidence supporting conclusions regarding which communication channels are most effective for reaching which technical audiences in which settings. Quasi-experimental matched comparison designs have been used to evaluate other kinds of public health practices outside of the emergency context (Rabarison et al., 2015) and could be employed to measure the effectiveness of communication channels used in different locations in a real (or simulated) public health emergency. Such designs, which, for example, could be used to identify agencies that are using communication strategy X and those that are not (or identify agencies that are using strategy X but not Y and those that are using strategy

Y but not X), may be more feasible to conduct in a real public health emergency relative to a randomized controlled trial.

It is important to recognize that there are many important aspects to communication with technical audiences, of which the implementation of communication channels is just one. Beyond a focus on communication channels, research is needed to address the influence of message format (e.g., text, infographic) and content (e.g., length of messages, presentation and/or framing) on the effectiveness of communication strategies for different technical audiences. This research would optimally include an evaluation of the most effective formats and approaches for highlighting new information and guidance as information changes during the course of response to an event. Such research could be informed by targeted monitoring and evaluation (M&E) in practice settings that examined where information was going and who was using it. One such channel that could be a good candidate for targeted M&E is CDC's HAN. In their review, Revere and colleagues (2011) note very few studies attempting to evaluate whether HAN messages were received and acted on by the intended recipients. Similarly, the committee, in its review, found that only case reports and AARs briefly mentioned HAN. As HAN is a strategy already in widespread use to communicate public health alerts and guidance with technical audiences, future research on HAN could benefit from implementation science methods.

The committee found qualitative studies useful for exploring the social factors, including those that create barriers and facilitators, involved in communicating public health alerts and guidance with technical audiences. However, only eight qualitative research studies met the committee's inclusion criteria, and of those, only three were directly relevant. The result was a weak basis for the study findings based on synthesized qualitative evidence. However, the study by Khan and colleagues (2017) provided an example of a high-quality qualitative research study exploring in-depth perspectives on effective communication between public health and health care stakeholders. These authors conducted a qualitative study guided by complexity theory to explore current practices, barriers, and facilitators, and to develop a framework for promoting effective communication that could eventually be validated and implemented. A gap identified throughout the corpus of studies was the uncertainty around whether some of the intermediate outcomes examined, such as message receipt and recall, translated to action and behavior change. Khan and colleagues (2017) recognized this issue at the outset of their study. Accordingly, they closely linked their objectives to principles of knowledge translation and knowledge to action (Graham et al., 2006) to ensure that the strategies they described would also be related to a rapid knowledge-to-action cycle. It would be valuable for future efforts to focus on ways of ensuring that evaluators adhere to rigorous protocols for data collection, analysis, and interpretation for qualitative research, as such protocols can be useful in developing the program theory for a potential intervention. This is an especially critical point for such topics as communicating public health alerts and guidance when an important consideration is user preference and access to technology (see Chapter 8 for additional detail regarding methodological improvements).

Technology is continuously evolving, and research studies can quickly become outdated. The body of research studies examined by the committee demonstrated that there is a considerable time gap between the adoption of new communication technologies for use in the field and the publication of research studies evaluating those technologies. For example, although text messaging– and Internet-based technologies (notably social media) have been in use for some time, there is relatively little research looking at their use or effectiveness in PHEPR, indicating an urgent need for more research on these channels. Moreover, as new modalities for communicating alerts and guidance become available, additional research will be needed to assess their effectiveness and their acceptability and feasibility for public health stakeholders. Given that communication channels are likely to continue to evolve, this topic might be considered for a living systematic review and guideline, which offers a mechanism for continuously updating evidence syntheses and recommendations as new evidence is published (Akl et al., 2017; Elliott et al., 2017).

The vast majority of available evidence related to this practice addresses communication with health care stakeholders during infectious disease epidemics. The committee found limited evidence for other technical audiences or public health emergencies, raising questions about the broad applicability of the existing evidence. The management of Ebola cases in the United States provides a recent example of a situation in which public health agencies needed to communicate with other technical audiences. Specifically, public health agencies had to communicate with hazardous material responders, transportation agencies, and other non-traditional technical audiences to manage potentially contaminated environments (CDC, 2019). Moreover, no studies examine communication channels (simulated or real) with tribal or territorial public health agencies and technical audiences, which the committee believes is a gap in understanding the effectiveness of this practice in these contexts. Future research will need to examine differences in effectiveness and preferences across the range of emergencies, settings, and technical audiences listed earlier in Table 6-1.

REFERENCES

References marked with an asterisk (*) are formally included in the mixed-method review. The full reference list of articles included in the mixed-method review can be found in Appendix B3.

Akl, E. A., J. J. Meerpohl, J. Elliott, L. A. Kahale, H. J. Schünemann, T. Agoritsas, J. Hilton, C. Perron, E. Akl, R. Hodder, et al. 2017. Living systematic reviews: Living guideline recommendations. *Journal of Clinical Epidemiology* 91:47–53.

*Baseman, J., D. Revere, I. Painter, M. Oberle, J. Duchin, H. Thiede, R. Nett, D. MacEachern, and A. Stergachis. 2016. A randomized controlled trial of the effectiveness of traditional and mobile public health communications with health care providers. *Disaster Medicine and Public Health Preparedness* 10(1):98–107.

CDC (Centers for Disease Control and Prevention). 2018a. *Public health emergency preparedness and response capabilities: National standards for state, local, tribal, and territorial public health.* Atlanta, GA: Centers for Disease Control and Prevention. https://www.cdc.gov/cpr/readiness/00_docs/CDC_PreparednesResponseCapabilities_OctOcto2018_Final_508.pdf (accessed March 16, 2020).

CDC. 2018b. *Crisis and emergency risk communication.* https://emergency.cdc.gov/cerc/manual/index.asp (accessed May 9, 2020).

CDC. 2019. *Ebola-associated waste management.* https://www.cdc.gov/vhf/ebola/clinicians/cleaning/waste-management.html (accessed Feburary 24, 2020).

Elliott, J., A. Synnot, T. Turner, M. Simmonds, E. Akl, S. McDonald, G. Salanti, J. Meerpohl, H. MacLehose, J. Hilton, I. Shemilt, J. Thomas, T. Agoritsas, R. Hodder, and J. Yepes-Nuñez. 2017. Living systematic review: Introduction: The why, what, when and how. *Journal of Clinical Epidemiology* 91.

Graham, I. D., J. Logan, M. B. Harrison, S. E. Straus, J. Tetroe, W. Caswell, and N. Robinson. 2006. Lost in knowledge translation: Time for a map? *Journal of Continuing Education in the Health Professions* 26(1):13–24.

*Khan, Y., S. Sanford, D. Sider, K. Moore, G. Garber, E. de Villa, and B. Schwartz. 2017. Effective communication of public health guidance to emergency department clinicians in the setting of emerging incidents: A qualitative study and framework. *BMC Health Services Research* 17(1).

Merchant, R. M., S. Elmer, and N. Lurie. 2011. Integrating social media into emergency-preparedness efforts. *New England Journal of Medicine* 365(4):289–291.

Rabarison, K. M., L. Timsina, and G. P. Mays. 2015. Community health assessment and improved public health decision-making: A propensity score matching approach. *American Journal of Public Health* 105(12):2526–2533.

Revere, D., K. Nelson, H. Thiede, J. Duchin, A. Stergachis, and J. Baseman. 2011. Public health emergency preparedness and response communications with health care providers: A literature review. *BMC Public Health* 11:337.

Savoia, E., F. Agboola, and P. D. Biddinger. 2012. Use of after action reports (AARs) to promote organizational and systems learning in emergency preparedness. *International Journal of Environmental Research and Public Health* 9(8):2949–2963.

*Staes, C. J., A. Wuthrich, P. Gesteland, M. A. Allison, M. Leecaster, J. H. Shakib, M. E. Carter, B. M. Mallin, S. Mottice, R. Rolfs, A. T. Pavia, B. Wallace, A. V. Gundlapalli, M. Samore, and C. L. Byington. 2011. Public health communication with frontline clinicians during the first wave of the 2009 influenza pandemic. *Journal of Public Health Management and Practice* 17(1):36–44.

*van Woerden, H. C., M. R. Evans, B. W. Mason, and L. Nehaul. 2007. Using facsimile cascade to assist case searching during a Q fever outbreak. *Epidemiology and Infection* 135(5):798–801.

WHO (World Health Organization). 2018. *Communicating risk in public health emergencies: A WHO guideline for emergency risk communication (ERC) policy and practice.* Geneva, Switzerland: World Health Organization.

7

Implementing Quarantine to Reduce or Stop the Spread of a Contagious Disease

Implementation of quarantine by state, local, tribal, and territorial public health agencies is recommended to reduce disease transmission and associated morbidity and mortality during an outbreak only after consideration of the best available science regarding the characteristics of the disease, the expected balance of benefits and harms, and the feasibility of implementation.

Finding Statements and Certainty of the Evidence

●●●● High ●●● Moderate ●● Low ● Very Low

Finding Statement	Certainty
Quarantine can be effective at reducing overall disease transmission in the community in certain circumstances	●●●●
Quarantine can reduce the time from symptom onset to diagnosis in quarantined individuals	●●
Congregate quarantine for influenza and agents with similar transmissibility can increase risk of infection among those in the shared setting	●●●●
Quarantine can result in psychological harms among quarantined individuals, including posttraumatic stress disorder, anxiety, and anger, the risk of which increases with the duration of quarantine	●●●
Quarantine can be associated with individual financial hardship for quarantined individuals	●●●●
Emphasis on health by those leading the outbreak response (i.e., health-promoting leadership) can reduce depression and anxiety symptoms in quarantined individuals	●
While adherence to quarantine measures can vary by culture, disease, and socioeconomic status, use of various strategies, including risk communication and messaging and access to employment leave can improve adherence	●●●

Implementation Guidance

Considerations for *when* to implement quarantine

- ☑ Early on in the outbreak, especially when there is a shortage or absence of available medical countermeasures
- ☑ Only after weighing the resources required for quarantine against the expected benefits
- ☑ When the basic reproductive number (R_0) of a given pathogen is in a range in which quarantine can be expected to reduce transmission importantly. Quarantine may be more effective for a pathogen with moderate R_0, or for a pathogen with a higher R_0 that has previously produced durable immunity in a population
- ☑ When quarantine can reliably separate identified individuals from the general population for durations commensurate with the expected duration of asymptomatic infectiousness
- ☑ When the asymptomatic infectious period is short or there is no asymptomatic infectious period
- ☑ When exposed individuals can be identified reliably and quickly
- ☑ When isolation of individuals once they become symptomatic is slow or unreliable without quarantine

Considerations for *how* to implement quarantine

- ☑ Consider voluntary before legally enforced quarantine
- ☑ Avoid congregate quarantine whenever possible to reduce the risk of disease transmission among those in the shared setting
- ☑ Implement quarantine at a smaller scale before considering implementation at a large scale
- ☑ Understand the population on which quarantine will be imposed. At-risk populations will require greater consideration because of the potential for greater harms
- ☑ Allow reasonable modifications of policies to suit the needs of the situation and the people placed under quarantine
- ☑ Ensure that a legal framework is in place and develop options for different levels of quarantine that are matched to the pathogen and risk of exposure

Considerations for *during* and *after* the implementation of quarantine

- ☑ Use culturally informed approaches to quarantine, and use an orientation of care approach rather than enforcement
- ☑ Ensure transparent risk communications. Provide clear messaging on the rationale for quarantine
- ☑ Provide financial, food, and social and psychological support to quarantined individuals
- ☑ Plan for what will happen as and after quarantine measures are lifted

Context Considerations

Setting

Settings reflected in this evidence review were primarily non-U.S. settings.

Population

Populations reflected in this evidence review were primarily general public and health care workers. Some studies examined quarantine and at-risk population groups.

Emergency Phase

The evidence review included primary response phase studies.

Emergency Type

Emergencies were primarily real events, with some simulated events, and covered all infectious disease events (Ebola, influenza, severe acute respiratory syndrome, Middle East respiratory syndrome, measles, Lassa fever).

Quarantine Setting

The quarantine settings primarily reflected in this evidence review were home quarantine and health care facility quarantine, not quarantine set in some other designated facility.

DESCRIPTION OF THE PRACTICE

Defining the Practice

The committee examined the evidence for the circumstances in which implementing quarantine is effective at reducing or stopping the spread of a contagious disease. It also examined potential undesirable effects or harms associated with quarantine and factors that may mediate its effectiveness (e.g., resources, setting, enforcement). Quarantine is one type of non-pharmaceutical intervention (NPI), and falls primarily under Capability 11: Non-Pharmaceutical Interventions (NPI Capability) in the Centers for Disease Control and Prevention's (CDC's) *Public Health Emergency Preparedness and Response Capabilities: National Standards for State, Local, Tribal, and Territorial Public Health* (CDC PHEPR Capabilities) (CDC, 2018).

At the time of this writing, the nation and the world were responding to a pandemic caused by the severe acute respiratory syndrome coronavirus 2 (SARS-CoV-2) (the causative agent of coronavirus disease 2019 [COVID-19]). The committee selected quarantine as one of its four review topics using the specific process described in Chapter 3 and Appendix A. This careful topic selection process and the committee's evidence review were conducted well in advance of the COVID-19 pandemic; therefore, the evidence review did not include studies examining applications of quarantine, social distancing strategies, or other NPIs implemented specifically in response to COVID-19. However, the committee reflects on its review in the context of COVID-19 at the end of this chapter.

Quarantine is the physical separation and restriction of movement of individuals who may have been exposed to a contagious disease, who may or may not be infected but are not ill, and who may become infectious to others (CDC, 2017). Thus, individuals who are quarantined are asymptomatic and may or may not be infected or pose any danger to others. This is in contrast to isolation, which is the sequestration of individuals known to be infected with a contagious disease, who often are symptomatic.

Quarantine is an NPI that falls under the general designation of social distancing (i.e., measures intended to reduce direct physical contact between individuals to reduce the transmission of contagious diseases). The NPI Capability, and specifically quarantine, is closely linked to other CDC PHEPR Capabilities (see Box 7-1).

The types and intensity of quarantine measures can differ. The decision to implement quarantine includes the following components:

- Who—determination of which asymptomatic individuals might have been exposed to the infectious agent and whether the likelihood of exposure and the consequences of transmission are great enough to warrant separation from the community.
- Where—decisions about whether the physical separation should occur at home, in a health care facility, or in some other designated facility.
- How—decisions about whether quarantine should be voluntary or mandatory, and if the latter, how to enforce it.
- Duration—determination as to the length of quarantine, which is generally based on the incubation period (if known) of the infectious agent to which the person has potentially been exposed.

In sum, quarantine is always implemented in a target population for which infection status is unknown but in which there is some increased probability of infection due to possible or known exposure.

BOX 7-1 HOW QUARANTINE RELATES TO THE CENTERS FOR DISEASE CONTROL AND PREVENTION'S PHEPR CAPABILITIES

Capability 3: Emergency Operations Coordination—involves, in part, the facilitation of improved coordination of resource deployment by response partners involved in a public health response such as quarantine.

Capability 4: Emergency Public Information and Warning—is the ability to develop, coordinate, and disseminate information, alerts, warnings, and notifications to the public and incident management personnel, which is vital in a situation involving quarantine.

Capability 6: Information Sharing—refers to the effective interagency exchange of health-related information and situational awareness among different government agencies and other partners, including political officials and lawyers, to enact measures such as quarantine.

Capability 7: Mass Care—includes coordination with and support by public health agencies and other partners to address the needs of the population placed under quarantine at home, in health care facilities, or in other designated facilities, including meeting their mental and behavioral health needs, among others.

Capability 11: Non-Pharmaceutical Interventions—includes multiple actions that people and communities can take to help slow the spread of a contagious disease, which are used in various combinations. In addition to quarantine, other NPIs include less invasive restrictions on movement or travel, decontamination, personal protective equipment, hygiene practices such as handwashing and cough etiquette, and other protective behaviors. The NPI Capability calls for public health to engage partners on NPIs, determine which to implement, do so, and then monitor them.

Capability 13: Public Health Surveillance and Epidemiological Investigation—is used to determine who might warrant placement in quarantine and often involves reporting of events (disease cases, possible exposures) by external partners (e.g., health care, police, transportation) to public health agencies.

Capability 14: Responder Safety and Health—is the ability to protect public health and other emergency responders during predeployment, deployment, and postdeployment. During a situation involving quarantine, responders and other medical personnel may be in contact with quarantined populations. Protection and control measures are needed to protect and support these care providers.

SOURCE: CDC, 2018.

Scope of the Problem Addressed by the Practice

NPIs are often used in efforts to reduce disease transmission. For novel infections or those without effective and available treatments or vaccines, NPIs are the only means available to curb the spread of the disease (Aiello et al., 2010; Aledort et al., 2007; Love et al., 2007). NPIs have played important roles in notable contagious disease emergencies, most notably in the 1918 pandemic influenza and the 2003 severe acute respiratory syndrome (SARS) coronavirus outbreak (Markel et al., 2006, 2007; Svoboda et al., 2004). Quarantining suspected asymptomatic carriers of an illness has been public health practice for centuries (Barbisch et al., 2015; Gensini et al., 2004); the term itself stems from the practice of keeping ships at harbor for 40 days ("una quarantina") during the great plagues of Europe in an effort to prevent the spread of disease between cities. In the 21st century, quarantine has been part of the response for multiple global infectious disease outbreaks:

- The novel coronavirus COVID-19 pandemic in 2019 (ongoing at the time of this writing). In January 2020, China attempted to institute city-level quarantine in Wuhan on a historically unprecedented level, prohibiting intercity movement and severely limiting intracity transportation (Lai et al., 2020). As the virus spread globally, countries, including the United States, and localities implemented quarantine and various social distancing measures as well (CDC, 2020; Nussbaumer-Streit et al., 2020).
- The Middle East respiratory syndrome (MERS) coronavirus in 2015 in Korea and the Middle East. Quarantine was implemented along with other NPI measures, as well as use of antiviral regimens (Oh et al., 2018).
- The Ebola virus in 2014. The outbreak resulted in the quarantine of individuals and communities in West Africa and of some travelers returning from West Africa to the United States (Sell et al., 2019).
- H1N1 in Australia and China, among other countries in 2009 (Binns et al., 2010; Chin et al., 2012). Quarantine was used along with school closures in the United States (Copeland et al., 2012).
- SARS in eastern Asia and Canada in 2003. Quarantine was employed along with mass screening of travelers and other control measures (Svoboda et al., 2004; Zhang et al., 2011).
- Smaller-scale outbreaks in which quarantine was used for control, such as localized measles epidemics (CDC, 2004; Collier et al., 2013; Gahr et al., 2014; Gastanaduy et al., 2016; Sugerman et al., 2010).
- Historical outbreaks during which quarantine was implemented (e.g., 1918–1919 influenza pandemic), with available data being applied to understand the effects of quarantine and other NPIs (MacDougall, 2007; Markel et al., 2006, 2007; Sattenspiel and Herring, 2003).

Questions raised by public health emergency preparedness and response (PHEPR) practitioners as critical to the use of quarantine surround its implementation, such as deciding when to implement it, whom to quarantine, and what operational supports to institute so that the quarantine is more likely to be successful (note that "success" in this context is usually measured by determining people's adherence to the quarantine's restrictions, not by documenting reduced transmission of disease). There can be significant political pressure to implement quarantine, as was seen with the 2014 Ebola epidemic and travelers returning from West Africa to the United States (Asgary et al., 2015; Miles, 2015), and there is a potential hypothetical social value associated with the practice as a means of calming public fears during an epidemic. On the other hand, there can be pressure not to quarantine, and implementing quarantine may also contribute to public fears during an epidemic.

CDC issued the Final Rule for Control of Communicable Diseases: Interstate and Foreign[1] in 2017, which enhanced the ability to prevent the introduction, transmission, and spread of communicable diseases in the United States. Each state also has its own legal authorities over

[1] See https://www.federalregister.gov/documents/2017/01/19/2017-00615/control-of-communicable-diseases (accessed June 25, 2020).

quarantine. In January 2020, in response to the ongoing COVID-19 outbreak, CDC issued federal quarantine orders for the first time in more than 50 years (CDC, 2020). In 2017, CDC published community mitigation guidelines for pandemic influenza and concluded, based on the available evidence, that voluntary home quarantine of exposed household members *might be recommended* (CDC, 2017). More recently, the World Health Organization (WHO) reviewed the evidence and provided guidance on the use of quarantine, among other NPI measures, for mitigating the risk and impact of pandemic influenza (*quarantine was not recommended*) (WHO, 2019).

The committee considered the implementation of different types of quarantine (not just household quarantine) as a strategy for reducing the spread of any contagious disease. Some of the findings discussed in the CDC guidelines and the WHO guidelines for pandemic influenza reflect issues similar to those considered by the committee and discussed in this chapter (e.g., the effectiveness of quarantine in reducing the burden of disease, the location of quarantine, its scale). Having clear guidelines as to when quarantine should improve outcomes and how best to implement it may help public health practitioners implement this practice so as to maximize its benefits and minimize its harms.

OVERVIEW OF THE KEY REVIEW QUESTIONS AND ANALYTIC FRAMEWORK

Defining the Key Review Questions

Theoretically, the benefit of quarantine is effective curbing of the spread of contagious diseases by preventing person-to-person transmission. Therefore, the primary question posed by the committee in this review is: "In what circumstances (e.g., based on biologic factors, risks, resource availability, legal authorities, social context) is quarantine effective at reducing or stopping the spread of a contagious disease?" To answer this primary question, the committee sought evidence on several sub-questions related to evidence on the pros and cons of specific adherence strategies, the documented benefits and harms of implementing quarantine, and the factors that create barriers to and facilitators of its implementation (see Box 7-2).

The evidence review focused on those aspects of quarantine that fall primarily under the jurisdiction of public health. In evaluating the effectiveness of quarantine, however, the committee considered studies from occupational health and hospital settings. The committee did

BOX 7-2 KEY REVIEW QUESTIONS

In what circumstances (e.g., based on biologic factors, risks, resource availability, legal authorities, social context) is quarantine effective at reducing or stopping the spread of a contagious disease?

- What strategies affect adherence to quarantine?
- What benefits and harms (desirable and/or undesirable impacts) of quarantine have been described or measured?
- What are the barriers to and facilitators of effective implementation of quarantine?

not include studies in which the effect of NPIs bundled together was examined (Markel et al., 2007), and instead focused its review on trying to tease out the impact of quarantine alone. The committee did not broaden its evidence search to include practices of self-quarantine intended to avoid potential exposures beyond a contagious disease scenario, such as people who choose to shelter in place following an environmental, chemical, or radiological event to limit exposure to potential toxins or radiation. Furthermore, the committee did not include evidence examining *cordon sanitaire* and shelter-in-place and stay-at-home orders, such as those that have been implemented among various localities, states, and countries in response to the COVID-19 pandemic. While the latter encompass types of quarantine under a broad definition of the term, these strategies had not been used until recently in modern public health responses to infectious disease outbreaks. Furthermore, such actions and others, such as travel bans, are intended to restrict the movement of all people in a geographic region, regardless of individual level of exposure risk. This makes these interventions qualitatively different from traditional quarantine, which is based on an assessment of likely individual exposure.

Analytic Framework

For the purposes of this review, the committee developed an analytic framework to present the causal pathway and interactions between quarantine and its components, populations, and outcomes of interest (see Figure 7-1). The mechanism by which quarantine can ultimately reduce or stop the spread of a contagious disease is well established and noncontroversial: there is a period of time (the incubation period) between when a person is exposed to a contagious illness and when that person, if infected, becomes contagious to others; if individuals who are exposed and become infected are not in contact with anyone else at the time they become contagious, they cannot spread the infection (Drews, 2013). As a practical matter, implementing quarantine entails determining which people are at higher risk of having been infected because of exposure but are not yet showing signs or symptoms of illness and are therefore presumed not yet to be contagious, and then physically segregating these people from others for a defined period of time, usually intended to exceed the incubation period of the illness (WHO, 2019). If any of these people become ill during their time under quarantine, they will have been prevented from being in contact with those not infected and spreading the infection more widely.

Quarantine relies on a number of important assumptions regarding the biology of the contagious disease at hand (e.g., How readily transmissible is the agent? Is it transmissible during the incubation period or only after symptoms arise?). Of particular note is that the value of quarantine in preventing the spread of contagion will vary based on when during the course of infection individuals become contagious. For example, if an infected person does not become contagious until some time after symptoms of the illness emerge, the theoretical value of quarantining asymptomatic people may be reduced (because the same benefit could be achieved by monitoring for early symptoms and isolating those who became ill). By contrast, if infected people become contagious while they are still asymptomatic, the value of quarantine is potentially much greater. But such biological factors are not the only factors that can alter the effectiveness of quarantine as a strategy for reducing or halting the spread of a contagious illness; the effectiveness of quarantine is also dependent on a number of social factors, including the extent to which exposed individuals can be contacted and their subsequent willingness and ability to adhere to quarantine. The outcomes of quarantine may hinge as well on its interaction with other NPIs.

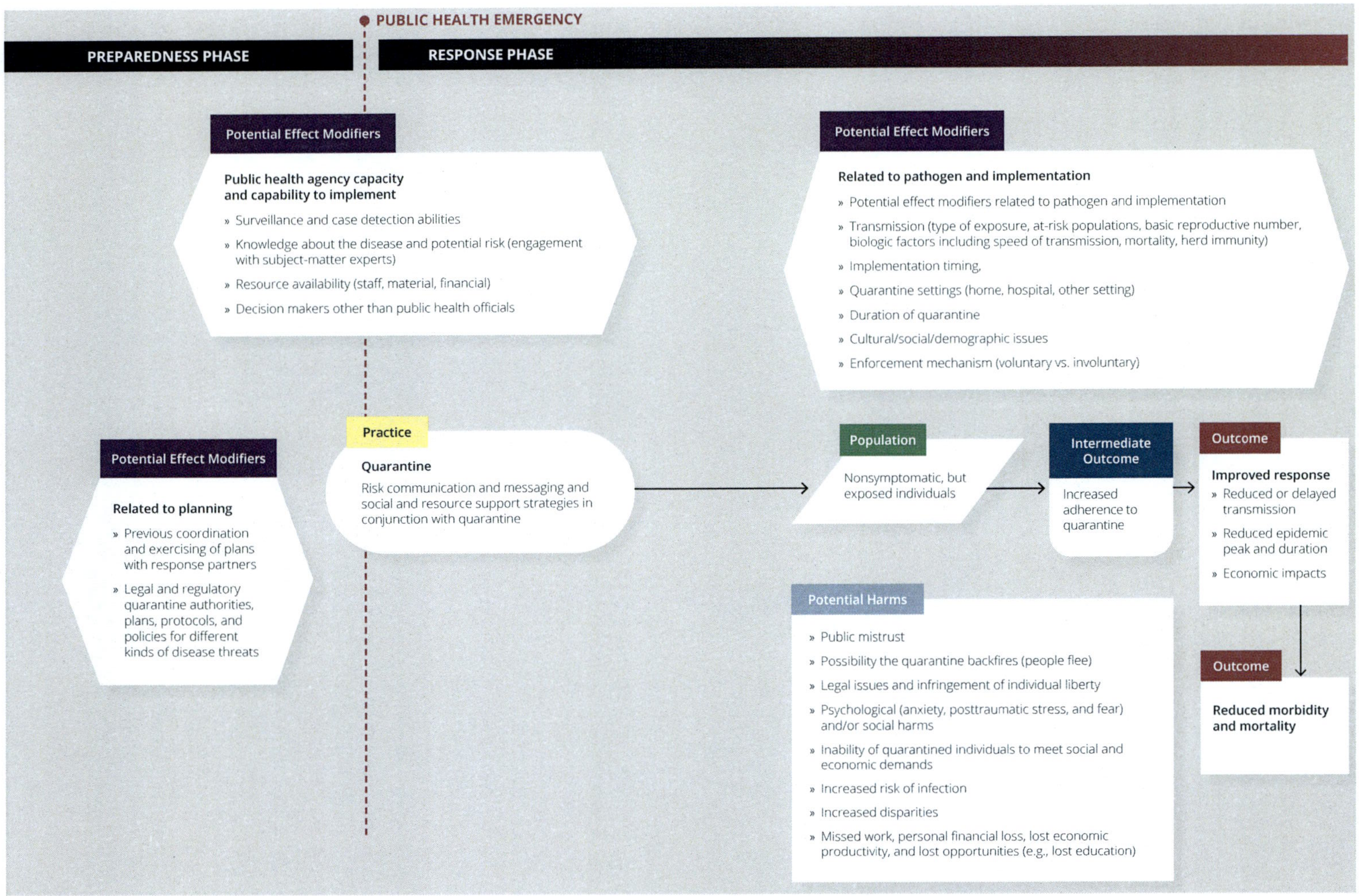

FIGURE 7-1 Analytic framework for implementing quarantine during a public health emergency.
NOTE: Arrows in the framework indicate hypothesized causal pathways between interventions and outcomes.

OVERVIEW OF THE EVIDENCE SUPPORTING THE PRACTICE RECOMMENDATION[2]

This section summarizes the evidence from the mixed-method review examining the implementation of quarantine to reduce or stop the spread of a contagious disease. Following the summary of the evidence of effectiveness, summaries are presented for each element of the Evidence to Decision (EtD) framework (encompassing balance of benefits and harms, acceptability and preferences, feasibility and PHEPR system considerations, resource and economic considerations, equity, and ethical considerations), which the committee considered in formulating its practice recommendation. Full details on the review strategy and findings can be found in the appendixes: Appendix A provides a detailed description of the study eligibility criteria, search strategy, data extraction process, and individual study quality assessment criteria; Appendix B4 provides a full description of the evidence, including the literature search results, evidence profile tables, and EtD framework for implementing quarantine; and Appendix C links to all the commissioned analyses that informed this review. Table 7-1 shows the types of evidence included in this review.

Effectiveness

Three quantitative comparative studies address the overarching key question regarding in what circumstances quarantine is effective at reducing or stopping disease transmission in the community. These three studies examine whether quarantine reduced disease transmission in response to three different contagious diseases: H1N1 pandemic influenza, SARS, and measles. Another six quantitative comparative studies and four quantitative noncomparative studies examine other potential benefits and harms of quarantine, as well as strategies that may be effective at improving adherence to quarantine. (Refer to Section 1, "Determining Evidence of Effect," in Appendix B4 for additional detail.)

Consistent with the methods described in Chapter 3, in making its final judgment on the evidence of effectiveness for quarantine, the committee considered other types of evidence that could inform a determination of what works for whom and in which contexts, ultimately reaching consensus on the certainty of the evidence (COE) for each outcome. Including other forms of evidence beyond quantitative comparative studies is particularly important when assessing evidence in settings where controlled studies are challenging to conduct and/or other forms of quantitative comparative data are difficult to obtain. Descriptive evidence from real-world implementation of practices offers the potential to corroborate research findings or explain differences in outcomes in practice settings, even if it has less value for causal inference. Moreover, qualitative studies can complement quantitative studies by providing additional useful evidence to guide real-world decision making, because well-conducted qualitative studies produce deep and rich understandings of how interventions are implemented, delivered, and experienced. Other forms of evidence considered for evaluation of effectiveness included mechanistic evidence, evidence from modeling studies, evidence from qualitative studies, and quantitative data reported in case reports that involved a real disaster or public health emergency.

The evidence suggests that quarantine can be effective at reducing overall disease transmission in the community in certain circumstances (high COE based on three quantitative studies, mechanistic evidence, modeling evidence, and case report evidence) and reducing

[2] To enhance readability for an end user audience, this section does not include references. Citations supporting the findings in this section appear in Appendix B4.

TABLE 7-1 Evidence Types Included in the Mixed-Method Review of Implementing Quarantine

Evidence Type[a]	Number of Studies (as applicable)[b]
Quantitative comparative	9
Quantitative noncomparative (postintervention measure only)	4
Qualitative	16
Modeling	12[c]
Descriptive surveys	13
Case reports	28
After action reports	N/A
Mechanistic[d]	Yes
Parallel (systematic reviews)	N/A

[a] Evidence types are defined in Chapter 3.
[b] Note that sibling articles (different results from the same study published in separate articles) are counted as one study in this table. Mixed-method studies may be counted in more than one category.
[c] The committee chose a sample of 12 studies out of 47 modeling studies for detailed review based on an assessment of their methodologic approach, data sources, relevance to the key questions for this practice, potential implications for public health practice, and disease condition studied. Given the time and resources available, the committee had to exclude a number of well-conducted modeling studies. Studies were excluded from detailed review if they reported major limitations to their model conclusions due to such factors as excessive uncertainty about modeling parameter values.
[d] For the purposes of this report, the committee defined mechanistic evidence as evidence that denotes relationships for which causality has been established—generally within other scientific fields, such as chemistry, biology, economics, and physics (e.g., the accelerating effect of the gravitational attraction of Earth and the slowing effect of air resistance)—and that can reasonably be applied to the PHEPR context through mechanistic reasoning. Mechanistic evidence is discussed further in Chapter 3.

the time from symptom onset to diagnosis in quarantined individuals (low COE based on one quantitative study, mechanistic evidence, modeling evidence, and case report evidence). However, quarantine can result in harms for those individuals on whom it is imposed, including increased risk of infection among those placed together in congregate quarantine settings[3] (high COE based on two quantitative studies and mechanistic evidence); psychological harms, the risk of which increases with the longer duration of quarantine (moderate COE based on six quantitative studies, qualitative evidence, and case report evidence); and individual financial hardship (high COE based on two quantitative studies, mechanistic evidence, and qualitative evidence). There is very low COE (based on one quantitative study and case report evidence) that an emphasis on health by those leading the outbreak response (i.e., health-promoting leadership) can reduce depression in quarantined individuals. The effectiveness of quarantine is also dependent on a number of social factors, some of which might be addressed through various implementation strategies. There is moderate COE that while adherence to quarantine measures can vary by culture, disease, and socioeconomic status, use of various strategies, including risk communication and messaging and access to employment leave, can improve adherence.

[3] A congregate quarantine setting is the sharing of the same room or facilities with an infected case. This is mainly applicable to individuals quarantined at home who fall ill and thereby increase the likelihood of another household member acquiring the illness.

Findings from a Synthesis of Modeling Studies: Quarantine Is More Effective Under Certain Circumstances

Across the 12 modeling studies considered, quarantine was found to be more or less likely to be effective depending on systematic and consistent factors related both to characteristics of the pathogen and to the population and setting (see Table 7-2). Understanding of these systematic relationships is aided specifically by one of the modeling studies included in this review (Peak et al., 2017), which contains analyses for a range of diseases and attempts to provide answers to this question within a common modeling framework.[4] (Refer to Section 2, "Findings from a Synthesis of Modeling Studies: Quarantine Is More Effective Under Certain Circumstances," in Appendix B4 for additional detail.)

Consistent with the findings of Peak and colleagues (2017), as well as the other modeling studies and the drivers of effectiveness they identify or imply, quarantine was more likely to be effective at reducing or stopping the spread of a contagious disease in the following circumstances:

- *Moderate basic reproductive number* (R_0)—when the R_0 of a given pathogen is in a range in which quarantine can be expected to reduce transmission importantly. Quarantine may be more effective for a pathogen with a moderate R_0, or for a pathogen with a higher R_0 that has previously produced durable immunity in a population (i.e., the population in question has been exposed previously) such that the effective reproductive number (R_e)[5] in the population even without intervention is relatively lower. If a pathogen has a high R_0, more transmission may occur before quarantine can be implemented, reducing quarantine's effectiveness at limiting the final size of the outbreak. As a practical matter, for pathogens with a very low R_0 (i.e., <1), disease transmission will not be sustained, making quarantine theoretically effective but perhaps practically unnecessary.
- *Shorter incubation period*—when quarantine can reliably separate identified individuals from the general population for durations commensurate with the expected duration of asymptomatic infectiousness. Quarantine may become infeasible or less effective as the result of reduced adherence if its duration must be very long because of a prolonged incubation period (the period between exposure and when infection becomes detectable).
- *Relatively short asymptomatic infectiousness period*—when the asymptomatic infectious period is short or there is no asymptomatic infectious period. When there is a long period of asymptomatic infectiousness, quarantine of recently infected people must be extremely rapid and comprehensive to prevent transmission by asymptomatic individuals, which may be so logistically challenging as to be practically infeasible. In addition, if the asymptomatic infectious period is long in absolute terms, quarantine may become infeasible or less effective because of reduced adherence (see the previous bullet).
- *Rapid identification*—when exposed individuals can be identified reliably and quickly.

---

[4] Peak et al. (2017) was selected as the scaffold for the synthesis of modeling studies because it considers factors for a range of diseases, whereas the other included modeling studies look at only one disease.

[5] Note that the pathogen's R_0 changes over time as the result of interventions and as the infection establishes immunity. The R_e (in this case in the presence of quarantine) is related conceptually to the ability of an infection to have persistent or growing prevalence in a population (when R_e is above 1, the disease will have growing prevalence; below 1, it will decline).

TABLE 7-2 Summary of Findings on the Effectiveness of Quarantine from 12 Modeling Studies

Disease	Quarantine Likely Effective?	Notes
Ebola	Yes	Two studies find quarantine can drive R_e <1[a] (D'Silva and Eisenberg, 2017; Peak et al., 2017).
Hepatitis A	Yes based on 1 study	One study finds quarantine can drive R_e <1 (Peak et al., 2017).
Influenza A/ H1N1	Maybe	Two studies. One study finds quarantine can drive R_e <1 (Peak et al., 2017). Another study focuses on delaying the epidemic peak and suggests that quarantine can possibly be effective depending on the specific features of the pathogen in the population and the level of intervention (An der Heiden et al., 2009).
Middle East respiratory syndrome (MERS)	Yes	Two studies find quarantine can drive R_e <1 (Ahn et al., 2018; Peak et al., 2017).
Pertussis	No based on 1 study	One study finds quarantine is unlikely to drive R_e <1 (Peak et al., 2017).
Severe acute respiratory syndrome (SARS)	Maybe	Seven studies. Three studies identify situations in which quarantine may not be effective in driving R_e <1, with effectiveness depending on the pathogen's basic reproductive number (R_0) in a given population (less likely with higher R_0), the likely effectiveness of isolation of symptomatic individuals as an alternative strategy, the likelihood of there being individuals who are asymptomatic but contagious and the fraction of those individuals, and the ability to quickly identify a large fraction of exposed individuals for quarantine (Day et al., 2006; Hsieh et al., 2007; Peak et al., 2017). Four studies find (or in essence assume [based on models of past limited outbreaks]) that sufficiently effective, properly scaled and targeted, or potentially dynamic quarantine policies can drive R_e <1 (Feng et al., 2009; Gupta et al., 2005; Mubayi et al., 2010; Podder et al., 2007).
Smallpox	Maybe	Two studies. One study finds quarantine is unlikely to drive R_e <1. Another study finds that early initiation of quarantine that removes a large fraction of exposed cases can likely avoid an epidemic resulting from a smallpox bioterrorism attack (Meltzer et al., 2001; Peak et al., 2017).
Measles	Yes/maybe based on 1 study	One study finds that despite measles having a high R_0, if there is a sufficient level of background immunity, it may be possible to use quarantine to end an outbreak quickly. However, with lower levels of background immunity, quarantine is unlikely to drive R_e <1 or to do so quickly (Enanoria et al., 2016).

[a] R_e = effective reproductive number (in this case in the presence of quarantine), which conceptually is related to the ability of an infection to have persistent or growing prevalence in a population (when R_e is above 1, the disease will have growing prevalence; when it is below 1, prevalence will decline).

- *To aid isolation*—when isolation of individuals once they become symptomatic is slow or unreliable without quarantine, quarantine may reduce transmission through its effects on facilitating more rapid isolation of ill and contagious individuals.

Balance of Benefits and Harms

Quarantine can be effective at reducing the transmission of contagious disease and has the possible additional benefit of reducing the time to diagnosis for infected patients who are being monitored while under quarantine. However, it also can result in a number of harms. In particular, quarantine has the potential to result in the abridging of individual or community rights of freedom, movement, and association. In addition, as noted above, there may be an increased risk of infection among those placed together in congregate quarantine settings. Quarantine can also create financial instability, social stigma, and compromised psychological well-being for quarantined individuals. Given these undesirable effects of quarantine, which can be both short and long term, the balance of benefits and harms is open to debate and should be assessed on a case-by-case basis. (Evidence source: synthesis of evidence of effect and qualitative evidence synthesis. Refer to Section 3, "Balance of Benefits and Harms," in Appendix B4 for additional detail.)

Acceptability and Preferences

Overall, the public understands and accepts the general concept of quarantine, but this understanding and acceptance is not uniform across all societies, and the acceptability of quarantine can vary depending on levels of social trust in the authorities implementing it. Moreover, fear of harms may make quarantine unacceptable in some communities. The acceptability of and preference for quarantine may differ as well across the multiple individuals and agencies that often must work together to implement quarantine, with some advocating for an emphasis on voluntary adherence and others seeking mandatory enforcement, which may include a militaristic response. In general, the evidence suggests that voluntary quarantine is more acceptable, and therefore can be more effective, than mandatory quarantine. (Evidence source: qualitative evidence synthesis, case report evidence synthesis, and descriptive survey study evidence. Refer to Section 4, "Acceptability and Preferences," in Appendix B4 for additional detail.)

Feasibility and PHEPR System Considerations

Quarantine is more effective at reducing or stopping the transmission of a contagious disease when exposed individuals can be identified reliably and quickly. To initiate quarantine in a timely manner requires accurate, up-to-date, and specific pre- and intra-outbreak surveillance, as well as preexisting organizational frameworks and linkages to rapid decision making, including an in-place legal framework. Feasibility is also related to the scale of quarantine; if quarantine is uncoordinated and implemented at an intense level in multiple geographic areas, there is greater potential for redundancy and excess effort and resource expenditures, as well as for flight of individuals beyond designated boundaries. In addition, quarantine may become infeasible or less effective because of reduced adherence when the proposed duration of quarantine is longer. Although staffing and operational capacities to implement quarantine currently exist in many agencies, operational limitations may arise when quarantine is implemented on a large scale. Home quarantine may be more feasible than providing designated facilities for quarantined individuals, but is not without concerns over such harms as increased risk of infection among those housed together and challenges with adherence. (Evidence source: synthesis of modeling studies, qualitative evidence synthesis, and case report evidence synthesis. Refer to Section 5, "Feasibility and PHEPR System Considerations," in Appendix B4 for additional detail.)

Resource and Economic Considerations

Implementing quarantine is highly resource intensive (e.g., the potential need to provide financial compensation, food, and social support). Therefore, factors that need to be considered when deciding whether to implement quarantine include resource availability, such as the ability to mobilize public health personnel to conduct contact tracing (to identify those who might warrant being placed in quarantine) and regular symptom monitoring of those in quarantine (to detect those who are becoming ill and require isolation and medical care). Resources related to the medical care of quarantined individuals include environmental decontamination, waste management, safe transportation, and availability of sufficient stocks of such supplies as masks and thermometers. Quarantine may be costly not only for response agencies but also for the individuals placed in quarantine, and has the potential to result in broad social and economic disruption. Quarantined individuals may incur both direct and indirect costs, including child care expenses and lost wages due to a lack of employer or government compensation. Thus, public health agencies need to consider the resources required for quarantine against its expected benefits. (Evidence source: qualitative evidence synthesis, case report evidence synthesis, and descriptive survey study evidence. Refer to Section 6, "Resource and Economic Considerations," in Appendix B4 for additional detail.)

Equity

People in quarantine may be publicly labeled as potential carriers of a contagious disease, which can lead others to develop toward them feelings of avoidance, suspicion, mistrust, and fear, and thus stigma. When people from already marginalized communities are quarantined, this stigmatization can exacerbate marginalization and discrimination, which can last well beyond the quarantine period.

When considering whether or how to impose quarantine on members of at-risk populations, public health leaders and agencies need to acknowledge that greater harms are likely to result for marginalized populations, creating a stronger obligation to protect them. At-risk populations can have additional needs affecting their ability to adhere to quarantine, and agencies need to consider the impact on various sub-populations based on demographics, socioeconomic considerations, and baseline access to resources. For example, potential challenges to quarantine arise when it involves transient populations such as people that are homeless, as they may be difficult to locate and monitor. Additionally, being forced to miss work can potentially exacerbate preexisting socioeconomic inequalities. The inequitable impacts of quarantine tend to be compounded over time such that the longer a quarantine lasts, the more sacrifice it requires of those being quarantined, and the more likely it is to exacerbate underlying societal, economic, and health care inequities. Finally, health care workers on whom quarantine is imposed may experience financial, social, and psychological harms, similar to those that occur to the general public; however, these harms may be amplified for health care workers for a number of reasons because of their responsibilities. (Evidence source: synthesis of evidence of effect, qualitative evidence synthesis, case report evidence synthesis, and descriptive survey study evidence. Refer to Section 7, "Equity," in Appendix B4 for additional detail.)

Ethical Considerations

When implemented correctly and in the proper setting, quarantine is ethically justified by the expectation that it will protect unexposed people from the harm of being exposed to and contracting a contagious disease—a notion that has been called the harm principle. Given this ethical justification (i.e., that quarantine prevents harm), one could say that any quarantine action that does not in fact reduce or stop the spread of a contagious disease is unethical. Of course, the problem with saying this is that one may not know whether a quarantine will be effective until it is tried. In reality, then, the core ethical obligation involved in considering whether to implement quarantine is to do the very best to determine in advance whether the quarantine will work, and to implement it in ways that will maximize its effectiveness while minimizing the extent to which it infringes on individual or group liberties and rights (principle of proportionality).

Another ethical consideration for quarantine is the need to recognize that people in quarantine are giving up their personal freedoms (whether voluntarily or not) in an effort to protect their community, and thus deserve gratitude and respect (principle of respect for persons and communities). Indeed, this consideration represents one justification for efforts to ensure that people in quarantine are well cared for, and that they do not suffer stigma later on. The other justification for such efforts is utilitarian (principle of harm reduction/benefit promotion): people who fear being placed in quarantine may flee the area, potentially spreading the contagion even farther than it might have spread without a threatened quarantine. This is not an entirely hypothetical concern; there are several real-world examples of quarantines that failed or even backfired when people threatened with quarantine fled the area. With regard to legal justifications, essentially all governments have laws and regulations that allow for the implementation of quarantine in some circumstances. In the United States, these laws are primarily at the state rather than the federal level, which means that it is important for public health professionals to be familiar with the specific legal requirements in their locality. (Evidence source: committee discussion drawing on key ethics and policy texts. Refer to Section 8, "Ethical Considerations," in Appendix B4 for additional detail.)

CONSIDERATIONS FOR IMPLEMENTATION

The following considerations for implementation were drawn from the syntheses of quantitative comparative studies, modeling studies, qualitative research studies, and case reports, as well as descriptive surveys, the findings of which are presented in Appendix B4. Note that this is not an exhaustive list of considerations; additional implementation resources should be consulted before the practice recommendation is implemented.

Facilitating Adherence to and Minimizing Harms from Quarantine Measures

Ensure Transparent and Strategic Risk Communication Using Clear Definitions

Communication strategies can increase adherence to quarantine, and frequent and transparent communication with the public is likely to ease fear and anxiety. Communication needs to take place over the full course of the event; strive to be bidirectional; and involve multiple channels, such as mass media and education campaigns via billboards and bus advertisements, and multiple sources. Effective communication will provide information about the contagious disease and the need and instructions for the quarantine measures. It is important in these communications not to arouse fear and anxiety, not to be stigmatizing, not to use terms with confusing meanings, and to include clear and consistent information about infection control and coping strategies. Anecdotal evidence shows that basic knowledge of the pathogen at hand is associated with willingness to adhere to quarantine measures and suggests that the higher the perception of risk, the more likely people are to do what they say they are going to do with respect to quarantine. Public health agencies need to consider these issues when developing communication strategies. (Evidence source: synthesis of evidence of effect, qualitative evidence synthesis, case report evidence synthesis, and descriptive survey study evidence. Refer to Section 9, "Facilitating Adherence to and Minimizing Harms from Quarantine Measures," in Appendix B4 for additional detail.)

Adapt Policy: Voluntary Versus Legally Enforced Quarantine

Some modeling studies indicate that adherence may be more likely with less strict quarantine procedures, leading to greater effectiveness. In other words, quarantine may be more effective when the people on whom it is imposed adhere voluntarily to the quarantine restrictions rather than adhering under the threat of legal enforcement, perhaps because people adhere out of an altruistic choice (of which they are proud) rather than an enforced obligation (of which they are resentful or ashamed). Another factor that may make quarantine restrictions more acceptable is allowing reasonable modifications of rules and procedures to suit the needs of the situation and those being placed under quarantine. These factors may be particularly relevant in societies that place greater value on individual liberties. In sum, while some legally enforceable quarantine strategies may be relevant in the U.S. context, more intrusive or aggressive measures may provoke greater resistance and make quarantine less effective. If quarantine is legally enforced, public health agencies need to ensure that a legal framework and a clear process for carrying out proposed enforcement measures are in place. (Evidence source: synthesis of modeling studies, qualitative evidence synthesis, and case report evidence synthesis. Refer to Section 9, "Facilitating Adherence to and Minimizing Harms from Quarantine Measures," in Appendix B4 for additional detail.)

Provide Financial Compensation, Food, and Social and Psychological Support

Factors that may make quarantine measures more acceptable include the provision of financial compensation for lost work or access to employment leave, provision of food and other basic necessities, and provision of social and psychological support by governmental or other agencies. This compensation may include partial or full income replacement for the duration of the quarantine; assurance of job security after the quarantine ends; and payment for child care, rent, water, electricity, and other utilities. The government and other agencies can deliver food and basic necessities directly to people in quarantine, or agencies can assist neighbors, friends, and volunteers with the purchase and delivery of such items. An important consideration is matching food support to the dietary needs and preferences of the people under quarantine. Social and psychological support can take many forms, including dedicated or preexisting general confidential telephone hotlines that provide professional counseling, in-person mental health services, provision of social services by local health or civic affairs departments, daycare, and community committees mobilizing for such gestures as comforting letters and prayer services. Engaging a wide range of community partners such as businesses, schools, charitable organizations, community and faith-based organizations, and mental health resources can help in preparing resources to meet potential needs in the event of a quarantine. (Evidence source: synthesis of evidence of effect, qualitative evidence synthesis, case report evidence synthesis, and descriptive survey study evidence. Refer to Section 9, "Facilitating Adherence to and Minimizing Harms from Quarantine Measures," in Appendix B4 for additional detail.)

Use Culturally and Contextually Relevant Approaches: A Community and Care Orientation

Agencies need to keep in mind that the impact of quarantine at the community level may be more important to the members of the community on which quarantine is imposed as opposed to the level of the individual or the abstract "common good." When quarantine is imposed on some individuals in a community, especially one with tight social bonds, the life of the whole community may be affected. Thus, to ensure that individuals on whom quarantine is imposed adhere to proposed restrictions, agencies need to understand the life circumstances, economic status, political history, level of trust in agencies and government, and cultural and religious customs of the community to which those individuals belong and work in cooperation with its existing power and leadership social structures. The approach adopted by agencies in their interactions with people under quarantine needs to embody care, showing concern for their needs and extending empathetic support. Such an approach stands in contrast to one that emphasizes control and enforcement. Trusted local leaders can help facilitate trust and act as liaisons between the community and district health authorities, and integrating them into response planning and allowing them to provide feedback before decisions related to public health interventions are made may promote adherence to quarantine measures. (Evidence source: qualitative evidence synthesis, case report evidence synthesis, and descriptive survey study evidence. Refer to Section 9, "Facilitating Adherence to and Minimizing Harms from Quarantine Measures," in Appendix B4 for additional detail.)

Other Implementation Considerations

The following conceptual findings inform the perspectives and approaches public health agencies could consider when implementing quarantine.

Define the Effectiveness of Quarantine More Broadly

Agencies and researchers often judge the effectiveness of quarantine from one of two perspectives: it is deemed effective (or not) either (1) if it reduces or stops the spread of a contagious disease, or (2) if people in quarantine adhere to its rules. Yet, because quarantine represents a significant restriction on individual liberty and is essentially always imposed on people who would rather not be subjected to it, at least two additional effectiveness criteria need to be considered when evaluating a quarantine action: the extent to which the quarantine measures succeed in (1) protecting the civil rights of quarantined individuals, including due process; and (2) protecting quarantined individuals from experiencing avoidable harms, including social, financial, psychological, and medical harms. (Evidence source: qualitative evidence synthesis and case report evidence synthesis. Refer to Section 10, "Other Implementation Considerations," in Appendix B4 for additional detail.)

Develop Options for Different Levels of Quarantine and Plans for Integration with Other NPIs

Agencies can enhance the effectiveness of quarantine by developing screening and monitoring criteria that allow for graded options for quarantine that are matched to the characteristics of the contagious disease at hand, its spread, and the risk of exposure. Modeling studies that explore quarantine efforts in various localities or focus differential quarantine efforts on locally exposed individuals and travelers entering an area suggest that the relative value of these efforts depends on the fraction of an epidemic or outbreak driven by local transmission versus imported cases. Local quarantine efforts can have direct and indirect spillover effects. If quarantine is used to help control an outbreak in one area, nearby areas may face fewer imported cases; hence, the need for implementing quarantine in these surrounding areas may be reduced (an example of direct spillover). Moreover, chains of such spillovers to areas not directly connected to the original area can occur, which may alter the need for or required level and speed of quarantine in these areas as well (indirect spillover). As a result, if quarantines are implemented in an uncoordinated manner in multiple areas, redundancy and excess effort and resource expenditure may occur. Additionally, modeling studies that compare quarantine with other, less invasive or intensive NPIs note that it may be possible to achieve similar levels of control using these alternatives without the potential social stigma of quarantine, its potential to cause social and economic disruption, and its potential large-scale use of resources. This may be especially true for less transmissible infections or those that have a very short or no asymptomatic infectious period. (Evidence source: synthesis of modeling studies and qualitative evidence synthesis. Refer to Section 10, "Other Implementation Considerations," in Appendix B4 for additional detail.)

Consider Implementing Quarantine Early, Especially When There Is a Shortage or Absence of Available Medical Countermeasures

At the start of a contagious disease outbreak, there may be a shortage or absence of countermeasures such as drugs and vaccines. Similarly, there may be regions in the country where the stockpile of drugs and vaccines is limited or the delivery of such supplies will take time because of remoteness. In these circumstances, NPIs, including quarantine, may be the only measures available to combat the outbreak. Modeling studies suggest that quarantine is more effective when implemented earlier in an outbreak, and even a relatively ineffective quarantine may help blunt or slow the epidemic curve, allowing more time for resources to arrive in the area. (Evidence source: synthesis of modeling studies, qualitative evidence synthesis, and case report evidence synthesis. Refer to Section 10, "Other Implementation Considerations," in Appendix B4 for additional detail.)

Integrate and Coordinate Response at the Systems Level

Multiple and often competing interests are involved in deciding whether, when, and how to implement quarantine. Agencies need to keep in mind that the planning and implementation of quarantine require interagency and multisectoral cooperation, encompassing both the legal and political systems. Planning also needs to consider the scalability of operations, as the number of people placed in quarantine may rise during the course of a contagious disease event. Robust preexisting organizational frameworks can enable efficient redirection of the resources necessary to implement quarantine. Collaborative agreements and coordinated incident command are essential for incidents involving multiple jurisdictions (e.g., civilian, military, federal, tribal). A strong sense of political will and a shared sense of urgency also facilitate the rapid establishment of command structures aimed at steering action and mobilizing relevant sectors and resources. The need for flexibility is important as well, as existing plans and predetermined control measures may need to be modified as the event evolves. Public health agencies also need to coordinate on and plan for when and how to lift quarantine measures and what will happen as and after quarantine measures are lifted. (Evidence source: qualitative evidence synthesis and case report evidence synthesis. Refer to Section 10, "Other Implementation Considerations," in Appendix B4 for additional detail.)

PRACTICE RECOMMENDATION, JUSTIFICATION, AND IMPLEMENTATION GUIDANCE

Practice Recommendation

Implementation of quarantine by state, local, tribal, and territorial public health agencies is recommended to reduce disease transmission and associated morbidity and mortality during an outbreak only after consideration of the best available science regarding the characteristics of the disease, the expected balance of benefits and harms, and the feasibility of implementation.

Justification for the Practice Recommendation

The practice recommendation is based on high certainty of the evidence (COE) that quarantine can be effective in certain circumstances, but evidence also points to substantial undesirable effects and harms. Quarantine specifically can result in increased risk of infection in congregate quarantine settings (high COE), psychological harms (moderate COE), and individual financial hardship (high COE).

The public understands and accepts the general concept of quarantine. However, concerns about undesirable effects and harms may make this practice unacceptable to some communities. Implementing quarantine effectively, especially at a large scale, is very challenging and resource intensive, and the evidence highlights several feasibility issues with respect to implementation. The evidence also highlights several strategies for improving adherence to quarantine measures, including frequent and transparent risk communication and messaging and access to employment leave (moderate COE).

The breadth of coverage across the studies included in this review is reasonably good, and overall findings are unlikely to be overly influenced by a focus on a single pathogen or population, strengthening the conclusions that can be drawn from those findings. Whether the evidence is applicable to diseases beyond those in which quarantine has been evaluated depends on many factors, including the characteristics of a disease's transmission and the circumstances of the outbreak.

Implementation Guidance

Considerations for *when* to implement quarantine:

- Early on in the outbreak, especially when there is a shortage or absence of available medical countermeasures.
- Only after weighing the resources (e.g., cost, staffing for contact tracing and monitoring) required for quarantine against the expected benefits.
- When the basic reproductive number (R_0) of a given pathogen is in a range in which quarantine can be expected to reduce transmission importantly. Quarantine may be more effective for a pathogen with a moderate R_0, or for a pathogen with a higher R_0 that has previously produced durable immunity in a population (i.e., the population in question has been exposed previously) such that the effective reproductive number (R_e) in the population even without intervention is relatively lower.
- When quarantine can reliably separate identified individuals from the general population for durations commensurate with the expected duration of asymptomatic infectiousness.
- When the asymptomatic infectious period is short or there is no asymptomatic infectious period. When there is a long period of asymptomatic infectiousness, quarantine of recently infected people must be extremely rapid and comprehensive to prevent transmission by asymptomatic individuals, which may be so logistically challenging as to be practically infeasible.
- When exposed individuals can be identified reliably and quickly.
- When isolation of individuals once they become symptomatic is slow or unreliable without quarantine.

Considerations for *how* to implement quarantine:

- Consider voluntary before legally enforced quarantine.
- Avoid congregate quarantine whenever possible to reduce the risk of disease transmission among those in the shared setting.
- Implement quarantine at a smaller scale before considering implementation at a large scale.
- Understand the population on which quarantine will be imposed, and consider that at-risk populations will require greater consideration because of the potential for greater harms.
- Allow reasonable modifications of rules and procedures to suit the needs of the situation and the people placed under quarantine.
- Consider the outcomes of protection of civil rights and protection from avoidable harms in addition to reduced disease transmission.
- Ensure that a legal framework is in place, and develop options for different levels of quarantine that are matched to the characteristics of the pathogen and based on the risk of exposure.

Considerations for *during* and *after* the implementation of quarantine:

- Use culturally and contextually informed approaches to quarantine, keeping in mind the community perspective and an orientation of care rather than enforcement.
- Ensure transparent and strategic risk communications, providing clear messaging on the rationale for quarantine.
- Provide financial compensation, food, and social and psychological support to quarantined individuals.
- Plan for what will happen as and after quarantine measures are lifted.

EVIDENCE GAPS AND FUTURE RESEARCH PRIORITIES

The committee noted several design limitations in the studies included in this review that could be addressed in future research. There have been few quantitative comparative studies of when quarantine is effective at reducing the spread of contagious disease, and of these, some relied on inadequate outcome measures; for example, the use of rapid diagnostic testing and clinical diagnosis rather than laboratory-confirmed disease may have resulted in greatly underestimated numbers of infections. Several of the quantitative studies of quarantine evaluated effectiveness only with regard to adherence (an intermediate outcome, measuring the effectiveness of implementation) and not with regard to the effects of quarantine on the course of the outbreak. Whenever possible, it is important for studies to include measures of the impact of quarantine on the outbreak. Additionally, the authors of some studies of effectiveness do not report whether any of the quarantined individuals ended up infected. This is an essential outcome to report since a quarantine that sequesters only healthy people is, by definition, ineffective at reducing disease transmission. Because it is difficult to evaluate quarantine using randomized controlled trials, researchers need to ensure that robust data are used in any future experimental studies.

During a pandemic, CDC has advised public health agencies (including the agency itself) to carry out monitoring and evaluation (M&E) of NPIs and collect data on

- the degree of transmission and the severity of the pandemic;
- the type and extent of NPI implementation;
- the level of adherence to NPI measures, the emergence of intervention fatigue, and the effectiveness of NPIs in mitigating a pandemic's impact (e.g., effects on virus transmission, hospitalizations, and deaths); and
- secondary negative effects of NPIs and the effectiveness of strategies for mitigating those effects (Qualls et al., 2017).

To capture these data, M&E systems, capacities, and capabilities need to be established before a pandemic occurs. Quasi-experimental designs could make use of these data to evaluate the effectiveness of quarantine.

In addition to measuring the impact of quarantine on the spread of illness and studying metrics related to the effectiveness of implementation (adherence), quarantine needs to be recognized as reflecting an infringement of basic human rights of freedom of movement and association. Accordingly, it is important to incorporate at least two additional outcomes into evaluations of quarantine actions: the extent to which the quarantine procedures succeed in (1) protecting the civil rights of quarantined individuals, including due process; and (2) protecting quarantined individuals from experiencing avoidable harms (including social, financial, mental health, and medical harms). Finally, because quarantine tends to affect many people in a community, not just those who are quarantined, the impact of implementing a quarantine on a community, and even states or the country as a whole, needs to be examined. In its review, the committee considered outcomes related to both psychological and financial harms. Many of the quantitative studies that addressed these outcomes were of poor methodological quality—they used a cross-sectional survey design, had sample size limitations, were conducted months after the implementation of quarantine (i.e., post-intervention), and used scales that may not have been validated. Future research on the secondary effects of quarantine, including harms, will need to apply more rigorous methods.

Future studies also will need to clearly define the quarantine protocol used and its components (e.g., type of quarantine, type of support provided, types of resources required). One challenge with reviewing evidence on quarantine is that NPIs are often implemented in bundles. Studies examining quarantine in real circumstances or in models often include effects from screening and isolation; vaccination programs (if possible); and social distancing or other behavioral changes, such as avoiding public transit, wearing masks, and increasing handwashing. The multifaceted nature of NPI use in real-world implementation makes it difficult to discern the specific impact of quarantine. Research on quarantine could benefit from advances in the study of complex interventions in the fields of health care and humanitarian aid (see Chapter 8 for additional detail regarding methodological improvements).

Much of the evidence on the effectiveness of quarantine is reliant on mathematical and statistical modeling and simulation studies. The committee found modeling studies using empirical data from actual outbreaks to be particularly useful. Real-time, rapid modeling during an outbreak or epidemic has proven valuable in guiding decision making during response (Rivers et al., 2019), and further efforts to expand the capability for and coordination and use of such real-time modeling would be helpful. Additional modeling research focused on identifying the impact on the effectiveness of quarantine of the pathogen involved, the host (if an animal vector), and population differences would also be beneficial.

As previously noted, many questions regarding quarantine relate to its implementation. The qualitative literature is useful in examining the barriers to and facilitators of the implementation of quarantine, but additional qualitative research is warranted to describe specific aspects of quarantine from the perspectives of both the agencies that implement it and the people on whom it is imposed. As multiple, and often competing, interests (e.g., political, the public) are involved in quarantine decision making, analysis and synthesis of findings from individual media reports could be informative. Indeed, a recent WHO guideline on emergency risk communications reflects the incorporation of a synthesis of media reports into the review on which the guideline is based (WHO, 2017). In addition, no studies included in the committee's review examined quarantine (simulated or real) implemented by tribal or territorial public health agencies or imposed upon those populations, which the committee believes is a significant gap in understanding the effectiveness of quarantine in these contexts. It will be important for future qualitative research to make a point of seeking out best practices in these areas. Moreover, there is a need for greater investment in implementation science methods and approaches for evaluating aspects of quarantine implementation.

Quarantine and the COVID-19 Pandemic

In response to COVID-19, states and localities have been implementing combinations of various NPIs, such as social distancing, cancellation of mass gatherings, school and business closures, isolation and quarantine, and shelter-in-place and stay-at-home orders, among others, at different intensities and speeds. At the time of this writing, WHO and CDC were recommending 14 days of quarantine for individuals having had close contact with a confirmed COVID-19 case (Jernigan, 2020; WHO, 2020). This duration was based on the virus's estimated incubation period. The committee concluded that many of the findings from its mixed-method review are transferrable to COVID-19, as the evidence was drawn from a number of different quarantine episodes, including similar severe coronavirus outbreaks (SARS and MERS).

Since the onset of the COVID-19 pandemic, several rapid reviews of the evidence have examined the effectiveness of quarantine alone or in combination with other public health measures, adherence to quarantine, and the psychological impact of quarantine (Brooks et al., 2020; Nussbaumer-Streit et al., 2020; Webster et al., 2020). Findings from these rapid reviews are consistent with those of the committee's review. Findings from a Cochrane review examining the effectiveness of quarantine during severe coronavirus outbreaks (which included 10 modeling studies on COVID-19) indicate that quarantine is important in reducing disease incidence and mortality and that early implementation of quarantine is important to ensuring its effectiveness (Nussbaumer-Streit et al., 2020). Webster and colleagues (2020) examined the published literature on reasons for and factors associated with adherence to quarantine and found that the main factors associated with adherence were the knowledge people had about the disease and quarantine procedures, social norms, perceived benefits and risks, and such practical issues as running out of supplies or financial consequences. A rapid review of the evidence on the psychological impacts of quarantine found that quarantine results in posttraumatic stress symptoms, confusion, and anger and that to reduce the psychological impacts, officials should quarantine individuals for no longer than required, provide a clear rationale for quarantine and information about protocols, and ensure the provision of sufficient supplies (Brooks et al., 2020). Brooks and colleagues also note that quarantine may have long-lasting psychological effects.

Given the rapid and evolving nature of the COVID-19 pandemic and the speed with which new studies are being published on non-peer-reviewed, preprint servers, the committee was unable to update its evidence review at the time of this writing to incorporate studies examining the implementation of quarantine as applied to COVID-19. Additionally, given that China was the first country to observe the novel coronavirus, relevant published data are more widely available from China, which implemented sweeping control measures, such as *cordon sanitaire,* that were beyond the scope of this review. However, it will be important to expand and update this review of quarantine once the field has rigorously collected, analyzed, and published such data.

The COVID-19 pandemic, like past epidemics, has illustrated gaps and themes related to designing and rapidly executing scientific research specifically on quarantine during the response phase. Chapter 8 addresses the importance of having in place in nonemergency times the infrastructure needed to be able to identify research priorities and support the deployment of rapid response teams with applied research expertise during a public health emergency. Perhaps not surprisingly, mathematical and statistical modeling, epidemiological models, and simulation studies have dominated the research on quarantine, further emphasizing the importance of continuing to improve review methodologies to evaluate and incorporate these types of studies into reviews of the evidence. As different geographic areas have been implementing quarantine and other NPIs in various combinations and at different intensities and speeds, comparing the effectiveness of these strategies (e.g., by using a matched comparison group design; see Chapter 8 for additional detail) will help inform preparedness and response efforts for future pandemics. Additionally, as a complement to effectiveness research, qualitative research is vital for understanding and capturing the social responses to and implications of quarantine and this pandemic.

Many of the issues discussed in the committee's review, including the timing of quarantine implementation; voluntary versus mandatory enforcement of quarantine; harms of quarantine; communication strategies; and financial, food, social, and psychological support for quarantined individuals, will require further examination in the context of the COVID-19 pandemic. A critical research gap highlighted by the pandemic is evidence on when and how to lift quarantine measures. During and following the COVID-19 pandemic, it will be crucial to coordinate research efforts to ensure that the priority questions related to quarantine are answered with appropriate and rigorous methods.

REFERENCES

References marked with an asterisk (*) are formally included in the mixed-method review. The full reference list of articles included in the mixed-method review can be found in Appendix B4.

*Ahn, I., S. Heo, S. Ji, K. H. Kim, T. Kim, E. J. Lee, J. Park, and K. Sung. 2018. Investigation of nonlinear epidemiological models for analyzing and controlling the MERS outbreak in Korea. *Journal of Theoretical Biology* 437:17–28.

Aiello, A. E., R. M. Coulborn, T. J. Aragon, M. G. Baker, B. B. Burrus, B. J. Cowling, A. Duncan, W. Enanoria, M. P. Fabian, Y. H. Ferng, E. L. Larson, G. M. Leung, H. Markel, D. K. Milton, A. S. Monto, S. S. Morse, J. A. Navarro, S. Y. Park, P. Priest, S. Stebbins, A. M. Stern, M. Uddin, S. F. Wetterhall, and C. J. Vukotich, Jr. 2010. Research findings from nonpharmaceutical intervention studies for pandemic influenza and current gaps in the research. *American Journal of Infection Control* 38(4):251–258.

Aledort, J. E., N. Lurie, J. Wasserman, and S. A. Bozzette. 2007. Non-pharmaceutical public health interventions for pandemic influenza: An evaluation of the evidence base. *BMC Public Health* 7:208.

*An der Heiden, M., U. Buchholz, G. Krause, G. Kirchner, H. Claus, and W. H. Haas. 2009. Breaking the waves: Modelling the potential impact of public health measures to defer the epidemic peak of novel influenza A/H1N1. *PLOS ONE* 4(12):e8356.

Asgary, R., J. A. Pavlin, J. A. Ripp, R. Reithinger, and C. S. Polyak. 2015. Ebola policies that hinder epidemic response by limiting scientific discourse. *American Journal of Tropical Medicine & Hygiene* 92(2):240–241.

*Barbisch, D., K. L. Koenig, and F. Y. Shih. 2015. Is there a case for quarantine? Perspectives from SARS to Ebola. *Disaster Medicine and Public Health Preparedness* 9(5):547–553.

*Binns, P. L., V. Sheppeard, and M. P. Staff. 2010. Isolation and quarantine during pandemic (H1N1) 2009 influenza in NSW: The operational experience of public health units. *New South Wales Public Health Bulletin* 21(1–2):10–15.

Brooks, S. K., R. K. Webster, L. E. Smith, L. Woodland, S. Wessely, N. Greenberg, and G. J. Rubin. 2020. The psychological impact of quarantine and how to reduce it: Rapid review of the evidence. *The Lancet* 395(10227):912–920.

*CDC (Centers for Disease Control and Prevention). 2004. Postexposure prophylaxis, isolation, and quarantine to control an import-associated measles outbreak—Iowa, 2004. *Morbidity and Mortality Weekly Report* 53(41):969–971.

CDC. 2017. *Quarantine and isolation.* https://www.cdc.gov/quarantine/index.html (accessed January 21, 2020).

CDC. 2018. *Public health emergency preparedness and response capabilities: National standards for state, local, tribal, and territorial public health.* Atlanta, GA: Centers for Disease Control and Prevention. https://www.cdc.gov/cpr/readiness/00_docs/CDC_PreparednesResponseCapabilities_OctOcto2018_Final_508.pdf (accessed March 19, 2020).

CDC. 2020. *CDC issues federal quarantine order to repatriated U.S. citizens at March Air Reserve Base.* https://www.cdc.gov/media/releases/2020/s0131-federal-quarantine-march-air-reserve-base.html (accessed May 21, 2020).

Chin, B. S., Y. T. Chae, H. K. Choi, J. H. Baek, S. J. Jin, S. Y. Shin, S. H. Han, J. Y. Choi, C. O. Kim, Y. G. Song, S. H. Jeong, and J. M. Kim. 2012. Viral shedding of 2009 pandemic H1N1 and evaluation of quarantine recommendations. *Japanese Journal of Infectious Diseases* 65(2):105–110.

*Collier, M. G., A. Cierzniewski, T. Duszynski, C. Munson, M. Wenger, B. Beard, R. Gentry, J. Duwve, P. K. Kutty, and P. Pontones. 2013. Measles outbreak associated with international travel, Indiana, 2011. *Journal of the Pediatric Infectious Diseases Society* 2(2):110–118.

Copeland, D. L., R. Basurto-Davila, W. Chung, A. Kurian, D. B. Fishbein, P. Szymanowski, J. Zipprich, H. Lipman, M. S. Cetron, M. I. Meltzer, and F. Averhoff. 2012. Effectiveness of a school district closure for pandemic influenza A (H1N1) on acute respiratory illnesses in the community: A natural experiment. *Clinical Infectious Diseases* 56(4):509–516.

*Day, T., A. Park, N. Madras, A. Gumel, and J. Wu. 2006. When is quarantine a useful control strategy for emerging infectious diseases? *American Journal of Epidemiology* 163(5):479–485.

*Drews, K. 2013. A brief history of quarantine. *The Virginia Tech Undergraduate Historical Review* 2. http://doi.org/10.21061/vtuhr.v2i0.16.

*D'Silva, J. P., and M. C. Eisenberg. 2017. Modeling spatial invasion of Ebola in West Africa. *Journal of Theoretical Biology* 428:65–75.

*Enanoria, W. T., F. Liu, J. Zipprich, K. Harriman, S. Ackley, S. Blumberg, L. Worden, and T. C. Porco. 2016. The effect of contact investigations and public health interventions in the control and prevention of measles transmission: A simulation study. *PLOS ONE* 11(12):e0167160.

*Feng, Z., Y. Yang, D. Xu, P. Zhang, M. M. McCauley, and J. W. Glasser. 2009. Timely identification of optimal control strategies for emerging infectious diseases. *Journal of Theoretical Biology* 259(1):165–171.

*Gahr, P., A. S. DeVries, G. Wallace, C. Miller, C. Kenyon, K. Sweet, K. Martin, K. White, E. Bagstad, C. Hooker, G. Krawczynski, D. Boxrud, G. Liu, P. Stinchfield, J. LeBlanc, C. Hickman, L. Bahta, A. Barskey, and R. Lynfield. 2014. An outbreak of measles in an undervaccinated community. *Pediatrics* 134(1):e220–e228.

*Gastanaduy, P. A., J. Budd, N. Fisher, S. B. Redd, J. Fletcher, J. Miller, D. J. McFadden, 3rd, J. Rota, P. A. Rota, C. Hickman, B. Fowler, L. Tatham, G. S. Wallace, S. de Fijter, A. Parker Fiebelkorn, and M. DiOrio. 2016. A measles outbreak in an underimmunized Amish community in Ohio. *New England Journal of Medicine* 375(14):1343–1354.

Gensini, G. F., M. H. Yacoub, and A. A. Conti. 2004. The concept of quarantine in history: From plague to SARS. *Journal of Infection* 49(4):257–261.

*Gupta, A. G., C. A. Moyer, and D. T. Stern. 2005. The economic impact of quarantine: SARS in Toronto as a case study. *Journal of Infection* 50(5):386–393.

*Hsieh, Y. H., C. C. King, C. W. Chen, M. S. Ho, S. B. Hsu, and Y. C. Wu. 2007. Impact of quarantine on the 2003 SARS outbreak: A retrospective modeling study. *Journal of Theoretical Biology* 244(4):729–736.

Jernigan, D. B. 2020. Update: Public health response to the coronavirus disease 2019 outbreak—United States. *Morbidity and Mortality Weekly Report* 69(8):216–219.

Lai, S., N. W. Ruktanonchai, L. Zhou, O. Prosper, W. Luo, J. R. Floyd, A. Wesolowski, M. Santillana, C. Zhang, X. Du, H. Yu, and A. J. Tatem. 2020. Effect of non-pharmaceutical interventions to contain COVID-19 in China. *Nature.* https://doi.org/10.1038/s41586-020-2293-x.

Love, E. G., K. N. Reed-Hirsch, and L. J. Kilborn. 2007. The role of nonpharmaceutical interventions during a pandemic. *Texas Medicine* 103(10):42–44.

MacDougall, H. 2007. Toronto's health department in action: Influenza in 1918 and SARS in 2003. *Journal of the History of Medicine & Allied Sciences* 62(1):56–89.

Markel, H., A. M. Stern, J. A. Navarro, J. R. Michalsen, A. S. Monto, and C. DiGiovanni. 2006. Nonpharmaceutical influenza mitigation strategies, U.S. communities, 1918–1920 pandemic. *Emerging Infectious Diseases* 12(12):1961–1964.

Markel, H., H. B. Lipman, J. A. Navarro, A. Sloan, J. R. Michalsen, A. M. Stern, and M. S. Cetron. 2007. Nonpharmaceutical interventions implemented by US cities during the 1918–1919 influenza pandemic. *Journal of the American Medical Association* 298(6):644–654.

*Meltzer, M. I., I. Damon, J. W. LeDuc, and J. D. Millar. 2001. Modeling potential responses to smallpox as a bioterrorist weapon. *Emerging Infectious Diseases* 7(6):959–969.

Miles, S. H. 2015. Kaci Hickox: Public health and the politics of fear. *American Journal of Bioethics* 15(4):17–19.

*Mubayi, A., C. K. Zaleta, M. Martcheva, and C. Castillo-Chavez. 2010. A cost-based comparison of quarantine strategies for new emerging diseases. *Mathematical Biosciences & Engineering* 7(3):687–717.

Nussbaumer-Streit, B., V. Mayr, A. I. Dobrescu, A. Chapman, E. Persad, I. Klerings, G. Wagner, U. Siebert, C. Christof, C. Zachariah, and G. Gartlehner. 2020. Quarantine alone or in combination with other public health measures to control COVID 19: A rapid review. *Cochrane Database of Systematic Reviews* 4(CD013574). doi: 10.1002/14651858.CD013574.

Oh, M.-D., W. B. Park, S.-W. Park, P. G. Choe, J. H. Bang, K.-H. Song, E. S. Kim, H. B. Kim, and N. J. Kim. 2018. Middle East Respiratory Syndrome: What we learned from the 2015 outbreak in the Republic of Korea. *The Korean Journal of Internal Medicine* 33(2):233–246.

*Peak, C. M., L. M. Childs, Y. H. Grad, and C. O. Buckee. 2017. Comparing nonpharmaceutical interventions for containing emerging epidemics. *Proceedings of the National Academy of Sciences of the United States of America* 114(15):4023–4028.

*Podder, C. N., A. B. Gumel, C. S. Bowman, and R. G. McLeod. 2007. Mathematical study of the impact of quarantine, isolation and vaccination in curtailing an epidemic. *Journal of Biological Systems* 15(02):185–202.

Qualls, N., A. Levitt, N. Kanade, N. Wright-Jegede, S. Dopson, M. Biggerstaff, C. Reed, and A. Uzicanin. 2017. Community mitigation guidelines to prevent pandemic influenza—United States, 2017. *Morbidity and Mortality Weekly Report* 66:1–34. http://dx.doi.org/10.15585/mmwr.rr6601a1external icon.

Rivers, C., J.-P. Chretien, S. Riley, J. A. Pavlin, A. Woodward, D. Brett-Major, I. Maljkovic Berry, L. Morton, R. G. Jarman, M. Biggerstaff, M. A. Johansson, N. G. Reich, D. Meyer, M. R. Snyder, and S. Pollett. 2019. Using "outbreak science" to strengthen the use of models during epidemics. *Nature Communications* 10(1):3102.

Sattenspiel, L., and D. A. Herring. 2003. Simulating the effect of quarantine on the spread of the 1918–19 flu in central Canada. *Bulletin of Mathematical Biology* 65(1):1–26.

Sell, T. K., M. P. Shearer, D. Meyer, M. Leinhos, E. G. Carbone, and E. Thomas. 2019. Influencing factors in the development of state-level movement restriction and monitoring policies in response to Ebola, United States, 2014–15. *Health Security* 17(5):364–371.

Sugerman, D. E., A. E. Barskey, M. G. Delea, I. R. Ortega-Sanchez, D. Bi, K. J. Ralston, P. A. Rota, K. Waters-Montijo, and C. W. Lebaron. 2010. Measles outbreak in a highly vaccinated population, San Diego, 2008: Role of the intentionally undervaccinated. *Pediatrics* 125(4):747–755.

Svoboda, T., B. Henry, L. Shulman, E. Kennedy, E. Rea, W. Ng, T. Wallington, B. Yaffe, E. Gournis, E. Vicencio, S. Basrur, and R. H. Glazier. 2004. Public health measures to control the spread of the severe acute respiratory syndrome during the outbreak in Toronto. *New England Journal of Medicine* 350(23):2352–2361.

Webster, R. K., S. K. Brooks, L. E. Smith, L. Woodland, S. Wessely, and G. J. Rubin. 2020. How to improve adherence with quarantine: Rapid review of the evidence. *Public Health* 182:163–169.

WHO (World Health Organization). 2017. *Communicating risk in public health emergencies.* Geneva, Switzerland: World Health Organization. https://apps.who.int/iris/bitstream/handle/10665/259807/9789241550208-eng.pdf;jsessionid=E5F98FC8DA6FB72F155C32FD528A7955?sequence=2 (accessed March 19, 2020).

WHO. 2019. *Non-pharmaceutical public health measures for mitigating the risk and impact of epidemic and pandemic influenza.* Geneva, Switzerland: World Health Organization. https://apps.who.int/iris/bitstream/handle/10665/329438/9789241516839-eng.pdf?ua=1 (accessed March 19, 2020).

WHO. 2020. *Considerations for quarantine of individuals in the context of containment for coronavirus disease (COVID-19).* Geneva, Switzerland: World Health Organization. www.who.int/internal-publications-detail/considerations-for-quarantineof-individuals-in-the-context-of-containment-for-coronavirusdisease-(covid-19) (accessed May 7, 2020).

Zhang, Y., P. Yang, S. Liyanage, H. Seale, Y. Deng, X. Pang, L. Tian, B. Liu, L. Zhang, and Q. Wang. 2011. The characteristics of imported cases and the effectiveness of outbreak control strategies of pandemic influenza A (H1N1) in China. *Asia Pacific Journal of Public Health* 24(6):932–939.

8

Improving and Expanding the Evidence Base for Public Health Emergency Preparedness and Response

As described in preceding chapters, despite investments in public health emergency preparedness and response (PHEPR) research in the past two decades, the corresponding PHEPR evidence base remains limited (Carbone and Thomas, 2018). Figure 8-1 shows the study design distribution of all articles included in a committee-commissioned scoping review focused on the 15 PHEPR Capabilities (see Chapter 2 and Appendix D for additional detail on the commissioned scoping review). Among the 1,692 articles included, approximately 35 percent were classified as opinion, concept, or position papers or literature reviews, while 65 percent reflected some form of systematic data collection and analysis that could potentially provide evidence regarding 1 of the 15 PHEPR Capabilities. The most common study design category was quantitative nonimpact studies, which accounted for 33 percent of all articles and 51 percent of evidentiary studies. The quantitative nonimpact category includes studies that describe and identify the magnitude, severity, and preventability of a PHEPR problem and could potentially be used to inform the development of PHEPR practices aimed at addressing that problem. The quantitative impact category, accounting for only about 6 percent of all articles, includes studies that evaluate specific PHEPR practices.

This distribution of study designs presents challenges for identifying evidence-based practices, and in Chapter 2, the committee presents the following conclusion:

> *Conclusion: With the increasing complexity of both public health emergencies and the PHEPR system, policy makers and practitioners have a crucial need for access to guidance based on robust evidence to support their decisions on practices, policies, and programs for saving lives during future public health emergencies. Therefore, a coordinated and comprehensive approach to prioritizing and aligning research efforts and ensuring that research is relevant and consistently connected to practice, along with investments in research infrastructure, is necessary to strengthen the PHEPR evidence base, thereby ensuring that PHEPR practitioners have the scientific evidence they need to guide and inform their actions. At the same time, PHEPR practitioners will require incentives to base their practices, policies, and programs on evidence.*

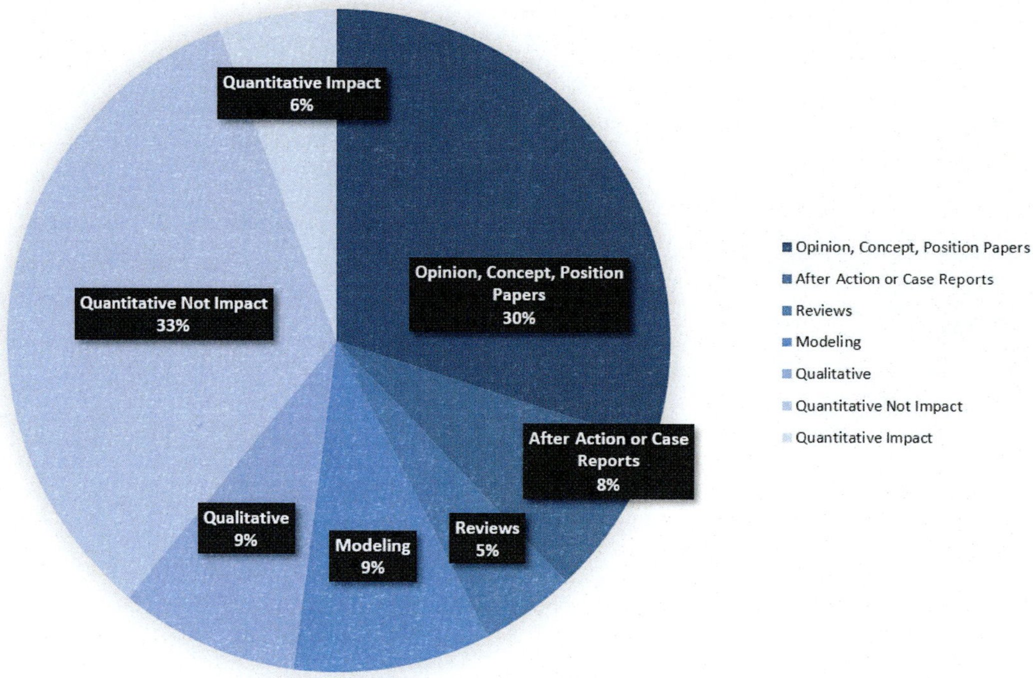

FIGURE 8-1 Distribution of all scoping review articles by study design (N = 1,692).

In this chapter, the committee describes a framework to support the systematic development of knowledge in the PHEPR field and sets forth the aspirations for high-quality, rigorous PHEPR research and evaluation.

A NATIONAL PHEPR SCIENCE FRAMEWORK

The generation of a PHEPR evidence base has been hindered by the inherent challenges of conducting research on public health emergencies, which can limit the opportunities to observe and proactively study the effects of practices used to mitigate harm before, during, and after such an event (see Chapter 2 for additional details). In addition to those challenges, federal partners and other stakeholders repeatedly have attempted to enhance PHEPR research capacity. However, many of these efforts have not been sustained or adequately resourced, and the result has been a limited infrastructure to support the generation and dissemination of PHEPR research.

Conclusion: Funding for and prioritization of research before, during, and following public health emergencies are currently fragmented and disorganized, spread across multiple funding agencies, inconsistent, and do not encourage the progression of quality research or the sustainable development of research expertise. This situation has contributed to a field based on long-standing rather than evidence-based practice.

Despite the implications of public health emergencies for the nation's health and economic security, there is currently no mechanism for ensuring the coordinated resourcing, monitoring, and execution of public- and private-sector PHEPR research.

Key Components of a National PHEPR Science Framework

The importance of developing a disaster research strategy has previously been underscored (Keim et al., 2019). The committee proposes that a comprehensive National PHEPR Science Framework could move the PHEPR field beyond the near-term goal of a research agenda toward a more coherent vision of coordinating and aligning efforts effectively to advance evidence-based practice in PHEPR (see Figure 8-2). The key components of this framework are discussed in the following sections.

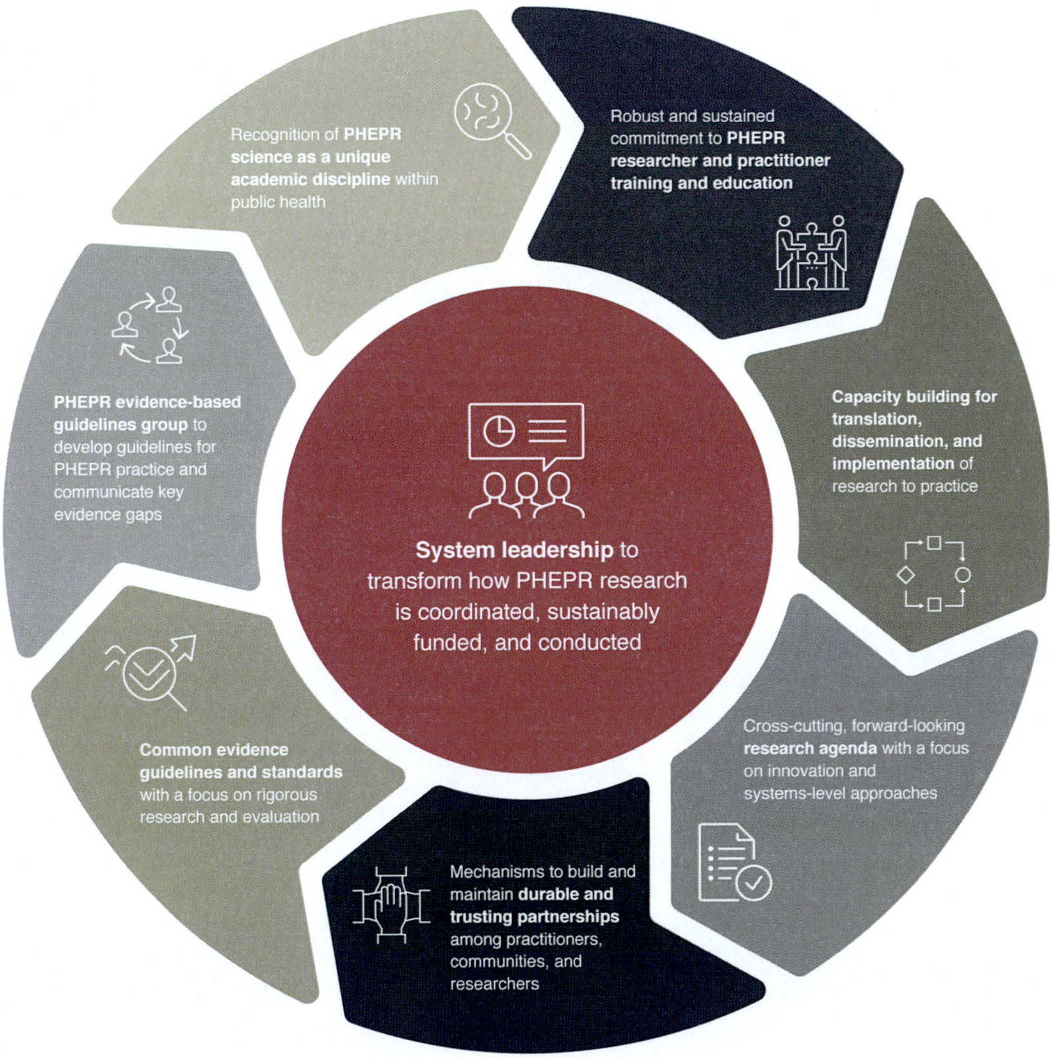

FIGURE 8-2 Key components of a National PHEPR Science Framework.

System Leadership to Transform the PHEPR Research Enterprise

The foundations of scientific progress in PHEPR lie in building and sustaining a research enterprise. Strong leadership at all levels, but especially at the federal level, is central to the framework and essential to support systems-level change and mobilize agencies to transform the way PHEPR research is coordinated, funded, and conducted. An interagency and multidisciplinary effort led by the Centers for Disease Control and Prevention (CDC) will be necessary to develop and implement a National PHEPR Science Framework; establish an authority and process for supporting research before, during, and following public health emergencies; and ensure that adequate research funding, capacities, and infrastructure are in place. CDC is the funding agency with the primary mission responsibility in PHEPR, and it is important that the agency responsible for supporting PHEPR planning and implementation also leads efforts to increase the scientific evidence base that supports the execution of that responsibility. However, the committee acknowledges that no one agency can accomplish this transformation of the PHEPR research enterprise, and it will be necessary to leverage the strengths of different partners, including funding partners, in these efforts. Given the complexity of the PHEPR system and the fact that it is nested within many integrated, larger systems (e.g., supply chain, transportation), it will be imperative for this effort to be carried out in cooperation with other fields, industries, and organizations. It will also be essential to provide CDC with adequate resources and expertise to support its lead role in these efforts and to encourage CDC to become a learning organization. Appropriation language will need to be explicit and clear that funding can be used for these research efforts.

An enterprise for coordinating medical countermeasure (MCM) efforts in the federal government could serve as a model for coordinating and funding PHEPR research (HHS, 2017a). The Public Health Emergency Medical Countermeasures Enterprise (PHEMCE), established by the U.S. Department of Health and Human Services (HHS) in 2006 and led by the Assistant Secretary for Preparedness and Response (ASPR), has the following core members: the director of CDC, the director of the National Institute of Allergy and Infectious Diseases within the National Institutes of Health (NIH), and the commissioner of the U.S. Food and Drug Administration. Key PHEMCE partners include senior leadership from other federal agencies and numerous nonfederal partners. Recognizing that the development of MCMs requires significant resources in terms of time and cost, the PHEMCE helps coordinate funding across portfolios and prioritize efforts through a coherent plan that spans several years (HHS, 2017b). PHEMCE members are motivated and guided by the need to develop responses and cost-efficient methods to protect the nation against novel threats. This enterprise has been successful in bringing attention to the issue of MCM development, generating additional research investment, and prompting government agencies and departments to coordinate their research efforts. Such a coordinated effort can bring common terminology and infrastructure to a fragmented research enterprise.

Recognition of PHEPR Science as a Unique Academic Discipline Within Public Health

PHEPR research is transdisciplinary and draws on the knowledge base from many different fields, from behavioral and social sciences and political science to systems science and operations research, among others. However, recognition that PHEPR science is a unique academic discipline within the broader public health field represents the first step in addressing the substantial need for research; qualified, well-trained researchers; and preexisting, durable, and reliable engagement and partnerships with PHEPR practitioners.

The nuances and complexity of the PHEPR field pose unique challenges for designing research studies that differ from those in the broader public health field (e.g., population health research), and the usual approach for clinical research—randomized controlled trials (RCTs)—is not always feasible. Researching public health emergencies requires specific knowledge and understanding of how the systems involved work, and public health scientists may lack the knowledge, experience, and credibility to conduct research before, during, or following a public health emergency. Given the nuances of PHEPR research, it can be especially important for researchers to be familiar with the strengths and limitations of various approaches to and methods for evaluation. These may include, for example, observational studies designed in real time with strong data collection, predesigned pragmatic trials ready for deployment, simulations and exercises that use RCT approaches, side-by-side qualitative research studies to supplement quantitative methods, and methods for capturing data from after action reports (AARs) in a way that supports knowledge generation.

Recognizing PHEPR science as a unique academic discipline within the broader public health field could generate the resources and efforts needed to better support current and new academic departments or centers focused on PHEPR; establish degree or certification programs; and support career mechanisms that would enhance the conduct of high-quality, rigorous PHEPR research. Training and career development for PHEPR researchers are discussed in greater depth in the section on workforce capacity development for PHEPR research and practitioners later in this chapter. With recognition of PHEPR as a distinct field of study, the PHEPR research community could develop its own unique culture with the support of scientific societies and associations, which currently is lacking.

A Forward-Looking PHEPR Research Agenda and Common Evidence Guidelines

A research agenda is necessary to galvanize the PHEPR research field to meet the needs and respond to the concerns of PHEPR practitioners and society at large (IOM, 2008). This agenda must be more than a simple inventory of research needs (see Box 8-1). It will require leadership, and an organizing entity will need to be identified and made responsible for aggregating research conducted in alignment with the agenda and for tracking progress on and updating the agenda. A component of the agenda could highlight what is and is not known or what PHEPR research is currently under way. PHEPR evidence gaps could, for example, be identified and communicated by the PHEPR evidence-based guidelines group proposed in Chapter 3. Another essential feature of the research agenda will be to describe a process for rapidly identifying and prioritizing research needs during a public health emergency and to establish a minimum set of data elements that would be sought by anyone collecting data during such an event (NBSB, 2011).

A formal research prioritization process will be necessary, including a top-down, bottom-up approach to setting the research agenda. An important consideration is for the process to be inclusive of governmental, nongovernmental, private, and academic organizations, as well as broad public input from practitioners, policy makers, researchers, and the community. Given that outcomes of interest in PHEPR also include process and system improvements (Carbone and Thomas, 2018), it will be valuable to engage in the research agenda development process experts in the fields of health services research; social science; implementation and improvement science; operations research; complex interventions; quality improvement; cost-effectiveness; and systems, policy, and organizational research. The National Institute of Environmental Health Sciences (NIEHS) has conducted a successful town hall model in communities across the country for bringing practitioners, researchers, and community members

BOX 8-1 COMPONENTS OF A PHEPR RESEARCH AGENDA

The committee identified the following essential components of a PHEPR research agenda:

- a convening or organizing entity with the authority to develop and update the research agenda;
- funding for development of the agenda, ongoing technical assistance for researchers, and aggregation of research conducted in alignment with the agenda;
- guidance for informing decisions about federal and nonfederal funding for research;
- a development process that employs various input strategies and is inclusive of governmental, nongovernmental, private, and academic organizations and based on broad public input from practitioners, researchers, and the community;
- a method for determining research needs and gaps and research questions based on an inclusive and rigorous process for identifying and categorizing the available literature and data;
- a specified, logical timeline that supports the progression from building an evidence base through the advancement of quality standards and methodological improvements, now and into the future; and
- a process for tracking research and evaluating progress toward meeting the priorities set forth in the research agenda.

together to participate in setting a research agenda, enhance practitioner–researcher partnerships, and foster greater awareness of community and public health needs (O'Fallon et al., 2003). O'Fallon and colleagues (2003) note several best practices for successful town halls:

- the meeting is held in a location that is convenient and comfortable for the participants;
- controversial topics are encouraged, and when such a topic is selected, it is important to ensure that both sides of the issue are presented;
- lecturing is minimized and audience participation is maximized; and
- the final agenda is determined by the host organization.

In addition to town hall models, workshops and leadership retreats for practitioners and researchers can be useful to identify new developments and research topics in PHEPR (O'Fallon et al., 2003).

It will be important for the research agenda to encompass a range of research questions that would be addressed through different methods of inquiry (see the section on common evidence guidelines for PHEPR later in this chapter), including and going beyond the topics covered within CDC's 15 PHEPR Capabilities. A good starting point for identifying research questions will be to examine previously developed research agendas for PHEPR (Acosta et al., 2009; IOM, 2008). Additional research priorities may be informed by the evidence gaps identified in the committee's commissioned scoping review (see Appendix D) and the committee's evidence reviews for practices within the Community Preparedness, Emergency Operations Coordination, Information Sharing, and Non-Pharmaceutical Interventions Capabilities (see the sections on future research priorities in Chapters 4–7).

Meaningful Partnerships Between PHEPR Practitioners and Researchers to Promote Knowledge

Crucial to a National PHEPR Science Framework will be ensuring a strong connection between PHEPR practitioners and researchers, as well as strong community partnerships. Understanding how to promote, improve, and sustain the engagement of PHEPR practitioners and communities in a thoughtful and inclusive process for generating research will be an essential element of a robust and effective PHEPR research field (Miller et al., 2016). With the proper incentives in place, PHEPR practitioners and researchers can be encouraged to engage in more meaningful partnerships to promote knowledge. Academic partners can help public health agencies by providing data and findings to inform practice (especially during a real public health emergency, when public health agencies may be challenged in conducting research), executing studies, facilitating stakeholder meetings, assessing training needs, providing technical assistance, and collaborating on publications (IOM, 2015). Specifying expectations related to the conduct, and subsequent publication, of research and evaluation in practitioner position descriptions, or even designating a dedicated "science" position within the agency, could provide an incentive for collaborating and partnering with researchers. Furthermore, partnerships between PHEPR practitioners and researchers could be strengthened by integrating expectations into Project Public Health Ready (PPHR), a criteria-based training and recognition program that assesses local health departments' PHEPR capacity, or the Public Health Accreditation Board (PHAB) accreditation process. Additionally, establishing the trust of the community before a public health emergency occurs is critical to ensuring that research can be conducted effectively and equitably. The community also has many resources to offer the PHEPR research enterprise, including its experiences and knowledge of its needs and existing networks that can be leveraged. Overall, PHEPR research requires the collaboration, insight, and trust of professionals from public health, other response agencies, academia, private entities, and members of the community prior to a public health emergency, and an effective National PHEPR Science Framework will support strategies for strengthening and maintaining these partnerships to promote successful PHEPR research. Collaboration and engagement among practitioners, researchers, and the community is a critical element that is highlighted throughout this chapter—from the development of a research agenda and funding of research programs to participation in the design and conduct of the research and translation, dissemination, and implementation of evidence-based practices.

PHEPR Evidence-Based Guidelines Group and Other Efforts to Facilitate the Translation, Dissemination, and Implementation of PHEPR Research

If the PHEPR field is to be grounded in evidence, the translation, dissemination, and implementation of research findings represent a crucial component of a National PHEPR Science Framework. The research and other evidence driven by this framework will need to be translated into clear evidence-based practices for public health agencies through an ongoing evidence review process. Accordingly, it will be important for the PHEPR evidence-based guidelines group proposed in Recommendation 1 in Chapter 3 to be integrated into the activities of the National PHEPR Science Framework, and to review relevant research and distill it into guidelines for the benefit of practitioners.

The use of sustainable strategies and mechanisms, such as training specialists in translation and implementation science, particularly for the PHEPR field, can help bridge the often daunting gap between practice and research (Carbone and Thomas, 2018). Researchers need to engage with potential users of their research, involving them in the research design and implementation process to increase the likelihood that results will be translatable and practiced (Jillson et al., 2019). At the same time, while practitioners' perspectives and needs are an important consideration in developing research projects, practitioners also need to be accepting of innovations that emerge from the research community (Carbone and Thomas, 2018). Workforce capacity development programs are necessary to improve the implementation capacity of public health agencies. These issues are explored in depth in the sections on workforce capacity development for PHEPR research and practitioners and on translation of research into practice and dissemination and implementation of evidence-based PHEPR practices later in this chapter.

Ensuring Adequate Infrastructure and Supporting Mechanisms to Facilitate the Conduct of PHEPR Research

To conduct research effectively before, during, and following a public health emergency, additional capacities, infrastructure, policies, and other elements must be strengthened or created. Adequate and sustained federal funding for PHEPR research is necessary to ensure the continual flow of scientific discoveries to mitigate the health impacts of public health emergencies.

Recognizing that this is an applied research field, there needs to be an emphasis on funding mechanisms that facilitate practice-based approaches and support the collection of experiential evidence from real-world practice and public health emergencies. It is imperative to ensure that funded research programs are relevant to practice, and in Chapter 2, the committee concludes that, in addition to investments in research infrastructure, **a coordinated and comprehensive approach to prioritizing and aligning research efforts and ensuring that research is relevant and consistently connected to practice is necessary to strengthen the PHEPR evidence base.**

The best practitioner-centered evaluations will be achieved through trusting and durable partnerships between practitioners and researchers. Some example practice-based approaches that could be supported include a researcher residency model, a practice-based research network (PBRN) model, and a research-oriented tabletop exercise model. A researcher residency model (i.e., researchers embedded in the PHEPR system) could enable researchers to attend and observe exercises, have a seat in the emergency operations center during a public health emergency, and participate in the after action reporting. In learning health care systems, it has increasingly been recognized that embedding researchers in the system offers multiple benefits, including the identification of practitioner- and systems-relevant research questions and the ability to close the research and practice gap (both of which are persistent challenges in PHEPR) (Forrest et al., 2018). CDC could also consider requiring the inclusion of PHEPR practitioners in research proposals or implementing a PBRN model within PHEPR that might enable important advances in these areas. PBRNs—groups of practitioners and researchers working together to answer community-based questions and translate research findings into practice—are a result of the increasing need for research conducted in real-world settings (AHRQ, 2019; DeVoe et al., 2012; Mays et al., 2013; RWJF and University of Kentucky College of Public Health, 2020). PBRNs have previously been supported in public health (such a program was supported by the Robert Wood Johnson Foundation [RWJF] from approximately 2007 to 2015) (RWJF, 2013), and some of this work focused on PHEPR (CTEC, 2016; Wimsatt, 2017). Additionally, research-oriented tabletop exercises can aid in developing practice-driven research. For example, Chandra and colleagues (2015) developed a community resilience tabletop exercise and administered it to stakeholders from multiple disciplines to assess progress in community resilience and provide an opportunity for quality improvement and capacity building. The NIEHS Disaster Research Response (DR2) program has previously conducted regional tabletop exercises for researchers and practitioners to facilitate the development of these partnerships and to educate practitioners on ways of incorporating data collection and research into disaster response (NIH, 2019b). Attention to emerging practice-based approaches is needed as well.

An equally important aspect of funding is mechanisms that allow for investigator-driven research, facilitate engagement and collaboration with researchers from different disciplines, and encourage the progression from development to intervention to secondary analysis to center grants—something that is currently lacking in the PHEPR field but is fundamental to any research enterprise. Several models for sustained funding programs for research series and multidisciplinary and collaborative research centers, as well research education and training projects (i.e., career development grants), currently exist at the National Science Foundation (NSF) and NIH and could be replicated for the PHEPR field (NIH, 2019c, 2020a; NSF, 2020b). CDC currently funds research through the use of grants and cooperative agreements (CDC, 2020b). Foundations, such as RWJF, the Alfred P. Sloan Foundation, the Bill & Melinda Gates Foundation, and the Open Philanthropy Project, among others, can support research programs when federal support is limited (Alfred P. Sloan Foundation, 2020; Bill & Melinda Gates Foundation, 2020; Open Philanthropy, 2020; RWJF, 2020a).

Addressing PHEPR knowledge gaps will require sustained lines of research, with multiple studies addressing similar research questions in different contexts and populations in nonemergency times and with the ability to refocus efforts or activate additional protocols, if warranted, in the event of a future public health emergency. Given the inherent challenges of conducting research during public health emergencies, it is important to give careful consideration to opportunities for advancing PHEPR science during nonemergency times and to the pre-event planning needed to enable research during and following future public health emergencies. Types of PHEPR research that could be supported in nondisaster times include modeling, simulations and exercises, and research on public health implementation issues that would likely translate in the event of a public health emergency. One of the challenging aspects of all PHEPR activities, including research, is the natural aversion to creating unused capacity. A solution to this challenge could be providing funding and resources for individuals conducting research in nonemergency times with the expectation—and support—that they will turn their attention to researching a public health emergency at hand. Research funders could consider requiring researchers to account for this possibility by describing such contingency processes in their proposals.

As mentioned above, deliberative planning during nonemergency times is necessary so that the resources and supporting mechanisms needed to rapidly conduct scientific research in the context of a public health emergency will be in place. Past efforts have made strides toward developing mechanisms to support scientific research in the context of a public health emergency, some of which have indeed been developed and even tested (e.g., rapid identification and prioritization of research needs and funding after Hurricane Sandy) (Lurie et al., 2013). In Table 8-1, Lurie and colleagues (2013) describe key components of an integrated approach to research before, during, and after an emergency and explicitly lay out actions that could be taken before as well as during the emergency. One consideration not included in this table is the action of developing metrics and outcome measures, an important component of the conduct of research and evaluation of practices. Future efforts to ensure adequate infrastructure and supporting mechanisms to facilitate the conduct of research during public health emergencies could be guided and informed by these past efforts.

To support research during a public health emergency, sustainable, rapid, and nimble funding mechanisms, together with award criteria and preapproved PHEPR research study

TABLE 8-1 Key Components of Research Response in the Context of Public Health Emergencies

Component	Actions Before the Event	Actions During the Event
Identify questions that will need to be addressed for common scenarios and develop generic study protocols	Identify experts in research design and in key topic areas Develop and gain approval from institutional review boards for key study protocols	Convene experts, and review and amend protocols as needed
Ensure that appropriate cadres of scientists are available to respond to events	Roster experts in research design and in topical areas of concern Develop an on-call research "ready reserve" of clinicians, scientists, and other experts in government, academia, and industry	Convene experts (and potentially others with concerns) to identify areas for priority research
Develop a process for activating research response	Incorporate the concept of an "incident commander for research" into response plans Determine criteria for activation of research response	Identify an "incident commander for research" and representatives from relevant science agencies that will be charged with supporting and conducting research Notify prerostered experts
Identify and prioritize research needs	Identify potential knowledge gaps and research questions	Convene experts and others, such as those in affected communities, to review previously identified gaps, identify unforeseen and emerging knowledge gaps, prioritize research and baseline data collection needs, and recommend to researchers and funders which to pursue in the short term
Ensure conditions for rapid data collection	Develop and preapprove generic protocols and survey instruments so that only changes to them require review when the event occurs Develop protocols for collecting and storing biospecimens	Modifying preexisting survey and other data collection tools for event-specific conditions
Ensure rapid and appropriate human subjects review	Establish a Public Health Emergency Research Review Board Promote a commitment to expedite review by grantee institutions and prepositioned research networks	Facilitate rapid review of protocols by national or local institutional review boards
Ensure mechanisms for rapid funding	Use prefunded research networks and preawarded but just-in-time funded research contracts Incorporate research response to public health emergencies in specific aims on grant awards to better facilitate administrative supplements Identify nongovernmental funders, both regionally and by sector, with an interest in addressing knowledge gaps	Convene potential governmental and nongovernmental funders Share prioritized research agenda

TABLE 8-1 Continued

Component	Actions Before the Event	Actions During the Event
Ensure that response workers and other exposed persons are identified and rostered	Develop and use a Rapid Response Registry Identify potential monitoring and tracking devices to facilitate exposure monitoring (e.g., among emergency responders)	Activate registry enrollment and designated data collection networks, including for biospecimens, when appropriate Deploy monitoring and tracking devices, when appropriate
Understand concerns of affected communities	Identify a generic list of concerns to address, drawing on community-based participatory research and experience with previous events	Engage community representatives in discussion of concerns and potential studies Ensure mechanisms to share findings with the community

SOURCE: Lurie et al., 2013. Reprinted with permission from Massachusetts Medical Society.

protocols, are needed. Several such mechanisms currently exist, but they are uncoordinated and focused disproportionately on infrastructure, engineering, and environmental health. An example is NSF's Rapid Response Researich funding mechanism, used when quick-response research on disasters is needed (NSF, 2018). Additionally, with the support of NSF, the National Hazards Center at the University of Colorado administers a Quick Response Research Grant Program that provides small grants to help researchers collect data following an event (National Hazards Center, 2019). This program can be mobilized quickly to put some of the necessary research infrastructure in place in the immediate aftermath of a disaster and could serve as a model for funders, although it is at a smaller scale than that needed for the PHEPR research enterprise. NIEHS's Time-Sensitive Research Grants Program is another example of a rapid funding mechanism for public health emergencies. Its aim is to receive, review, and fund research applications within 90–120 days, and it supports research to characterize initial exposures, collect human biological samples, and collect human health and exposure data (Miller et al., 2016). Other agencies could replicate these rapid response funding models specifically for PHEPR research. Additionally, partnerships with foundations that are interested in addressing the needs of communities and health-related research could help fill gaps in funding.

Rapid funding to support research in the event of a public health emergency is not enough, however; efforts are also needed to enhance capacities to conduct the research and improve data collection capabilities. Such efforts might include establishing formalized academic–public health agency research partnerships and a cadre of researchers and preassembled teams embedded in the response system—specifically within the incident management structure—and available to respond rapidly to public health emergencies (Lurie et al., 2013). In 2012, for example, the U.S. Department of the Interior's Strategic Sciences group was created to meet the immediate need for scientific information during an environmental disaster (DOI, 2020). In the case of PHEPR, CDC could build research expertise into the training for Epidemic Intelligence Service (EIS) officers, a subset of whom could then be deployed for the sole purpose of conducting PHEPR research during public health emergencies (CDC, 2020a). A benefit of doing so would be that EIS officers are often most knowledgeable about needs and opportunities in communities and have the relationships to carry out the necessary research and evaluations in real time. They can be mobilized quickly and are positioned to have their results incorporated rapidly into guidance, funding, and translation efforts. With respect to data collection, the NIEHS DR2 program has a central repository[1] of publicly available data collection tools, such as surveys, questionnaires, and protocols, that could be used to establish early baselines and cohorts for research.

Also important is to synergize and catalog past, ongoing, and future PHEPR-related research to avoid duplication (unless warranted) and reduce participant burden when research is conducted during or following a public health emergency. A database of PHEPR research studies categorized to facilitate analysis could be created, which would help foster research that would progressively improve PHEPR. Establishing and incentivizing partnerships and networks across research teams and institutions, other disciplines, and other organizations could also help coordinate research efforts.

Research involving human subjects during or following public health emergencies may pose ethical and data sharing challenges (Packenham et al., 2017). The Public Health Emergency Research Review Board was established in 2012 to provide centralized, rigorous, and expeditious reviews of human subject protections for HHS-conducted, -supported, or -regulated research studies addressing public health emergencies (HHS and NIH, 2020). This entity is currently under the auspices of the NIH network of institutional review boards (IRBs), and an IRB Authorization Agreement between NIH and the institutions conducting research is required (IOM, 2015). The NIEHS Best Practices Working Group for Special IRB Considerations in the Review of Disaster-Related Research has also been making progress in this area. The DR2 program has developed a pre-event generic protocol, the Rapid Acquisition of Pre- and Post-Incident Disaster Data (RAPIDD) protocol, for provisional approval by IRBs, which has been used by several universities. The objective of the RAPIDD protocol is to facilitate the collection of epidemiologic information and laboratory test results and the collection and storage of human biospecimens (Miller et al., 2016).

When it comes to research, public health agencies have different sets of concerns from researchers and institutions. A key issue is the security of confidential data and the privacy of subjects. Research during or following public health emergencies can also raise ethical challenges, including the burden on the population, potential harms, and the potential for therapeutic misconception (IOM, 2015). Further guidance and support are needed for academic entities and public health agencies to develop effective and efficient means for reviewing and addressing unique ethical issues in the conduct of PHEPR research, such as through pre-emergency review of standard protocols, training of IRB members on unique aspects of PHEPR research, and the establishment of specific review mechanisms for this research.

Conclusion and Recommendations

Conclusion: A National PHEPR Science Framework can establish the goals and objectives necessary to improve coordination, integration, and alignment among existing PHEPR research efforts, but will require adequate resourcing and oversight.

RECOMMENDATION 3: Develop a National Public Health Emergency Preparedness and Response (PHEPR) Science Framework

To enhance and expand the evidence base for PHEPR practices and translation of the science to the practice community, the Centers for Disease Control and Prevention should work with other relevant funding agencies; state, local, tribal, and territorial public health agencies; academic researchers; professional associations; and other stake-

[1] See https://dr2.nlm.nih.gov/tools-resources (accessed March 10, 2020).

holders to develop a National PHEPR Science Framework so as to ensure resourcing, coordination, monitoring, and execution of public- and private-sector PHEPR research. The National PHEPR Science Framework should do the following:

- Build on and improve coordination, integration, and alignment among existing PHEPR research efforts (e.g., the National Institute of Environmental Health Sciences' Disaster Research Response Program), and ensure integration of these efforts with the activities of the PHEPR evidence-based guidelines group proposed in Recommendation 1.
- Recognize and support PHEPR science as a unique academic discipline within the broader public health field to address the substantial need for research and diverse and qualified researchers.
- Create a common, robust, and forward-looking PHEPR research agenda that supports advancement beyond traditional epidemiological research to include research in the fields of social science, implementation science, complex interventions, and quality improvement, as well as intervention, operations, systems, and cost-effectiveness research.
- Support meaningful partnerships between PHEPR practitioners and researchers, and develop strategies to better ensure that PHEPR research is relevant to practice.
- Prioritize sustainable strategies and mechanisms for the translation, dissemination, and implementation of PHEPR research.

RECOMMENDATION 4: Ensure Infrastructure and Funding to Support Public Health Emergency Preparedness and Response (PHEPR) Research
The Centers for Disease Control and Prevention (CDC), in collaboration with other relevant funding agencies, should ensure adequate and sustained oversight, coordination, and funding to support a National PHEPR Science Framework and to further develop the infrastructure necessary to support more efficient production of and better-quality PHEPR research. Such infrastructure should include

- sustained funding for practice-based and investigator-driven research that allows for the progression from exploratory to effectiveness to scale-up research and encourages researcher diversity;
- support for partnerships (e.g., with academic institutions, hospital systems, and state, local, tribal, and territorial public health agencies) to facilitate collaboration in research on the preparedness, response, and recovery phases of a public health emergency;
- development of a rapid research funding mechanism and interdisciplinary rapid response teams with applied research expertise (similar to CDC's Epidemic Intelligence Service) for deployment to conduct just-in-time studies related to the implementation of PHEPR practices at the time of events; and
- enhanced mechanisms to enable routine, standardized, efficient data collection with minimal disruption to delivery of services (including preapproved, adaptable research and institutional review board protocols and a research arm within the response structure).

SUPPORTING METHODOLOGICAL IMPROVEMENTS FOR PHEPR RESEARCH

The results of the committee's four evidence reviews highlight the paucity of research that has generated credible evidence to inform PHEPR practice (see Chapters 4–7). In some cases, the committee found few to no studies with which to address the questions of interest (e.g., no quantitative studies were included in the review for emergency operations coordination). In other cases, a sizable body of research exists, but the committee noted limitations in study designs (e.g., lack of baseline measurements or comparison groups, use of unvalidated or subjective and self-reported measures), execution (e.g., underpowered studies, high loss to follow-up), analysis (e.g., failure to conduct statistical tests or lack of statistical adjustment), or reporting of information (e.g., lack of details on the methodology, the PHEPR practice, population characteristics, other contextual factors, and outcomes). Some research methods were also poorly matched to the research questions they were intended to address. To help ensure that future studies yield results from which stronger conclusions can be drawn about the effectiveness of PHEPR practices, future investments in PHEPR research will need to remedy these common methodological shortcomings. Standards, guidance, and incentives can help raise the quality and evidentiary value of research in the PHEPR field.

Common Evidence Guidelines

Federal agencies can have a significant influence on the generation of the evidence base for practice (Maynard, 2018). In fields other than PHEPR setting priorities and standards for research and using them to guide funding decisions has improved the quality and usefulness of the evidence base. An example is the response of the education research field to shifts in funding priorities to align with agency evidence agendas and guidelines, which began in 2002 with the creation of the Institute of Education Sciences (IES) within the U.S. Department of Education.[2] Early on, IES established evidence guidelines for causal inference studies; a system for sourcing, grading, and synthesizing evidence; a web-based clearinghouse for evidence reviews; and an active program of funding for professional development (pre- and postdoctoral training grants; professional meetings and association development). These efforts resulted in a dramatic shift in the methodological rigor of education evaluations (Whitehurst, 2018).

Similar improvements could be achieved in PHEPR by drawing on these experiences in other fields to enact policies and practices that can improve how PHEPR research is conducted, disseminated, and used (IES and NSF, 2013). The goal is to ensure that scarce evaluation dollars are used most productively to advance the evidence available to inform policy and practice. Achieving this goal necessitates careful balancing of several factors: the importance of the questions studied, the rigor with which the questions can and will be studied, the timeliness of the research findings, and the accessibility and usability of the findings. Tiered evidence standards for grantmaking can be a useful mechanism to guide funding decisions, as they allow federal agencies to award smaller amounts to promising concepts and larger amounts to practices grounded in strong evidence of success, encouraging innovation while still rewarding programs with robust research backing (GAO, 2016).

Going forward, the PHEPR research field will need to have clear guidelines and standards for evaluation methods and study designs that will produce credible answers to various types of questions of importance to the field. The objective is to encourage a balance

[2] Education Sciences Reform Act. HR 3801, Section 116. 107th Cong. (January 23, 2002).

of research throughout the knowledge-building continuum, from basic science through effectiveness trials and modeling studies, and to foster rather than stifle research innovation.

Guiding the Use of Different Types of Research Methods and Approaches

Well-crafted guidance will incorporate the full spectrum of research methods, which may range from exploratory case studies to RCTs and modeling studies for evaluating PHEPR practices. The PHEPR research field would be strengthened by creating a unified taxonomy of research methods, accompanied by guidelines for judging the credibility of study findings intended to address various types of questions. A first step in developing this guidance will be to identify the various genres of PHEPR research, and for each genre describe its purpose (i.e., how that type of research contributes to the evidence base) (see Annex 8-1). It will also be important for each genre of research to be supported by theoretical and empirical justifications when possible, and to adhere to established expectations for research design, methods, and products of the research. Expectations will need to be established as well for review of the products of each type of research (i.e., what information is required to judge the credibility and applicability of the findings and how that information can be judged).

While acknowledging the value of randomization for demonstrating a causal link between interventions and outcomes, the committee recognizes that it is difficult, if not infeasible or inappropriate, to implement RCTs for some PHEPR practices, particularly in the context of a real public health emergency. As discussed in Chapter 3, other study types (e.g., quasi-experimental study designs) may provide credible estimates of a causal impact (or lack thereof) when PHEPR practices are evaluated. Table 8-2 describes the strengths and limitations of common study designs for quantitative impact evaluation with applicability to PHEPR.

Other experimental study designs have begun to emerge that may also present opportunities for PHEPR research. Adaptive platform trial designs, such as the vaccine trial proposed during the 2014–2015 Ebola outbreak, allow for flexibility along the timeline of an event, with interim analysis of data to enable investigators to determine whether to continue moving forward, change course, or divest more rapidly from interventions that are not showing promise (Berry et al., 2016). Pragmatic trials evaluate the effectiveness of interventions in real-life routine practice rather than the highly controlled conditions typical of experimental research studies (Ford and Norrie, 2016; Patsopoulos, 2011). This design incorporates more real-world evidence into controlled trials, allowing for a broader environment for testing, as well as greater generalizability of findings. A stepped wedge cluster design is a type of pragmatic trial used to evaluate the efficacy of service delivery interventions. This type of design may be a good option when operating within logistical or political constraints and has been used in a variety of areas, ranging from vaccine development to social policy and criminal justice (Hemming et al., 2015).

On the other hand, the committee encourages the PHEPR field to move beyond experimental study designs and consider a broader range of methods for exploring what works (and when, why, and for whom). Many PHEPR practices are designed to improve outcomes, particularly systems-level outcomes, in complex settings in response to unpredictable events. PHEPR practitioners and researchers are often interested in whether a practice made a difference or what would have happened had it not been implemented (e.g., what would have happened had the public health emergency operations center not been activated). Qualitative research methodologies (e.g., ethnographic observations, interviews, and focus group discussions) can inform why and how PHEPR practices may or may not be effective (Teti et

TABLE 8-2 A Brief Overview of Strengths and Limitations of Study Designs for Quantitative Impact Evaluation for PHEPR

Study Design	Strengths	Limitations
Randomized controlled trial (RCT)	Provides the most unbiased, robust, and reliable estimates of the effectiveness of a PHEPR practice, which gives confidence that any measured differences between groups are due to the intervention. Depending on the sample size and diversity, it may be possible to conduct sub-group analysis to determine whether impacts vary by conditions in the implementing sites (e.g., urban and rural, diversity of languages spoken by residents) that influence the effectiveness of the PHEPR practice.	It is often difficult to conduct an RCT at the community or national level, which is often the target of PHEPR practices. Results from a simulated trial may not mirror those in a true emergency, and it may not be feasible to conduct an RCT during a public health emergency. If there is a desire to conduct an RCT during an emergency, completing the study requires waiting for emergencies to occur. Testing the differential effectiveness of strategies in real emergencies introduces uncertainties in the timeframe, cost, and context for the study. It may be costly to recruit the sample for the study, and it may be difficult to persuade decision makers of the benefits of this design given political and ethical issues concerning randomization.
Quasi-experimental study (matched comparison group study, interrupted time series, regression discontinuity design, multivariate analysis)	Provides reasonably strong evidence of the relationship between the PHEPR practice and outcomes measured. It is a powerful method for exploring the impact of a PHEPR practice when randomization is not possible. It can be applied to large communities, and launching such a study may be more feasible than an RCT close to the time of an emergency, which would improve the ability to collect reliable data prior to the emergency.	There could be systematic differences between the jurisdictions implementing the PHEPR practice that are not captured in the data, and therefore that cannot be controlled for in the analysis. This could result in less reliable findings. Matching techniques require a great deal of data, and the study could require considerable resources (time and cost) to identify jurisdictions that had implemented the PHEPR practices of interest and collect the data. These designs require complex analytical work and specialized knowledge.
Pre-post comparison design	For studies based on simulated emergency situations, comparison of outcomes pre and post provides plausible indications of whether the PHEPR practice was implemented and whether outcomes changed as a result. In cases in which it is possible to measure outcomes for multiple time periods prior to and after implementation of the PHEPR practice, it is possible to compare not only differences in outcomes immediately before and after the event but also differences in trends before and after. This design may be the most feasible option given that it requires relatively little time and money, depending on the outcomes of interest and the cooperation of practitioners in the jurisdictions selected for study. Some outcomes of interest may be sufficiently predictable over time that observed shifts after implementation of the PHEPR practice will have high credibility.	There are significant threats to internal validity, but a study of this type could provide preliminary evidence of effectiveness. Changes may be occurring in the study sites between the pre and post periods, such as the adoption of other PHEPR practices or staff turnover. For some outcomes, there is likely to be considerable variation that cannot be explained by contextual factors, and it may be difficult or impossible to obtain reliable and consistent measures of the outcomes of interest through existing records or recall and reconstruction.

al., 2020). A range of approaches are gaining recognition, such as realist evaluations[3] and qualitative comparative analyses,[4] that acknowledge the complexity of causality (Blanchet et al., 2018). There is also defined guidance for evaluating complex interventions (e.g., the UK Medical Research Council, the Patient-Centered Outcomes Research Institute), but these concepts have yet to be fully adopted by the PHEPR research field (AcademyHealth, 2017; MRC, 2019; PCORI, 2019). Furthermore, as PHEPR research is transdisciplinary, design methodologies used in such fields as public health services and systems research, operations research, behavioral and social sciences, organizational research, and quality improvement can also provide evidence for understanding PHEPR practices. In particular, simulation-based research methods (e.g., tabletop exercises), systematic expert opinion methodologies (e.g., Delphi), and systems science approaches (e.g., social network analyses, causal process diagrams, adaptive systems theories, modeling, machine learning, and big data analyses) can provide insight on systems-level outcomes and the interdependent relationships among the many components of the PHEPR system. Overall, there are many rigorous methodologies from diverse fields that could be used to evaluate PHEPR practices, and the key takeaway is to match the study design appropriately to the research question to produce credible answers. Annex 8-1 provides a brief summary of genres of research, example research questions, and some appropriate methods.

Comprehensive guidance would include suggestions for strategically mixing methods to improve both the design of intervention studies (e.g., through baseline studies conducted before a PHEPR practice is implemented) and understanding of the findings, including their breadth and limitations (postintervention). An example of such a strategic mixed-method approach in PHEPR is the Los Angeles County Community Disaster Resilience (LACCDR) project[5] (see Figure 8-3). The PHEPR field could benefit from conducting sequential or parallel studies focused on particular aspects of PHEPR practices. It is also important to note that the LACCDR project used community participatory methods, and the committee's evidence review on engaging with and training community-based partners (see Chapter 4) found that community and stakeholder involvement in research and programmatic efforts from conceptualization to implementation may correspond with more effective engagement and training through enhanced inclusion, cultural acceptability, shared ownership, and capacity building of community members. Comprehensive guidance would incorporate such participatory methods, and also refer to their use in such emerging fields as engagement science (Dungan et al., 2019).

Standards for Reporting of Study Information

It is essential for all intervention studies to have well-articulated research plans that, when possible, are published before the analysis itself begins (Burlig, 2018; Lupia and Alter, 2014; Moravcsik, 2014). Such plans describe the study design, identify the primary and supplemental research questions to be addressed, provide background on the study setting,

---

[3] "Realist evaluations are based on an assumption that projects and programs work under certain conditions and are influenced by the way that different stakeholders respond to them. Realist evaluations attempt to answer questions such as what works, for whom, in which circumstances, and why. They are designed to improve understanding about how development interventions work in different contexts" (INTRAC, 2017b).

[4] "Qualitative Comparative Analysis (QCA) is a methodology that enables the analysis of multiple cases in complex situations. It can help explain why change happens in some cases but not others. QCA is designed for use with an intermediate number of cases, typically between 10 and 50. It can be used in situations where there are too few cases to apply conventional statistical analysis" (INTRAC, 2017a).

[5] See http://www.laresilience.org (accessed May 11, 2020).

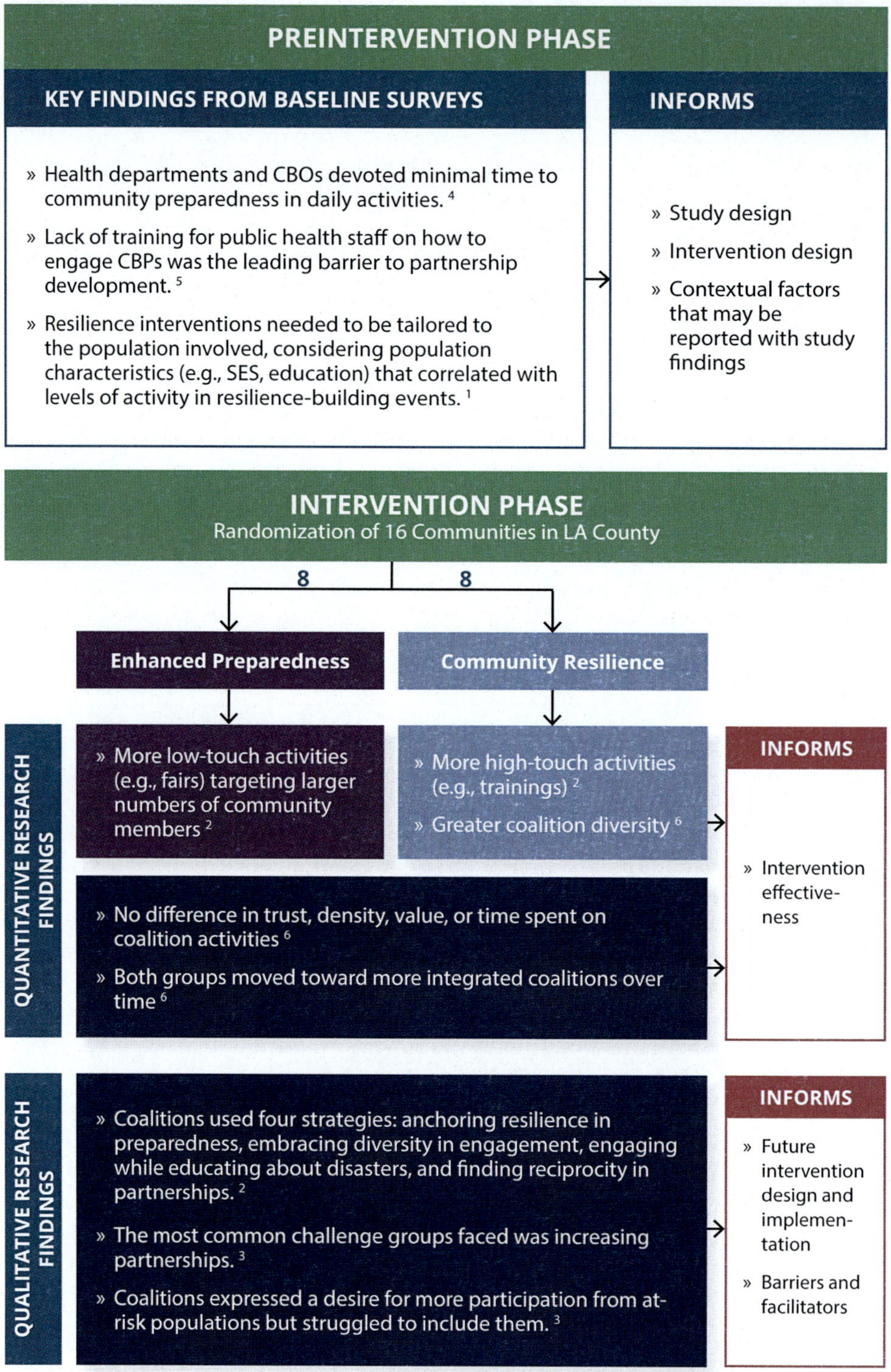

FIGURE 8-3 Los Angeles County Community Disaster Resilience mixed-method research study.
NOTES: The numbers shown on the figure denote the following sources: [1]Adams et al., 2017; [2]Bromley et al., 2017; [3]Cha et al., 2016; [4]Chandra et al., 2013; [5]Chi et al., 2015; [6]Williams et al., 2018. CBO = community-based organization; CBP = community-based partner; SES = socioeconomic status.

define the target population(s), and explain why the proposed program may change practice and improve decision making and outcomes for PHEPR practitioners or the community. They also detail the data collection plan, including measures to be used, and describe the analysis and reporting plans.

Given that PHEPR research funding and prioritization efforts are currently fragmented, disorganized, and inconsistent, there is no standardized peer-reviewed grant process, and as a result there are currently no specific standard guidelines or benchmarks for reporting the results of evaluations of the effectiveness of PHEPR practices. Reporting guidelines for health-related research have been developed for RCTs (Begg et al., 1996), observational studies in epidemiology (von Elm et al., 2007), systematic reviews of complex interventions (Guise et al., 2017a,b), studies of diagnostic accuracy (Bossuyt et al., 2015), qualitative research (O'Brien et al., 2014; Tong et al., 2007), implementation studies (Pinnock et al., 2015), and quality improvement studies (Ogrinc et al., 2016), among others (Hoffmann et al., 2014; Simera et al., 2008). Given the experience with a wide range of other types of research, it appears likely that developing, publishing, and disseminating tailored guidelines for PHEPR evaluations might well improve the reporting of such studies.

Federal agencies can support standardized reporting (e.g., through the development of guidance and standards and requirements linked to grants), which improves the usability of results and may over time result in efficiencies and cost savings (Maynard, 2018). Professional associations and journals also have important roles in the adoption of and commitment to reporting standards. PHEPR professional associations could establish the need and advocate for well-defined reporting standards, gather and review standards developed by other fields, draft standards for use by journals, and ensure that standards are shared and understood by the PHEPR research and practice fields. Journals play a vital role in communicating research findings to practitioners, as well as making information available to those in other sectors. By requiring the use of reporting standards, they can also promote the transparency and reproducibility of scientific research.

Conclusion and Recommendation

Conclusion: The lack of formal guidance and expectations regarding the various genres of PHEPR research has led to variable levels of credibility of the evidence produced. Given that evidence-based practices are dependent on existing research, efforts to delineate common expectations for PHEPR research need to be a priority to enhance the conduct of high-quality research and evaluation and help organize research investments.

RECOMMENDATION 5: Improve the Conduct and Reporting of Public Health Emergency Preparedness and Response (PHEPR) Research

The Centers for Disease Control and Prevention, the Office of the Assistant Secretary for Preparedness and Response, the National Institutes of Health, the U.S. Department of Homeland Security, the National Science Foundation, and other relevant PHEPR research funders should use funding requirements to drive needed improvements in the conduct and reporting of research on the effectiveness and implementation of PHEPR practices. Such efforts should include

- developing guidance on and incorporating into funding decisions the use of appropriate research methods as determined by the level of research (e.g., exploratory, effectiveness, scale-up) and type of research question(s) being addressed, includ-

ing but not limited to encouraging the use of concurrent comparison groups when feasible and assessment of baseline measures;
- establishing guidelines for evaluations using different designs and evidence streams and concepts from emerging evaluation approaches, such as complex intervention evaluations; and
- developing reporting guidelines, including essential reporting elements (e.g., addressing contextual factors, confounding factors, and negative results), in partnership with professional associations, journal editors, researchers, and methodologists for PHEPR intervention studies.

IMPROVING SYSTEMS TO GENERATE HIGH-QUALITY EXPERIENTIAL EVIDENCE FOR PHEPR

Public health agencies typically conduct after action reviews following real or simulated (exercise) public health emergencies in an effort to identify lessons learned and strengths and weaknesses of the response, and ultimately to improve emergency preparedness and response capabilities (Davies et al., 2019). The after action review process is an important source of experiential evidence in PHEPR and is the primary approach used by public health agencies to evaluate public health emergency response. In evaluation of the effectiveness of PHEPR practices, AARs offer the potential for improved understanding of context and implementation considerations that could be difficult to obtain through research. AARs can also be used to develop theories and logic models to inform future research. However, because they are not designed to be research, they are not without their methodological limitations. To help ensure that future AARs result in more useful and meaningful information for the evaluation of PHEPR practices (including the establishment of credible baselines for evaluation), it will be necessary to focus on strengthening methodological approaches, establishing mechanisms for analysis and dissemination of lessons learned from the reviews, and fostering a culture of improvement.

In the United States, several agencies and organizations that fund or oversee aspects of PHEPR, including CDC and ASPR, formally require after action reviews. The Federal Emergency Management Agency's (FEMA's) Homeland Security Exercise and Evaluation Program (HSEEP) developed a framework for agencies, including public health agencies, to use when developing, executing, and evaluating exercises. This program provides AAR templates and guidance to inform agencies in documenting strengths, areas for improvement, and corrective actions (FEMA, 2013). Because the framework is not organized according to the CDC PHEPR Capabilities, however, public health agencies have had to make major adaptations, such that the potential advantages of a standardized AAR have not been realized (Barnett et al., 2020). Thus, current reporting requirements and methodological standards for AARs lack clarity and uniformity. Moreover, evaluations are rarely conducted by independent evaluators with appropriate expertise (Davies et al., 2019; Gossip et al., 2017). AARs are typically reviewed and vetted throughout the agency or agencies that produced them before being submitted or shared with partners or the public, which may limit the candor of the information they contain (Gossip et al., 2017). The result is significant variability in the quality and reliability of AARs. The lack of consistent reporting requirements and variable report structures, together with limited CDC and public health agency resources, impedes the aggregation of AAR data and thus their use as a potential source of evidence for evaluating the effectiveness of PHEPR practices.

Limitations of AARs as a Source of Experiential Evidence for Mixed-Method Evidence Reviews

In recognition of the potential of AARs to inform the effectiveness and implementation of PHEPR practices in different contexts, the committee considered evidence from AARs in two of its evidence reviews. Davies and colleagues (2019) recently developed an appraisal tool with which to compare methodological reporting and document validity for AARs (see Box 8-2). To inform efforts focused on improvements needed to enhance the evidentiary

BOX 8-2 11-ITEM TOOL FOR ASSESSING THE METHODOLOGICAL RIGOR OF AFTER ACTION REPORTS

- **Prolonged engagement with the subject of inquiry**—Has the review included lengthy and perhaps repeated interviews with respondents, and/or days and weeks of engagement within a case study site or group?
- **Use of theory**—Has theory been used to guide sample selection, data collection, and analysis?
- **Data selection**—Has purposive selection been used to allow prior theory and initial assumptions to be tested or to examine "average" or unusual experience?
- **Information sampling**—Has the review gathered views from a wide range of perspectives and respondents rather than letting one viewpoint (person, organization, or specialty) dominate? Has it sampled enough people, places, times, etc., to ensure that the influence of these factors on the behavior and views of those people providing the information is minimized? Has sampling been expanded in the light of early findings?
- **Multiple data sources**—Has the review sought multiple information sources (documents, personal testimony, site visits) and collated multiple examples of each? For example, have duplicate formal interviews with all sampled staff been undertaken? Has the review used researcher observation and informal discussion, and have interviews been conducted with people in different roles and levels of seniority?
- **Triangulation**—Has the review looked for patterns of convergence and divergence by comparing results across multiple sources of evidence (e.g., across interviewees, and between interview and other data), among researchers, and across different methodological approaches? Has it also made comparisons within data (e.g., comparing different interview accounts)?
- **Negative case analysis**—Has the review looked for evidence that contradicts its initial findings, explanations, and theory, and refined them accordingly?
- **Peer debriefing and support**—Has the review included a step whereby the findings and reports have been reviewed by other researchers or investigators?
- **Respondent validation**—Have findings and reports been reviewed by respondents to check investigators' interpretation of their input?
- **Clear report of methods of data collection and analysis (audit trail)**—Has the review kept and reported a full record of activities that is available to others and presented a full account of how methods evolved and were applied?
- **Depth and insight**—Has the review established the direct and indirect root causes and underlying contributory factors linked to errors, inaction, or latent failures?

SOURCES: Davies et al., 2019; ECDC, 2018.

value of AARs for future use, the committee commissioned a quality assessment of the 38 AARs included in its evidence reviews using this 11-item appraisal tool (Patel, 2019).[6,7]

Overall, the application of the tool to 38 AARs yielded low scores. Notably, consultants wrote two of the three highest-quality AARs, and AARs based on real events were of better quality on average than those based on exercises. The vast majority of AARs failed to provide a rationale for data selection, and more than half provided no detail on information sampling or multiple data sources, making it difficult to ascertain the appropriateness of the sample or sources used to inform the AAR findings. Practitioners were often surveyed for comments and observations, but the sample size of those practitioners, the timeline for data collection (immediate postevent versus after a reflection period), the information collected, and the format for collection varied widely and were rarely documented. Limiting samples to response leadership potentially skewed findings toward a leadership perspective at the cost of including feedback from staff engaged more directly in response operations. The grouping of leadership with general staff in feedback sessions could have discouraged staff from fully expressing any critiques they may have had regarding how leadership handled a response. Excluding communities from the after action review process also represented a missed opportunity to hear from diverse voices that might not have been reflected in the demographics of the leadership or staff. None of the AARs mentioned negative case analysis or respondent validation. Only three described peer debriefing and support; two of these were written by consultants, and one validated regional findings at the state level.

Overall, findings from applying the AAR quality assessment tool indicate a significant need to improve both after action review processes and the level of detail included in the reports themselves. It is unclear whether AAR authors omitted basic methodological information in a process that was otherwise rigorous, or if the reports would have scored low even if the requisite categories had been included.

In addition to these methodological shortcomings, the committee noted several other gaps and biases in its review of AARs and the AAR generation process that will need to be addressed moving forward:

- local political pressures and fear of judgment or retribution for reporting errors or negative outcomes;
- retrospective, subjective reporting based on the recall of participants, which may be influenced by the experience itself, pressures to "move on" and resume usual workflow, and limited roles in and siloed views of the activities;
- lack of methodological standards and tools for collecting, aggregating, analyzing, and disseminating information and reports;
- limited access to and the variable quality of data, information, and reports; and
- limited formal training, infrastructure, and resources to develop specialized personnel and/or programs to critically analyze AAR data and information in a culture of quality improvement.

[6] This section draws heavily on a report commissioned by the committee on "Quality Assessment of After Action Reports: Findings and Recommendations," by Sneha Patel.

[7] The committee included 38 AARs in its evidence reviews. Approximately 61 percent of those reports were based on real events, and full-scale and functional exercises accounted for 16 percent and 21 percent of the reports, respectively. Hazards and threats included infectious diseases (e.g., H1N1, Ebola, hepatitis A), natural disasters, and human-made disasters (e.g., oil spills, explosions). Incident years ranged from 2009 to 2017 in 20 U.S. states. The AARs were all published either in the same year or the year following the real event or exercise.

Strengthening Methodological Approaches

Given the shortcomings discussed above, there is a clear need for CDC, in collaboration with ASPR and FEMA, to develop after action review policies and guidance that will ensure the capture of data relevant to the evolving response to a public health emergency and allow for in-depth analysis of the response. After action reviews can serve multiple purposes, including continuous quality improvement and, in some cases, accountability as part of grant requirements (Savoia et al., 2012; Stoto et al., 2013), and these purposes often require different methodological approaches to data collection, aggregation, and analysis. After action reviews are frequently completed by public health agencies themselves, and the methods used to collect information and data for the reports vary widely from agency to agency. In general, though, after action reviews use a wide variety of fairly common qualitative and quantitative methods, including surveys, interviews, focus groups or hotwashes, workshops, public forums, document reviews, and site visits (ECDC, 2018).

There is broad agreement that an after action review should seek to establish more than the immediate cause of response and recovery issues, and should analyze the factors behind the immediate causes, aiming to get to the root causes (Barnett et al., 2020; Davies et al., 2019; ECDC, 2018; Piltch-Loeb et al., 2014b; Singleton et al., 2014; Stoto et al., 2015, 2019) (see Figure 8-4 for an example depicting the steps of root-cause analysis). This systematic approach to root-cause analysis forms the basis of most approaches, such as peer assessment approaches[8] and facilitated look-backs.[9] Gossip and colleagues (2017) note that public health agencies frequently utilize partner agencies and academic centers in the evaluation of exercises, but only rarely utilize this same expertise during or after a real-life response. Furthermore, while there is consensus that after action reviews should identify root causes, gaps remain in public health agencies' use of this approach. An analysis of AARs conducted by Barnett and colleagues (2020) found several cases in which stated recommendations did not identify an underlying problem; an earlier analysis by Singleton and colleagues (2014) also highlighted the frequent failure of recommendations and corrective actions to include root-cause analysis.

AARs are at risk of the same biases as the qualitative and quantitative methods on which they rely, and findings from the committee's commissioned quality assessment of AARs indicate that the reports typically omit the majority of important validity categories that could foster greater confidence in after action findings. Guidance aimed at improving after action review methods and the level of detail included in AAR methods sections is needed for both transparency and quality purposes, and AARs need to meet some minimum criteria concerning methods and reporting (Davies et al., 2019). The PHEPR field could benefit from drawing on the broader public health field to apply more rigorous evaluation processes when assessing lessons learned from public health emergencies. Training for evaluation participants, including academic programs in HSEEP certification and evaluation design, need to be encouraged and supported, if not required (Stoto et al., 2019). Standards and expectations regarding AARs could be strengthened by being integrated into PPHR (Summers and Ferraro, 2017). Similarly, PHAB could shape the evaluation of PHEPR by modifying its standards and measures to specifically include those that relate to PHEPR, thereby fostering efforts at quality improvement and evaluation (Brownson et al., 2018). Most important is for CDC and state,

---

[8] The peer assessment approach employs an evaluation conducted by peers in similar jurisdictions. This approach offers the potential for objective analyses by PHEPR professionals and knowledge of the particularities of the system being assessed (Piltch-Loeb et al., 2014b).

[9] The facilitated look-back approach uses a neutral facilitator and a no-fault approach to probe the nuances of decision making through moderated discussions (Piltch-Loeb et al., 2014b).

1. Define the story arc by summarizing the context and pivotal nodes (events, decisions, time points) when events could have unfolded differently and could have led to a substantially different outcome.
2. Identify the public health system's major organizational goals or objectives in responding to the incident, including which PHEP Capabilities and IHR (2005) core capacities that were stressed.
3. Identify the major response challenges that had a qualitative impact on permitting achievement of the public health system's goals or at least had the potential to do so.
4. Define the immediate causes of the challenges and the factors that contributed to the challenges, whether modifiable (within the jurisdiction's influence) or not modifiable (not within the jurisdiction's influence); note pre-event decisions and factors beyond the system's control.
5. Identify factors that, if not addressed, are likely to limit the public health system in future incidents. With these steps in mind, RCA can help those conducting the AAR to include the deepest level of analysis within their review.

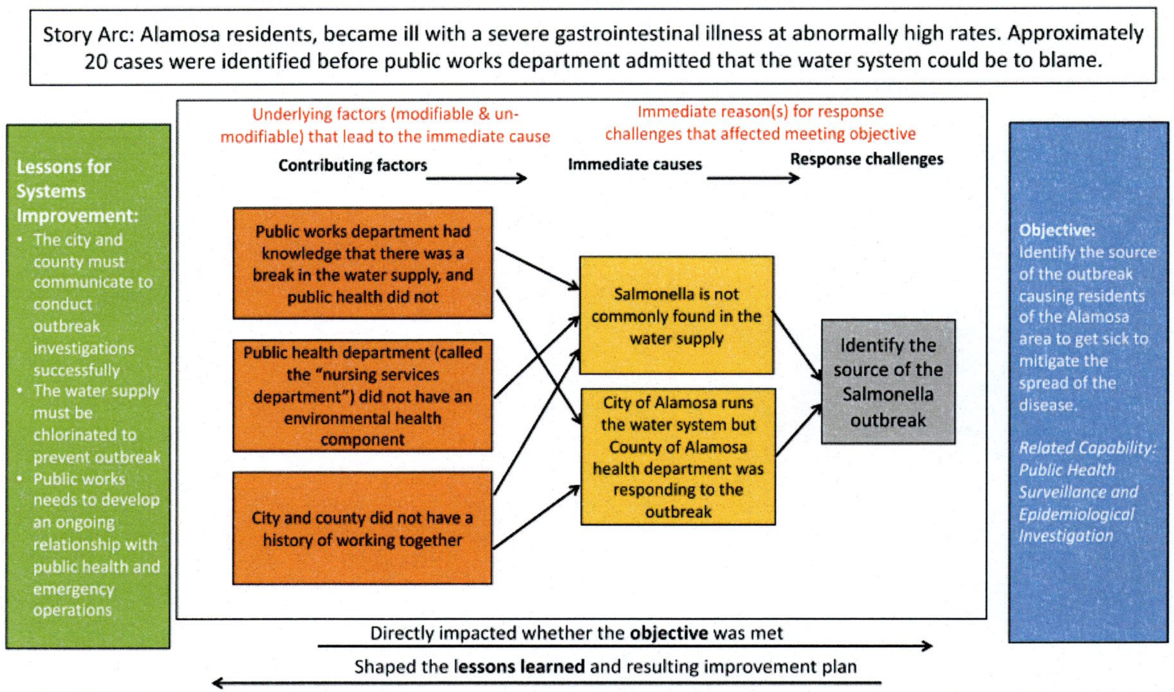

FIGURE 8-4 Root-cause analysis: Steps and examples.
NOTE: AAR = after action report; IHR = International Health Regulations; PHEP = public health emergency preparedness; RCA = root-cause analysis
SOURCE: Reprinted with permission from Stoto et al., 2019.

local, tribal, and territorial (SLTT) public health agencies, in addition to approaching AARs as an administrative requirement, to begin viewing them as a source of experiential evidence that could inform the development of evidence-based PHEPR practices and providing the necessary training, infrastructure, and resources to improve the quality of AARs produced.

Independent After Action Review Panel

According to Gossip and colleagues (2017), partnering with external organizations (e.g., peer agencies, consultants, academic centers) improves the depth and quality of documentation and assessments, as external organizations often have the requisite expertise and skills and capacity (e.g., time and personnel) to conduct or guide more rigorous evaluations. The United States has a strong history of creating objective, independent review panels (e.g., the National Transportation Safety Board and the National Institute of Standards and Technology's National Construction Safety Team Advisory Committee), consisting of collaborative partners to develop guidelines, evaluate data and findings, and investigate incidents. These objective bodies have been proposed as a model for the PHEPR field (Barnett et al., 2020; Keim et al., 2019; Kirsch et al., 2018). These types of processes ensure objective expertise by eliminating the inherent biases of self-assessment and make use of consistent methods so that findings are comparable over time. Such a panel could review all events reaching the threshold of a Stafford Act or Public Health Service Act event. This process could be conducted by a newly established group, through existing professional associations, accrediting bodies, or regional academic partnerships and networks.

Essential Core Elements of a PHEPR AAR

To enable aggregation and analysis of AAR data for use as a potential source of evidence on the effectiveness of PHEPR practices, it is essential to define the core elements of a PHEPR AAR that builds on the existing HSEEP format but embraces more of a public health perspective. These elements would include a standardized core dataset and root-cause analysis framework that ultimately could be used not only by one jurisdiction, but also across jurisdictions for purposes of aggregation, trend analysis, and systemwide comparison (see Box 8-3 for the committee's suggested elements for such an AAR template). Focusing on system-level root causes rather than specific problems would help make the experience more broadly applicable (i.e., enhance generalizability) (Stoto et al., 2019). An executive summary with high-level findings for each AAR would aid further in developing the empirical evidence base. An online platform prepopulating evaluation forms for practitioner-specific reporting objectives could also be developed (Agboola et al., 2015). Such a platform, with standardized questions at the national level, would assist practitioners in completing evaluations, integrate consistent measures into the review process, and aid in conducting trend analyses over time.

Establishing Mechanisms for Analysis and Dissemination of Lessons Learned from AARs

Proper conditions for establishing the utility and credibility of AARs as a less biased source are needed to improve the utility of these reports in evidence reviews and guidance for practical decision making. Improved mechanisms for public sharing of lessons learned from AARs, such as an enhanced national AAR repository, that specifically preclude the use of the reports for punitive purposes would foster more accurate and reliable information.

BOX 8-3 THE COMMITTEE'S SUGGESTED ELEMENTS FOR A PHEPR AFTER ACTION REPORT TEMPLATE

- a structured executive summary focused on what agency leadership would find most useful for decision making to inform current and future responses (and designed to be database searchable with a maximum word count);
- a word-limited abstract to provide an overview of the incident, important contextual factors, the tested PHEPR Capabilities, and key findings;
- an acronym and definition list, as jurisdictions often use terms differently;
- a background section that provides enough information for someone with an outsider's perspective to understand the context of the situation and event without being overburdened by unnecessary details;
- a methods section that describes the sampling, data sources, and other elements from the European Centre for Disease Prevention and Control's 11-item validity tool;
- a section for root-cause analysis of the system response, with specific assessments of the PHEPR Capabilities and explicit interventions used in the event;
- specific fields for the reporting of standardized information, such as a defined list of outcomes and corrective actions; and
- inclusion of the tools used to conduct the review for the after action report (e.g., surveys, hotwash guides, focus group guides) as an appendix, so that jurisdictions need not reinvent the wheel.

Currently, finding relevant and publicly available AARs that can serve as reliable sources of information and identifying useful observations within them is a notably labor-intensive process with variable yield. With the proper incentives and standards in place to encourage submission of AARs (e.g., formal recognition from the user community or appropriate agencies or qualification for additional exercise funding), an enhanced national AAR repository could be a useful tool for improving PHEPR (Kearns, 2010; Piltch-Loeb et al., 2014a; Turner et al., 2018).

FEMA's Lessons Learned Information Sharing (LLIS) platform was developed to serve as a protected repository of AARs, reports of best practices, and lessons learned for all emergency response communities (HSDL, 2020). In 2015, LLIS was consolidated with the Homeland Security Digital Library (HSDL). Presently, the HSDL serves as the only repository for AARs, but submission of AARs to this database is voluntary, AARs include those submitted by sectors other than public health, other documents are also submitted, and the database is not easily searchable. These factors make it difficult to locate public health AARs to include in analyses.

A national AAR repository would ideally include indexed and searchable executive summaries and searchable high-level findings derived from AARs of federal- and state-supported exercises and tabletops, as well as responses to real events. This information would be organized and referenced by thematic content, findings, and type of event. To ensure a national AAR repository that is both feasible and useful, it is important to consider the following issues:

- the required resources and barriers to overcome for the creation, establishment, and curating of such a repository;
- the necessary infrastructure and protocols, which may include the creation and the adoption and assurance of submission standards, technology-based capture of key information from submitted AARs, and automated data aggregation and analysis;

- the incorporation of wide-ranging and user-friendly capabilities, which at a minimum would need to include systematic searchable parameters enabling identification of specific examples and details likely to emerge as themes across AARs;
- the ability to support analysis by verified users by providing channels for sharing anonymous or deidentified data;
- the ability to routinely audit and review entries, coupled with technical support to ensure accuracy and relevance; and
- mechanisms for response to user feedback and other continuous quality improvement measures.

Fostering a Culture of Quality Improvement

PHEPR programs reside in SLTT public health agencies, and because they are government entities, their reports are open to public access through local and state freedom of information laws. Reports filed with CDC are open to access through the Freedom of Information Act. Sensitivity to the release of security issues captured in reports, as well as concern about the exposure of vulnerabilities or weaknesses, has resulted in a reluctance to publish or even complete these reports. PHEPR practitioners are hesitant to report problems or weaknesses observed during a response because of the potential political ramifications and fear of punitive action (Gossip et al., 2017). Therefore, current agency culture leads to overlooking AARs as critical for informing evidence-based decision making. This situation stands in contrast to data used for health care quality assurance and protected in most states by "safe harbor" laws, data that have been cited as pivotal in participation in quality improvement initiatives by health care entities and practitioners (Gliklich et al., 2014). The PHEPR field would similarly benefit from a more open, structured, and meaningful culture of quality improvement that would enable the ongoing reporting and analysis of successes and challenges.

Conclusions and Recommendation

Conclusion: Unclear reporting requirements, a lack of methodological standards, and disincentives for accurate reporting of problems experienced during response operations limit the evidentiary value of AARs for the development of evidence-based guidelines. These issues represent a significant lost opportunity to learn from practice and to leverage real-world experience to develop such guidelines.

Conclusion: Unless protection is ensured for sensitive data collected in AARs, information on shortcomings during public health emergency responses will remain hidden, and similar errors will be repeated. Improved systems for public sharing of AARs that specifically preclude their use for punitive purposes would foster access to more accurate and reliable information, supporting the utility of the reports in evidence reviews and guidance for practical decision making.

RECOMMENDATION 6: Pursue Efforts to Further a Process of Quality Improvement to Enhance the Quality and Utility of After Action Reports (AARs)
The Centers for Disease Control and Prevention, in collaboration with the Office of the Assistant Secretary for Preparedness and Response and the Federal Emergency Management Agency, should convene an expert panel of relevant federal agencies; state, local, tribal, and territorial public health agencies; and professional associations to advance

a process for quality improvement at the local, regional, state, and national levels to enhance the quality and utility of AARs and support their use as sources of evidence for evaluating the effectiveness of public health emergency preparedness and response (PHEPR) practices. This process should foster a culture of improvement in public health emergency response and include, but not be limited to, discussions aimed at

- raising standards and expectations regarding the quality of information reported in AARs by defining the essential core elements of a PHEPR AAR;
- establishing an independent review panel with a standardized after action reporting process, with the aims of reducing bias and increasing the utility of AARs produced following public health emergency responses;
- establishing and maintaining a national repository of AARs or of reports based on analysis of AARs that is readily accessible to support the dissemination of key findings, lessons learned, and best practices for public health emergency response; and
- exploring the relevant privacy issues and the protection of information in AARs from use in legal proceedings or other punitive actions against practitioners and organizations, as has been done for "peer-review" data in other fields (medicine, aviation, and occupational health).

WORKFORCE CAPACITY DEVELOPMENT FOR RESEARCHERS AND PRACTITIONERS IN PHEPR

A robust and sustained commitment to workforce capacity development for both PHEPR researchers and practitioners is essential to advancing evidence-based practice in PHEPR. Investigators will have to produce research that is relevant to practitioners, and practitioners will have to turn routinely to research when making important decisions about implementing practices. Although there exists a network of researchers capable of conducting high-quality research on public health emergencies, these researchers require additional and ongoing training to design and implement studies and analyze and report study findings in a rigorous manner. It will also be important for practitioners to participate in or conduct evaluations. New skills, some going beyond traditional public health training, are often needed for practitioners to successfully conduct evaluations and identify and implement evidence-based practices (Brownson et al., 2018). Currently, the PHEPR workforce comprises both researchers and practitioners who often are educated and trained in schools of public health, but many other disciplines are represented as well, including physicians, nurses, social workers, veterinarians, and social scientists. Yet, there is little evidence that the graduate education and training these individuals receive in their respective domains is designed or tailored to address the unique challenges of conducting research in disaster-affected communities or during public health emergencies.

Researchers

Academic disaster research centers proliferated after the events of September 11, 2001, and funding for training for disaster researchers was readily available (see Chapter 2). Given the ongoing reduction in funding over the past several years, however, workforce attrition is likely. Academic researchers who moved into PHEPR research from public health and other related fields when funding was readily available may have left the PHEPR field when funding became more limited.

There exists today virtually no investment in the developmental pipeline for PHEPR researchers, a gap that corresponds to the relative dearth of funding opportunities for related research. The scarcity of PHEPR research and training grants inhibits the training of a new generation of researchers in the PHEPR field. In addition to funding for research awards, it is important to consider funding for training grants and career development awards. In the past, CDC has funded Mentored Research Scientist Development Awards (K01) to provide support for intensive research career development under the guidance of a mentor in areas addressing bioterrorism, other infectious disease outbreaks, and other public health threats and emergencies, among other areas (CDC, 2007). To ensure diverse, adequately trained, and sufficiently available disaster researchers, it will be necessary to invest in improved and sustained researcher training programs and grants (e.g., NIH career development K awards, RWJF leadership development programs), particularly those aimed at increasing PHEPR research capacity in the areas of implementation science and evaluation of complex interventions (NIH, 2020b; RWJF, 2020b). Researcher training programs can help direct training toward specific important areas; provide support for training in other, emerging areas; and establish research standards.

Additionally, special attention is essential to recruiting and supporting underrepresented minority researchers, including those who understand critical race theory, indigenous research methods, and other relevant frameworks, so that PHEPR science can advance equitably. Efforts are needed to connect doctoral and postdoctoral students early on in their careers so as to build relationships, connections, and teams to carry out ongoing PHEPR research projects. In a similar vein, mentoring programs involving senior and early-career researchers can support training for future generations. Many fields have recognized that providing means of supporting a steady infusion of highly trained researchers with new ideas is necessary to advance the quality of research (DHS, 2020; NCER, 2020; NIH, 2019a; NSF, 2020a).

Practitioners

As previously mentioned, PHEPR practitioners require the knowledge and skills not only to identify and implement evidence-based practices but also to conduct and participate in research and evaluation. In general, the public health workforce varies greatly in terms of job descriptions, education requirements, and experience, which are not standardized across public health agencies. A recent study found that having a public health degree was significantly associated with reduced odds of reporting a skill gap in identifying and applying evidence-based approaches to address a public health issue (Maddock, 2018; Taylor and Yeager, 2019).

A barrier to PHEPR practitioners working effectively with researchers may be that practitioners do not have the training or experience to identify programmatic and practice challenges that could be studied by researchers (Carbone and Thomas, 2018). Renewable certification programs, similar to the certified emergency manager program (IAEM, 2020), and a standardized training program for CDC project officers and state preparedness directors, as well as practitioners working in PHEPR more broadly, could ensure familiarity with evidence-based practices and promote the consistent creation and evaluation of real-world evidence as captured in AARs. CDC's TRAIN Learning Network; ASPR's Technical Resources, Assistance Center, and Information Exchange; and FEMA's Emergency Management Institute provide a wealth of trainings and resources for PHEPR practitioners that could be leveraged and enhanced to provide practitioners with the knowledge and skills needed to identify and implement evidence-based practices and to conduct and participate in research and evaluation (ASPR, 2020; FEMA, 2020; PHF, 2020).

A number of other policy and operational barriers, including workload and responsibilities and priorities during a response, impede PHEPR practitioners' abilities to conduct and participate in evaluations. Another model for addressing these barriers is to give practitioners access to external contractors with evaluation expertise that can provide tailored evaluation tools, appropriate training, and feedback on program evaluation plans and products (Maynard, 2018).

Recognizing that not everyone is equally suited or professionally able to be both a practitioner and researcher, it is necessary to develop stronger systems, infrastructure, and norms around the notion of an integrated PHEPR research and practice system that includes both those who are focused on advancing the science and those applying this knowledge. Platforms to provide ongoing technical assistance, peer networking, and collaboration across disciplines for both practitioners and researchers could ensure an interconnected workforce. Individuals who perceived themselves as part of this new interconnected PHEPR undertaking would share the mission of improving population health outcomes during public health emergencies and would be better positioned to interact with their colleagues across the traditional divides of practice and research.

Conclusion and Recommendation

Conclusion: Training, education, and technical assistance programs to provide PHEPR researchers and practitioners with the knowledge, skills, and competencies to conduct rigorous and relevant PHEPR research and evaluation and implement evidence-based practices are seriously deficient. Comprehensive efforts to support workforce capacity development are necessary to ensure that a qualified and competent PHEPR researcher and practitioner workforce is developed and sustained to address increasingly complex public health emergencies.

RECOMMENDATION 7: Support Workforce Capacity Development and Technical Assistance Programs for Public Health Emergency Preparedness and Response (PHEPR) Researchers and Practitioners

The Centers for Disease Control and Prevention (CDC) and the Office of the Assistant Secretary for Preparedness and Response should work with professional and academic organizations that represent multiple disciplines to guide and support the creation of the workforce capacity development and technical assistance programs necessary to ensure the conduct of quality PHEPR research and evaluation and improve the implementation capacity of state, local, tribal, and territorial public health agencies. Such efforts should include

- developing a research training infrastructure and career development grants—institutional and individual predoctoral, postdoctoral, loan repayment, and career awards—to develop and support researchers in PHEPR in order to address research gaps in the field;
- providing training grants so that PHEPR researcher and practitioner teams can learn how to develop PHEPR practices that are grounded in science and theory and to evaluate the effectiveness and implementation of PHEPR practices using rigorous and appropriate designs;
- providing ongoing technical assistance and peer networking for both PHEPR researchers and practitioners; and

- creating a training and certification program for CDC project officers and state preparedness directors to ensure their familiarity with evidence-based practices and promote consistent creation and evaluation of real-world evidence as captured in after action reports.

TRANSLATION, DISSEMINATION, AND IMPLEMENTATION OF PHEPR RESEARCH TO PRACTICE

While there is a clear need to strengthen the evidence base for PHEPR practices through improvements in research and quality improvement processes, an equally pressing challenge is the translation, dissemination, and implementation of the evidence to practice (Carbone and Thomas, 2018). Numerous barriers impede the uptake of evidence-based practice, including varying awareness of the existing evidence base and lack of coordination between researchers and practitioners, lack of time, inadequate funding, inability to analyze and interpret evidence, and absence of cultural and managerial support (Brownson et al., 2018; Siegfried et al., 2017). Nonetheless, the absence of incentives has been found to be the greatest barrier, compounded by the disincentive of the time required (Jacobs et al., 2010). Such challenges are not unique to PHEPR. For example, the cultural shift toward evidence-based practice in health care evolved over decades, driven in part by financial and reputational liabilities for institutions and practitioners and increased accountability for clinical outcomes (Carbone and Thomas, 2018). While the adoption of evidence-based practices has been an ongoing challenge in the PHEPR field, significant investments made in implementation science more broadly across public health, health care, and other disciplines could guide the translation and implementation of research to practice for PHEPR (Brown et al., 2017; Brownson et al., 2012).

Recognizing the importance of this issue, CDC in 2015 initiated the Translation, Dissemination, and Implementation of Public Health Preparedness and Response Research and Training Initiative (TDI Initiative), a 2-year effort to consolidate and synthesize the research produced by the Preparedness and Emergency Response Research Centers and Preparedness and Emergency Response Learning Centers and translate that research into practice (Qari et al., 2018) (see Chapter 2). Table 8-3 describes best practices for the translation, dissemination, and implementation of PHEPR tools and resources that emerged from this initiative. Despite these efforts, however, barriers to the adoption of evidence-based PHEPR practices persist, related largely to capacity issues.

Building Implementation Capacity

Successful implementation requires that public health agencies have sufficient capacity to identify and translate scientific knowledge into practice (Brownson et al., 2018). Uneven infrastructure and capacity represent a long-standing challenge for public health systems (Baker and Koplan, 2002), and many SLTT public health agencies lack sufficient capacity (i.e., resources, infrastructure, and workforce) to identify and translate research and implement evidence-based practices. Fluctuations in public health funding are common and often result in smaller public health entities having to prioritize "keeping the doors open" and ensuring that critical public health services remain functional, leaving them with little to no financial means for investing in PHEPR training and implementation efforts (NORC at the University of Chicago, 2017). Furthermore, best practices currently are often not developed

TABLE 8-3 Best Practices for the Translation, Dissemination, and Implementation of Evidence-Based PHEPR Practices

Area	Best Practices
Translation	• Engage the end user (i.e., public health practice community) from the start to ensure that evidence-based practices are appropriate and relevant • Create training webinars to acquaint PHEPR practitioners with new skills or processes to improve performance • Include real-world and local community scenarios and examples to demonstrate how to use practices, processes, tools, and resources
Dissemination	• Word of mouth and personal recommendation • Conferences and national meetings • Radio stations, to present and translate important information (especially for tribes) • In-person meetings, which provide an opportunity for direct communication • The Internet, including websites, blog posts, email newsletters, gaming techniques, distribution lists, and social media • Trusted public health agencies and public health professional organizations, such as the Association of State and Territorial Health Officials and the National Association of County & City Health Officials • Publication of evidence-based practices in the Centers for Disease Control and Prevention (CDC) communication platforms (e.g., *Morbidity and Mortality Weekly Report*, blogs) • Peer-to-peer learning through existing networks • State health departments, which receive information and resources from CDC and share them with local health departments • Health care coalitions that exist within various states and localities
Implementation	• Ensure that products and tools can be implemented by different agency and organization types (health care, public health, emergency management agencies, others) • Provide implementation support for a new tool or resource, as it can be challenging for public health agencies to gain momentum for implementation • Identify an advocate within the agency who will ensure that the tool remains a priority during planning and implementation • Provide support to bring staff together to review and practice implementing evidence-based practices • Create products that are ready to use, because practitioners have limited time to review, modify, and adapt resources for local use • Build in-person trainings into existing grant structures

SOURCES: Adapted from NORC at the University of Chicago, 2017; Qari et al., 2018.

with smaller or tribal or territorial public health agencies in mind, which frequently leads to implementation issues.

Addressing these barriers will require a multipronged and coordinated approach involving a combination of training, technical assistance, tools, and incentives (e.g., grant and funding requirements). The Interactive Systems Framework for Dissemination and Implementation offers a model for building public health agencies' capacity to use best practices (Wandersman et al., 2008). The TDI Initiative utilized this framework, incorporating prevention support systems, which "provide information, training, technical assistance, or other support for practitioners," to enhance program implementation efforts (Qari et al., 2018, p. S359).

Creating and Disseminating Practice-Ready Resources and Tools

Researchers are often ill equipped to translate research and resources for practitioners' implementation. There is a clear need for tools and resources that are ready for "on the ground" use and disseminated in accordance with practitioner demand. Engaging translation and implementation specialists in the development of such tools and resources could help ensure that they are practice ready and can be implemented by practitioners at all levels

(Carbone and Thomas, 2018). For example, understanding that a translation gap persists between the availability of PHEPR tools and their adoption within public health agencies, Revere and colleagues (2018) explored with practitioners a process for identifying communication products to be considered as the highest implementation priority to improve communications in public health agencies. To increase awareness of existing resources and knowledge, CDC could provide dissemination support by deploying field agents to champion and disseminate evidence-based practices and tools across the PHEPR practice community (Carbone and Thomas, 2018).

Facilitating Tailoring of Evidence-Based Practices to Fit Local Contexts

Given differences among public health jurisdictions, including variability in contexts and capacity, it is essential for any implementation effort to recognize the importance of local needs and allow for the tailoring of practices to those needs (Arora et al., 2018; Baseman et al., 2018; Eisenman et al., 2018; Revere et al., 2018; Testa et al., 2018). Practitioners need appropriate training and a robust public health knowledge base to make appropriate and effective modifications to a practice so that it suits new settings or contexts (Eisenman et al., 2018). Eisenman and colleagues (2018) recently implemented a two-component intervention involving training and technical assistance and the creation and use of a guidebook to enhance the capacity of local public health agencies to translate and implement evidence-based practices in emergency preparedness. Evaluation of this program showed that after it was implemented, practitioners' skills had significantly increased, indicating that such a program could be useful to other public health agencies. Existing tools are also available to decision makers to facilitate the implementation of evidence-based policies. For example, the SUPporting POlicy relevant Reviews and Trials tools are designed to help decision makers consider the applicability of evidence-based practices to their local conditions and tailor implementation strategies accordingly to address identified barriers and facilitators (Lavis et al., 2009; Lewin et al., 2009).

When a PHEPR practice is being considered for implementation in different contexts, identifying its core components can help determine what should remain intact and what can be modified without jeopardizing outcomes. An intervention's core components are the basic principles and activities deemed necessary to generate desired outcomes, and they are rooted in its theoretical drivers of change (ASPE, 2013). Identifying specific core components can thus help practitioners tailor existing evidence-based practices to the local context. This tailoring is based on answers to such operational questions as: What activities are we going to conduct? Who is going to carry out the activity? What must people learn? and What resources are required? Additional research into the identification of core components of PHEPR practices would improve understanding of which components are essential for evidence-based practices to produce desired outcomes and how this is moderated by differences in population, setting, and other contextual factors, thus enabling practitioners to better operationalize interventions in their local setting. Encouraging the inclusion of core components in descriptions of evidence-based practices could also help ensure ongoing fidelity over time (ASPE, 2013). Funding for the translation, dissemination, and implementation of these identified core components would promote the replication and scalability of practices and the associated tools and resources across a variety of settings.

Incentivizing Adoption of Evidence-Based PHEPR Practices

Other changes to federal programming and policy could facilitate the implementation of evidence-based PHEPR practices. As discussed in Chapter 2, CDC's Public Health Emergency Preparedness (PHEP) Cooperative Agreement represents the primary mechanism for funding by the federal government for SLTT public health agencies, accounting for the overwhelming majority of any preparedness funds at the SLTT level. However, current programmatic grant requirements do not sufficiently emphasize or support the generation of PHEPR evidence or the use of evidence-based practices, and PHEPR practitioners generally have no incentive to use evidence-based practices in their planning (CDC, 2019). To begin to bridge the gap between research and practice, CDC could incorporate the use of evidence-based practices (e.g., those identified by the PHEPR evidence-based guidelines group proposed in Recommendation 1 in Chapter 3) into the PHEP Cooperative Agreement, with linkage to CDC's PHEPR Capabilities, asking grantees to use evidence-based practices where available and to justify why they are not doing so when they are not. It will be important to engage with state health officials as well as other key stakeholders with regard to this proposed strategy. Accreditation bodies such as PHAB and recognition programs such as PPHR are also positioned to act as drivers for embedding evidence-based practices into PHEPR programs, and could be leveraged to facilitate the translation, dissemination, and implementation of research to practice (Brownson et al., 2018; Summers and Ferraro, 2017).

Conclusion and Recommendation

Conclusion: Evidence derived from PHEPR research and evaluation efforts will improve response outcomes in the event of a public health emergency only if it is translated to and implemented by PHEPR practitioners. Ensuring the translation, dissemination, and implementation of evidence-based PHEPR practices will require the infrastructure not only to produce evidence but also to summarize, synthesize, and disseminate it and ensure its effective use.

RECOMMENDATION 8: Ensure the Translation, Dissemination, and Implementation of Public Health Emergency Preparedness and Response (PHEPR) Research to Practice
The Centers for Disease Control and Prevention (CDC) should use a coordinated implementation science approach to ensure that the evidence-based practice recommendations resulting from the PHEPR evidence-based guidelines group proposed in Recommendation 1 achieve broad reach and become the standard of practice of the target audience. Strategies to this end include

- incorporating evidence-based practices into the *Public Health Emergency Preparedness and Response Capabilities: National Standards for State, Local, Tribal, and Territorial Public Health* guidance document;
- building evidence-based practices into the design of and funding decisions for the Public Health Emergency Preparedness Cooperative Agreement program;
- incentivizing and requiring state, local, tribal, and territorial public health agencies to test and evaluate new or adapted practices and embed program evaluations into routine operations to help better understand whether evidence-based practices worked, under what conditions, with what impacts and consequences, and at what cost;

- publishing evidence-based practices in CDC communication platforms (e.g., the *Morbidity and Mortality Weekly Report,* blogs) and partnering with public health professional organizations, such as the Association of State and Territorial Health Officials and the National Association of County & City Health Officials (NACCHO), to disseminate evidence-based practices;
- incorporating the requirement of utilizing evidence-based PHEPR practices into such processes as the Public Health Accreditation Board accreditation and such recognition programs as NACCHO's Project Public Health Ready; and
- incorporating implementation science principles, such as the conduct of research to understand core components required for intervention effectiveness, into PHEPR research.

ANNEX 8-1
GENRES OF RESEARCH TO INFORM PUBLIC HEALTH EMERGENCY PREPAREDNESS AND RESPONSE PRACTICES

TABLE ANNEX 8-1 Genres of Research to Inform PHEPR Practices: Purpose, Example Research Questions, and Appropriate Methods

Genre of Research*	Purpose	Example Research Question(s)	Appropriate Methods and Theoretical Perspectives
Priority Setting and Clarifying the Problem and Causes	To understand the cause and magnitude of the problem and to determine that something should be done. These studies can also provide evidence of relationships between emergency events and consequences in a particular context and/or for particular population groups. To understand the PHEPR system challenges and stakeholders' views and experiences, and to provide contextual information relevant to other forms of research.	What are the nature, magnitude, and appropriate framing of the problem, as well as contributing factors, that together indicate the need for intervention? What PHEPR practices are needed, and what would they look like? What outcomes are important, and for whom?	Epidemiological studies (cohort and case control), community surveys, and analyses of data systems Qualitative studies (focus groups, interviews, observations, documentary analysis) Quantitative, qualitative, and mixed-method synthesis methods Rapid review methods, research priority-setting methods

TABLE ANNEX 8-1 Continued

Genre of Research*	Purpose	Example Research Question(s)	Appropriate Methods and Theoretical Perspectives
Design and Development, Including Feasibility and Pilot Testing	To inform the design and development of new or improved PHEPR practices that will address particular problems in PHEPR. These studies can also help develop the intervention program theory (theory of change), core components, and selected outcomes of interest. To test the feasibility of implementing the intervention in specific contexts, recruitment of participants, and the availability and feasibility of collecting data. To establish the sample size calculation if needed; clarify the program theory; and determine primary outcomes, whether a complexity perspective would be useful, and what cost data are required and available. The information from such studies is often used to identify evidence that suggests potential causal relationships (or the lack thereof) for a PHEPR practice. To determine how best to implement the PHEPR practice, such as what strategies (e.g., training and resources) are required and what approaches could be used.	What is the PHEPR practice, how is it intended to work, and what outcomes is it designed to achieve and with whom? What outcome measures are appropriate? Which stakeholders need to be involved in the implementation of a preparedness training program for community-based partners? How feasible is the PHEPR practice to implement? What aspects of complexity appear important when implementing this PHEPR practice (e.g., system adaptivity and feedback loops)? Does the PHEPR practice need further development or adaptation? Does the pilot trial work as intended in this setting with this PHEPR practice? What implementation strategy works best with whom and in which context?	Qualitative studies (focus groups, interviews, observations) Community-based participatory research, mixed methods, case studies Qualitative and mixed-method process evaluations, realist synthesis methods Feasibility studies, health economic methods, pilot trials Implementation science methods Other considerations: Consider the use of existing intervention development frameworks for complex intervention development (e.g., UK Medical Research Council Framework). Also, sociobehavioral research is needed to lay the theoretical and empirical foundation for PHEPR practices (e.g., it is challenging to have an effective program for delivering vaccines or countermeasures without knowing about such sociobehavioral domains as trust and mistrust; risk perceptions and health behaviors; and the effects of racism, both historical and everyday or ordinary, on health care access)

continued

TABLE ANNEX 8-1 Continued

Genre of Research*	Purpose	Example Research Question(s)	Appropriate Methods and Theoretical Perspectives
Quantitative Impact Evaluation	To determine whether PHEPR practices are effective or work as intended to achieve the desired outcomes; to understand the benefits and harms of PHEPR practices. Impact evaluations are typically conducted in cases where there exist a well-developed theory of change and a well-defined PHEPR practice that is being tested. In some cases, the impact evaluation will be testing the intervention in a well-controlled setting and with high-fidelity implementation, while in other cases, it may be tested under routine conditions of practice.	Is activating public health emergency operations centers [specify components] more effective than the status quo approach (commonly referred to as "business as usual") in achieving Y [specified outcomes]? Is strategy A [specify] for communicating public health guidance and alerts with technical audiences during a public health emergency more effective than strategy B [specify] in achieving Y [specified outcomes]? What core components of public health emergency operations centers are critical to their effectiveness? What are the comparative costs of strategy A and strategy B?	Randomized controlled trials, quasi-experimental studies (matched comparison group studies, interrupted time series, regression discontinuity design, multivariate analyses), pre-post comparison design
Process Evaluation	To determine what happened when a PHEPR practice was implemented (e.g., what worked for whom in which contexts). To learn about the relationships between PHEPR-related practices and outcomes in various contexts and gather implementation knowledge (e.g., adoption, fidelity, barriers, facilitators, scale-up costs, equity). To identify variation among impacts across implementation contexts and explore potential mediators and moderators of the impacts.	What worked for whom in which contexts? What would have happened if the practice had not been implemented? Is the PHEPR practice acceptable and feasible for recipients and key stakeholders? What are the barriers to and facilitators of effective engagement and training of community-based partners?	Realist trials and process evaluation methods Qualitative and mixed-method process evaluations Qualitative comparative analysis Equity frameworks and methods Case studies, after action reviews

TABLE ANNEX 8-1 Continued

Genre of Research*	Purpose	Example Research Question(s)	Appropriate Methods and Theoretical Perspectives
Systems and Operations Research	To use quantitative approaches to analyze strategic, tactical, and operational aspects of public health emergency response to improve preparedness policies or practices. Models typically use historical or simulated data to estimate expected responses to emergency conditions under varying preparedness conditions, controlling for or varying potential confounding or complicating factors.	In what circumstances (e.g., based on biologic factors, risks, resource availability, legal authorities, social context) is quarantine effective at reducing or stopping the spread of a contagious disease?	Statistical and mathematical modeling, simulation modeling, queueing theory, optimization
Implementation, Adaptation, and Scale-Up	To determine how best to adapt and tailor PHEPR practices to specific populations and contexts. To determine how best to scale up interventions for widespread adoption.	What needs adapting and how? Is the scaled-up version as effective as the original version? What does it cost to scale up an intervention?	Randomized controlled trials, quasi-experimental studies (matched comparison group studies, interrupted time series, regression discontinuity design, multivariate analyses), pre-post comparison design Realist trials and process evaluation methods Qualitative and mixed-method process evaluations Implementation science methods Health economic methods

* For all genres of research, engaging end users and other stakeholders is advised when feasible.

REFERENCES

AcademyHealth. 2017. *Evaluating complex health interventions: A guide to rigorous research designs.* https://www.academyhealth.org/sites/default/files/AH_Evaluation_Guide_FINAL.pdf (accessed March 10, 2020).

Acosta, J. D., C. Nelson, E. B. Beckjord, S. R. Shelton, E. Murphy, K. L. Leuschner, and J. Wasserman. 2009. *A national agenda for public health systems research on emergency preparedness.* Santa Monica, CA: RAND Health.

Adams, R. M., H. Rivard, and D. P. Eisenman. 2017. Who participates in building disaster resilient communities: A cluster-analytic approach. *Journal of Public Health Management & Practice* 23(1):37–46.

Agboola, F., D. Bernard, E. Savoia, and P. D. Biddinger. 2015. Development of an online toolkit for measuring performance in health emergency response exercises. *Prehospital and Disaster Medicine* 30(5):503–508.

AHRQ (Agency for Healthcare Research and Quality). 2019. *Pratice-based research networks: Research in everyday practice.* https://pbrn.ahrq.gov (accessed February 21, 2020).

Alfred P. Sloan Foundation. 2020. *Biosecurity.* https://sloan.org/programs/completed-programs/biosecurity (accessed May 13, 2020).

Arora, M., B. Granillo, T. K. Zepeda, and J. L. Burgess. 2018. Experiential adult learning: A pathway to enhancing medical countermeasures capabilities. *American Journal of Public Health* 108(S5):S378–S380.

ASPE (Office of the Assistant Secretary for Planning and Evaluation). 2013. *Core intervention components: Identifying and operationalizing what makes programs work.* https://aspe.hhs.gov/report/core-intervention-components-identifying-and-operationalizing-what-makes-programs-work (accessed February 21, 2020).

ASPR (Assistant Secretary for Preparedness and Response). 2020. *Welcome to ASPR TRACIE.* https://asprtracie.hhs.gov (accessed May 13, 2020).

Baker, E. L., Jr., and J. P. Koplan. 2002. Strengthening the nation's public health infrastructure: Historic challenge, unprecedented opportunity. *Health Affairs (Project Hope)* 21(6).

Barnett, D. J., K. Strauss-Riggs, V. L. Klimczak, A. J. Rosenblum, and T. D. Kirsch. 2020. An analysis of after action reports from Texas hurricanes in 2005 and 2017. *Journal of Public Health Management and Practice* (prepublication).

Baseman, J., D. Revere, H. Karasz, and S. Allan. 2018. Implementing innovations in public health agency preparedness and response programs. *American Journal of Public Health* 108(S5):S369–S371.

Begg, C., M. Cho, S. Eastwood, R. Horton, D. Moher, I. Olkin, R. Pitkin, D. Rennie, K. F. Schulz, D. Simel, and D. F. Stroup. 1996. Improving the quality of reporting of randomized controlled trials: The consort statement. *Journal of the American Medical Association* 276(8):637–639.

Berry, S. M., E. A. Petzold, P. Dull, N. M. Thielman, C. K. Cunningham, G. R. Corey, M. T. McClain, D. L. Hoover, J. Russell, J. M. Griffiss, and C. W. Woods. 2016. A response adaptive randomization platform trial for efficient evaluation of ebola virus treatments: A model for pandemic response. *Clinical Trials* 13(1):22–30.

Bill & Melinda Gates Foundation. 2020. *How we work—Grant opportunities.* https://www.gatesfoundation.org/how-we-work/general-information/grant-opportunities (accessed May 13, 2020).

Blanchet, K., C. Allen, J. Breckon, P. Davies, D. Duclos, J. Jansen, H. Mthiyane, and M. Clarke. 2018. *Using research evidence in the humanitarian sector: A practice guide.* London: Evidence Aid, London School of Hygiene and Tropicla Medicine and Nesta (Alliance for Useful Evidence). https://www.evidenceaid.org/wp-content/uploads/2018/10/Evidence_Aid_Practice_Guide_52pp_DIGITAL-FINAL-VERSION-2018-10-22.pdf (accessed March 10, 2020).

Bossuyt, P. M., J. B. Reitsma, D. E. Bruns, C. A. Gatsonis, P. P. Glasziou, L. Irwig, J. G. Lijmer, D. Moher, D. Rennie, H. C. W. de Vet, H. Y. Kressel, N. Rifai, R. M. Golub, D. G. Altman, L. Hooft, D. A. Korevaar, and J. F. Cohen. 2015. STARD 2015: An updated list of essential items for reporting diagnostic accuracy studies. *Radiology* 277(3):826–832.

Bromley, E., D. P. Eisenman, A. Magana, M. Williams, B. Kim, M. McCreary, A. Chandra, and K. B. Wells. 2017. How do communities use a participatory public health approach to build resilience? The Los Angeles County Community Disaster Resilience Project. *International Journal of Environmental Research and Public Health* 14(10).

Brown, C. H., G. Curran, L. A. Palinkas, G. A. Aarons, K. B. Wells, L. Jones, L. M. Collins, N. Duan, B. S. Mittman, A. Wallace, R. G. Tabak, L. Ducharme, D. A. Chambers, G. Neta, T. Wiley, J. Landsverk, K. Cheung, and G. Cruden. 2017. An overview of research and evaluation designs for dissemination and implementation. *Annual Review of Public Health* 38(1):1–22.

Brownson, R. C., G. A. Colditz, and E. K. Proctor. 2012. *Dissemination and implementation research in health: Translating science to practice.* Oxford: Oxford University Press.

Brownson, R. C., J. E. Fielding, and L. W. Green. 2018. Building capacity for evidence-based public health: Reconciling the pulls of practice and the push of research. *Annual Review of Public Health* 39(1):27–53.

Burlig, F. 2018. Improving transparency in observational social science research: A pre-analysis plan approach. *Economics Letters* 168:56–60.

Carbone, E. G., and E. V. Thomas. 2018. Science as the basis of public health emergency preparedness and response practice: The slow but crucial evolution. *American Journal of Public Health* 108(S5):S383–S386.

CDC (Centers for Disease Control and Prevention). 2007. *CDC mentored public health research scientist development award (K01).* https://grants.nih.gov/grants/guide/rfa-files/RFA-CD-07-003.html#PartII (accessed February 12, 2020).

CDC. 2019. *Public health emergency preparedness (PHEP) cooperative agreement. CDC-RFA-TP19-1901.* https://www.grants.gov/web/grants/view-opportunity.html?oppId=310318 (accessed May 14, 2020).

CDC. 2020a. *Epidemic intelligence service.* https://www.cdc.gov/eis/index.html (accessed March 13, 2020).

CDC. 2020b. *Grants.* https://www.cdc.gov/grants/index.html (accessed May 13, 2020).

Cha, B. S., R. I. Lawrence, J. C. Bliss, K. B. Wells, A. Chandra, and D. P. Eisenman. 2016. The road to resilience: Insights on training community coalitions in the Los Angeles County Community Disaster Resilience Project. *Disaster Medicine and Public Health Preparedness* 10(6):812–821.

Chandra, A., M. Williams, A. Plough, A. Stayton, K. B. Wells, M. Horta, and J. Tang. 2013. Getting actionable about community resilience: The Los Angeles County Community Disaster Resilience Project. *American Journal of Public Health* 103(7):1181–1189.

Chandra, A., M. V. Williams, C. Lopez, J. Tang, D. Eisenman, and A. Magana. 2015. Developing a tabletop exercise to test community resilience: Lessons from the Los Angeles County Community Disaster Resilience Project. *Disaster Medicine and Public Health Preparedness* 9(5):484–488.

Chi, G. C., M. Williams, A. Chandra, A. Plough, and D. Eisenman. 2015. Partnerships for community resilience: Perspectives from the Los Angeles County Community Disaster Resilience Project. *Public Health.* http://www.escholarship.org/uc/item/30f4f1kf (accessed March 10, 2020).

CTEC (California Tribal Epidemiology Center). 2016. *Health policy brief—Barriers to collaboration between tribal and county governments: Planning for major disasters and other emergencies.* Sacramento, CA: California Tribal Epidemiology Center. http://www.publichealthsystems.org/sites/default/files/PHS4/72458GPreport_06.pdf (accessed May 14, 2020).

Davies, R., E. Vaughan, G. Fraser, R. Cook, M. Ciotti, and J. E. Suk. 2019. Enhancing reporting of after action reviews of public health emergencies to strengthen preparedness: A literature review and methodology appraisal. *Disaster Medicine and Public Health Preparedness* 13(3):618–625.

DeVoe, J. E., S. Likumahuwa, P. Eiff, C. A. Nelson, J. E. Carroll, C. N. Hill, R. Gold, and P. A. Kullberg. 2012. Developing a new practice-based research network (PBRN): Lessons learned and challenges ahead. *Journal of the American Board of Family Medicine* 25(5).

DHS (U.S. Department of Homeland Security). 2020. *Welcome to the Centers of Excellence.* https://www.dhs.gov/science-and-technology/centers-excellence (accessed February 21, 2020).

DOI (U.S. Department of the Interior). 2020. *Strategic sciences group.* https://www.doi.gov/strategicsciences (accessed May 22, 2020).

Dungan, R., R. Angove, E. Cope, and H. Peay. 2019. *Engagement science: Introducing inclusive research practices and potential impacts.* AcademyHealth. https://www.academyhealth.org/blog/2019-01/engagement-science-introducing-inclusive-research-practices-potential-impacts (accessed May 13, 2020).

ECDC (European Centre for Disease Prevention and Control). 2018. *Best practice recommendations for conducting after action reviews to enhance public health preparedness.* Solna, Sweden: European Centre for Disease Prevention and Control. https://www.ecdc.europa.eu/sites/default/files/documents/public-health-preparedness-best-practice-recommendations.pdf (accessed March 10, 2020).

Eisenman, D. P., R. M. Adams, C. M. Lang, M. Prelip, A. Dorian, J. Acosta, D. Glik, and M. Chinman. 2018. A program for local health departments to adapt and implement evidence-based emergency preparedness programs. *American Journal of Public Health* 108(S5):S396–S398.

FEMA (Federal Emergency Management Agency). 2013. *Homeland security exercise and evaluation program.* https://www.fema.gov/media-library-data/20130726-1914-25045-8890/hseep_apr13_.pdf (accessed April 1, 2019).

FEMA. 2020. *Emergency management institute: Distance learning.* https://training.fema.gov/is (accessed May 13, 2020).

Ford, I., and J. Norrie. 2016. Pragmatic trials. *New England Journal of Medicine* 375(5):454–463.

Forrest, C. B., F. D. Chesley, Jr., M. L. Tregear, and K. B. Mistry. 2018. Development of the learning health system researcher core competencies. *Health Services Research* 53(4):2615–2632.

GAO (U.S. Government Accountability Office). 2016. *Tiered evidence grants: Opportunities exist to share lessons from early implementation and inform future federal efforts.* Washington, DC: GAO. https://www.gao.gov/assets/680/679917.pdf (accessed March 10, 2020).

Gliklich, R., N. Dreyer, and M. Leavy. 2014. Protecting data: Confidentiality and legal concerns of providers, manufacturers, and health plans. In *Registries for evaluating patient outcomes: A user's guide, 3rd ed.* Rockville, MD: Agency for Healthcare Research and Quality.

Gossip, K., H. Gouda, Y. Y. Lee, S. Firth, R. Bermejo, 3rd, W. Zeck, and E. Jimenez Soto. 2017. Monitoring and evaluation of disaster response efforts undertaken by local health departments: A rapid realist review. *BMC Health Services Research* 17(1):450.

Guise, J.-M., M. E. Butler, C. Chang, M. Viswanathan, T. Pigott, and P. Tugwell. 2017a. AHRQ series on complex intervention systematic reviews—Paper 6: PRISMA-CI extension statement and checklist. *Journal of Clinical Epidemiology* 90:43–50.

Guise, J.-M., M. Butler, C. Chang, M. Viswanathan, T. Pigott, and P. Tugwell. 2017b. AHRQ series on complex intervention systematic reviews—Paper 7: PRISMA-CI elaboration and explanation. *Journal of Clinical Epidemiology* 90:51–58.

Hemming, K., T. P. Haines, P. J. Chilton, A. J. Girling, and R. J. Lilford. 2015. The stepped wedge cluster randomised trial: Rationale, design, analysis, and reporting. *BMJ* 350:h391.

HHS (U.S. Department of Health and Human Services). 2017a. *Public health emergency medical countermeasures enterprise (PHEMCE) strategy and implementation plan.* https://www.phe.gov/Preparedness/mcm/phemce/Pages/strategy.aspx (accessed March 10, 2020).

HHS. 2017b. *Public health emergency medical countermeasures enterprise multiyear budget: Fiscal years 2016–2020.* https://www.phe.gov/Preparedness/mcm/phemce/phemce-myb/Pages/default.aspx (accessed March 10, 2020).

HHS and NIH (National Institutes of Health). 2020. *Public health emergency research review board (PHERRB).* https://ohsr.od.nih.gov/pherrb.php (accessed February 21, 2020).

Hoffmann, T. C., P. P. Glasziou, I. Boutron, R. Milne, R. Perera, D. Moher, D. G. Altman, V. Barbour, H. Macdonald, M. Johnston, S. E. Lamb, M. Dixon-Woods, P. McCulloch, J. C. Wyatt, A. W. Chan, and S. Michie. 2014. Better reporting of interventions: Template for intervention description and replication (TIDieR) checklist and guide. *BMJ* 348:g1687.

HSDL (Homeland Security Digital Library). 2020. *Lessons learned information sharing.* https://www.hsdl.org/c/llis-in-the-hsdl (accessed May 13, 2020).

IAEM (International Association of Emergency Managers). 2020. *Certification introduction.* https://www.iaem.org/certification/intro (accessed May 13, 2020).

IES and NSF (Institute of Education Sciences and National Science Foundation). 2013. *Common guidelines for education research and development.* https://www.nsf.gov/pubs/2013/nsf13126/nsf13126.pdf?WT.mc_id=USNSF_124 (accessed February 21, 2020).

INTRAC (International NGO Training and Research Centre). 2017a. *Qualitative comparative analaysis (QCA).* https://www.intrac.org/wpcms/wp-content/uploads/2017/01/Qualitative-comparative-analysis.pdf (accessed March 10, 2020).

INTRAC. 2017b. *Realist evaluation.* https://www.intrac.org/wpcms/wp-content/uploads/2017/01/Realist-evaluation.pdf (accessed March 10, 2020).

IOM (Institute of Medicine). 2008. *Research priorities in emergency preparedness and response for public health systems: A letter report.* Washington, DC: The National Academies Press.

IOM. 2015. *Enabling rapid and sustainable public health research during disasters: Summary of a joint workshop by the Institute of Medicine and the U.S. Department of Health and Human Services.* Washington, DC: The National Academies Press.

Jacobs, J. A., E. A. Dodson, E. A. Baker, A. D. Deshpande, and R. C. Brownson. 2010. Barriers to evidence-based decision making in public health: A national survey of chronic disease practitioners. *Public Health Reports* 125(5):736–742.

Jillson, I. A., M. Clarke, C. Allen, S. Waller, T. Koehlmoos, W. Mumford, J. Jansen, K. McKay, and A. Trant. 2019. Improving the science and evidence base of disaster response: A policy research study. *BMC Health Services Research* 19(1):274.

Kearns, S. 2010. *Good Catch program encourages reporting near-miss medical errors.* https://www.healthleadersmedia.com/clinical-care/good-catch-program-encourages-reporting-near-miss-medical-errors (accessed March 10, 2020).

Keim, M. E., T. D. Kirsch, O. Alleyne, G. Benjamin, L. DeGutis, D. Dyjack, and F. M. Burkle, Jr. 2019. The need for a national strategy to assess and reduce disaster-related mortality in the United States. *American Journal of Public Health* 109(4):539–540.

Kirsch, T. D., G. Benjamin, P. D. Kivela, D. T. Dyjack, and M. Keim. 2018. *National Disaster Safety Board: Objective measures, improved outcomes.* https://www.healthaffairs.org/do/10.1377/hblog20180720.168527/full (accessed March 10, 2020).

Lavis, J. N., A. D. Oxman, S. Lewin, and A. Fretheim. 2009. SUPPORT tools for evidence-informed health policymaking (STP). *Health Research Policy and Systems* 7(Suppl 1):I1. https://health-policy-systems.biomedcentral.com/articles/supplements/volume-7-supplement-1 (accessed March 10, 2020).

Lewin, S., A. D. Oxman, J. N. Lavis, A. Fretheim, S. Garcia Marti, and S. Munabi-Babigumira. 2009. SUPPORT tools for evidence-informed policymaking in health 11: Finding and using evidence about local conditions. *Health Research Policy and Systems* 7(Suppl 1):S11. https://health-policy-systems.biomedcentral.com/articles/10.1186/1478-4505-7-S1-S11 (accessed March 10, 2020).

Lupia, A., and G. Alter. 2014. Data access and research transparency in the quantitative tradition. *Political Science and Politics* 47(1):54–59.

Lurie, N., T. Manolio, A. P. Patterson, F. Collins, and T. Frieden. 2013. Research as a part of public health emergency response. *New England Journal of Medicine* 368(13):1251–1255.

Maddock, J. E. 2018. Preparing public health for the unexpected. *American Journal of Public Health* 108(S5):S348.

Maynard, R. A. 2018. The role of federal agencies in creating and administering evidence-based policies. *The Annals of the American Academy of Political and Social Science* 678(1):134–144.

Mays, G. P., R. A. Hogg, D. M. Castellanos-Cruz, A. G. Goover, and L. C. Fowler. 2013. Engaging public health settings in research implementation and translation activities: Evidence from practice-based research networks. *American Journal of Preventive Medicine* 45(6):752–762.

Miller, A., K. Yeskey, S. Garantziotis, S. Arnesen, A. Bennett, L. O'Fallon, C. Thompson, L. Reinlib, S. Masten, J. Remington, C. Love, S. Ramsey, R. Rosselli, B. Galluzzo, J. Lee, R. Kwok, and J. Hughes. 2016. Integrating health research into disaster response: The new NIH disaster research response program. *International Journal of Environmental Research and Public Health* 13(7).

Moravcsik, A. 2014. Transparency: The revolution in qualitative research. *Political Science and Politics* 47(1):48–53.

MRC (Medical Research Council). 2019. *Developing and evaluating complex interventions.* https://mrc.ukri.org/documents/pdf/complex-interventions-guidance (accessed February 21, 2020).

National Hazards Center. 2019. *Quick Response research grant program.* https://hazards.colorado.edu/research/quick-response (accessed January 9, 2020).

NBSB (National Biodefense Science Board). 2011. *Call to action: Include scientific investigations as an integral component of disaster planning and response.* https://www.phe.gov/Preparedness/legal/boards/nbsb/Documents/nbsbrec14.pdf (accessed March 10, 2020).

NCER (National Center for Education Research). 2020. *Predoctoral interdisciplinary research training programs in the education sciences.* https://ies.ed.gov/ncer/projects/program.asp?ProgID=16 (accessed March 10, 2020).

NIH (National Institutes of Health). 2019a. *About the Division of Biomedical Research Workforce (DBRW).* https://researchtraining.nih.gov/dbrw (accessed February 21, 2020).

NIH. 2019b. *NIH disaster research response training and exercises.* https://dr2.nlm.nih.gov/training-exercises#NIEHS_Disaster_Research_Response_Tabletop_Exercise_Assessment (accessed February 21, 2020).

NIH. 2019c. *Types of grant programs.* https://grants.nih.gov/grants/funding/funding_program.htm#RSeries (accessed May 13, 2020).

NIH. 2020a. *P30 center core grant.* https://www.niddk.nih.gov/research-funding/process/apply/funding-mechanisms/p30 (accessed May 13, 2020).

NIH. 2020b. *Research career development awards.* https://researchtraining.nih.gov/programs/career-development (accessed May 13, 2020).

NORC at the University of Chicago. 2017. *Evaluation of the translation, dissemination, and implementation of public health preparedness response research and training project.* Bethesda, MD: NORC at the University of Chicago. https://s3.amazonaws.com/ASPPH_Media_Files/Docs/CDC_Preparedness_Evaluation_Report (accessed March 10, 2020).

NSF (National Science Foundation). 2018. *Proposal preparation instructions: Rapid research (RAPID) proposal.* https://www.nsf.gov/pubs/policydocs/pappg18_1/pappg_2.jsp#IIE1 (accessed January 9, 2020).

NSF. 2020a. *Accelerating discovery: Educating the future STEM workforce.* https://nsf.gov/funding/pgm_summ.jsp?pims_id=505552&org=EHR&sel_org=EHR&from=fund (accessed February 21, 2020).

NSF. 2020b. *About funding.* https://www.nsf.gov/funding/aboutfunding.jsp (accessed May 13, 2020).

O'Brien, B. C., I. B. Harris, T. J. Beckman, D. A. Reed, and D. A. Cook. 2014. Standards for reporting qualitative research: A synthesis of recommendations. *Academic Medicine* 89(9):1245–1251.

O'Fallon, L. R., G. M. Wolfle, D. Brown, A. Dearry, and K. Olden. 2003. Strategies for setting a national research agenda that is responsive to community needs. *Environmental Health Perspectives* 111(16):1855–1860.

Ogrinc, G., L. Davies, D. Goodman, P. Batalden, F. Davidoff, and D. Stevens. 2016. Squire 2.0 (Standards for QUality Improvement Reporting Excellence): Revised publication guidelines from a detailed consensus process. *BMJ Quality and Safety* 25(12):986–992.

Open Philanthropy. 2020. *Grants database.* https://www.openphilanthropy.org/giving/grants (accessed May 13, 2020).

Packenham, J. P., R. T. Rosselli, S. K. Ramsey, H. A. Taylor, A. Fothergill, J. Slutsman, and A. Miller. 2017. Conducting science in disasters: Recommendations from the NIEHS working group for special IRB considerations in the review of disaster related research. *Environmental Health Perspectives* 125(9):094503.

Patel, S. 2019. *Quality assessment of after action reports: Findings and recommendations.* Paper commissioned by the Committee on Evidence-Based Practices for Public Health Emergency Preparedness and Response.

Patsopoulos, N. A. 2011. A pragmatic view on pragmatic trials. *Dialogues in Clinical Neuroscience* 13(2):217–224.

PCORI (Patient-Centered Outcomes Research Institute). 2019. *PCORI methodology standards.* https://www.pcori.org/research-results/about-our-research/research-methodology/pcori-methodology-standards#Complex (accessed February 21, 2020).

PHF (Public Health Foundation). 2020. *Welcome to the TRAIN learning network.* https://www.train.org/main/welcome (accessed May 13, 2020).

Piltch-Loeb, R., J. D. Kraemer, C. Nelson, and M. A. Stoto. 2014a. A public health emergency preparedness critical incident registry. *Biosecurity and Bioterrorism: Biodefense Strategy, Practice, and Science* 12(3).

Piltch-Loeb, R. N., C. D. Nelson, J. D. Kraemer, E. Savoia, and M. A. Stoto. 2014b. A peer assessment approach for learning from public health emergencies. *Public Health Reports* 129(Suppl 4):28–34.

Pinnock, H., E. Epiphaniou, A. Sheikh, C. Griffiths, S. Eldridge, P. Craig, and S. J. Taylor. 2015. Developing standards for reporting implementation studies of complex interventions (STaRI): A systematic review and e-Delphi. *Implementation Science* 10(42).

Qari, S. H., M. R. Leinhos, T. N. Thomas, and E. G. Carbone. 2018. Overview of the translation, dissemination, and implementation of public health preparedness and response research and training initiative. *American Journal of Public Health* 108(S5):S355–S362.

Revere, D., S. Allan, H. Karasz, and J. Baseman. 2018. Expanding methodologies to identify high-priority emergency preparedness tools for implementation in public health agencies. *American Journal of Public Health* 108(S5):S372–S374.

RWJF (Robert Wood Johnson Foundation). 2013. *Robert Wood Johnson Foundation practice-based research networks in public health.* https://www.rwjf.org/en/library/research/2013/06/robert-wood-johnson-foundation-practice-based-research-networks-.html (accessed May 13, 2020).

RWJF. 2020a. *Grants and grant programs.* https://www.rwjf.org/en/how-we-work/grants-and-grant-programs.html (accessed May 13, 2020).

RWJF. 2020b. *Leadership for better health.* https://www.rwjf.org/en/our-focus-areas/focus-areas/health-leadership.html (accessed May 13, 2020).

RWJF and University of Kentucky College of Public Health. 2020. *The national coordinating center for public health services and systems research and public health practice-based research networks.* http://www.publichealthsystems.org (accessed May 13, 2020).

Savoia, E., F. Agboola, and P. D. Biddinger. 2012. Use of after action reports (AARs) to promote organizational and systems learning in emergency preparedness. *International Journal of Environmental Research and Public Health* 9(8):2949–2963.

Siegfried, A. L., E. G. Carbone, M. B. Meit, M. J. Kennedy, H. Yusuf, and E. B. Kahn. 2017. Identifying and prioritizing information needs and research priorities of public health emergency preparedness and response practitioners. *Disaster Medicine and Public Health Preparedness* 11(5):552–561.

Simera, I., D. G. Altman, D. Moher, K. F. Schulz, and J. Hoey. 2008. Guidelines for reporting health research: The Equator Network's survey of guideline authors. *PLOS Medicine* 5(6):e139.

Singleton, C. M., S. Debastiani, D. Rose, and E. B. Kahn. 2014. An analysis of root cause identification and continuous quality improvement in public health H1N1 after-action reports. *Journal of Public Health Management and Practice* 20(2):197.

Stoto, M. A., C. Nelson, M. A. Higdon, J. Kraemer, L. Hites, and C. M. Singleton. 2013. Lessons about the state and local public health system response to the 2009 H1N1 pandemic: A workshop summary. *Journal of Public Health Management and Practice* 19(5):428–435.

Stoto, M., A., R. Piltch-Loeb, and E. Savoia. 2015. *The public health system response to the 2014 West Virginia water crisis.* https://cdn1.sph.harvard.edu/wp-content/uploads/sites/1609/2015/01/WV-water-crisis-report-final.pdf (accessed March 10, 2020).

Stoto, M. A., C. Nelson, R. Piltch-Loeb, L. N. Mayigane, F. Copper, and S. Chungong. 2019. Getting the most from after action reviews to improve global health security. *Globalization and Health* 15(1):58. http://creativecommons.org/licenses/by/4.0 (accessed June 17, 2020).

Summers, S. K., and M. J. Ferraro. 2017. Project Public Health Ready: History and evolution of a best practice for public health preparedness planning. *American Journal of Public Health* 107(S2):S138–S141.

Taylor, H. L., and V. A. Yeager. 2019. Core competency gaps among governmental public health employees with and without a formal public health degree. *Journal of Public Health Management Practice.* [Epub ahead of print.]

Testa, M. A., E. Savoia, M. Su, and P. D. Biddinger. 2018. Social media learning collaborative for public health preparedness. *American Journal of Public Health* 108(S5):S375–S377.

Teti, M., E. Schatz, and L. Liebenberg. 2020. Methods in the time of COVID-19: The vital role of qualitative inquiries. *International Journal of Qualitative Methods* 19(1–5).

Tong, A., P. Sainsbury, and J. Craig. 2007. Consolidated Criteria for Reporting Qualitative Research (COREQ): A 32-item checklist for interviews and focus groups. *International Journal for Quality in Health Care* 19(6):349–357.

Turner, D. A., J. Bae, G. Cheely, J. Milne, T. A. Owens, and C. M. Kuhn. 2018. Improving resident and fellow engagement in patient safety through a graduate medical education incentive program. *Journal of Graduate Medicine Education* 10(6):671–675.

von Elm, E., D. G. Altman, M. Egger, S. J. Pocock, P. C. Gotzsche, and J. P. Vandenbroucke. 2007. The Strengthening the Reporting of OBservational studies in Epidemiology (STROBE) statement: Guidelines for reporting observational studies. *Annals of Internal Medicine* 147(8):573–577.

Wandersman, A., J. Duffy, P. Flaspohler, R. Noonan, K. Lubell, L. Stillman, M. Blachman, R. Dunville, and J. Saul. 2008. Bridging the gap between prevention research and practice: The interactive systems framework for dissemination and implementation. *American Journal of Community Psychology* 41(3–4):171–181.

Whitehurst, G. J. 2018. The Institute of Education Sciences: A model for federal research offices. *The Annals of the American Academy of Political and Social Science* 678(1):124–133.

Williams, M. V., A. Chandra, A. Spears, D. Varda, K. B. Wells, A. L. Plough, and D. P. Eisenman. 2018. Evaluating community partnerships addressing community resilience in Los Angeles, California. *International Journal of Environmental Research and Public Health* 15(4).

Wimsatt, M. A. 2017. Cross-jurisdictional sharing for emergency management-related public health: Exploring the experiences of tribes and counties in California. *Frontiers in Public Health* 5(254). https://doi.org/10.3389/fpubh.2017.00254.

A

Detailed Description of the Committee's Methods for Formulating the Scope of the Reviews and Capturing the Evidence

The committee was charged with conducting a systematic review of the evidence base for selected public health emergency preparedness and response (PHEPR) practices from the 15 PHEPR Capabilities defined in the Centers for Disease Control and Prevention's (CDC's) *Public Health Emergency Preparedness and Response Capabilities: National Standards for State, Local, Tribal, and Territorial Public Health* (CDC, 2018). This appendix provides additional detail on some aspects of the committee's evidence review methods, which are briefly described in Chapter 3. Specifically, this appendix details the committee's review methods only to the point of data extraction and quality assessment of individual studies. The committee's evidence synthesis and grading methodology is described in detail in Chapter 3. For examples of how the methods were applied to the review topics, see Chapters 4–7.

To develop its evidence review and evaluation methodology, the committee reviewed the standards, protocols, and best practices from several prominent guideline groups and their relevant publications (see Box A-1), although other sources were also consulted. Recognizing the complexity of PHEPR practices, the committee focused substantial effort up front on formulating the scope of the reviews and adapting review methods that would take into account practice and system complexity. Additional information regarding the complexity perspective that guided the committee's approach to its task can be found in Chapter 3.

FORMULATING THE SCOPE OF THE REVIEWS

Selecting the Review Topics

In response to its charge, the committee developed a process for identifying which of the CDC PHEPR Capabilities would be the focus of its systematic literature reviews. Recognizing that the PHEPR Capabilities are broad, overarching topics, the committee gradually focused the scope of its reviews to specific PHEPR practices within the selected PHEPR Capabilities.

BOX A-1 SEMINAL LITERATURE SOURCES FOR THE COMMITTEE'S EVIDENCE REVIEW METHODOLOGY

- Institute of Medicine's *Finding What Works in Health Care: Standards for Systematic Reviews*[a]
- Centers for Disease Control and Prevention's The Guide to Community Preventive Services (The Community Guide)[b]
- U.S. Preventive Services Task Force Procedure Manual[c]
- Agency for Healthcare Research and Quality series on Complex Intervention Systematic Reviews[d]
- Cochrane series *Considering Complexity in Systematic Reviews of Interventions*[e]
- The BMJ Global Health supplemental *Complex Health Interventions in Complex Systems: Concepts and Methods for Evidence-Informed Health Decisions*[f]

---

[a] See https://www.nap.edu/catalog/13059/finding-what-works-in-health-care-standards-for-systematic-reviews (accessed June 18, 2020).

[b] See https://www.thecommunityguide.org/about/our-methodology (accessed June 18, 2020).

[c] See https://www.uspreventiveservicestaskforce.org/uspstf/procedure-manual (accessed June 18, 2020).

[d] See https://effectivehealthcare.ahrq.gov/products/interventions-tools-guidance/abstract (accessed June 18, 2020).

[e] See https://www.jclinepi.com/content/jce-considering-complexity-in-systematic-reviews-of-intervention (accessed June 18, 2020).

[f] See https://gh.bmj.com/content/4/Suppl_1 (accessed June 18, 2020).

The evidence review topics were scoped through iterative stages with input from the literature, key stakeholders, and the committee's expertise.

Preliminary Literature Review

To better understand the current evidence base for PHEPR practices, the committee conducted a preliminary literature review. This preliminary review helped formulate the scope of the final reviews and frame the key review questions that governed the committee's systematic searches of the evidence. The committee focused its efforts on reviewing published scoping and literature reviews on the PHEPR literature (Abramson et al., 2007; Acosta et al., 2009; Challen et al., 2012; Khan et al., 2015; Savoia et al., 2017; Yeager et al., 2010) to get a sense of the research gaps in the field, as well as PHEPR practitioner and program assessments, when relevant, to understand the type of research that would be relevant and important to practitioners (CDC, 2016; Center for Public Health Systems and Services Research, 2018; Horney et al., 2017; Murthy et al., 2017; Siegfried et al., 2017).

Engaging with Stakeholders to Meet Practitioner Needs

To ensure that its report would be relevant and useful to key stakeholders, the committee appointed nine diverse state, local, tribal, and territorial (SLTT) PHEPR practitioners as consultants to advise on the systematic literature review process. The members of this group were suggested by practitioner associations, such as the National Association of County & City Health Officials (NACCHO) and the Association of State and Territorial Health Officials (ASTHO), and selected based on such criteria as jurisdiction type and demographics, size of public health agency, individual tenure and experience, number of emergencies during tenure, the Federal Emergency Management Agency (FEMA) region, and state governance, as well as meeting conflict-of-interest requirements. The committee engaged with these PHEPR practitioner consultants throughout the review process on the refinement of its conceptual approach and the selection, development, and refinement of review topics, and solicited their feedback on the review findings and the committee's recommendations. The PHEPR practitioner consultants provided real-world input and assisted in focusing the review topics on issues relevant to decision makers.

Selection Criteria and Selected Review Topics

In making decisions about the scope of its reviews, the committee, which included individuals with diverse expertise in evidence review and evaluation methodologies and the PHEPR subject matter (see Appendix F for biosketches of the committee members), considered criteria adapted from The Community Guide (Zaza et al., 2000) and the U.S. Preventive Services Task Force (USPSTF, 2015). These criteria are described in Box A-2.

BOX A-2 SELECTION CRITERIA FOR REVIEW TOPICS

Relevance and importance to national health security: This criterion acknowledges the current priorities for national health security and the potential for advancing public health emergency preparedness and response (PHEPR) capabilities.

Current needs among key stakeholders, including practitioners and policy makers: This criterion recognizes the current needs of PHEPR practitioners and policy makers for evidence-based guidance and areas in which stakeholders believe additional research is needed to inform practice.

Potential to affect PHEPR practice: This criterion addresses the notion that a knowledge gap exists between the evidence and the PHEPR practice (whether that gap exists because of insufficient dissemination, ineffective implementation, or a lack of existing research). In thinking about the potential to affect PHEPR practice, the committee considered the potential to increase the implementation of effective practices and phase out widely used but less effective practices.

Methodological diversity: This criterion was specific to the committee's task of developing an evidence review and evaluation methodology for generating recommendations for evidence-based PHEPR practices, and is something that likely would not be considered in selecting topics for future reviews. Given the context-sensitive, heterogeneous nature of PHEPR practices and their focus on systems and processes, the committee considered how the type of research might vary across the Centers for Disease Control and Prevention's PHEPR Capabilities and the characteristics that might differ across PHEPR practices that are important to interpreting the evidence. By selecting PHEPR practices that engage different parts of the PHEPR system for its review, the committee aimed to develop an evidence review and evaluation methodology that would be flexible enough to accommodate the diverse range of PHEPR practices that may be reviewed in the future. For future reviews, this element could evolve into what the U.S. Preventive Services Task Force calls the "balance of portfolio" (i.e., whether the review topic overlaps with current or in-process recommendations; whether the review topic balances the overall portfolio of recommendations) (USPSTF, 2015).

NOTE: The criteria for selecting review topics did not include the perceived feasibility of a review and the likelihood of available evidence.

Selected review topics The committee determined that, to develop an evidence review and evaluation methodology and demonstrate its feasibility, the task of selecting review topics needed to be approached from a "proof-of-concept" perspective. Therefore, for the initial development of its methodology for generating recommendations for evidence-based PHEPR practices, the committee applied the selection criteria discussed in Box A-2 and narrowed the scope of its reviews to four PHEPR Capabilities: Community Preparedness, Emergency Operations Coordination, Information Sharing, and Non-Pharmaceutical Interventions. In consultation with the PHEPR practitioner consultant group, the committee further focused its reviews on four topic areas within each of these four PHEPR Capabilities:

- engaging with and training community-based partners to improve the outcomes of at-risk populations after public health emergencies (falls under Capability 1, Community Preparedness);
- activating a public health emergency operations center (Capability 3, Emergency Operations Coordination);
- communicating public health alerts and guidance with technical audiences during a public health emergency (Capability 6, Information Sharing); and
- implementing quarantine to reduce or stop the spread of a contagious disease (Capability 11, Non-Pharmaceutical Interventions).

The process of focusing the selected broad PHEPR Capabilities into more precise topics was a considerable challenge because the Capabilities are standards, not practices; thus, to achieve each Capability requires many different practices, which are not always evident. To guide the selection process, the committee developed a comprehensive list of potential PHEPR practices by breaking down the functions and tasks within the PHEPR Capabilities into more manageable topics.

Selection justification It is important to note that the committee's process for selecting review topics was systematic and based on classifying the topics on a number of key dimensions and criteria. The committee acknowledges that a different group might have chosen a different set of topics. Given that the committee was able to conduct reviews for only a very small subset of PHEPR practices, it sought to inform future priorities for review topics by commissioning a scoping review and evidence map to examine and describe the extent and the nature of research conducted on practices within all of the CDC PHEPR Capabilities (see Chapter 2 and Appendix D). The discussion below describes how the committee applied the criteria listed in Box A-2 to select review topics.

Relevance and importance to national health security In thinking more broadly about the strategies, priorities, strengths, and weaknesses in PHEPR for the nation, the committee reviewed the 2018 *National Health Security Preparedness Index;*[1] Trust for America's Health 2017 *Ready or Not?: Protecting the Public's Health from Diseases, Disasters, and Bioterrorism Report;*[2] CDC's *Public Health Preparedness and Response 2018 National Snapshot;*[3] CDC's Public Health Emergency Preparedness (PHEP) Cooperative Agreement funding announcement;[4] and the Assistant Secretary for Preparedness and Response's

[1] See https://nhspi.org (accessed June 18, 2020).

[2] See https://www.tfah.org/report-details/ready-or-not-2017 (accessed June 18, 2020).

[3] See https://www.cdc.gov/cpr/pubs-links/2018/documents/2018_Preparedness_Report.pdf (accessed June 18, 2020).

[4] See https://www.cdc.gov/cpr/readiness/phep.htm (accessed June 18, 2020).

(ASPR's) *National Health Security Strategy*.[5] The committee deliberated as to where a review and evaluation of the evidence might advance the capacity of the nation to prepare for and respond to disasters and public health emergencies.

Current needs among key stakeholders In considering the current needs for research to support practices among key stakeholders, including practitioners and policy makers, the committee reviewed the research domains and questions deemed a priority by practitioners in Siegfried et al. (2017) and the findings from the 2016 practitioner assessment of the CDC PHEPR Capabilities (CDC, 2016). Siegfried and colleagues' findings provided crucial insight into where PHEPR practitioners perceived knowledge gaps and where future research studies would provide the information they need to enhance their capacity. One key finding was that the research question within the community resilience domain related to appropriate methods and procedures for identifying and mapping at-risk populations received the highest importance rating from the practitioners surveyed. As described later in this appendix, the committee leveraged this important work in conducting a structured priority-setting activity to identify priority topics for future systematic evidence reviews (refer to the section below on "Prioritization of Future Systematic Evidence Review Topics").

The committee also considered the input offered by CDC in its remarks to the committee at the outset of this study, as well as input from the PHEPR practitioner consultants. In the 2016 practitioner assessment of the CDC PHEPR Capabilities, it was noted that such Capabilities as Mass Care, Fatality Management, Community Recovery, and Medical Surge are often the responsibilities of agencies other than public health (CDC, 2016). In its remarks, CDC also noted that Volunteer Management is less critical for public health than other PHEPR Capabilities and that it should be of lower priority in the allocation of resources for review (Carbone, 2018). Public Health Laboratory Testing and Public Health Surveillance and Epidemiological Investigation are considered well-established public health functions (Carbone, 2018; CDC, 2016). Furthermore, the evidence supporting Emergency Public Information and Warning, Responder Safety and Health, and Medical Materiel Management and Distribution is derived primarily from disciplines other than public health. Therefore, the committee decided not to focus its efforts and resources on reviewing these Capabilities because an aim of the study was to develop PHEPR-specific methods.

Potential to affect PHEPR practice Siegfried and colleagues (2017) note that knowledge gaps identified by the practice community may result from insufficient dissemination, ineffective implementation, or a lack of existing research. Abramson and colleagues (2007) state that it is fundamental for potential research questions to question assumptions (e.g., asking whether the way in which response systems have been organized using an incident command system is effective). The committee deliberated about those areas in which a review and evaluation of the evidence would have the highest potential to increase the implementation of effective practices and phase out widely used but less effective practices.

Methodological diversity The committee approached its reviews as a proof of concept for its methodology for generating recommendations for evidence-based PHEPR practices. Therefore, the committee assigned this criterion more weight than the others to ensure that the methodology it developed would be flexible enough to accommodate the range of PHEPR practices that may be reviewed in the future. Through an initial review of the literature

[5] See https://www.phe.gov/Preparedness/planning/authority/nhss/Documents/NHSS-Strategy-508.pdf (accessed June 18, 2020).

and its members' expertise, the committee considered how the type of research required to support evidence-based practice recommendations might vary across the CDC PHEPR Capabilities. The type of research that falls within the Community Preparedness and Information Sharing Capabilities aligns more with traditional research designs, such as randomized controlled trials (RCTs) and quasi-experimental studies, whereas the type of research that falls within Emergency Operations Coordination aligns more with noncomparative studies and experience-based evidence, including case reports and after action reports (AARs), as well as organizational theory, systems, and processes. The committee was also interested in developing a methodology that would accommodate modeling studies and qualitative evidence, and the research within the Non-Pharmaceutical Interventions Capability includes a considerable number of such studies.

Additionally, the committee considered characteristics of the PHEPR practices within these four Capabilities that might differ in ways important to interpreting the evidence. For example, the Emergency Operations Coordination Capability is inward facing, with the aim of supporting the ongoing response effort, while the Non-Pharmaceutical Interventions Capability is outward facing, with the aim of helping the public. Likewise, practices within Information Sharing may need to be implemented more quickly than those within Community Preparedness in order to be effective. These characteristics, defined by the committee as classification dimensions (listed in Figure 3-1 in Chapter 3) were examined for each PHEPR Capability to aid in the selection of practices that were diverse with respect to those characteristics.

Developing the Analytic Frameworks and Key Review Questions

Once the four review topics had been selected, the committee focused on further describing and constraining the scope of its reviews through the development of a detailed analytic framework and set of key review questions for each topic. The analytic frameworks and key review questions for each of the four review topics can be found in Chapters 4–7 and Appendixes B1–B4.

Analytic Frameworks

The purpose of developing analytic frameworks is to present clearly in visual format the causal pathway and interactions between a practice and its components, populations, and outcomes of interest (i.e., a logic model). As described in Chapter 3, the analytic frameworks also facilitated a mixed-method approach to the committee's systematic reviews by serving as a construct that enabled integration of the findings from separate syntheses of quantitative, qualitative, and case report and AAR evidence.

The committee developed analytic frameworks using its members' experiential knowledge, feedback from the PHEPR practitioner consultants, and the available research. The primary results of this process are focused on the identification of the outcomes of a practice, its postulated harms, and key factors to examine for potential effect modification and applicability of the results to other contexts (e.g., populations, settings).

For the purposes of this review, the committee adapted The Community Guide approach for developing analytic frameworks (Briss et al., 2000). The committee used the analytic frameworks for the four practices to conceptualize their relationship to outcomes of interest. In addition to health outcomes (e.g., reduced morbidity and mortality), other outcomes of interest included intermediate outcomes (e.g., knowledge, behaviors), as well as system- and process-level outcomes (e.g., accelerated recovery and cohesive and effective operations, respectively). These frameworks were not simple, linear models, and represented both direct pathways to outcomes (e.g., a study that directly assessed the impact of an intervention on the outcomes of interest), and indirect pathways (e.g., the intermediate steps or intermediate outcomes that led to an effect on the final outcomes of interest).

The committee had to make explicit judgments about the extent to which PHEPR practices are grouped together and considered in the same body of evidence because PHEPR practices are carried out in different settings and populations, and often implemented in different ways. If practices are defined very narrowly, there may not be sufficient evidence to evaluate effectiveness. However, when practices are grouped together, the available evidence may be heterogeneous. While that possibility poses a different kind of challenge for analyzing the evidence, it also makes it possible to assess generalizability and consistency across different contexts. Thus, the committee discussed the degree to which the grouping of PHEPR practices was needed to achieve a balance between sufficiency and heterogeneity of evidence. Similarly, the committee had to make judgments about how to define outcomes for its evidence synthesis, given the significant variation in the measures used in the studies included in its review. For example, rather than evaluating preparedness behaviors related to stockpiling supplies and developing a family communication plan separately, these outcome measures were grouped together into an outcome category of preparedness behavior.

Key Review Questions

As the committee generated an initial list of review questions for each review topic, it became clear that beyond questions about a practice's effectiveness (i.e., what works), it was also important to consider questions about how and why it works, for whom, and under what circumstances. The initial question lists were then reviewed and prioritized in collaboration with the PHEPR practitioner consultants. The committee drafted an overarching question for each of the four topics, which was further broken down into several sub-questions that were addressed in the review as well (see Chapters 4–7 and Appendixes B1–B4). These sets of key review questions specified the logic and scope of the review of each topic and were critical in guiding the literature searches, data extraction, and evidence analyses.

The committee then applied the PICOTS (population, intervention/phenomena of interest, comparators, outcomes, timing, and setting) question formulation framework (Butler et al., 2017). The committee added timing and setting to the traditional PICO in an effort to capture important contextual factors. The PICOTS framework helped specify the committee's search parameters and define the inclusion and exclusion criteria.

Throughout the process of framing questions, the committee returned to the issues of complexity and the need to answer questions that go beyond the effectiveness of a practice. These questions also relate to practitioners' needs for recommendations that are practicable and evidence that can help them make informed decisions about response activities.

Topic Refinement: Iterative Process

When addressing such complex topics, finalizing analytic frameworks and key review questions a priori is often not a suitable approach. Therefore, the committee refined the analytic frameworks and key review questions iteratively as it explored the evidence and engaged with stakeholders.

LITERATURE SEARCH

Multicomponent Approach to Searching the Evidence

Recognizing that evaluations of PHEPR practices may be published not only as intervention research studies but also as organizational reports, white papers, or program evaluations, including AARs, the committee adopted a multicomponent approach to searching the evidence. This approach included searching bibliographic databases and gray literature sources, as well as issuing a call for reports.

A professional librarian worked closely with the committee to plan the literature search strategies, ensure the appropriate translation of the key review questions into relevant and accurate terms, and conduct the searches so as to identify relevant research. Specific details regarding the search strategies and article selection process for each of the four review topics can be found at the end of this appendix.

Bibliographic Database Search

The committee conducted a series of searches in four databases—PubMed, Scopus, Medline (Ovid), and Embase (Ovid)—between December 2017 and January 2019 to identify peer-reviewed literature for the four selected PHEPR practices. The committee applied a date limit of 2001 to the present, limited the literature to the English language, and excluded editorials from the search results. The first search, conducted in December 2017, captured 14 of the 15 CDC PHEPR Capabilities (excluding Community Recovery, which is out of scope) and leveraged search strategies from existing scoping reviews. The searches conducted in July 2018 and December 2018 (and updated in June 2019) focused on the selected four review topics. In January 2019, the committee conducted two expanded searches on Information Sharing and Emergency Operations Coordination in subject-specific databases. The complete search syntax and search terms for each topic can be found at the end of this appendix.

Gray Literature Search

The committee identified gray literature published by relevant domestic and international organizations and agencies. These entities included the Association of Public Health Laboratories, ASPR, ASTHO, CDC, the Center for Health Security, the Council of State and Territorial Epidemiologists, the European Centre for Disease Prevention and Control, the Disaster Information Management Research Center at the National Library of Medicine in the National Institutes of Health (NIH), the U.S. Department of Homeland Security, FEMA, the U.S. Government Accountability Office, NACCHO, the National Center for Disaster Medicine and Public Health (NCDMPH), Preparedness and Emergency Response Research Centers (PERRCs), Public Health Canada, Public Health England, RAND Corporation, and the World Health Organization. In addition, the committee obtained 370 AARs published from 2009 to 2019 from the Homeland Security Digital Library.[6]

Call for Reports

In addition to online searching, the committee proactively solicited reports, both published and unpublished, through a request for documents via internal listservs at the National Academies and external mechanisms. An online request was published on the webpage for

[6] See https://www.hsdl.org/c (accessed May 26, 2020).

this study,[7] and the National Academies' Board on Health Sciences Policy distributed the call for reports through the Forum on Medical and Public Health Preparedness for Disasters and Emergencies and the Disaster Science Action Collaborative. Staff contacted CDC, the study sponsor, for document suggestions, and also asked the agency to disseminate the announcement to its networks, particularly the former PERRC and Preparedness and Emergency Response Learning Centers networks. Additionally, staff sent targeted emails to PHEPR practitioner associations (e.g., NACCHO and ASTHO) and disaster science organizations (e.g., NIH's Disaster Research Response system, NCDMPH, and the Association of Schools and Programs of Public Health). Submissions were accepted through March 8, 2019. This proved to be an effective way of collecting AARs, theses, and white papers.

Article Selection Method

Selecting which articles to include in the committee's reviews was a multistep process that involved developing inclusion and exclusion criteria, conducting an initial screening of titles and abstracts, and retrieving and reviewing selected full-text articles. Deciding which articles were relevant to the analytic frameworks and key review questions required significant judgment and thorough documentation. Preferred Reporting Items for Systematic Reviews and Meta-Analyses flowcharts for each review topic can be found in Chapters 4–7.

Inclusion and Exclusion Criteria

The committee developed specific inclusion and exclusion criteria based on the PICOTS framework for each of the four review topics. Generally, the committee did not exclude based on study design, lack of comparison groups, or lack of explicit outcomes (i.e., it included articles that describe lessons learned or present conclusions). Articles were excluded if they were editorials, opinion pieces, or commentaries with no indication of empirical evidence. A common set of inclusion and exclusion criteria was used for screening articles (see Box A-3).

Initial Screening and Full-Text Review

One staff member conservatively screened titles and abstracts for relevance to the four topic areas. Additional articles were identified for inclusion in the review through reference mining.

The next step was to review the full-text articles that had passed the first screen. Prior to that review, the process was pilot tested on a sample of articles, with screeners participating in a calibration training call. Two individuals, one committee member and one staff, then worked independently to review all selected full-text articles against the inclusion and exclusion criteria (see Box A-3). Discrepant articles were adjudicated primarily by the committee chair and in some instances by staff, and committee members were given the opportunity to review and object if necessary to the decisions made during the adjudication process. Articles on studies that used a clear research method were categorized as Tier 1, and articles that did not, including case reports, as Tier 2; both tiers were selected for extraction of key findings. Articles that were excluded but contained information that could provide background information for the review were categorized as background and kept for potential use at a later date. The committee used EndNote to manage its references and maintained in real time a detailed account of study selections and decisions.

---

[7] See https://www.nationalacademies.org/our-work/evidence-based-practices-for-public-health-emergency-preparedness-and-response-assessment-of-and-recommendations-for-the-field (accessed May 26, 2020).

BOX A-3 PICOTS CRITERIA FOR INCLUSION AND EXCLUSION OF ARTICLES

- **Eligible Study Designs**
  - Any study design, including primary quantitative studies, qualitative research studies, surveys, simulation models, after action reports, case reports, and related narrative descriptive studies
  - Any study duration or length of follow-up
  - Any sample size, including case reports without clear sample sizes
  - *Excluded:* existing systematic reviews and nonprimary studies (e.g., commentaries, editorials, opinion pieces)
- **Eligible Populations**
  - Any people, organizations, or other entities responding to or preparing for any event with public health ramifications that may impact a locality, region, or wider geographic area
    - — May include the general public or national, state, local, territorial, or tribal public health agencies; other public health practitioners or researchers; and other professionals (e.g., emergency management, health care)
    - — May include disasters and public health emergencies (e.g., hurricanes, epidemics) or other major events that may impact public health (e.g., the Pope's visit to Philadelphia)
    - — May include events that are real (e.g., Hurricane Sandy), simulated (e.g., a viral pandemic or toxic spill), theorized (e.g., a future hurricane), or implied (e.g., unknown events for which a community may prepare)
  - Events (if real) or studies since September 11, 2001
    - — Simulation and related models if they, in part, used data from older events (e.g., 1918 Spanish influenza pandemic data used to inform a simulation of a future viral pandemic)
- **Eligible Interventions and Comparators***
  - Community Preparedness Capability
    - — Practices used to engage with and train community-based partners to assess and plan for the access and functional needs of at-risk populations that may be disproportionately impacted by a public health emergency
  - Emergency Operations Coordination Capability
    - — Strategies or criteria used by public health agencies to determine when to activate public health emergency operations, with a focus on determining when public health should have a lead response role, a supporting role, or no role based on identified or potential public health consequences
  - Information Sharing Capability
    - — Practices used by public health agencies to communicate public health alerts and guidance with technical audiences during a public health emergency that include actions to increase awareness and understanding of information

DATA EXTRACTION AND STUDY QUALITY ASSESSMENT

Studies captured in the literature searches for each review topic were placed in six categories:

- quantitative comparative studies,
- quantitative noncomparative (single-group) studies of specific interventions,
- surveys (descriptive only),

- Non-Pharmaceutical Interventions Capability
  - Strategies used by public health agencies to implement quarantine, including strategies to increase adherence and reduce harms
  - *Excluded:* studies of isolating unexposed people (reverse quarantine) or true isolation (of ill patients, usually in hospitals or equivalent)
- Comparators
  - Not required, but analyses of interest included comparisons of a practice with one or more alternative practices or with no practice (e.g., usual practice)

- **Eligible Outcomes**
  - Overall, included
    - Health outcomes: impacts on health, morbidity, mortality, health disparities, and other clinical outcomes
    - Intermediate outcomes: intermediate or surrogate outcomes that are plausibly related to health outcomes (e.g., knowledge, participation in activities, coordination, information exchange, quarantine adherence)
    - Harms (nonhealth)
    - Other outcomes (e.g., equity)
- **Eligible Settings**
  - In general, countries deemed to be most generalizable to the United States, taking into consideration the likely sources of relevant data
  - Variable across review topics
    - Notably, included studies from any country regarding quarantine
    - *Excluded:* for Community Preparedness and Information Sharing, studies from an international setting, except those from the United Kingdom, Western Europe, Canada, Australia, and New Zealand
    - *Excluded:* for Emergency Operations Coordination, studies from any international setting, except those from the United Kingdom, Western Europe, Canada, Mexico, Panama, Australia, New Zealand, and Israel
  - Any geographic or civic setting, including urban, suburban, or rural; federal, national, state, regional, city, or neighborhood; general or focused community (e.g., Latinos, Navajo); or other settings

---

* For qualitative evidence, the "I" in PICOTS refers to phenomenon of interest rather than intervention. The committee did not use a question formulation framework that is specific to qualitative evidence synthesis. However, for the qualitative evidence syntheses, phenomena of interest included what worked or did not work; what happened; what benefits or harms resulted; what are barriers to and facilitators of implementation (e.g., acceptability and preferences, feasibility, resource and economic considerations); and what are the equity issues.

- simulation (and related) models,
- qualitative research studies, and
- AARs and case reports.

Mixed-method studies (having both quantitative and qualitative components) were included in both the quantitative and qualitative study categories, as appropriate. Data extraction and the quality assessment process were tailored as necessary to these categories of study types.

Data extraction and quality assessment for individual quantitative studies were performed by the Center for Evidence Synthesis in Health at Brown University, an evidence-based practice center (EPC) that conducts reviews for the Agency for Healthcare Research and Quality and others. Data extraction and quality assessment for the qualitative studies were performed by a commissioned team at Wayne State University. Prioritization of case reports and AARs for inclusion in the systematic reviews and data extraction for these reports were conducted by a PHEPR expert in evaluation at Columbia University. The evaluation and extraction of findings from selected modeling studies were performed by a modeling expert at Stanford University, as described further in Chapter 3.

Data Extraction

Data extracted from each study included the description of the practice being reviewed, elements needed to make determinations about the effect of the practice, and contextual

BOX A-4 DATA EXTRACTION ELEMENTS FOR QUANTITATIVE STUDIES

For all articles, the following data were extracted:

- Primary aim (hypothesis testing, descriptive)
- Study design
- Whether quantitative outcomes are reported
- Country
- Dates of intervention
- Target population (e.g., general population, vulnerable population, specific occupation or role, specific racial/ethnic group)
- Enrolled entities (e.g., general population, health care setting, public health setting, emergency organization)
- Entity that delivered the intervention (e.g., public health team, health care provider, emergency management)
- Disaster life cycle phase (preparedness, response, recovery, not reported)
- Format of "emergency" (real event, simulated event [including hypothetical, exercises, models], no event [e.g., for preparedness], not reported)
- Intervention components tested (based on The Community Guide[a])
  - Provision of information only[b]
  - Training and/or education[c]
  - Behavioral interventions[d]
  - Environmental interventions[e]
  - Public health or medical system interventions[f]
  - Legislation, regulation, and/or enforcement[g]
  - Other, none, not applicable, or unclear
- Topics of interest
  - Community Preparedness Capability (engaging with and training community-based partners)
  - Emergency Operations Coordination Capability (activating public health emergency operations)

elements that would contribute to an assessment of the applicability of its results to other contexts (e.g., populations, settings). Extracted data elements for quantitative studies are listed in Box A-4.

Qualitative studies, AARs, and case reports were coded in accordance with the framework synthesis method (Barnett-Page and Thomas, 2009; Pope et al., 2000), as described in Chapter 3. The codebook for extracting study characteristics and findings was developed in consultation with the committee and National Academies staff. Training sessions for the use of the codebook were conducted with the research team, and a pilot test of the codebook portion on extracting study characteristics and findings was conducted to refine the process.

Individual Study Quality Assessment

The quality assessment methodology was determined based on study design. Many standardized tools are available for assessing quality or risk of bias (RoB), each with its own

- Information Sharing Capability (communicating public health alerts and guidance with technical audiences)
- Non-Pharmaceutical Interventions Capability (quarantine)
- Outcome domains, per topic; specific domain (e.g., health disparities) within
  - Health outcomes
  - Intermediate outcomes
  - Harms
  - Values and preferences
  - Resource use
  - Equity
  - Acceptability
  - Feasibility
  - Other

[a] See The Community Guide for further details: https://www.thecommunityguide.org/sites/default/files/assets/abstractionform.pdf (accessed June 25, 2020).

[b] Provision of information only: These interventions are aimed at changing knowledge, attitudes, or norms.

[c] Training and education methods might involve instruction (e.g., classes, assemblies), small media (e.g., brochures, leaflets, posters, letters, newsletters), or large media (e.g., television, radio, newspapers, billboards).

[d] Behavioral interventions: These interventions are aimed at changing behaviors by providing necessary skills or materials.

[e] Environmental interventions: These interventions are aimed at changing the physical and/or social environment to promote health or prevent disease.

[f] Public health or medical care system interventions: These interventions are aimed at changing the public health or clinical care system to increase or improve the delivery of services (system focused).

[g] Legislation, regulation, and/or enforcement: These interventions are aimed at changing behaviors or altering disease risk factors by legislating particular behaviors, regulating risk factors, and enforcing those laws and regulations.

merits and shortcomings, and new tools continue to be developed. Described here is the approach taken by the committee and the groups commissioned to assess study quality and RoB; however, different tools and methods could reasonably be applied in future PHEPR evidence reviews.

Quantitative Studies

For quantitative comparative studies, an assessment tool was developed by the Brown University EPC[8] by drawing selected RoB domains from existing tools, including the Cochrane Risk of Bias version 2.0 tool (Higgins et al., 2019), Cochrane's suggested risk-of-bias criteria for Effective Practice and Organisation of Care reviews (Cochrane, 2017), and the Cochrane Risk of Bias in Non-Randomized Studies of Interventions (ROBINS-I) tool (Sterne et al., 2016). The selection of RoB domains reflected the dual goals of adequately addressing important potential methodological concerns and being mindful of the resources and time available for assessing the methodological quality of studies with a wide range of potential study designs. The final set of domains and their assessment criteria are as follows:

- **Study population (eligibility criteria):** Was the included sample prespecified, clearly specified, defined, and uniformly applied? Low RoB if yes; High RoB if no. This domain is consistent across outcomes.
- **Allocation concealment (and randomization method):** For RCTs, was there a problem with the randomization method or allocation concealment? High RoB if yes; Low RoB if explicitly no problem; Unclear RoB if insufficient reporting to judge. For nonrandomized comparative studies (NRCSs) of different interventions, High RoB unless analytic methods were used to account adequately for inherent baseline differences in compared groups or if it is otherwise reasonable to assume that compared groups are sufficiently similar. If pre-post study (of a single group), then "None." This domain is consistent across outcomes.
- **Comparator group:** Was the comparator group chosen from the same population, with the same general eligibility criteria, as the intervention group? For RCTs, Low RoB. For NRCSs, there is overlap between this assessment and the assessment of "Allocation" (see above). If pre-post study (of a single group), Low RoB (unless there is an indication that groups differed pre- and postintervention). This domain is consistent across outcomes.
- **Sample size:** Is there a justification of the sample size or power/analysis per outcome? High RoB if no; Low RoB if yes (and the sample size was reached) or if the analysis was statistically significant. This domain may differ for each outcome.
- **Loss to follow-up:** Was there high loss to follow-up, arbitrarily set at 20 percent, or was there unequal loss to follow-up between groups? This criterion is largely based on comparisons between enrolled (or randomized) individuals and the numbers analyzed. High RoB if yes; Low RoB if no. This domain may differ for each outcome.
- **Outcome measurement or ascertainment bias:** Was there a problem with how each outcome was measured? High RoB if unvalidated subjective outcome. For studies comparing different interventions, includes whether an outcome was measured differently in the different intervention groups. This domain may differ for each outcome.
- **Group similarity at baseline:** Were the groups (intervention and comparator) similar at baseline? If similar, Low RoB. If there was a (nonminor) difference, was the difference

[8] See Appendix C.

statistically accounted for for each outcome? Judgment of whether a difference was "nonminor" depended on both statistical and clinical significance. Unclear RoB only if baseline descriptions were omitted or were too sparse to evaluate for possible differences. If pre-post study (of a single group), Low RoB (unless there is an indication that groups differed pre- and postintervention). This domain may differ for each outcome (based primarily on whether adequate statistical adjustment was conducted).

- **Outcome assessor blinding:** Regardless of study design, was the outcome assessor blinded, or were methods used to minimize biased outcome assessment? "Hard" outcomes (unambiguous, potentially like death) or outcomes based on objective measurements (e.g., laboratory measurements or government records, such as number quarantined) generally qualified as Low RoB, as did outcomes that were explicitly blinded. Other outcomes from observational studies were assumed to have High RoB unless otherwise indicated. Self-reported outcomes were typically High RoB unless the participants were blinded to their intervention. This domain may differ for each outcome.
- **Group differences and confounders:** Did the analyses account for potential group differences or confounders, for example, by multivariable adjustment or propensity score analysis? For RCTs, Low RoB was assumed absent a suggestion of a lack of similarity between groups (despite randomization). For NRCSs, regardless of whether groups were similar at baseline, High RoB if there was no adjustment for potential differences or if adjustment was made only for something minor or insufficient (e.g., only sex across disparate populations). For pre-post studies, Low RoB (unless there was an indication that groups differed pre- and postintervention). This domain may differ for each outcome.
- **Other important limitations** per data extractor or as reported by study authors. This domain may differ for each outcome.

Each outcome of each quantitative comparative study was evaluated for all of the above domains. Then an overall assessment of the study (or outcome) methodology (rated as good, moderate, or poor) was made based on the judgment of the evaluators after considering the various bias domains, which were weighted differently for different study designs. Each study (and outcome) was assessed for methodological quality by the Brown team's senior researcher and was reviewed by at least one other experienced team member and was altered in discussion as needed.

The Brown University EPC developed and applied a separate tool for the assessment of descriptive surveys, drawing on published methods (Bennett et al., 2010; Davids and Roman, 2014). Descriptive surveys were assessed using the following domains and assessment criteria:

- **Adequacy of survey tool development:** Low RoB: A priori methodology with group development and pretesting reported that survey has been validated and/or found reliable. High RoB: Lack of structured methodology for developing questions, single person or group developed, and/or no outside input or pilot, field, or pretesting of questions (or prior use). Unclear RoB: No or incomplete description of development process.
- **Study population eligibility criteria prespecified and uniformly applied:** Low RoB: Explicitly reported, clear, and no major deviations from protocol. High RoB: Not prespecified or major deviation from protocol. Unclear RoB: Not reported whether prespecified or deviation.

- **Adequacy and appropriateness of polling/sampling methodology:** Low RoB: Everyone who met criteria (universe, census); probability sampling (e.g., random selection of telephone, email, and text of population with high access to these technologies); other unbiased sampling of population of interest. High RoB: Problems such as that sampling was likely biased (e.g., texting may miss individuals of low socioeconomic status or those difficult to reach), nonprobability sample (e.g., for focus group, convenience sample); if sample of general population, no attempt to capture difficult-to-reach individuals (e.g., those with no phone, email). Unclear RoB: Not adequately described.
- **Respondents nonrepresentative of the target population:** Low RoB: Respondents representative of target population and not different from nonrespondents. High RoB: Explicitly nonrepresentative; respondents differed from nonrespondents or target population. Unclear RoB: No description of target population or nonrespondents (and not High RoB).
- **Percentage who responded:** The actual response rate, without a judgment of its adequacy.
- **Information on margin of error reported:** Low RoB: If margin-of-error calculations made and reported, the reported values were extracted. Unclear RoB: No information on margin-of-error calculations. (While margin of error is a concept related to precision and not bias, the same terminology [High, Low, Unclear] was used for clarity and consistency.)

Qualitative Studies

Quality assessment for qualitative studies was undertaken as a component of a qualitative evidence synthesis commissioned to Wayne State University. The qualitative studies meeting the inclusion criteria for each review topic were appraised individually using the Critical Appraisal Skills Programme (CASP, 2018) checklist, which is applicable to assessing qualitative research. Areas of appraisal by CASP include appropriateness of qualitative methodology, data collection, relationship between research and participants, ethics, rigor of data analysis, clarity of findings, and value of research. Each area was assessed using "yes," "no," or "can't tell." In line with the Grading of Recommendations Assessment, Development and Evaluation Confidence in the Evidence from Reviews of Qualitative Research (GRADE-CERQual) approach for assessing methodological limitations (Lewin et al., 2018), each study received a final overall quality rating of "no or very minor concerns" (no significant methodological limitations), "minor concerns" (minor methodological limitations not impacting the credibility and validity of findings), "moderate concerns" (some methodological limitations likely to impact the credibility and validity of findings), or "serious concerns" (serious methodological limitation impacting the credibility and validity of findings).

After Action Reports

An appraisal tool for evaluating the methodological rigor of AARs was published in 2018 (ECDC, 2018) and was applied by a commissioned PHEPR expert to the AARs included in the committee's analyses. The 11-item tool is designed to assist with the systematic documentation of methods used in AARs, compare validity, and potentially inform best practices for a standard template. The tool includes the following criteria:

- prolonged engagement with the subject of inquiry,
- use of theory,

- data selection,
- information sampling,
- multiple data sources,
- triangulation,
- negative case analysis,
- peer debriefing and support,
- respondent validation,
- clear report of methods of data collection and analysis (audit trail), and
- depth and insight.

PRIORITIZATION OF FUTURE SYSTEMATIC EVIDENCE REVIEW TOPICS

The committee engaged with a second diverse group of 10 PHEPR practitioners, also representing SLTT agencies, in an open session to identify knowledge gaps that matter to practitioners and assess the relative priority, from their perspective, of potential evidence review topics encompassed within the CDC PHEPR Capabilities. This practitioner engagement activity was conducted after the committee's four evidence review topics had been selected and therefore did not inform the selection process. The activity was intended to inform the identification of priorities for future PHEPR evidence reviews, as well as future research needs, to address critical knowledge gaps in PHEPR practice. For this prioritization activity, the committee modified an existing group judgment process originally developed to assess the appropriateness of medical procedures, but since modified for many other uses (i.e., modified Delphi-like process) (Shekelle, 2004; Sloss et al., 2000). This process involved the selection of this group of SLTT PHEPR practitioners, a review of the literature, and multiple rounds of group voting with feedback between rounds. This process was led by an experienced moderator.

This second group of PHEPR practitioners was identified through a process similar to that used to select the PHEPR practitioner consultants. The list of PHEPR topics included in this activity was adapted from an existing list of 44 research questions deemed by PHEPR practitioners to be priority areas (Siegfried et al., 2017). Building from that list, the committee combined several research questions into one topic area, removed several research questions that did not lend themselves to a review of the evidence, and added several questions that the committee derived from a review of the literature. This process resulted in 39 topic areas across the six PHEPR domains identified by Siegfried and colleagues: community resilience, incident management, information management, countermeasures and mitigation, surge management, and biosurveillance.

In January 2019, the committee engaged with these PHEPR practitioners in an open session in a virtual premeeting for the first round of voting and at an in-person meeting for the second round of voting. All 10 PHEPR practitioners participated in both rounds. The committee used Sli.Do, an online polling software, to conduct this activity.

The PHEPR practitioners were asked to rank the importance of the 39 topic areas on the committee's list by rating each on a 5-point Likert rating scale—highest priority, high priority, moderate priority, low priority, and not a priority—as well as to provide any other comments or suggestions. They were provided with the following guidance with regard to rating the priority of topics:

> These ratings should reflect the need for a systematic review of the evidence, not necessarily the importance of the practice. All of the topics are certainly important, but rating everything as the highest priority will not be helpful. Furthermore, the evidence for some practices with

very high importance to PHEPR may be well established, and a review of the evidence for those topics may be less valuable than a review of other topics for which there are important knowledge gaps.

Results from the first round (virtual premeeting) were compiled for the second round (in-person meeting), during which the PHEPR practitioners received feedback on the results from the first round, discussed those results, and revoted if doing so was warranted. The outcome of this process was a set of PHEPR review topics classified into the five Likert scale categories: highest priority, high priority, moderate priority, low priority, and not a priority (see Box A-5). This information, along with the published literature, aided the committee in identifying priorities for future evidence reviews, as well as future research needs, to address critical knowledge gaps in PHEPR practice.

BOX A-5 PRIORITY TOPICS FOR FUTURE PHEPR EVIDENCE REVIEWS

The committee engaged with state, local, tribal, and territorial practitioners to assess the relative priority (from the practitioner perspective) of potential evidence review topics encompassed within the 15 Centers for Disease Control and Prevention Public Health Emergency Preparedness and Response Capabilities. Building on the work of Siegfried and colleagues (2017), the committee used a modified Delphi-like process that yielded the following results after two rounds of voting.

Topics that at least 66 percent of the panel rated as "highest priority" or "high priority":

- Engaging, educating, training, and motivating communities to prepare for, withstand, and recover from emergencies
- Strategies for engaging at-risk populations in community preparedness activities and in protective actions during and immediately after an emergency
- Strategies for integrating preparedness activities into routine public health practice
- Effective message formats for information sharing with at-risk populations (e.g., populations that rely on oral traditions, those with limited English proficiency, and individuals without Internet access or smartphones)
- Information management strategies for public risk perception during an emergency
- Monitoring and tracking health issues (physical safety and mental and behavioral health) of responders prior to, during, and following response

Topics that at least 50 percent of the panel rated as "highest priority" or "high priority":

- Resources and tools (e.g., data collection templates, methods for summarizing and sharing information, and/or data systems) to capture critical information during an emergency that involves public health
- Effective training and exercises for public health staff whose usual role is not emergency response
- Use of social media for communicating with the public during emergencies
- Use of multifunctional (e.g., environmental health, epidemiology) public health strike teams to respond to public health events

Topics that at least 50 percent of the panel rated as "low priority" or "not a priority":

- Use of simulation and modeling to inform planning, preparedness, and response
- Locating and mapping locations of at-risk populations before, during, and after an emergency
- Ensuring continuity-of-operations readiness of public health agencies and their workforces

BOX A-5 CONTINUED

- Strategies for ensuring that the emergency operations center (EOC) is not overwhelmed during a response and has appropriate levels of redundancy of planning and operations
- Strategies for building capacity to ensure a fully staffed EOC during a response (e.g., elimination of cross-jurisdictional barriers to mutual aid)
- Strategies for public health departments to coordinate with entities both within and outside the EOC
- Use of web-based command and control platforms (e.g., WebEOC), protocols, and trainings for EOC operations
- Methods for communicating within and between EOCs
- Leadership characteristics of incident commanders that influence the response system's performance to achieve optimal health outcomes
- Strategies for ensuring adoption of best practices in emergency risk communication
- Roles for public health departments in medical surge activities
- Strategies for facilitating collaboration in the management and staffing of medical countermeasure (MCM) dispensing points for optimal speed and coverage
- Use of surveillance systems to detect public health threats and support situational awareness during a response
- Operational planning and response over the course of short- and long-term incidents (to include the ability to scale up and scale down)
- Initiating a response in coordination with incident management teams beyond the local health system (e.g., Disaster Medical Assistance Teams)
- Quality and quantity of trainings suggested for key personnel on public health preparedness and response
- Minimum public health staffing standards for responses (i.e., what are the key positions)
- Strategies for optimal logistics management, including medical materiel warehousing and distribution
- Strategies for evaluating MCM and non-pharmaceutical intervention courses of action

Topics in the middle:

- Data sources (e.g., existing public health, historical, geological, ecological, and sociological data) and methods for centralized data compilation to inform jurisdictional risk assessments and real-time decision making
- Use of jurisdictional risk assessment–based planning to mitigate the impact of identified risks related to public health, health and human services, and infrastructure
- Elements of successful implementation of a continuity-of-operations plan for a health department
- Management structures that influence response system performance
- Strategies for optimizing use of information in leadership and management decision making
- Strategies for and barriers to sharing data and information among states, territories, and localities and for handling surge-related needs
- Practices, procedures, and strategies for isolation and quarantine for disease control
- Strategies and infrastructure for assessing and addressing mental health issues and needs during emergencies
- Metrics for assessing medical surge activities and operations (e.g., services, management processes, and standards of care)
- Strategies for facilitating preparedness in rural, isolated, or health professional shortage areas
- Strategies for facilitating medical surge capacity in rural, isolated, or health professional shortage areas

continued

BOX A-5 CONTINUED

- Strategies for dispensing MCMs, including the optimal mix of closed versus open points of dispensing
- Strategies for the public health and health care sectors to ensure readiness to activate and support surge activities
- Strategies and systems for facilitating collaboration and communication across agencies that support medical surge and mass care activities (e.g., regional planning, health care coalitions)
- Application of specific disease support and expertise (e.g., pediatric, bariatric, and chronic disease) to medical support, sheltering, and evacuation activities
- Processes and protocols for interjurisdictional epidemiological investigation during an emergency
- Data-sharing and data-use practices for public health surveillance to ensure the privacy, confidentiality, and security of personal health information in an emergency
- Communication and information-sharing methods for epidemiological response among public health and external partners
- Administrative preparedness procedures, including disaster finance procedures and tracking prior to, during, and after a response
- Best practices for working with jurisdictional officials to implement authority and processes for public health orders, including coordination with necessary law enforcement and health care partners
- Volunteer involvement, accrual, and retainment
- Factors that determine MCM adherence over time
- Use of "big data" to rapidly identify, characterize, and forecast the probable trajectory, duration, and magnitude of threats
- Essential elements of public health emergency response readiness specific to tribal communities
- Strategies for successful operational collaboration and mutual agreements between tribal governments and nontribal public health emergency preparedness and response partners during public health emergency responses

DATABASE SEARCH STRATEGIES

Initial searches were run on December 3, 2018, covering 2001–December 2018. Final update searches were performed on June 5, 2019, covering December 2018–June 2019.

Community Preparedness

Search Parameters:
Date: 2001–Present
Language: English
Document Type: Exclude commentaries, editorials, letters, and notes
Databases: Medline (Ovid), Embase (Ovid), Scopus

Search Syntax:

Medline (Ovid):

Search No.	Syntax	Results
1	((natural adj (disaster? or hazard?)) or (hurricane? or flood$ or typhoon? or earthquake$ or fire? or cyclon$ or heatwave? or freezing or ((ice or snow or lightning) adj storm?) or blizzard? or "heat wave" or (extreme adj (temperature? or heat or cold)) or tsunami? or "tidal wave")).tw.	75,331
2	("mass migration*" or SARS or ebola or smallpox or plague or measles).tw.	46,567
3	(firesetting or arson or explosion? or bomb$ or outbreak? or refugee* or (explo$ adj device?) or blackout? or brownout? or ((power or equipment) adj (loss or failure)) or radioactive or radiation or (nuclear adj (disaster or meltdown or catastrophe or fail$))).tw.	427,623
4	(((chemical or biological) adj warfare) or riot$ or influenza or flu or (civil adj (disorder? or defense or unrest))).tw.	89,156
5	cyclonic storms/ or droughts/ or floods/ or tidal waves/ or tsunami/ or snow/ or rain/ or avalanches/ or volcanic eruptions/ or earthquakes/ or landslides/ or fires/ or ice/ or tornadoes/ or extreme cold/ or extreme heat/ or lightning/ or cold temperature/ or hot temperature/ or wind/ or firesetting behavior/ or explosions/ or blackout/ or equipment failure/ or radioactive hazard release/ or influenza/ or refugees/ or riots/ or civil disorders/ or civil defense/ or communicable diseases/ or Severe Acute Respiratory Syndrome/ or SARS VIRUS/ or HEMORRHAGIC FEVER, EBOLA/ or MEASLES/ or SMALLPOX/ or PLAGUE/	341,253
6	or/1–5	859,584
7	(("public health" adj (practice or administration or incident* or emergenc*)) or "preventive medicine").tw. or "public health".ti,ab.	171,417
8	public health/ or preventive medicine/ or public health practice/ or public health administration/	101,802
9	"health department*".tw.	8,009
10	((public or local or state or tribal or territorial or multi) adj health adj (department* or agenc*or jurisdiction)).ti,ab.	3,961
11	or/7–10	232,661
12	6 and 11	21,249
13	(epidemic? or pandemic? or terroris$ or bioterroris$ or "mass casualt*").tw.	105,665
14	epidemics/ or pandemics/ or disease outbreaks/ or disasters/ or emergencies/ or mass casualty incidents/ or terrorism/ or bioterrorism/ or chemical terrorism/ or "september 11 terrorist attacks"/	152,746
15	((emergency adj (prepare* or response* or management or incident*)) or (disaster adj (plan$ or prepare* or mitigation or recover* or cycle or medicine or resilienc* or incident* or response* or management* or readiness))).tw.	8,725
16	emergency preparedness/ or emergency response/ or emergency management/ or disaster planning/ or disaster medicine/ or disaster resilience/	15,465
17	or/13–16	230,361
18	12 or 17	241,051
19	Vulnerable Populations/ or Minority Groups/ or "Sexual and Gender Minorities"/ or "Emigrants and Immigrants"/ or "Transients and Migrants"/ or African Americans/ or Hispanic Americans/ or Indians, North American/ or Asian Americans/ or Poverty/ or Socioeconomic Factors/ or "Aged, 80 and over"/ or Aged/ or INFANT/ or INFANT, NEWBORN/	4,051,798
20	Pregnant Women/ or DIABETES MELLITUS/ or Heart Diseases/ or DEAF-BLIND DISORDERS/ or BLINDNESS/ or Deafness/ or Persons With Hearing Impairments/ or Vision Disorders/ or Disabled Persons/ or Animal Assisted Therapy/ or Self-Help Devices/ or Autistic Disorder/	312,323
21	DEMENTIA/ or ANXIETY/ or ANXIETY DISORDERS/ or "Transportation of Patients"/ or Homeless Persons/ or Rural Population/ or ELECTRICITY/ or CHILD/ or Health Literacy/ or Educational Status/ or Communication Barriers/	1,835,230

Search No.	Syntax	Results
22	Alcoholism/ or Substance-Related Disorders/ or Mental Disorders/ or Stress Disorders, Post-Traumatic/ or Depressive Disorder/ or SCHIZOPHRENIA/ or Psychotic Disorders/	486,844
23	(vulnerable adj (population* or person* or individual*)).tw.	7,372
24	("at risk" adj (individual* or population* or person*)).tw.	4,905
25	"functional need*".tw.	327
26	vulnerability.tw.	40,340
27	(elderly or disabled).tw.	216,777
28	((racial or ethnic or sexual or gender) adj minorit*).tw.	10,036
29	("older adult*" or pediatric* or child*).tw.	1,288,450
30	(limited adj (english or language)).tw.	801
31	(migrant* or "low income" or "under resourced" or tribal or "dialysis patient*" or "electricity dependent" or "medically vulnerable").tw.	56,111
32	("pregnant wom*n" or "pre existing condition*" or "chronic condition*" or diabetes or "heart disease*" or blind* or deaf* or "assistive device*" or "service animal*" or "personal assistance service provider*" or autism or dementia or anxiety or "transportation need*" or homeless* or "lift equipped" or "oxygen tank*").tw.	1,108,388
33	"language barrier*".tw.	1,435
34	((low or limited) adj "health literacy").tw.	894
35	("mental health disorder*" or "group home patient*" or "substance abuse disorder*").tw.	2,989
36	(alcoholism or "substance disorder*" or "mental disorder*" or "stress disorder*" or PTSD or depression or "depressive disorder*" or schizophrenia or "psychotic disorder*").tw.	405,450
37	or/19–36	6,603,197
38	Community Health Planning/ or Community-Institutional Relations/ or Community Participation/ or Community Health Services/ or Community Networks/ or Community-Based Participatory Research/	66,327
39	Home Care Services/ or Hospices/ or Home Care Services/ or Hospice Care/ or Assisted Living Facilities/ or Skilled Nursing Facilities/ or Home Nursing/ or Local Government/	55,665
40	Emergency Shelter/ or Voluntary Health Agencies/ or Red Cross/	6,403
41	(community adj4 (engagement or outreach or preparedness or partner* or partnership* or train* or toolkit or education or plan*)).tw.	20,161
42	(community adj2 (stakeholder* or spokesperson* or spokespeople or gathering* or venue*)).tw.	848
43	"town hall meeting*".tw.	58
44	"faith based organization*".tw.	213
45	("animal service agenc*" or "childcare organization*" or "chronic disease program*" or "communicable disease program*" or "community coalition*" or "emergency management agenc*" or "emergency medical service*" or "environmental health agenc*" or "fire department*" or "fire and rescue" or "health care coalition*" or "health care organization*" or "health care system*" or "health care provider*" or "infection control program*" or "housing authorit*" or "shelter* authorit*" or "human service provider*" or "immunization program*" or "jurisdictional strategic advisory council*" or "law enforcement" or "media organization*" or "local media" or "metal health provider*" or "behavioral health provider*" or "public health preparedness program*" or "school agenc*" or "education agenc*" or "social service*" or "state office of aging" or "surveillance program*" or "volunteer organization*").tw.	88,794

Search No.	Syntax	Results
46	"community based participatory research".tw.	1,707
47	("C MIST" or "communication medical independence supervision transportation"). tw.	0
48	(sovi or "social vulnerability index").tw.	50
49	("at risk" adj (database* or registr* or map*)).tw.	3
50	"social capital".tw.	2,396
51	((medicare or medicaid or "health measure*") adj data).tw.	1,375
52	"empower initiative".tw.	0
53	("emergency shelter*" or NGO* or "red cross" or "local business*").tw.	6,186
54	("home care" or "hospice care" or hospice* or "home hospice" or "assisted living facilit*" or "skilled care facilit*").tw.	25,222
55	or/38–54	239,867
56	18 and 37 and 55	4,047
57	limit 56 to (english language and yr="2001-Current")	2,857
58	limit 57 to (comment or editorial or letter)	38
59	57 not 58	2,819

Embase (Ovid):

Search No.	Syntax	Results
1	((natural adj (disaster? or hazard?)) or (hurricane? or flood$ or typhoon? or earthquake$ or fire? or cyclon$ or heatwave? or freezing or ((ice or snow or lightning) adj storm?) or blizzard? or "heat wave" or (extreme adj (temperature? or heat or cold)) or tsunami? or "tidal wave")).tw.	87,057
2	("mass migration*" or SARS or ebola or smallpox or plague or measles).tw.	38,502
3	(firesetting or arson or explosion? or bomb$ or outbreak? or refugee* or (explo$ adj device?) or blackout? or brownout? or ((power or equipment) adj (loss or failure)) or radioactive or radiation or (nuclear adj (disaster or meltdown or catastrophe or fail$))).tw.	468,844
4	(((chemical or biological) adj warfare) or riot$ or influenza or flu or (civil adj (disorder? or defense or unrest))).tw.	93,578
5	hurricane/ or drought/ or flooding/ or tsunami/ or snow/ or rain/ or ice/ or avalanche/ or volcano/ or earthquake/ or landslide/ or fire/ or tornado/ or cold/ or heat/ or lightning/ or wind/ or arson/ or explosion/ or device failure/ or nuclear accident/ or civil disorder/ or influenza/ or communicable disease/ or severe acute respiratory syndrome/ or Ebola hemorrhagic fever/ or measles/ or smallpox/ or Smallpox virus/ or plague/ or refugee/	228,653
6	or/1–5	800,537
7	(("public health" adj (practice or administration or incident* or emergenc*)) or "preventive medicine").tw. or "public health".ti,ab.	213,782
8	"health department*".tw.	7,711
9	((public or local or state or tribal or territorial or multi) adj health adj (department* or agenc*or jurisdiction)).ti,ab.	3,708
10	public health/ or preventive medicine/ or public health service/	191,406
11	or/7–10	330,666
12	6 and 11	30,320
13	(epidemic? or pandemic? or terroris$ or bioterroris$ or "mass casualt*").tw.	114,929

Search No.	Syntax	Results
14	((emergency adj (prepare* or response* or management or incident*)) or (disaster adj (plan$ or prepare* or mitigation or recover* or cycle or medicine or resilienc* or incident* or response* or management* or readiness))).tw.	10,779
15	epidemic/ or pandemic/ or disaster/ or mass disaster/ or nuclear terrorism/ or terrorism/ or chemical terrorism/ or bioterrorism/ or disaster planning/ or disaster planning/ or disaster medicine/	121,985
16	or/13–15	191,448
17	12 or 16	208,880
18	vulnerable population/ or minority group/ or "sexual and gender minority"/ or undocumented immigrant/ or immigrant/ or migrant/ or African American/ or Hispanic/ or American Indian/ or Asian American/ or poverty/ or socioeconomics/ or very elderly/ or infant/ or newborn/	995,819
19	pregnant woman/ or diabetes mellitus/ or heart disease/ or deafblindness/ or blindness/ or hearing impairment/ or visual disorder/ or disabled person/ or animal assisted therapy/ or self help device/ or autism/ or mental deficiency/	728,645
20	dementia/ or anxiety/ or anxiety disorder/ or patient transport/ or homeless person/ or homeless man/ or homeless youth/ or homeless woman/ or rural population/ or electricity/ or health literacy/ or educational status/ or communication barrier/	430,145
21	alcoholism/ or substance abuse/ or mental disease/ or alcoholism/ or drug abuse/ or drug dependence/ or addiction/ or schizophrenia/ or psychosis/	468,019
22	(vulnerable adj (population* or person* or individual*)).tw.	11,533
23	("at risk" adj (individual* or population* or person*)).tw.	7,977
24	"functional need*".tw.	400
25	vulnerability.tw.	54,524
26	(elderly or disabled).tw.	267,455
27	((racial or ethnic or sexual or gender) adj minorit*).tw.	13,879
28	("older adult*" or pediatric* or child*).tw.	1,422,928
29	(limited adj (english or language)).tw.	1,192
30	(migrant* or "low income" or "under resourced" or tribal or "dialysis patient*" or "electricity dependent" or "medically vulnerable").tw.	68,197
31	("pregnant wom*n" or "pre existing condition*" or "chronic condition*" or diabetes or "heart disease*" or blind* or deaf* or "assistive device*" or "service animal*" or "personal assistance service provider*" or autism or dementia or anxiety or "transportation need*" or homeless* or "lift equipped" or "oxygen tank*").tw.	1,513,411
32	"language barrier*".tw.	2,429
33	((low or limited) adj "health literacy").tw.	1,636
34	("mental health disorder*" or "group home patient*" or "substance abuse disorder*").tw.	5,015
35	(alcoholism or "substance disorder*" or "mental disorder*" or "stress disorder*" or PTSD or depression or "depressive disorder*" or schizophrenia or "psychotic disorder*").tw.	518,753
36	or/18–35	4,505,232
37	community care/ or community program/ or community/ or emergency shelter/ or red cross/ or home care/ or hospice/ or hospice care/ or home for the aged/ or nursing home/ or assisted living facility/	210,785
38	(community adj4 (engagement or outreach or preparedness or partner* or partnership* or train* or toolkit or education or plan*)).tw.	25,460
39	(community adj2 (stakeholder* or spokesperson* or spokespeople or gathering* or venue*)).tw.	1,371

Search No.	Syntax	Results
40	"town hall meeting*".tw.	81
41	"faith based organization*".tw.	307
42	("animal service agenc*" or "childcare organization*" or "chronic disease program*" or "communicable disease program*" or "community coalition*" or "emergency management agenc*" or "emergency medical service*" or "environmental health agenc*" or "fire department*" or "fire and rescue" or "health care coalition*" or "health care organization*" or "health care system*" or "health care provider*" or "infection control program*" or "housing authorit*" or "shelter* authorit*" or "human service provider*" or "immunization program*" or "jurisdictional strategic advisory council*" or "law enforcement" or "media organization*" or "local media" or "metal health provider*" or "behavioral health provider*" or "public health preparedness program*" or "school agenc*" or "education agenc*" or "social service*" or "state office of aging" or "surveillance program*" or "volunteer organization*").tw.	112,450
43	"community based participatory research".tw.	2,259
44	("C MIST" or "communication medical independence supervision transportation"). tw.	0
45	(sovi or "social vulnerability index").tw.	67
46	("at risk" adj (database* or registr* or map*)).tw.	7
47	"social capital".tw.	3,029
48	((medicare or medicaid or "health measure*") adj data).tw.	2,567
49	"empower initiative".tw.	0
50	("emergency shelter*" or NGO* or "red cross" or "local business*").tw.	8,621
51	("home care" or "hospice care" or hospice* or "home hospice" or "assisted living facilit*" or "skilled care facilit*").tw.	29,249
52	or/37–51	349,425
53	17 and 36 and 52	5,222
54	limit 53 to (english language and yr="2001-Current")	4,712
55	limit 54 to (editorial or letter or note)	187
56	54 not 55	4,525

Scopus:
TITLE-ABS-KEY(((natural W/1 (disaster* or hazard*)) or hurricane* or flood* or typhoon* or earthquake* or fire* or cyclon* or heatwave* or freezing or ((ice or snow or lightning) W/1 storm*) or blizzard* or "heat wave" or (extreme W/1 (temperature* or heat or cold)) or tsunami* or drought* or "tidal wave" or epidemic* or pandemic* or terrorism or bioterrorism or "mass casualt*" or (firesetting or arson or explosion? or bomb* or (explo* W/1 device*) or blackout* or tornado* or brownout* or ((power or equipment) W/1 (loss or failure)) or radioactive or radiation or (nuclear W/1 (disaster or meltdown or catastrophe or fail*)) or (refugee* or "mass migration*" or SARS or ebola or smallpox or plague or measles or riot* or influenza or "communicable disease*" or ((chemical or biological) W/1 warefare) or (civil W/1 (disorder* or defense or unrest)))) AND (("public health" W/1 (practice or administration)) or "preventive medicine" or "health department" or ((public or local or state or tribal or territorial or multi) W/1 health W/1 (department* or agenc* or jurisdiction)))) OR ((emergency W/1 (preparedness or response or management)) or (disaster W/1 (plan* or preparedness or mitigation or recovery or cycle or medicine or resilience or readiness or ready))) AND ("vulnerable population*" or "minority group*" or {sexual and gender minorities} or "disabled person*" or immigrant* or emigrant* or transient* or refugee* or migrant* or "african ameri-

can*" or black or "hispanic American*" or hispanic or latin* OR indian* or "native american*" or "asian american*" or Asian* or poverty or "socioeconomic factor*" or ("at risk" w/1 (individual* or population*)) or "functional need*" or (vulnerable w/1 (individual* or population*)) or vulnerability or elderly or disabled or ((racial or ethnic or sexual or gender) w/1 minorit*) or "older adult" or pediatric* or child* or (limited w/1 (English or language)) or migrant* or immigrant* or "low income" or "under resourced" or tribal or "dialysis patient*" or "electricity dependent" or "medically vulnerable" or infant* or newborn* or {aged 80 and over} or "pregnant wom*n" or "pre existing condition*" or "chronic condition*" or diabetes or "heart disease*" or blind* or deaf* or "assistive device*" or "service animal*" or "personal assistance service provider*" or autism or dementia or anxiety or "transportation need*" or homeless* or "lift equipped" or "oxygen tank*" or "language barrier*" or ((low or limited) W/1 "health literacy") or "mental health disorder*" or "group home patient*" or "substance abuse disorder*" or alcoholism or "substance disorder*" or "mental disorder*" or "stress disorder*" or PTSD or depression or "depressive disorder*" or schizophrenia or "psychotic disorder*") AND ("community preparedness" OR "community partners" OR "community partnerships" OR "community engagement" OR "Community Health Planning" OR "Community Networks" OR "Community-Institutional Relations" or "cooperative behavior" or "risk assessment*" or "social capital" or "social support" or {community based participatory research} or (community w/2 (engagement or outreach or preparedness or partner* or partnership* or train* or toolkit or education or plan*)) or toolkit* or ("at risk" w/1 (database* or registr* or map*)) or "social capital" or CMIST OR "communication medical independence supervision transportation" or sovi or "social vulnerability index" or ("health measure*" w/1 data) or "empower initiative" or (community W/2 (stakeholder* or spokesperson* or spokespeople or gathering* or venue*)) or "town hall meeting*" or "faith based organization*" or "animal service agenc*" or "childcare organization*" or "chronic disease program*" or "communicable disease program*" or "community coalition*" or "emergency management agenc*" or "emergency medical service*" or "environmental health agenc*" or "fire department*" or {fire and rescue} or "health care coalition*" or "health care organization*" or "health care system*" or "health care provider*" or "infection control program*" or "housing authorit*" or "shelter* authorit*" or "human service provider*" or "immunization program*" or "jurisdictional strategic advisory council*" or "law enforcement" or "media organization*" or "local media" or "metal health provider*" or "behavioral health provider*" or "public health preparedness program*" or "school agenc*" or "education agenc*" or "social service*" or "state office of aging" or "surveillance program*" or "volunteer organization*" or "emergency shelter*" or NGO* or "red cross" or "local business*" or "home care" or "hospice care" or hospice* or "home hospice" or "assisted living facilit*" or "skilled care facilit*")) AND PUBYEAR AFT 2000
Exclude: Note, editorials, letters, and notes
Results: **3,406**

Emergency Operations Coordination

Search Parameters:
Date: 2001–Present
Language: English
Document Type: Exclude commentaries, editorials, letters, and notes
Databases: Medline (Ovid), Embase (Ovid), Scopus

Search Syntax:

Medline (Ovid):

Search No.	Syntax	Results
1	((natural adj (disaster? or hazard?)) or (hurricane? or flood$ or typhoon? or earthquake$ or fire? or cyclon$ or heatwave? or freezing or ((ice or snow or lightning) adj storm?) or blizzard? or "heat wave" or (extreme adj (temperature? or heat or cold)) or tsunami? or "tidal wave")).tw.	75,331
2	("mass migration*" or SARS or ebola or smallpox or plague or measles).tw.	46,567
3	(firesetting or arson or explosion? or bomb$ or outbreak? or refugee* or (explo$ adj device?) or blackout? or brownout? or ((power or equipment) adj (loss or failure)) or radioactive or radiation or (nuclear adj (disaster or meltdown or catastrophe or fail$))).tw.	427,623
4	(((chemical or biological) adj warfare) or riot$ or influenza or flu or (civil adj (disorder? or defense or unrest))).tw.	89,156
5	cyclonic storms/ or droughts/ or floods/ or tidal waves/ or tsunami/ or snow/ or rain/ or avalanches/ or volcanic eruptions/ or earthquakes/ or landslides/ or fires/ or ice/ or tornadoes/ or extreme cold/ or extreme heat/ or lightning/ or cold temperature/ or hot temperature/ or wind/ or firesetting behavior/ or explosions/ or blackout/ or equipment failure/ or radioactive hazard release/ or influenza/ or refugees/ or riots/ or civil disorders/ or civil defense/ or communicable diseases/ or Severe Acute Respiratory Syndrome/ or SARS VIRUS/ or HEMORRHAGIC FEVER, EBOLA/ or MEASLES/ or SMALLPOX/ or PLAGUE/	341,253
6	or/1-5	859,584
7	(("public health" adj (practice or administration or incident* or emergenc*)) or "preventive medicine").tw. or "public health".ti,ab.	171,417
8	public health/ or preventive medicine/ or public health practice/ or public health administration/	101,802
9	"health department*".tw.	8,009
10	((public or local or state or tribal or territorial or multi) adj health adj (department* or agenc*or jurisdiction)).ti,ab.	3,961
11	or/7-10	232,661
12	6 and 11	21,249
13	(epidemic? or pandemic? or terroris$ or bioterroris$ or "mass casualt*").tw.	105,665
14	epidemics/ or pandemics/ or disease outbreaks/ or disasters/ or emergencies/ or mass casualty incidents/ or terrorism/ or bioterrorism/ or chemical terrorism/ or "september 11 terrorist attacks"/	152,746
15	((emergency adj (prepare* or response* or management or incident*)) or (disaster adj (plan$ or prepare* or mitigation or recover* or cycle or medicine or resilienc* or incident* or response* or management* or readiness))).tw.	8,725
16	emergency preparedness/ or emergency response/ or emergency management/ or disaster planning/ or disaster medicine/ or disaster resilience/	15,465
17	or/13-16	230,361
18	12 or 17	241,051
19	"emergency operations coordination".tw.	4
20	"operation* center*".tw.	152
21	"emergency operations center*".tw.	67
22	"public health emergency operations center*".tw.	3
23	"national incident management system*".tw.	35
24	"incident management".tw.	219
25	Safety Management/	19,133
26	"safety management".tw.	818

Search No.	Syntax	Results
27	"emergency operation*".tw.	3,470
28	"unified command".tw.	12
29	"incident command".tw.	213
30	"incident management team*".tw.	16
31	"situational awareness".tw.	459
32	Cooperative Behavior/	40,680
33	"management infrastructure".tw.	101
34	"public health coordination*".tw.	7
35	"threshold criteria".tw.	291
36	"situational awareness".tw.	459
37	(essential adj (function* or personnel*)).tw.	4,635
38	Public Health Practice/st [Standards]	612
39	"delineation of service*".tw.	2
40	((tabletop or functional or "full scale" or trigger* or activat* or hypothetical or "stand up" or assessment) adj2 (drill or mobilize or mobilization or deploy* or exercise* or scenario* or incident* or event* or plan* or procedure* or protocol* or policy or policies)).tw.	28,387
41	"ESF-8".tw.	4
42	"incident management system*".tw.	78
43	"public health emergency operation*".tw.	6
44	"disaster* operation* center*".tw.	2
45	or/19–44	97,811
46	18 and 45	3,700
47	limit 46 to (english language and yr="2001–Current")	2,791
48	limit 47 to (comment or editorial or letter)	116
49	47 not 48	2,675

Embase (Ovid):

Search No.	Syntax	Results
1	((natural adj (disaster? or hazard?)) or (hurricane? or flood$ or typhoon? or earthquake$ or fire? or cyclon$ or heatwave? or freezing or ((ice or snow or lightning) adj storm?) or blizzard? or "heat wave" or (extreme adj (temperature? or heat or cold)) or tsunami? or "tidal wave")).tw.	106,875
2	("mass migration*" or SARS or ebola or smallpox or plague or measles).tw.	50,215
3	(firesetting or arson or explosion? or bomb$ or outbreak? or refugee* or (explo$ adj device?) or blackout? or brownout? or ((power or equipment) adj (loss or failure)) or radioactive or radiation or (nuclear adj (disaster or meltdown or catastrophe or fail$))).tw.	602,188
4	(((chemical or biological) adj warfare) or riot$ or influenza or flu or (civil adj (disorder? or defense or unrest))).tw.	111,443

Search No.	Syntax	Results
5	hurricane/ or drought/ or flooding/ or tsunami/ or snow/ or rain/ or ice/ or avalanche/ or volcano/ or earthquake/ or landslide/ or fire/ or tornado/ or cold/ or heat/ or lightning/ or wind/ or arson/ or explosion/ or device failure/ or nuclear accident/ or civil disorder/ or influenza/ or communicable disease/ or severe acute respiratory syndrome/ or Ebola hemorrhagic fever/ or measles/ or smallpox/ or Smallpox virus/ or plague/ or refugee/	274,496
6	or/1–5	1,010,732
7	(("public health" adj (practice or administration or incident* or emergenc*)) or "preventive medicine").tw. or "public health".ti,ab.	238,311
8	"health department*".tw.	9,525
9	((public or local or state or tribal or territorial or multi) adj health adj (department* or agenc*or jurisdiction)).ti,ab.	4,481
10	public health/ or preventive medicine/ or public health service/	231,842
11	or/7–10	387,664
12	6 and 11	32,828
13	(epidemic? or pandemic? or terroris$ or bioterroris$ or "mass casualt*").tw.	132,027
14	((emergency adj (prepare* or response* or management or incident*)) or (disaster adj (plan$ or prepare* or mitigation or recover* or cycle or medicine or resilienc* or incident* or response* or management* or readiness))).tw.	12,084
15	epidemic/ or pandemic/ or disaster/ or mass disaster/ or nuclear terrorism/ or terrorism/ or chemical terrorism/ or bioterrorism/ or disaster planning/ or disaster planning/ or disaster medicine/	138,280
16	or/13–15	221,710
17	12 or 16	241,171
18	"emergency operations coordination".tw.	6
19	"operation* center*".tw.	207
20	"emergency operations center*".tw.	78
21	"public health emergency operations center*".tw.	3
22	"national incident management system*".tw.	38
23	"incident management".tw.	330
24	"safety management".tw.	1,585
25	"emergency operation*".tw.	4,746
26	"unified command".tw.	19
27	"incident command".tw.	271
28	"incident management team*".tw.	25
29	"situational awareness".tw.	810
30	"management infrastructure".tw.	153
31	"public health coordination*".tw.	7
32	"threshold criteria".tw.	436
33	"situational awareness".tw.	810
34	(essential adj (function* or personnel*)).tw.	5,885
35	"delineation of service*".tw.	6

Search No.	Syntax	Results
36	((tabletop or functional or "full scale" or trigger* or activat* or hypothetical or "stand up" or assessment) adj2 (drill or mobilize or mobilization or deploy* or exercise* or scenario* or incident* or event* or plan* or procedure* or protocol* or policy or policies)).tw.	43,159
37	"ESF-8".tw.	5
38	"incident management system*".tw.	113
39	"public health emergency operation*".tw.	6
40	"disaster* operation* center*".tw.	2
41	cooperation/	40,559
42	or/18–41	97,713
43	17 and 42	2,404
44	limit 43 to (english language and yr="2001-Current")	2,141
45	limit 44 to (editorial or letter or note)	156
46	44 not 45	1,985

Scopus:
TITLE-ABS-KEY(((natural W/1 (disaster* or hazard*)) or hurricane* or flood* or typhoon* or earthquake* or fire* or cyclon* or heatwave* or freezing or ((ice or snow or lightning) W/1 storm*) or blizzard* or "heat wave" or (extreme W/1 (temperature* or heat or cold)) or tsunami* or drought* or "tidal wave" or epidemic* or pandemic* or terrorism or bioterrorism or "mass casualt*" or (firesetting or arson or explosion? or bomb* or (explo* W/1 device*) or blackout* or tornado* or brownout* or ((power or equipment) W/1 (loss or failure)) or radioactive or radiation or (nuclear W/1 (disaster or meltdown or catastrophe or fail*)) or (refugee* or "mass migration*" or SARS or ebola or smallpox or plague or measles or riot* or influenza or "communicable disease*" or ((chemical or biological) W/1 warefare) or (civil W/1 (disorder* or defense or unrest)))) AND (("public health" W/1 (practice or administration)) or "preventive medicine" or "health department" or ((public or local or state or tribal or territorial or multi) W/1 health W/1 (department* or agenc* or jurisdiction)))) OR ((emergency W/1 (preparedness or response or management)) or (disaster W/1 (plan* or preparedness or mitigation or recovery or cycle or medicine or resilience or readiness or ready))) AND PUBYEAR AFT 2000
Exclude: Editorials, letters, and notes
Results: **2,813**

Information Sharing

Search Parameters:
Date: 2001–Present
Language: English
Document Type: Exclude commentaries, editorials, letters, and notes
Databases: Medline (Ovid), Embase (Ovid), Scopus

Search Syntax:

Medline (Ovid):

Search No.	Syntax	Results
1	((natural adj (disaster? or hazard?)) or (hurricane? or flood$ or typhoon? or earthquake$ or fire? or cyclon$ or heatwave? or freezing or ((ice or snow or lightning) adj storm?) or blizzard? or "heat wave" or (extreme adj (temperature? or heat or cold)) or tsunami? or "tidal wave")).tw.	75,331
2	("mass migration*" or SARS or ebola or smallpox or plague or measles).tw.	46,567
3	(firesetting or arson or explosion? or bomb$ or outbreak? or refugee* or (explo$ adj device?) or blackout? or brownout? or ((power or equipment) adj (loss or failure)) or radioactive or radiation or (nuclear adj (disaster or meltdown or catastrophe or fail$))).tw.	427,623
4	(((chemical or biological) adj warfare) or riot$ or influenza or flu or (civil adj (disorder? or defense or unrest))).tw.	89,156
5	cyclonic storms/ or droughts/ or floods/ or tidal waves/ or tsunami/ or snow/ or rain/ or avalanches/ or volcanic eruptions/ or earthquakes/ or landslides/ or fires/ or ice/ or tornadoes/ or extreme cold/ or extreme heat/ or lightning/ or cold temperature/ or hot temperature/ or wind/ or firesetting behavior/ or explosions/ or blackout/ or equipment failure/ or radioactive hazard release/ or influenza/ or refugees/ or riots/ or civil disorders/ or civil defense/ or communicable diseases/ or Severe Acute Respiratory Syndrome/ or SARS VIRUS/ or HEMORRHAGIC FEVER, EBOLA/ or MEASLES/ or SMALLPOX/ or PLAGUE/	341,253
6	or/1–5	859,584
7	(("public health" adj (practice or administration or incident* or emergenc*)) or "preventive medicine").tw. or "public health".ti,ab.	171,417
8	public health/ or preventive medicine/ or public health practice/ or public health administration/	101,802
9	"health department*".tw.	8,009
10	((public or local or state or tribal or territorial or multi) adj health adj (department* or agenc*or jurisdiction)).ti,ab.	3,961
11	or/7–10	232,661
12	6 and 11	21,249
13	(epidemic? or pandemic? or terroris$ or bioterroris$ or "mass casualt*").tw.	105,665
14	epidemics/ or pandemics/ or disease outbreaks/ or disasters/ or emergencies/ or mass casualty incidents/ or terrorism/ or bioterrorism/ or chemical terrorism/ or "september 11 terrorist attacks"/	152,746
15	((emergency adj (prepare* or response* or management or incident*)) or (disaster adj (plan$ or prepare* or mitigation or recover* or cycle or medicine or resilienc* or incident* or response* or management* or readiness))).tw.	8,725
16	emergency preparedness/ or emergency response/ or emergency management/ or disaster planning/ or disaster medicine/ or disaster resilience/	15,465
17	or/13–16	230,361
18	12 or 17	241,051
19	Health Personnel/	35,245
20	Medical Staff/ or Public Health Administration/	17,520
21	Emergency Responders/ or Emergency Medical Technicians/	6,006
22	Physicians/ or Pharmacists/ or NURSES/ or Dental Staff/ or Nursing Staff/ or Local Government/ or "Coroners and Medical Examiners"/	156,181
23	(physician* or doctor* or nurse* or responder* or pharmacist* or "health worker*").tw.	671,000
24	"technical audience*".tw.	9
25	"health department*".tw.	8,009

Search No.	Syntax	Results
26	"public health agenc*".tw.	1,750
27	(provider* or "homeless service provider*" or veterinar* or "environmental health provider*").tw.	161,383
28	"Hazardous Materials Response Teams".tw.	1
29	("hazardous material*" adj4 (responder* or team*)).tw.	25
30	clinician*.tw.	162,346
31	(coroner* or "medical examiner*").tw.	4,641
32	((federal or state* or local or tribal or territorial) adj government*).tw.	8,525
33	"private sector".tw.	6,136
34	("first responder*" or "Program for Monitoring Emerging Diseases" or "Top Officials Three Exercise").tw.	1,476
35	or/19–34	1,061,369
36	Emergency Medical Service Communication Systems/	1,725
37	Electronic Mail/	2,469
38	Text Messaging/	2,062
39	Online Systems/ or Internet/ or Social Media/	77,266
40	COMMUNICATION/	77,527
41	Information Systems/ or Health Information Systems/ or "Surveys and Questionnaires"/ or Public Health Informatics/	431,884
42	Telefacsimile/	239
43	Telecommunications/	4,696
44	Computer Communication Networks/	13,375
45	"health alert network*".tw.	8
46	"public health alert*".tw.	30
47	"public health messag*".tw.	655
48	"emergency alert*".tw.	34
49	("joint information" adj (center* or system*)).tw.	2
50	"communication system*".tw.	3,984
51	(warning* or notification* or messag* or dissemination).tw.	117,401
52	((crisis or risk) adj communication*).tw.	1,958
53	"communication channel*".tw.	1,044
54	"community health information exchange".tw.	1
55	(email* or "text messag*" or "conference call*" or "provider access line*" or website* or "guidance document*" or "threshold criteria" or webinar* or webex or webcast* or "new technolog*" or "proprietary technolog*" or "bi directional information" or "data exchange*").tw.	44,575
56	("communication plan*" or "communication protocol*").tw.	474
57	(alert* adj (activation or trigger*)).tw.	53
58	((activation or trigger*) adj alert*).tw.	56
59	telefacsimile.tw.	10
60	or/36–59	724,798

Search No.	Syntax	Results
61	18 and 35 and 60	3,860
62	limit 61 to (english language and yr="2001-Current")	3,055
63	limit 62 to (comment or editorial or letter)	31
64	62 not 63	3,024

Embase (Ovid):

Search No.	Syntax	Results
1	((natural adj (disaster? or hazard?)) or (hurricane? or flood$ or typhoon? or earthquake$ or fire? or cyclon$ or heatwave? or freezing or ((ice or snow or lightning) adj storm?) or blizzard? or "heat wave" or (extreme adj (temperature? or heat or cold)) or tsunami? or "tidal wave")).tw.	106,875
2	("mass migration*" or SARS or ebola or smallpox or plague or measles).tw.	50,215
3	(firesetting or arson or explosion? or bomb$ or outbreak? or refugee* or (explo$ adj device?) or blackout? or brownout? or ((power or equipment) adj (loss or failure)) or radioactive or radiation or (nuclear adj (disaster or meltdown or catastrophe or fail$))).tw.	602,188
4	(((chemical or biological) adj warfare) or riot$ or influenza or flu or (civil adj (disorder? or defense or unrest))).tw.	111,443
5	hurricane/ or drought/ or flooding/ or tsunami/ or snow/ or rain/ or ice/ or avalanche/ or volcano/ or earthquake/ or landslide/ or fire/ or tornado/ or cold/ or heat/ or lightning/ or wind/ or arson/ or explosion/ or device failure/ or nuclear accident/ or civil disorder/ or influenza/ or communicable disease/ or severe acute respiratory syndrome/ or Ebola hemorrhagic fever/ or measles/ or smallpox/ or Smallpox virus/ or plague/ or refugee/	274,496
6	or/1-5	1,010,732
7	(("public health" adj (practice or administration or incident* or emergenc*)) or "preventive medicine").tw. or "public health".ti,ab.	238,311
8	"health department*".tw.	9,525
9	((public or local or state or tribal or territorial or multi) adj health adj (department* or agenc*or jurisdiction)).ti,ab.	4,481
10	public health/ or preventive medicine/ or public health service/	231,842
11	or/7-10	387,664
12	6 and 11	32,828
13	(epidemic? or pandemic? or terroris$ or bioterroris$ or "mass casualt*").tw.	132,027
14	((emergency adj (prepare* or response* or management or incident*)) or (disaster adj (plan$ or prepare* or mitigation or recover* or cycle or medicine or resilienc* or incident* or response* or management* or readiness))).tw.	12,084
15	epidemic/ or pandemic/ or disaster/ or mass disaster/ or nuclear terrorism/ or terrorism/ or chemical terrorism/ or bioterrorism/ or disaster planning/ or disaster planning/ or disaster medicine/	138,280
16	or/13-15	221,710
17	12 or 16	241,171
18	health care personnel/	140,648
19	medical staff/	33,299
20	public health service/	60,866
21	rescue personnel/	7,179
22	physician assistant/ or emergency physician/ or hospital physician/ or physician/	273,932

Search No.	Syntax	Results
23	pharmacist/	68,847
24	nurse/	108,515
25	dentist/	21,686
26	coroner/	2,341
27	(physician* or doctor* or nurse* or responder* or pharmacist* or "health worker*").tw.	1,004,960
28	"technical audience*".tw.	18
29	"health department*".tw.	9,525
30	"public health agenc*".tw.	2,263
31	(provider* or "homeless service provider*" or veterinar* or "environmental health provider*").tw.	250,619
32	"Hazardous Materials Response Teams".tw.	1
33	("hazardous material*" adj4 (responder* or team*)).tw.	30
34	clinician*.tw.	270,866
35	(coroner* or "medical examiner*").tw.	5,765
36	((federal or state* or local or tribal or territorial) adj government*).tw.	11,742
37	"private sector".tw.	8,311
38	("first responder*" or "Program for Monitoring Emerging Diseases" or "Top Officials Three Exercise").tw.	2,370
39	or/18–38	1,726,738
40	e-mail/	17,690
41	mobile phone/ or text messaging/ or reminder system/	19,052
42	Internet/	100,103
43	online system/	23,460
44	data base/	229,820
45	social media/	13,229
46	information system/	35,460
47	fax/	718
48	telecommunication/	22,813
49	computer network/	13,665
50	"health alert network*".tw.	10
51	"public health alert*".tw.	45
52	"public health messag*".tw.	947
53	"emergency alert*".tw.	56
54	("joint information" adj (center* or system*)).tw.	7
55	"communication system*".tw.	5,606
56	(warning* or notification* or messag* or dissemination).tw.	175,676
57	((crisis or risk) adj communication*).tw.	2,765
58	"communication channel*".tw.	1,535

Search No.	Syntax	Results
59	"community health information exchange".tw.	2
60	(email* or "text messag*" or "conference call*" or "provider access line*" or website* or "guidance document*" or "threshold criteria" or webinar* or webex or webcast* or "new technolog*" or "proprietary technolog*" or "bi directional information" or "data exchange*").tw.	85,158
61	("communication plan*" or "communication protocol*").tw.	818
62	(alert* adj (activation or trigger*)).tw.	130
63	((activation or trigger*) adj alert*).tw.	114
64	telefacsimile.tw.	10
65	or/40–64	659,896
66	17 and 39 and 65	3,673
67	limit 66 to (english language and yr="2001-Current")	3,230
68	limit 67 to (editorial or letter or note)	186
69	67 not 68	3,044

Scopus:
TITLE-ABS-KEY(((natural W/1 (disaster* or hazard*)) or hurricane* or flood* or typhoon* or earthquake* or fire* or cyclon* or heatwave* or freezing or ((ice or snow or lightning) W/1 storm*) or blizzard* or "heat wave" or (extreme W/1 (temperature* or heat or cold)) or tsunami* or drought* or "tidal wave" or epidemic* or pandemic* or terrorism or bioterrorism or "mass casualt*" or (firesetting or arson or explosion? or bomb* or (explo* W/1 device*) or blackout* or tornado* or brownout* or ((power or equipment) W/1 (loss or failure)) or radioactive or radiation or (nuclear W/1 (disaster or meltdown or catastrophe or fail*)) or (refugee* or "mass migration*" or SARS or ebola or smallpox or plague or measles or riot* or influenza or "communicable disease*" or ((chemical or biological) W/1 warefare) or (civil W/1 (disorder* or defense or unrest)))) AND (("public health" W/1 (practice or administration)) or "preventive medicine" or "health department" or ((public or local or state or tribal or territorial or multi) W/1 health W/1 (department* or agenc* or jurisdiction)))) OR ((emergency W/1 (preparedness or response or management)) or (disaster W/1 (plan* or preparedness or mitigation or recovery or cycle or medicine or resilience or readiness or ready))) AND (physician* or doctor* or nurse* or responder* or pharmacist* or "health worker*" or "technical audience*" or "health department*" or "public health agenc*" or provider* or "homeless service provider*" or veterinarian* or "environmental health provider*" or "Hazardous Materials Response Teams" or ("hazardous material*" W/4 (responder* or team*)) or clinician* or coroner* or "medical examiner*" or ((federal or state* or local or tribal or territorial) W/1 government*) or "private sector" or "first responder*" or "Program for Monitoring Emerging Diseases" or "Top Officials Three Exercise") AND ("health alert network*" or "public health alert*" or "public health messag*" or "emergency alert*" or ("joint information" W/1 (center* or system*)) or "communication system*" or warning* or notification* or "community health information exchange" or messag* or dissemination or ((crisis or risk) W/1 communication*) or "communication channel*" or email* or "text messag*" or "conference call*" or "provider access line*" or website* or "guidance document*" or "threshold criteria" or webinar* or webex or webcast* or "new technolog*" or "proprietary technolog*" or "bi directional information" or "data exchange*" or "communication plan*" or "communication protocol*" or (alert* W/1 (activation or trigger*)) or ((activation or trigger*) W/1 alert*) or telefacsimile)) AND PUBYEAR > 2000

Exclude: Editorials, letters, and notes
Results: **1,198**

Non-Pharmaceutical Interventions: Quarantine

Search Parameters:
Date: 2001–Present
Language: English
Document Type: Exclude commentaries, editorials, letters, and notes
Databases: Medline (Ovid), Embase (Ovid), Scopus

Search Syntax:

Medline (Ovid):

Search No.	Syntax	Results
1	((natural adj (disaster? or hazard?)) or (hurricane? or flood$ or typhoon? or earthquake$ or fire? or cyclon$ or heatwave? or freezing or ((ice or snow or lightning) adj storm?) or blizzard? or "heat wave" or (extreme adj (temperature? or heat or cold)) or tsunami? or "tidal wave")).tw.	75,331
2	("mass migration*" or SARS or ebola or smallpox or plague or measles).tw.	46,567
3	(firesetting or arson or explosion? or bomb$ or outbreak? or refugee* or (explo$ adj device?) or blackout? or brownout? or ((power or equipment) adj (loss or failure)) or radioactive or radiation or (nuclear adj (disaster or meltdown or catastrophe or fail$))).tw.	427,623
4	(((chemical or biological) adj warfare) or riot$ or influenza or flu or (civil adj (disorder? or defense or unrest))).tw.	89,156
5	cyclonic storms/ or droughts/ or floods/ or tidal waves/ or tsunami/ or snow/ or rain/ or avalanches/ or volcanic eruptions/ or earthquakes/ or landslides/ or fires/ or ice/ or tornadoes/ or extreme cold/ or extreme heat/ or lightning/ or cold temperature/ or hot temperature/ or wind/ or firesetting behavior/ or explosions/ or blackout/ or equipment failure/ or radioactive hazard release/ or influenza/ or refugees/ or riots/ or civil disorders/ or civil defense/ or communicable diseases/ or Severe Acute Respiratory Syndrome/ or SARS VIRUS/ or HEMORRHAGIC FEVER, EBOLA/ or MEASLES/ or SMALLPOX/ or PLAGUE/	341,253
6	or/1–5	859,584
7	(("public health" adj (practice or administration or incident* or emergenc*)) or "preventive medicine").tw. or "public health".ti,ab.	171,417
8	public health/ or preventive medicine/ or public health practice/ or public health administration/	101,802
9	"health department*".tw.	8,009
10	((public or local or state or tribal or territorial or multi) adj health adj (department* or agenc*or jurisdiction)).ti,ab.	3,961
11	or/7–10	232,661
12	6 and 11	21,249
13	(epidemic? or pandemic? or terroris$ or bioterroris$ or "mass casualt*").tw.	105,665
14	epidemics/ or pandemics/ or disease outbreaks/ or disasters/ or emergencies/ or mass casualty incidents/ or terrorism/ or bioterrorism/ or chemical terrorism/ or "september 11 terrorist attacks"/	152,746
15	((emergency adj (prepare* or response* or management or incident*)) or (disaster adj (plan$ or prepare* or mitigation or recover* or cycle or medicine or resilienc* or incident* or response* or management* or readiness))).tw.	8,725

Search No.	Syntax	Results
16	emergency preparedness/ or emergency response/ or emergency management/ or disaster planning/ or disaster medicine/ or disaster resilience/	15,465
17	or/13–16	230,361
18	12 or 17	241,051
19	"nonpharmaceutical intervention*".tw.	78
20	QUARANTINE/	2,031
21	Social Distance/	2,465
22	(quarantine* or "social distanc*").tw.	4,091
23	"self isolation".tw.	56
24	"voluntary quarantine*".tw.	6
25	"involuntary quarantine*".tw.	2
26	"home quarantine*".tw.	21
27	"hospital quarantine*".tw.	3
28	((adherence or compliance) adj4 (quarantine* or "control measure*")).tw.	176
29	"restricted movement*".tw.	316
30	(separation adj4 expose*).tw.	107
31	or/19–30	7,962
32	18 and 31	1,589
33	32	1,589
34	limit 33 to (english language and yr="2001-Current")	1,167
35	limit 34 to (comment or editorial or letter)	48
36	34 not 35	1,119

Embase (Ovid):

Search No.	Syntax	Results
1	((natural adj (disaster? or hazard?)) or (hurricane? or flood$ or typhoon? or earthquake$ or fire? or cyclon$ or heatwave? or freezing or ((ice or snow or lightning) adj storm?) or blizzard? or "heat wave" or (extreme adj (temperature? or heat or cold)) or tsunami? or "tidal wave")).tw.	106,875
2	("mass migration*" or SARS or ebola or smallpox or plague or measles).tw.	50,215
3	(firesetting or arson or explosion? or bomb$ or outbreak? or refugee* or (explo$ adj device?) or blackout? or brownout? or ((power or equipment) adj (loss or failure)) or radioactive or radiation or (nuclear adj (disaster or meltdown or catastrophe or fail$))).tw.	602,188
4	(((chemical or biological) adj warfare) or riot$ or influenza or flu or (civil adj (disorder? or defense or unrest))).tw.	111,443
5	hurricane/ or drought/ or flooding/ or tsunami/ or snow/ or rain/ or ice/ or avalanche/ or volcano/ or earthquake/ or landslide/ or fire/ or tornado/ or cold/ or heat/ or lightning/ or wind/ or arson/ or explosion/ or device failure/ or nuclear accident/ or civil disorder/ or influenza/ or communicable disease/ or severe acute respiratory syndrome/ or Ebola hemorrhagic fever/ or measles/ or smallpox/ or Smallpox virus/ or plague/ or refugee/	274,496
6	or/1–5	1,010,732
7	(("public health" adj (practice or administration or incident* or emergenc*)) or "preventive medicine").tw. or "public health".ti,ab.	238,311

Search No.	Syntax	Results
8	"health department*".tw.	9,525
9	((public or local or state or tribal or territorial or multi) adj health adj (department* or agenc*or jurisdiction)).ti,ab.	4,481
10	public health/ or preventive medicine/ or public health service/	231,842
11	or/7–10	387,664
12	6 and 11	32,828
13	(epidemic? or pandemic? or terroris$ or bioterroris$ or "mass casualt*").tw.	132,027
14	((emergency adj (prepare* or response* or management or incident*)) or (disaster adj (plan$ or prepare* or mitigation or recover* or cycle or medicine or resilienc* or incident* or response* or management* or readiness))).tw.	12,084
15	epidemic/ or pandemic/ or disaster/ or mass disaster/ or nuclear terrorism/ or terrorism/ or chemical terrorism/ or bioterrorism/ or disaster planning/ or disaster planning/ or disaster medicine/	138,280
16	or/13–15	221,710
17	12 or 16	241,171
18	"nonpharmaceutical intervention*".tw.	111
19	quarantine/	431
20	social distance/	2,047
21	(quarantine* or "social distanc*").tw.	5,139
22	"self isolation".tw.	82
23	"voluntary quarantine*".tw.	6
24	"involuntary quarantine*".tw.	3
25	"home quarantine*".tw.	25
26	"hospital quarantine*".tw.	6
27	((adherence or compliance) adj4 (quarantine* or "control measure*")).tw.	247
28	"restricted movement*".tw.	501
29	(separation adj4 expose*).tw.	168
30	or/18–29	7,740
31	17 and 30	1,441
32	limit 31 to (english language and yr="2001-Current")	1,165
33	limit 32 to (editorial or letter or note)	49
34	32 not 33	1,116

Scopus:
TITLE-ABS-KEY(((natural W/1 (disaster* or hazard*)) or hurricane* or flood* or typhoon* or earthquake* or fire* or cyclon* or heatwave* or freezing or ((ice or snow or lightning) W/1 storm*) or blizzard* or "heat wave" or (extreme W/1 (temperature* or heat or cold)) or tsunami* or drought* or "tidal wave" or epidemic* or pandemic* or terrorism or bioterrorism or "mass casualt*" or (firesetting or arson or explosion? or bomb* or (explo* W/1 device*) or blackout* or tornado* or brownout* or ((power or equipment) W/1 (loss or failure)) or radioactive or radiation or (nuclear W/1 (disaster or meltdown or catastrophe or fail*)) or (refugee* or "mass migration*" or SARS or ebola or smallpox or plague or measles or riot* or influenza or "communicable disease*" or ((chemical or biological) W/1 warefare) or (civil

W/1 (disorder* or defense or unrest)))) AND (("public health" W/1 (practice or administration)) or "preventive medicine" or "health department" or ((public or local or state or tribal or territorial or multi) W/1 health W/1 (department* or agenc* or jurisdiction)))) OR ((emergency W/1 (preparedness or response or management)) or (disaster W/1 (plan* or preparedness or mitigation or recovery or cycle or medicine or resilience or readiness or ready))) AND ("nonpharmaceutical intervention*" or "non-pharmaceutical intervention*" or quarantine* or "social distance*" or "self isolation*" or "voluntary quarantine*" or "involuntary quarantine*" or "home quarantine*" or "hospital quarantine*" or ((adherence or compliance) W/4 (quarantine* or "control measure*")) or "restricted movement*" or (separation W/4 expos*)))
AND PUBYEAR AFT 2000
Exclude: Editorials, letters, and notes
Results: **245**

REFERENCES

Abramson, D. M., S. S. Morse, A. L. Garrett, and I. Redlener. 2007. Public health disaster research: Surveying the field, defining its future. *Disaster Medicine and Public Health Preparedness* 1(1):57–62.

Acosta, J. D., C. Nelson, E. B. Beckjord, S. R. Shelton, E. Murphy, K. L. Leuschner, and J. Wasserman. 2009. *A national agenda for public health systems research on emergency preparedness.* Santa Monica, CA: RAND Health.

Barnett-Page, E., and J. Thomas. 2009. Methods for the synthesis of qualitative research: A critical review. *BMC Medical Research Methodology* 9(1):59.

Bennett, C., S. Khangura, J. C. Brehaut, I. D. Graham, D. Moher, B. K. Potter, and J. M. Grimshaw. 2010. Reporting guidelines for survey research: An analysis of published guidance and reporting practices. *PLOS Medicine* 8(8):e1001069.

Briss, P. A., S. Zaza, M. Pappaioanou, J. Fielding, L. K. Wright-De Aguero, B. I. Truman, D. P. Hopkins, P. Dolan Mullen, R. S. Thompson, S. H. Woolf, V. G. Carande-Kulis, L. Andersin, A. R. Hinman, D. V. McQueen, S. M. Teutsch, J. R. Harris, and The Task Force on Community Preventive Services. 2000. Developing an evidence-based guide to community preventive services—Methods. *American Journal of Preventive Medicine* 18(1S):35–43.

Butler, M., R. A. Epstein, A. Totten, E. P. Whitlock, M. T. Ansari, L. J. Damschroder, E. Balk, E. B. Bass, N. D. Berkman, S. Hempel, S. Iyer, K. Schoelles, and J.-M. Guise. 2017. AHRQ series on complex intervention systematic reviews—Paper 3: Adapting frameworks to develop protocols. *Journal of Clinical Epidemiology* 90:19–27.

Carbone, E. G. 2018 (unpublished). *Charge to committee: CDC talking points.* Atlanta, GA: Centers for Disease Control and Prevention.

CASP (Critical Appraisal Skills Programme). 2018. *CASP qualitative checklist.* http://casp-uk.net/casp-tools-checklists (accessed July 2, 2019).

CDC (Centers for Disease Control and Prevention). 2016. *Assessment of the public health preparedness capabilities: National standards for state and local planning final report.* Atlanta, GA: Centers for Disease Control and Prevention. https://www.cdc.gov/cpr/readiness/00_docs/PHEP-Final-Report_508_9_20_16.pdf (accessed March 26, 2020).

CDC. 2018. *Public health emergency preparedness and response capabilities: National standards for state, local, tribal, and territorial public health.* Atlanta, GA: Centers for Disease Control and Prevention. https://www.cdc.gov/cpr/readiness/00_docs/CDC_PreparednesResponseCapabilities_OctOcto2018_Final_508.pdf (accessed March 26, 2020).

Center for Public Health Systems and Services Research. 2018. *National health security preparedness index 2018 realease summary of key findings.* Lexington, KY: Center for Public Health Systems and Services Research. https://nhspi.org/wp-content/uploads/2018/04/2018-Key-Findings.pdf (accessed March 26, 2020).

Challen, K., A. C. Lee, A. Booth, P. Gardois, H. B. Woods, and S. W. Goodacre. 2012. Where is the evidence for emergency planning? A scoping review. *BMC Public Health* 12(542).

Cochrane. 2017. *Suggested risk of bias criteria for EPOC reviews.* https://epoc.cochrane.org/sites/epoc.cochrane.org/files/public/uploads/Resources-for-authors2017/suggested_risk_of_bias_criteria_for_epoc_reviews.pdf (accessed April 20, 2020).

Davids, E. L., and N. V. Roman. 2014. A systematic review of the relationship between parenting styles and children's physical activity. *African Journal for Physical, Health Education, Recreation and Dance* 228–246.

ECDC (European Centre for Disease Prevention and Control). 2018. *Best practice recommendations for conducting after-action reviews to enhance public health preparedness.* Solna, Sweden. https://www.ecdc.europa.eu/sites/default/files/documents/public-health-preparedness-best-practice-recommendations.pdf (accessed March 26, 2020).

Higgins, J. P. T., J. Savovic, M. J. Page, J. Sterne, and ROB2 Development Group. 2019. *Revised Cochrane risk-of-bias tool for randomized trials (ROB2).* https://sites.google.com/site/riskofbiastool/welcome/rob-2-0-tool/current-version-of-rob-2 (accessed March 26, 2020).

Horney, J. A., E. G. Carbone, M. Lynch, Z. J. Wang, T. Jones, and D. A. Rose. 2017. How health department contextual factors affect public health preparedness (PHP) and perceptions of the 15 PHP Capabilities. *American Journal of Public Health* 107(S2):S153–S160.

Khan, Y., G. Fazli, B. Henry, E. de Villa, C. Tsamis, M. Grant, and B. Schwartz. 2015. The evidence base of primary research in public health emergency preparedness: A scoping review and stakeholder consultation. *BMC Public Health* 15(432).

Lewin, S., A. Booth, C. Glenton, H. Munthe-Kaas, A. Rashidian, M. Wainwright, M. A. Bohren, O. Tuncalp, C. J. Colvin, R. Garside, B. Carlsen, E. V. Langlois, and J. Noyes. 2018. Applying GRADE-CERQual to qualitative evidence synthesis findings: Introduction to the series. *Implementation Science* 13(Suppl 1):2.

Murthy, B. P., N. M. Molinari, T. T. LeBlanc, S. J. Vagi, and R. N. Avchen. 2017. Progress in public health emergency preparedness: United States, 2001–2016. *American Journal of Public Health* 107(S2):S180–S185.

Pope, C., S. Ziebland, and N. Mays. 2000. Qualitative research in health care: Analysing qualitative data. *BMJ (Clinical Research)* 320(7227):114–116.

Savoia, E., L. Lin, D. Bernard, N. Klein, L. P. James, and S. Guicciardi. 2017. Public health system research in public health emergency preparedness in the United States (2009–2015): Actionable knowledge base. *American Journal of Public Health* 107(S2):e1–e6.

Shekelle, P. 2004. The appropriateness method. *Medical Decision Making* 24(2):228–231.

Siegfried, A. L., E. G. Carbone, M. B. Meit, M. J. Kennedy, H. Yusuf, and E. B. Kahn. 2017. Identifying and prioritizing information needs and research priorities of public health emergency preparedness and response practitioners. *Disaster Medicine and Public Health Preparedness* 11(5):552–561.

Sloss, E. M., D. H. Solomon, P. G. Shekelle, R. T. Young, D. Saliba, C. H. MacLean, L. Z. Rubenstein, J. F. Schnelle, C. J. Kamberg, and N. S. Wenger. 2000. Selecting target conditions for quality of care improvement in vulnerable older adults. *Journal of the American Geriatrics Society* 48(4):363–369.

Sterne, J. A., M. A. Hernan, B. C. Reeves, J. Savovic, N. D. Berkman, M. Viswanathan, D. Henry, D. G. Altman, M. T. Ansari, I. Boutron, J. R. Carpenter, A. W. Chan, R. Churchill, J. J. Deeks, A. Hrobjartsson, J. Kirkham, P. Juni, Y. K. Loke, T. D. Pigott, C. R. Ramsay, D. Regidor, H. R. Rothstein, L. Sandhu, P. L. Santaguida, H. J. Schunemann, B. Shea, I. Shrier, P. Tugwell, L. Turner, J. C. Valentine, H. Waddington, E. Waters, G. A. Wells, P. F. Whiting, and J. P. Higgins. 2016. ROBINS-I: A tool for assessing risk of bias in non-randomised studies of interventions. *BMJ* 355:i4919.

USPSTF (U.S. Preventive Services Task Force). 2015. *U.S. Preventive Services Task Force procedure manual.* https://www.uspreventiveservicestaskforce.org/Page/Name/procedure-manual (accessed March 4, 2020).

Yeager, V. A., N. Menachemi, L. C. McCormick, and P. M. Ginter. 2010. The nature of the public health emergency preparedness literature 2000–2008: A quantitative analysis. *Journal of Public Health Management and Practice* 16(5):441–449.

Zaza, S., R. S. Lawrence, C. S. Mahan, M. Fullilove, D. Fleming, G. J. Isham, and M. Pappaioanou. 2000. Scope and organization of the Guide to Community Preventive Services: The task force on community preventive services. *American Journal of Preventive Medicine* 18(1 Suppl):27–34.

B Mixed-Method Reviews of Selected Topics

INTRODUCTION TO THE MIXED-METHOD REVIEWS

This appendix details the mixed-method review process and evidence for each of the four review topics. Each review followed a similar process (see Chapter 3 and Appendix A), which was conducted by the committee, National Academies staff, and several commissioned groups. This appendix is broken down into four parts, describing the mixed-method reviews for the four following topic areas:

- engaging with and training community-based partners to improve the outcomes of at-risk populations after public health emergencies (Capability 1, Community Preparedness);
- activating a public health emergency operations center (Capability 3, Emergency Operations Coordination);
- communicating public health alerts and guidance with technical audiences during a public health emergency (Capability 6, Information Sharing); and
- implementing quarantine to reduce or stop the spread of a contagious disease (Capability 11, Non-Pharmaceutical Interventions).

B1 Mixed-Method Review of Strategies for Engaging with and Training Community-Based Partners to Improve the Outcomes of At-Risk Populations

This appendix provides a detailed description of the methods for and the evidence from the mixed-method review examining strategies for engaging with and training community-based partners (CBPs) to improve the outcomes of at-risk populations, which is summarized in Chapter 4.[1]

KEY REVIEW QUESTIONS AND ANALYTIC FRAMEWORK

The overarching question that guided this review addresses the effectiveness of different strategies for engaging with and training CBPs to improve the outcomes of at-risk populations after public health emergencies. Engaging with CBPs to meet the needs of at-risk populations may take place in the preparedness, response, and recovery phases of the emergency cycle. Recovery practices were outside the committee's scope of work, but separate key review sub-questions were formulated for the preparedness and response phases. The committee also posed sub-questions related to documented benefits and harms of CBP engagement and training strategies and the factors that create barriers to and facilitators of the implementation of such strategies (see Box B1-1).

The theory behind this public health emergency preparedness and response (PHEPR) practice is that when public health agencies adequately engage with and train CBPs who have established relationships with and/or serve at-risk populations on preparedness and response knowledge and concepts, the result is an increased capacity to reach at-risk populations before and during a public health emergency and the potential to reduce disaster-associated morbidity and mortality and ameliorate health disparities for those populations.

[1] This appendix draws heavily on three reports commissioned by the committee: (1) "Data Extraction and Quality Assessment: Methodology and Evidence Tables" by the Brown University Center for Evidence Synthesis in Health; "Engaging with and Training Community-Based Partners for Public Health Emergencies: Qualitative Research Evidence Synthesis" by Julie Novak and Pradeep Sopory; and "Engaging with and Training Community-Based Partners to Improve the Outcomes of At-Risk Populations After Public Health Emergencies: Findings from Case Reports" by Sneha Patel (see Appendix C).

BOX B1-1 KEY REVIEW QUESTIONS

What is the effectiveness of different strategies for engaging with and training community-based partners (CBPs) to improve the outcomes of at-risk populations after public health emergencies?

- What is the effectiveness of strategies for engaging with and training CBPs before a public health emergency?
- What is the effectiveness of strategies for engaging with and leveraging existing CBPs during a public health emergency?
- What benefits and harms (desirable and/or undesirable impacts) of different strategies for engaging with and training CBPs have been described or measured?
- What are the barriers to and facilitators of effective engagement and training of CBPs?

Engaging with and training CBPs may improve the outcomes of at-risk populations following a public health emergency through a number of presumed pathways (see the analytic framework in Figure B1-1). Such pathways generally focus on ensuring at-risk individuals' postdisaster access to critical services and/or resources (e.g., food, medication, information). CBP intermediaries may provide such services and resources directly or may assist public health agencies (or other emergency responders) in reaching at-risk populations to deliver these services and resources before or after an emergency. CBPs also can be well positioned to help ensure the cultural appropriateness of preparedness and response materials, services, and training so that they are functionally accessible (e.g., available in different languages for non-English-speaking individuals) and likely to be well received.

EVIDENCE SUPPORTING THE PRACTICE RECOMMENDATION

This section summarizes the evidence from the mixed-method review examining strategies for engaging with and training CBPs to improve the outcomes of at-risk populations. It begins with a description of the results of the literature search and then summarizes the evidence of effectiveness. In formulating its practice recommendation, the committee considered evidence beyond effectiveness, which was compiled using an Evidence to Decision (EtD) framework encompassing balance of benefits and harms, acceptability and preferences, feasibility and PHEPR system considerations, resource and economic considerations, equity, and ethical considerations. The evidence from each methodological stream applicable to each of the EtD criteria is discussed; a synthesis is provided in Table B1-10 later in this appendix and in Chapter 4. Graded finding statements from evidence syntheses are italicized in the narrative below.

Full details about the study eligibility criteria, search strategy, and processes for data extraction and individual study quality assessment are available in Appendix A. Appendix C links to all of the commissioned analyses informing this review.

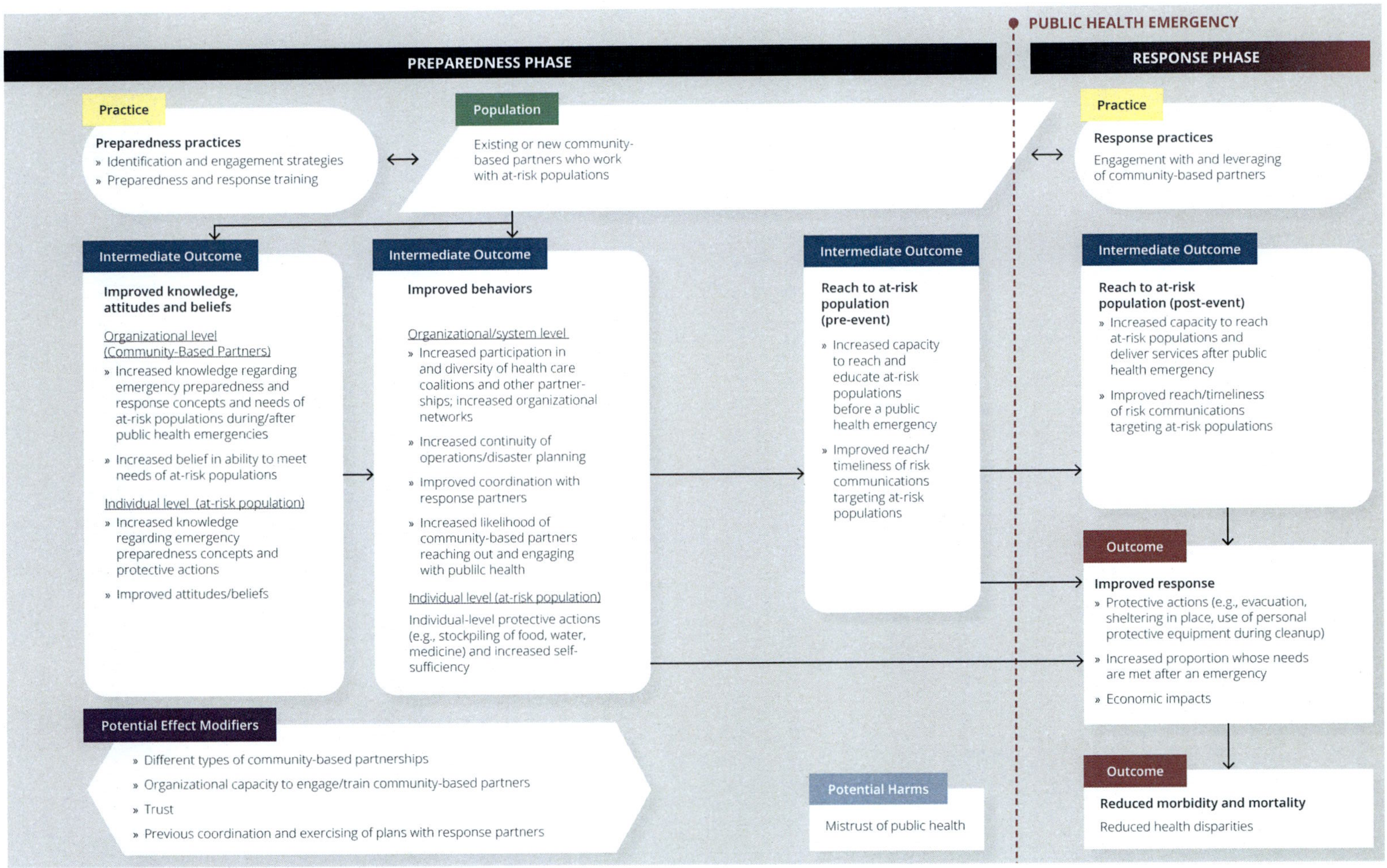

FIGURE B1-1 Analytic framework for engaging with and training community-based partners to improve the outcomes of at-risk populations.
NOTES: Arrows in the framework indicate hypothesized causal pathways between interventions and outcomes. Double-headed arrows indicate feedback loops.

Results of the Literature Search

The searches of bibliographic databases identified a total of 8,395 potentially relevant citations (deduplicated) for the mixed-method review of strategies for engaging with and training CBPs to improve the outcomes of at-risk populations. A search of the gray literature, reference mining, and a call for reports contributed an additional 269 articles. All 8,664 citations were imported into EndNote and were included in title and abstract screening. During screening, 8,548 articles were excluded because their abstracts did not appear to answer any of the key questions or they indicated that the articles were commentaries, editorials, or opinion pieces. After the abstracts had been reviewed, 116 full-text articles were reviewed and assessed for eligibility for inclusion in the mixed-method review. The committee considered 64 articles for data extraction and ultimately included 55 articles in the mixed-method review. Figure B1-2 depicts the literature flow, indicating the number of articles included and excluded at each screening stage. Table B1-1 indicates the types of evidence included in this review.

A separate targeted search was conducted to identify relevant systematic reviews of the effectiveness of community engagement strategies and cultural tailoring of interventions from outside the PHEPR context. This search was conducted in Google Scholar, PubMed, the Office of Minority Health Knowledge Center, and the U.S. Department of Health and Human Services' Think Cultural Health Resource Library. This parallel evidence (as described in Chapter 3) was considered in determining the certainty of the evidence (COE) for strategies for engaging with and training CBPs to improve the outcomes of at-risk populations. The search was limited to systematic reviews published in the past 5 years (2015–2019). Reviews of interventions implemented only in low- and middle-income countries were excluded. Search terms included systematic, meta-analysis, community engagement, community partner, vulnerable, minority, marginalized, indigenous groups, disabilities, community intervention, intervention review, intervention evaluation, cultural tailoring, cultural targeting, community engagement, and cultural competency. Additionally, the seminal report *Principles of Community Engagement* (NIH et al., 2011) was reference mined. The targeted search yielded 13 systematic reviews that the committee considered.

1. Determining Evidence of Effect

Seven quantitative comparative and four quantitative noncomparative studies directly addressed the overarching key question regarding the effectiveness of different strategies for engaging with and training CBPs to improve the outcomes of at-risk populations after public health emergencies. All 11 studies examined strategies for engaging with or training CBPs *before* a public health emergency (preparedness phase). The committee found no quantitative research studies addressing the key question regarding the effectiveness of strategies for engaging with and leveraging existing CBPs *during* a public health emergency (response phase). Ten of these 11 studies evaluated strategies that involve both engaging and training CBPs.

Strategies identified by the committee in the body of evidence fall into two broad categories: (1) those aimed at training and/or engaging individual CBPs, with a goal of reaching particular at-risk populations (training programs may be targeted solely to CBPs or to both CBPs and members of the at-risk populations they serve); and (2) those aimed at engaging multiple CBPs in a coalition or other multistakeholder partnership. From these two categories, three strategies for training and/or engaging CBPs were identified and evaluated separately:

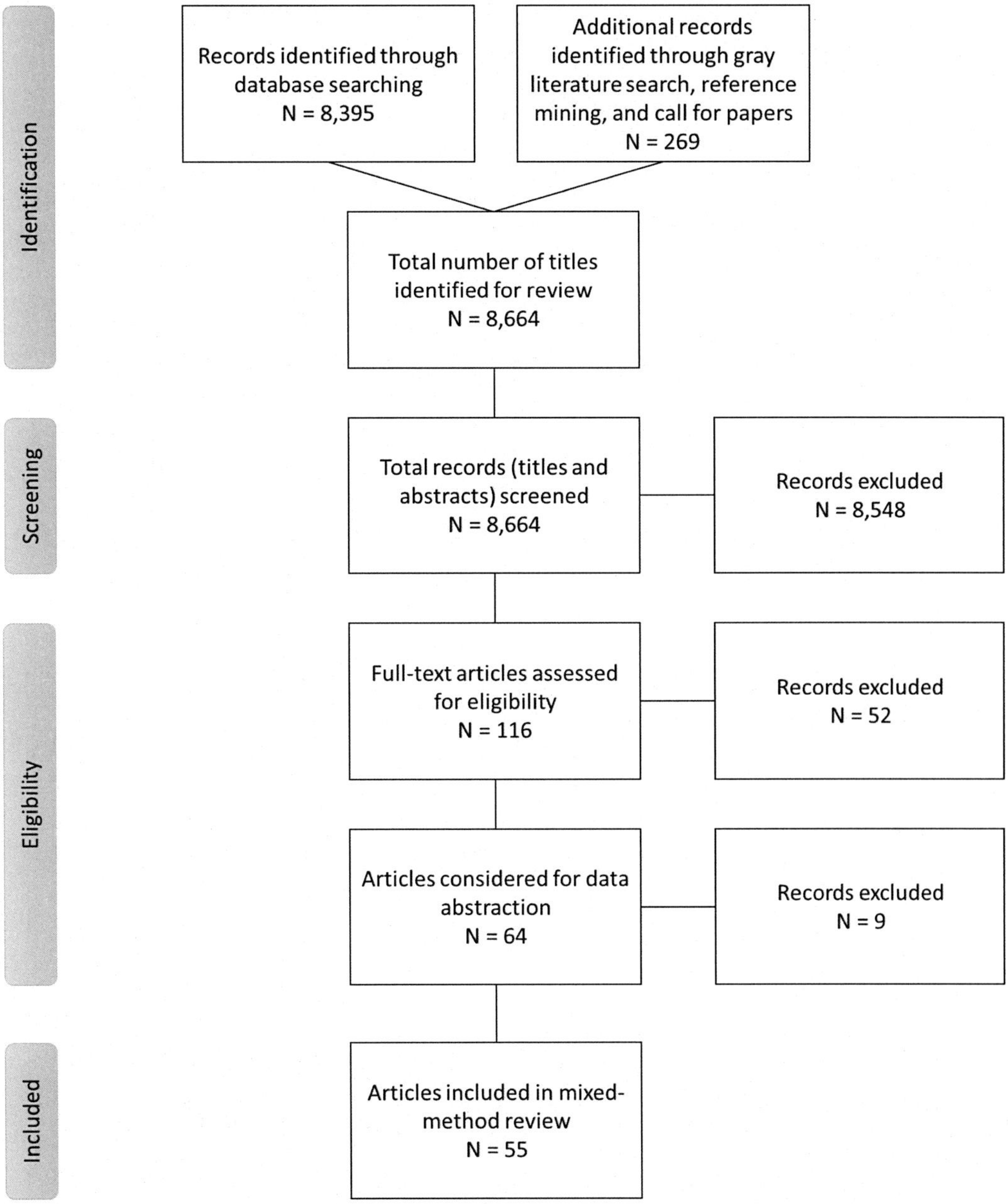

FIGURE B1-2 Preferred Reporting Items for Systematic Reviews and Meta-Analyses diagram for the mixed-method review of strategies for engaging with and training community-based partners to improve the outcomes of at-risk populations.

TABLE B1-1 Evidence Types Included in the Mixed-Method Review of Strategies for Engaging with and Training Community-Based Partners to Improve the Outcomes of At-Risk Populations

Evidence Type[a]	Number of Studies (as applicable)[b]
Quantitative comparative	7
Quantitative noncomparative (postintervention measure only)[c]	4
Qualitative	23
Modeling	0
Descriptive surveys	7
Case reports	15[d]
After action reports	N/A
Mechanistic	N/A
Parallel (systematic reviews)[e]	13

[a] Evidence types are defined in Chapter 3.
[b] Note that sibling articles (different results from the same study published in separate articles) are counted as one study in this table. Mixed-method studies may be counted in more than one category.
[c] Quantitative noncomparative studies were considered separately for the purpose of evaluating evidence of effect but were included in the case report evidence synthesis (or qualitative evidence synthesis in the case of mixed-method studies) to identify themes relevant to the Evidence to Decision (EtD) framework.
[d] A sample of case reports was prioritized for inclusion in this review based on relevance to the key questions, as described in Chapter 3.
[e] Parallel evidence for the purposes of this review was derived from existing systematic reviews of similar practices from outside the PHEPR context.

- implementation of culturally tailored preparedness[2] training programs for CBPs and at-risk populations they serve,
- engagement of CBPs in preparedness outreach activities targeting at-risk populations, and
- engagement and training of CBPs in coalitions addressing public health preparedness/resilience.

A meta-analysis of the evidence for the effectiveness of these strategies was not feasible, so the committee conducted a synthesis without meta-analysis (as described in Chapter 3). Consistent with the methods described in Chapter 3, in making its final judgment on the evidence of effectiveness for strategies for engaging with and training CBPs to improve the outcomes of at-risk populations, the committee considered other types of evidence that could inform a determination of what works for whom and in which contexts, ultimately reaching consensus on the COE for each outcome. Including forms of evidence beyond quantitative comparative studies is particularly important when assessing evidence in settings where controlled studies are challenging to conduct and/or other forms of quantitative comparative data are difficult to obtain. As discussed in Chapter 3, descriptive evidence from real-world implementation of practices offers the potential to corroborate research findings or explain differences in outcomes in practice settings, even if it has lesser value for causal inference. Moreover, qualitative studies can complement quantitative studies by providing additional useful evidence to guide real-world decision making, because well-conducted qualitative studies produce deep and rich understandings of how interven-

[2] The committee uses the term "culturally tailored" to describe an intervention that is targeted and/or tailored to ensure that it meets the unique needs of the target group by incorporating their experiences and norms and values.

tions are implemented, delivered, and experienced. Other forms of evidence considered for evaluation of effectiveness included quantitative data reported in case reports of real disasters or public health emergencies, and parallel evidence from systematic reviews on community engagement and cultural tailoring of interventions outside the PHEPR context. The parallel evidence was considered recognizing that the engagement and training of CBPs to better reach and improve outcomes for individuals with social vulnerabilities has much broader application in public health beyond the PHEPR context, and the committee believes this broader body of evidence may have some applicability to the PHEPR practices evaluated in this review.

Implementation of Culturally Tailored Preparedness Training Programs for CBPs and At-Risk Populations They Serve

Evidence from quantitative research studies Five quantitative comparative studies examined the effects of culturally tailored preparedness training programs for CBPs and at-risk populations they serve. Three of these studies employed a train-the-trainer approach whereby CBP representatives were trained in emergency preparedness concepts and skills and subsequently trained at-risk populations. Outcomes of interest reported by the authors include PHEPR knowledge of CBP representatives, attitudes and beliefs of CBP representatives regarding their preparedness to meet needs of at-risk individuals, and CBP disaster planning. Additionally, for studies in which training programs also targeted at-risk populations, outcomes of interest include knowledge of trained at-risk populations regarding PHEPR and protective actions, attitudes and beliefs of at-risk populations regarding their preparedness, and preparedness behaviors of at-risk populations.

A community-based randomized controlled trial (RCT) conducted by Eisenman and colleagues (2009) evaluated the effect on household disaster preparedness of participation in a program with *promotoras* (community health workers), who, after being trained in disaster preparedness, held face-to-face discussions about disaster preparedness with low-income Latino participants in Los Angeles County, California (Platica group). The media control group received culturally tailored mailings with preparedness information. Among participants who did not have disaster preparedness plans at baseline, household preparedness had significantly increased in both groups 3 months after the intervention, but those in the Platica group (N = 87) were more likely to increase household preparedness as measured by having a communication plan ($p = 0.002$) and a supply of numerous specific household preparedness items, including food ($p = 0.013$) and water ($p = 0.003$), relative to those in the media control group (N = 100). However, there were some concerns about the potential for social desirability bias and the generalizability of the study. Overall, the study (and each outcome) was deemed to be of moderate methodological quality.

Eisenman and colleagues (2014) also evaluated a train-the-trainer emergency preparedness program that was developed for and in consultation with adults with intellectual and developmental disabilities (IDDs). Clients (with IDDs) of a community-based organization (CBO) in Los Angeles, California, that serves adults with IDDs were trained as peer mentors. In an RCT, adults with IDDs who received the peer-mentored emergency preparedness training (N = 42) reported statistically significantly greater improvements in disaster preparedness behaviors ($p = 0.003$) and marginally better earthquake preparedness knowledge ($p = 0.052$) at 1-month follow-up relative to those in a waitlist (delayed intervention) control group (N = 40). Adults with IDDs in the experimental group increased preparedness activities by 19 percent and preparedness knowledge by 8 percent (as compared with 5 percent and 1 percent in the control group, respectively). The measures were not validated, and there was some concern about social desirability bias. Overall, the study (and each outcome) was deemed to be of moderate methodological quality.

The Montgomery County Department of Health and Human Services (2008) evaluated an intervention similar to that examined by Eisenman and colleagues (2009) using a prospective pre-post design (a single group study for which outcome data are available pre- and postintervention). After receiving training in emergency preparedness, six experienced *Vías de la Salud* health promoters conducted group educational sessions with Latino residents in Montgomery County, Maryland. Statistical analyses are not reported, but among the health promoters, knowledge improved from baseline immediately after their training and after the community education sessions regarding emergency plans, emergency shelters, evacuation, emergency preparation, and emergency supply kits. Except for knowledge about evacuation, promoters' knowledge (N = 5–6) was stable (mostly at 100 percent correct) from immediately after training until after the community education sessions. Among community members who participated in the educational sessions (N = 29–39), compared with before the course, there were improvements in feelings regarding their preparedness (from 8 percent before the educational sessions to 69 percent after completing all three sessions) and in self-reported household preparedness practices (e.g., having an emergency plan and stockpiling emergency supplies). After the third educational session, 100 percent of participants reported having an emergency plan (as compared with 23 percent before the training), and stockpiling of food and water had been completed by 93 percent and 97 percent, respectively (as compared with 21 percent and 10 percent at baseline). There were concerns about the validity of the study's outcomes. Overall, the study (and each outcome) was deemed to be of moderate methodological quality.

Hites and colleagues (2012) evaluated the effectiveness of a culturally tailored training program (for CBPs only) using a prospective pre-post study design. This program, adapted for community health representatives who serve tribal populations in the Navajo Nation (in Arizona), was shown to increase PHEPR-related knowledge as measured by scores for six Centers for Disease Control and Prevention–defined bioterrorism competencies. Compared with testing prior to training, the community health representatives (N = 83) scored statistically significantly better after the training on five of the six competencies, although the median number of correct answers rose by only one or two questions (out of one to seven questions per competency). The outcome was not validated, and overall, the study (and each outcome) was deemed to be of moderate methodological quality.

McCabe and colleagues (2014a,b) examined companion training interventions—implemented though a partnership comprising an academic health center, local health departments, and faith-based organizations (FBOs)—aimed at improving mental health preparedness and community resilience. The authors used a prospective pre-post design to assess the outcomes of sequential 1-day workshops in psychological first aid (PFA) and guided preparedness planning (GPP). FBO partners recruited members of their congregation and local communities (rural and urban) to receive PFA training, and subsequently designated small teams to represent their FBO in GPP and to develop draft disaster plans for their organization and community. Statistically significant improvements were observed after the training in objectively measured knowledge, as well as self-reported knowledge, skills, and some measures of attitudes (e.g., perceived self-efficacy, willingness to deliver PFA during an emergency) for PFA and GPP trainees (including at-risk rural cohorts). On average, approximately 80 percent of teams representing their FBO submitted a same-day draft of disaster plans following GPP, with average completeness scores ranging from 83.5 to 98.7 (out of 100).

At 1-year follow up, greater than 80 percent of respondent trainees were willing and confident in their ability to provide PFA following a disaster or public health emergency, and approximately 20 percent had provided PFA at least once following a disaster or other public health emergency (nearly two-thirds had provided it to someone experiencing a personal crisis). Because FBO representatives and community members were trained together (approximately 70 percent of participants were community members) and outcomes were not measured separately for these different populations, the study findings could not be applied to the outcomes related to knowledge and attitudes and beliefs for CBP representatives. With the trained FBO representatives themselves considered to be members of the at-risk population (residents of rural areas), the study was deemed to be applicable to at-risk population outcomes (knowledge, attitudes and beliefs, behavior). For the GPP component of the intervention, trained teams were selected by FBOs to generate disaster plans for their organization. Consequently, the committee also deemed the study results applicable to the CBP disaster planning outcome. There were concerns about measures that were not validated and about self-reporting for some outcomes. Methodological quality was moderate for the outcomes of objectively measured knowledge and completion of disaster plans and poor for all other outcomes.

In addition to the quantitative comparative studies described above, four cross-sectional studies (postintervention measurements only) addressed questions related to the effectiveness of culturally tailored preparedness training programs for CBPs and at-risk populations they serve. In a pilot of the earlier-described PFA training program implemented by McCabe and colleagues (2014a,b), the study team used a train-the-trainer model to provide culturally tailored PFA training to clergy members from urban areas in Maryland with large African American and Latino populations (McCabe et al., 2008). Self-reported self-efficacy with PFA among clergy following the training was high, ranging from 77.1 to 91.5 percent, depending on the evaluation item (e.g., accessing psychosocial and psychiatric resources, recognizing signs and symptoms of stress and acute stress disorder).

In a subsequent iteration of the culturally tailored PFA training program, the study team evaluated PFA training in a mixed cohort of FBO representatives and community residents from four rural counties in Maryland (McCabe et al., 2011). Following the training, 97–99 percent of trainees agreed or strongly agreed that training objectives related to acquisition of knowledge about the principles and practices of disaster mental health, PFA, at-risk populations, and self-care had been met. Additionally, 93–98 percent of trainees agreed or strongly agreed that their perceived self-efficacy for applying PFA techniques in a real-world disaster setting had improved. Immediately following the workshop, 31.5 percent of trainees submitted applications to be members of the Maryland Medical Professional Volunteer Corp, indicating a willingness to respond as a PFA provider.

McCabe and colleagues (2013) also trained FBO representatives and community members from the same rural Maryland counties in GPP. Following the training, 93–98 percent of participants agreed or strongly agreed that the program objectives had been met, core planning concepts had been learned, and the course had been a valuable experience. Depending on the evaluation item, 90–100 percent of participants agreed or strongly agreed that they had a better understanding of knowledge and skills required to create a disaster mental health plan following the training. Ninety-five percent of individual participants reported enhanced confidence (perceived self-efficacy) in their ability to execute disaster planning strategies and techniques (McCabe et al., 2013). All participants were able to generate partial disaster plan drafts by the end of the training, and by the end of the project, 15 out of 100 FBOs (all from a single county) had submitted completed disaster plans on behalf of their organizations and communities.

Laborde and colleagues (2013) similarly describe the results of a cross-sectional study evaluating a pilot disaster mental health training program, which was implemented as a train-the-trainer program tailored to black community leaders and clinical providers in rural and coastal areas of North Carolina with high poverty levels. The mean posttest knowledge score for CBO leaders was 61 percent, and individual competency scores ranged from 42 to 82 percent (pretest scores were not measured).

Other evidence that may inform effectiveness As noted earlier, in addition to the above direct evidence on tailored strategies for engaging with and training CBPs, the committee considered parallel evidence consisting of systematic reviews of community engagement and culturally tailored interventions used outside the PHEPR context to improve the outcomes of at-risk or disadvantaged populations (primarily populations of low socioeconomic status and racial/ethnic minorities).

The search for relevant systematic reviews yielded four broad reviews (all from the health field but not specific to a single population or health condition)—three on community engagement models (Cyril et al., 2015; O'Mara-Eves et al., 2015; Viswanathan et al., 2004) and one on cultural competence and tailoring of health care interventions (Butler et al., 2016). There was minimal overlap in primary studies across these four systematic reviews. Taken together, the systematic reviews provide promising evidence of a beneficial effect of community engagement and cultural tailoring on the outcomes that were evaluated, including knowledge of health risks and mitigation strategies, health behaviors (e.g., physical activity, healthy eating, smoking cessation, cancer screening), and health-related outcomes (e.g., hypertension, mental health conditions). The outcomes from the systematic reviews related to knowledge of health risks and health behaviors align reasonably with the outcomes related to PHEPR knowledge of trained populations and preparedness behaviors in the present review. Despite the beneficial effects described in the systematic reviews, however, authors of two of the four broad reviews—one on community engagement (Viswanathan et al., 2004) and one on culturally tailored interventions (Butler et al., 2016)—concluded that they could not determine the effectiveness of these broad classes of interventions, in part because of the heterogeneity of the included studies and the challenges of attributing the observed effects to one component of what is usually a multicomponent intervention.

In addition to the four broad systematic reviews, the committee's search captured nine population- and health condition–specific systematic reviews of culturally tailored interventions targeting at-risk populations—many of which were educational—that were published after those broader reviews (DeRose and Rodriguez, 2019; Florez et al., 2019; Kim et al., 2016; McCall et al., 2019; McCallum et al., 2017; McCurley et al., 2017; Nasir et al., 2016; Schroeder et al., 2018; Shommu et al., 2016). All but one of these nine reviews (McCall et al., 2019) involve engagement of CBOs, FBOs, or community health workers. Overall, the more specific systematic reviews focus on adult populations of low socioeconomic status and/or racial and ethnic minorities. The majority address community-based participatory research intervention models utilizing cultural tailoring and community partnership methodology. Relevant outcomes discussed in these nine systemic reviews include knowledge of health risks (DeRose and Rodriguez, 2019; Kim et al., 2016; McCallum et al., 2017; Nasir et al., 2016; Shommu et al., 2016), health behavior (DeRose and Rodriguez, 2019; Florez et al., 2019; Kim et al., 2016; McCurley et al., 2017; Shommu et al., 2016), and health conditions (DeRose and Rodriguez, 2019; Florez et al., 2019; Kim et al., 2016; McCall et al., 2019; McCallum et al., 2017; McCurley et al., 2017; Schroeder et al., 2018; Shommu et al., 2016). All of the reviews report beneficial effects for at least some outcome measures. The authors of the reviews generally offer conclusions similar to those of the four broader systematic reviews described above: that community engagement and cultural tailoring are promising intervention methods, but that further rigorous study—including more RCTs, better measurement of health outcomes and effect sizes, and more consistent study populations to reduce bias—is needed to provide higher-quality evidence with which to compare and contrast engagement methods.

One challenge when looking at these systematic reviews as parallel evidence on strategies for engaging with and training CBPs in PHEPR stems from the breadth of community engagement strategies covered in the reviews, not all of which involve CBPs as the committee has defined them. For example, some engagement strategies involve assembling a community advisory board comprising individual community members, which may not be comparable to a model whereby CBPs are engaged in co-designing and co-delivering interventions. Moreover, the authors of the reviews could not always distinguish the contribution of CBP engagement to the intervention effects. Additionally, the committee recognized that the motivation of at-risk populations to improve knowledge and behavior related to known health risks (e.g., diabetes, obesity) may not reflect their motivation to address risks from low-probability public health emergencies. As a result, the committee considered parallel evidence to be supportive[3] rather than very supportive.

Summary of the evidence: PHEPR knowledge of CBP representatives The committee concluded that *there is low COE that culturally tailored preparedness training programs for CBPs and at-risk populations they serve improve PHEPR knowledge of CBP representatives.* Two of the five quantitative comparative studies (Hites et al., 2012; Montgomery County Department of Health and Human Services, 2008) and one of the four cross-sectional (postintervention) studies (Laborde et al., 2013) provide low COE regarding the effects of culturally tailored preparedness training programs on PHEPR knowledge of trained CBP representatives (see Table B1-2). Despite supportive parallel evidence (described above) and the absence of studies with discordant results, the weight of the evidence was insufficient to upgrade the COE.

[3] As described in Chapter 3, the committee reviewed other evidence that informed the COE (e.g., mechanistic evidence, experiential evidence from case reports and after action reports, qualitative evidence) for coherence with the findings from the quantitative research studies and classified that evidence as very supportive, supportive, inconclusive (no conclusion can be drawn on coherence, either because results are mixed or the data are insufficient), or unsupportive (discordant with the findings from the quantitative research studies). The distinction between supportive and very supportive is based on the magnitude of the reported effect and the directness of the evidence to the question of interest.

TABLE B1-2 Effect of Culturally Tailored Preparedness Training Programs on Improved PHEPR Knowledge of Community-Based Partner Representatives

Quality Assessment	Number of Studies	3
	Study Infomation	Montgomery County Department of Health and Human Services, 2008 Prospective pre-post, moderate methodological quality (▲) Hites et al., 2012 Prospective pre-post, moderate methodological quality (▲) Laborde et al., 2013 Cross-sectional (postintervention), poor methodological quality (▲)
	Risk of Bias	Serious
	Inconsistency	Not serious
	Indirectness	Not serious
	Imprecision	Not serious
	Publication Bias	Unlikely
	Upgrade for Large Effect, Dose Response, Plausible Confounding	Large effect (Montgomery County Department of Health and Human Services, 2008)
Summary of Findings	Initial Certainty of the Evidence (COE)	Low
	Other Evidence	Supportive parallel evidence, no discordant studies
	COE	Low (improves PHEPR knowledge of CBP representatives)

NOTE: Effect direction: upward arrow (▲) = improvement/beneficial effect; downward arrow (▼) = harm/negative effect; sideways arrows (◄►) = no effect; up and down arrows (▲▼) = mixed effect/conflicting findings.

Summary of the evidence: Attitudes and beliefs of CBP representatives The committee concluded that *there is very low COE that culturally tailored preparedness training programs for CBPs and at-risk populations they serve improve attitudes and beliefs of CBP representatives regarding their preparedness to meet needs of at-risk individuals.* One cross-sectional (postintervention) study (McCabe et al., 2008) provides very low COE regarding the effects of culturally tailored preparedness training programs on attitudes and beliefs of CBP representatives (see Table B1-3), and no supporting evidence from other sources was identified.

TABLE B1-3 Effect of Culturally Tailored Preparedness Training Programs on Improved Attitudes and Beliefs of Community-Based Partner Representatives Regarding Their Preparedness to Meet Needs of At-Risk Individuals

Quality Assessment	Number of Studies	1
	Study Infomation	McCabe et al., 2008 Cross-sectional (postintervention), poor methodological quality (▲)
	Risk of Bias	Very serious
	Inconsistency	Not applicable
	Indirectness	Not serious
	Imprecision	Serious
	Publication Bias	Unlikely
	Upgrade for Large Effect, Dose Response, Plausible Confounding	No
Summary of Findings	Initial Certainty of the Evidence (COE)	Very low
	Other Evidence	No
	COE	Very low (improves preparedness attitudes and beliefs of CBP representatives)

NOTE: Effect direction: upward arrow (▲) = improvement/beneficial effect; downward arrow (▼) = harm/negative effect; sideways arrows (◄►) = no effect; up and down arrows (▲▼) = mixed effect/conflicting findings.

Summary of the evidence: CBP disaster planning The committee concluded that *there is very low COE that culturally tailored preparedness training programs for CBPs and at-risk populations they serve increase CBP disaster planning.* One quantitative comparative study (McCabe et al., 2014a,b) and one cross-sectional (postintervention) study (McCabe et al., 2013) provide very low COE regarding the effects of culturally tailored preparedness training programs on CBP disaster planning (see Table B1-4), and no supporting evidence from other sources was identified.

TABLE B1-4 Effect of Culturally Tailored Preparedness Training Programs on Community-Based Partner Disaster Planning

Quality Assessment	Number of Studies	2
	Study Infomation	McCabe et al., 2014a,b Prospective pre-post, moderate methodological quality (▲) McCabe et al., 2013 Cross-sectional (postintervention), moderate methodological quality (▲)
	Risk of Bias	Serious
	Inconsistency	Not serious
	Indirectness	Not serious
	Imprecision	Not serious
	Publication Bias	Unlikely
	Upgrade for Large Effect, Dose Response, Plausible Confounding	No
Summary of Findings	Initial Certainty of the Evidence (COE)	Very low
	Other Evidence	No
	COE	Very low (increases CBP disaster planning)

NOTE: Effect direction: upward arrow (▲) = improvement/beneficial effect; downward arrow (▼) = harm/negative effect; sideways arrows (◄►) = no effect; up and down arrows (▲▼) = mixed effect/conflicting findings.

Summary of the evidence: PHEPR knowledge of trained at-risk populations The committee concluded that *there is moderate COE that culturally tailored preparedness training programs for CBPs and at-risk populations they serve improve the PHEPR knowledge of trained at-risk populations.* Two quantitative comparative studies (Eisenman et al., 2014; McCabe et al., 2014a,b) and two cross-sectional (postintervention) studies (McCabe et al., 2011, 2013) provide moderate COE regarding the effects of culturally tailored preparedness training programs on PHEPR knowledge of trained at-risk representatives (see Table B1-5). Despite supportive parallel evidence (described above) and the absence of studies with discordant results, the weight of the evidence was insufficient to upgrade the COE.

TABLE B1-5 Effect of Culturally Tailored Preparedness Training Programs for Community-Based Partners and At-Risk Populations They Serve on Improved PHEPR Knowledge of Trained At-Risk Populations

Quality Assessment	Number of Studies	4
	Study Infomation	Eisenman et al., 2014 Randomized controlled trial (RCT), moderate methodological quality (▲) McCabe et al., 2014a,b Prospective pre-post, moderate methodological quality (▲) McCabe et al., 2011 Cross-sectional (postintervention), poor methodological quality (▲) McCabe et al., 2013 Cross-sectional (postintervention), poor methodological quality (▲)
	Risk of Bias	Serious
	Inconsistency	Not serious
	Indirectness	Not serious
	Imprecision	Not serious
	Publication Bias	Unlikely
	Upgrade for Large Effect, Dose Response, Plausible Confounding	No
Summary of Findings	Initial Certainty of the Evidence (COE)	Moderate
	Other Evidence	Supportive parallel evidence, no discordant studies
	COE	Moderate (improves PHEPR knowledge of at-risk populations)

NOTE: Effect direction: upward arrow (▲) = improvement/beneficial effect; downward arrow (▼) = harm/negative effect; sideways arrows (◀▶) = no effect; up and down arrows (▲▼) = mixed effect/conflicting findings.

Summary of the evidence: Preparedness attitudes and beliefs of trained at-risk populations
The committee concluded that *there is low COE that culturally tailored preparedness training programs for CBPs and at-risk populations they serve improve attitudes and beliefs of trained at-risk populations regarding their preparedness.* Two quantitative comparative studies (McCabe et al., 2014a,b; Montgomery County Department of Health and Human Services, 2008) and one cross-sectional (postintervention) study (McCabe et al., 2011) provide low COE regarding the effects of culturally tailored preparedness training programs on preparedness attitudes and beliefs of trained at-risk representatives (see Table B1-6), and no supporting evidence from other sources was identified.

TABLE B1-6 Effect of Culturally Tailored Preparedness Training Programs for Community-Based Partners and At-Risk Populations They Serve on Improved Attitudes and Beliefs of Trained At-Risk Populations Regarding Their Preparedness

Quality Assessment	Number of Studies	3
	Study Infomation	Montgomery County Department of Health and Human Services, 2008 Prospective pre-post, moderate methodological quality (▲) McCabe et al., 2014a,b Prospective pre-post, poor methodological quality (▲) McCabe et al., 2011 Cross-sectional (postintervention), poor methodological quality (▲)
	Risk of Bias	Serious
	Inconsistency	Not serious
	Indirectness	Not serious
	Imprecision	Not serious
	Publication Bias	Unlikely
	Upgrade for Large Effect, Dose Response, Plausible Confounding	Large effect (Montgomery County Department of Health and Human Services, 2008)
Summary of Findings	Initial Certainty of the Evidence (COE)	Low
	Other Evidence	No
	COE	Low (improves attitudes and beliefs of at-risk populations)

NOTE: Effect direction: upward arrow (▲) = improvement/beneficial effect; downward arrow (▼) = harm/negative effect; sideways arrows (◄►) = no effect; up and down arrows (▲▼) = mixed effect/conflicting findings.

Summary of the evidence: Preparedness behaviors of trained at-risk populations The committee concluded that *there is moderate COE that culturally tailored preparedness training programs for CBPs and at-risk populations they serve improve preparedness behaviors of trained at-risk populations.* Four quantitative comparative studies (Eisenman et al., 2009, 2014; McCabe et al., 2014a,b; Montgomery County Department of Health and Human Services, 2008) provide moderate COE regarding the effects of culturally tailored preparedness training programs on preparedness behaviors of trained at-risk representatives (see Table B1-7). Despite supportive parallel evidence (described above) and the absence of studies with discordant results, the weight of the evidence was insufficient to upgrade the COE.

TABLE B1-7 Effect of Culturally Tailored Preparedness Training Programs for Community-Based Partners and At-Risk Populations They Serve on Improved Preparedness Behaviors of Trained At-Risk Populations

Quality Assessment	Number of Studies	4
	Study Infomation	Eisenman et al., 2009 Randomized controlled trial (RCT), moderate methodological quality (▲) Eisenman et al., 2014 RCT, moderate methodological quality (▲) Montgomery County Department of Health and Human Services, 2008 Prospective pre-post, moderate methodological quality (▲) McCabe et al., 2014a,b Prospective pre-post, poor methodological quality (▲)
	Risk of Bias	Serious
	Inconsistency	Not serious
	Indirectness	Not serious
	Imprecision	Not serious
	Publication Bias	Unlikely
	Upgrade for Large Effect, Dose Response, Plausible Confounding	No
Summary of Findings	Initial Certainty of the Evidence (COE)	Moderate
	Other Evidence	Supportive parallel evidence, no discordant studies
	COE	Moderate (improves preparedness behaviors of at-risk populations)

NOTE: Effect direction: upward arrow (▲) = improvement/beneficial effect; downward arrow (▼) = harm/negative effect; sideways arrows (◀▶) = no effect; up and down arrows (▲▼) = mixed effect/conflicting findings.

Engagement of CBPs in Preparedness Outreach Activities Targeting At-Risk Populations

Evidence from quantitative research studies One quantitative comparative study examined the effect of engaging CBPs in preparedness outreach activities targeting at-risk populations. The study conducted by Coady and colleagues (2008) used a community-based participatory research (CBPR) approach to engage CBPs in the design and implementation of a community-based intervention aimed at increasing interest in influenza vaccination in economically disadvantaged, difficult-to-reach populations (e.g., substance abusers, undocumented immigrants) residing in urban settings. Although the intervention was implemented in the context of seasonal influenza, it was developed with the intent that it could be used to increase vaccination rates during a pandemic influenza scenario, and the committee mapped interest in influenza vaccination to its analytic framework for this practice (see Figure B1-1) as a measure of at-risk population attitudes toward preparedness behaviors. In addition to CBPs' engagement in the design of the rapid vaccination intervention, CBP venues were leveraged during implementation as sites for information dissemination and vaccination to increase access to difficult-to-reach populations (vaccination and information dissemination also occurred door to door and at street-based venues). The study, which used a nonconcurrent nonrandomized comparative design (the same individuals were not sampled before and during the intervention), showed that interest in vaccination was higher in populations queried during the program (N = 3,082) compared with interest levels in the population (N = 3,744) queried prior to the program (adjusted odds ratio 2.69, 95 percent confidence interval 2.17 to 3.33) (Coady et al., 2008).

Other evidence that may inform effectiveness Although the committee considered parallel evidence, the studies included in the systematic reviews of community engagement strategies generally did not address outcomes related to improved attitudes and beliefs. Therefore, this evidence could not be applied to the assessment of the effect of CBP engagement in preparedness outreach activities on attitudes and beliefs of at-risk populations. The committee also considered evidence from a single case report addressing the effects of CBP inclusion in outreach activities on at-risk population attitudes toward preparedness behaviors (vaccination). Plough and colleagues (2011) describe the development of partnerships with CBPs in Los Angeles County, California, to address low vaccination rates among African American populations during the H1N1 outbreak and associated trust issues. The authors indicate that 31,166 vaccinations were administered at 580 vaccination outreach events conducted by the public health department and community partners. CBPs also provided information and referred 6,000 clients to free or low-cost vaccination providers. There were no studies with discordant results.

Summary of the evidence: Engagement of CBPs in preparedness outreach activities targeting at-risk populations The committee concluded that *there is very low COE that CBP engagement in preparedness outreach activities improves the attitudes and beliefs of at-risk populations toward preparedness behaviors.* One quantitative comparative study (Coady et al., 2008) provides very low COE regarding the effect of CBP engagement in preparedness outreach activities on the attitudes and beliefs of at-risk populations (see Table B1-8), and the evidence from the single very supportive case report (Plough et al., 2011) was insufficient to upgrade the COE.

TABLE B1-8 Effect of Community-Based Partner Engagement in Preparedness Outreach Activities Targeting At-Risk Populations on Improved Attitudes and Beliefs of At-Risk Populations Toward Preparedness Behaviors

Quality Assessment	Number of Studies	1
	Study Infomation	Coady et al., 2008 Nonrandomized comparative study (NRCS), poor methodological quality (▲)
	Risk of Bias	Very serious
	Inconsistency	Not applicable
	Indirectness	Not serious
	Imprecision	Serious
	Publication Bias	Unlikely
	Upgrade for Large Effect, Dose Response, Plausible Confounding	No
Summary of Findings	Initial Certainty of the Evidence (COE)	Very low
	Other Evidence	One very supportive case report, no discordant studies
	COE	Very low (improves attitudes and beliefs of at-risk populations)

NOTE: Effect direction: upward arrow (▲) = improvement/beneficial effect; downward arrow (▼) = harm/negative effect; sideways arrows (◄►) = no effect; up and down arrows (▲▼) = mixed effect/conflicting findings.

Engagement and Training of CBPs in Coalitions Addressing Public Health Preparedness/Resilience

Evidence from quantitative research studies One quantitative comparative study examined the effect of engaging multiple CBPs in coalitions and training them in PHEPR concepts on system-level outcomes related to improving outcomes for at-risk populations. Williams and colleagues (2018) describe results from an RCT in which 16 community coalitions in Los Angeles County, California, were randomized to use and receive training in either community resilience or enhanced standard preparedness as an organizing frame for engagement activities. The trial was conducted starting in 2013–2014 and followed for 1–2 years through 2015.

Over the course of the trial, various apparently post hoc analyses were conducted. Reported outcomes of interest include size and diversity of coalitions and coordination among coalition members. Differences in coalition diversity (number of sectors represented) and size favored the resilience group, but the difference was not statistically significant for coalition size. Process activities decreased and integrated activities (greater degree of coordination among coalition members) increased over the first year for both coalition types, although the effect was greater for the preparedness group (no statistical analysis) (Williams et al., 2018). A separately published article on the study shows that both types of coalitions pursued activities focused on reaching and educating vulnerable populations, another outcome of interest, although there is no statistical analysis to support conclusions regarding the relative effects of the two training strategies on this outcome. As evidenced by frequency count data, resilience coalitions focused more on intensive but lower-reach trainings, while preparedness coalitions relied more on "low-touch" fairs. The resilience coalitions conducted five times as many trainings for vulnerable groups (20 versus 4) (Bromley et al., 2017).

Other evidence that may inform effectiveness There was no supporting evidence from other sources for this practice.

Summary of the evidence: Engagement and training of CBPs in coalitions The committee concluded that *there is very low COE that CBP engagement and training in coalitions addressing public health preparedness/resilience increases the diversity of coalitions, the coordination of CBPs with other response partners, or the capacity to reach and educate at-risk populations before an emergency.* One quantitative comparative study (results described in Bromley et al., 2017, and Williams et al., 2018) provides very low COE regarding the effects of engagement and training of CBPs in preparedness/resilience coalitions on diversity of coalitions, coordination of CBPs with response partners, and the capacity to reach and educate at-risk populations (see Table B1-9), and no supporting evidence from other sources was identified.

TABLE B1-9 Effect of Engagement and Training of Community-Based Partners in Coalitions Addressing Public Health Preparedness/Resilience

Quality Assessment	Number of Studies	1
	Study Infomation	Bromley et al., 2017; Williams et al., 2018 Randomized controlled trial (RCT), poor methodological quality (▲)
	Risk of Bias	Very serious
	Inconsistency	Not applicable
	Indirectness	Not serious
	Imprecision	Serious
	Publication Bias	Unlikely
	Upgrade for Large Effect, Dose Response, Plausible Confounding	No
Summary of Findings	Initial Certainty of the Evidence (COE)	Very low
	Other Evidence	No
	COE	Very low (increases diversity of coalitions, coordination of CBPs with response partners, or capacity to reach at-risk populations)

NOTES: For each outcome, the effects for the two interventions evaluated in the two randomized controlled trial study arms were considered together given the similarity of the interventions (preparedness and resilience training). Effect direction: upward arrow (▲) = improvement/beneficial effect; downward arrow (▼) = harm/negative effect; sideways arrows (◄►) = no effect; up and down arrows (▲▼) = mixed effect/conflicting findings.

2. Balance of Benefits and Harms

Synthesis of Evidence of Effect

Engagement and culturally tailored training of CBPs may have benefits related to improved PHEPR-related knowledge among CBP representatives, particularly knowledge related to at-risk populations (low COE). Training of at-risk populations by or alongside CBP representatives may in turn improve the PHEPR knowledge of those populations (moderate COE) and may prompt at-risk individuals to engage in protective behaviors (e.g., stockpiling critical supplies, developing a communication plan, expanding social networks) (moderate COE). Such training may also improve the attitudes and/or beliefs of at-risk populations regarding their preparedness (low COE). However, there is little evidence linking preparedness phase outcomes (e.g., improved knowledge, attitudes and beliefs, and preparedness behaviors) with health and other outcomes for at-risk populations after an event. No evidence of harms is reported in the quantitative studies.

Qualitative Evidence Synthesis

Twenty qualitative studies (Andrulis et al., 2011; Bromley et al., 2017; Cha et al., 2016; Charania and Tsuji, 2012; Cordasco et al., 2007; Cuervo et al., 2017; Gagnon et al., 2016; Gin et al., 2016, 2018; Hipper et al., 2015; Ingham and Redshaw, 2017; Kamau et al., 2017; Laborde et al., 2011; Messias et al., 2012; Miller et al., 2015; Peterson et al., 2019; Rowel et al., 2012; Schoch-Spana et al., 2013; Shih et al., 2018; Stajura et al., 2012) supported a finding that *engagement of community-based partners corresponded almost entirely to collaborations (coalitions and partnerships). The effectiveness of such collaborations appears to depend on inclusive membership—which helps members manage capacity constraints—and cooperative and shared goals (high confidence in the evidence).* Collaborations with CBPs facilitate (1) inclusion of community organizations (formal or informal) in emergency preparedness and response efforts (Charania and Tsuji, 2012; Gagnon et al., 2016; Gin et al., 2018; Ingham and Redshaw, 2017; Miller et al., 2015); and (2) awareness and appreciation of the varied community and cultural perspectives and operating characteristics of those organizations (including language, leadership, and decision-making styles) (Bromley et al., 2017; Gagnon et al., 2016; Peterson et al., 2019; Rowel et al., 2012; Schoch-Spana et al., 2013). Expanding the number and/or size of collaborations through the inclusion of diverse CBPs better embeds their perspectives in community efforts and strengthens commitments to improving outcomes for all community members, including traditionally at-risk populations (Charania and Tsuji, 2012; Cordasco et al., 2007; Miller et al., 2015; Peterson et al., 2019; Stajura et al., 2012). Engaging those CBPs traditionally underrepresented in community collaborations also helps extend the reach of response partners to some of the highest-risk populations (Ingham and Redshaw, 2017). Inclusive and purposeful collaborations prompted by goals for community-wide emergency preparedness and response may achieve additional benefits, such as cultural sensitivity and appropriateness and shared ownership of community efforts (Charania and Tsuji, 2012; Cordasco et al., 2007; Miller et al., 2015; Peterson et al., 2019). Inclusive approaches to CBP engagement may also serve to enhance trust in government initiatives (Cordasco et al., 2007; Gin et al., 2016; Peterson et al., 2019; Rowel et al., 2012).

A frequently noted perceived benefit of collaborations is improved awareness among public health departments of the CBPs in the community and the services they provide, as well as improved understanding among CBPs of the services and activities of public health agencies (Bromley et al., 2017; Cuervo et al., 2017; Gagnon et al., 2016; Gin et al., 2016;

Laborde et al., 2011; Schoch-Spana et al., 2013; Shih et al., 2018). *Collaborations appear to provide all members with a means of learning and understanding each other's roles during routine operations. Such shared knowledge in turn provides the basis for leveraging and coordinating existing services when emergency events occur. Similarly, such knowledge is foundational for identifying and developing strategies for covering gaps in services, which may improve preparedness and coordination of response related to community-wide public health emergencies* (high confidence in the evidence). This finding is supported by nine qualitative studies (Andrulis et al., 2011; Bromley et al., 2017; Cuervo et al., 2017; Gagnon et al., 2016; Gin et al., 2018; Ingham and Redshaw, 2017; Laborde et al., 2011; Schoch-Spana et al., 2013; Shih et al., 2018). Collaborations may also help CBPs integrate preparedness efforts into their core services (Ingham and Redshaw, 2017; Shih et al., 2018).

Collaborations with CBPs provide an opportunity for relationship building for nonemergency purposes. Collaborations appear to nurture relationships developed through preparedness efforts that may not lead immediately to leveraging or developing services, but may assist with informal and emergent responses during an emergency (Bromley et al., 2017; Cha et al., 2016; Cuervo et al., 2017, Gin et al., 2016; Ingham and Redshaw, 2017; Shih et al., 2018; Stajura et al., 2012). Successes experienced by collaborations may foster ongoing and new multisectoral collaborative efforts, as well as member commitment (Gagnon et al., 2016; Gin et al., 2016; Ingham and Redshaw, 2017; Peterson et al., 2019).

Participatory approaches to CBP engagement may improve the capacity of stakeholders (Andrulis et al., 2011; Charania and Tsuji, 2012; Gagnon et al., 2016; Miller et al., 2015). For example, collaborations may be effective at finding ways to bypass administrative constraints experienced by CBPs or may assist with obtaining funding using collective rather than competing strategies among members (Gagnon et al., 2016; Ingham and Redshaw, 2017). These are likely to be perceived and experienced as benefits.

At the same time, the body of qualitative studies notes several potential harms and/or undesirable impacts of CBP engagement. Participatory approaches to CBP engagement may be risky in that implicit biases may surface as explicit biases. Miller and colleagues (2015) report that this occurred when discussion included "issues that often go unsaid in communities," and some typically marginalized members challenged assumptions that may privilege certain populations or perspectives over others. Although some may welcome the opportunity to confront this terrain, the process involved in addressing such biases constructively is often difficult and resisted (Miller et al., 2015). When approaches are less than participatory, foundational elements of what is valued, what is considered knowledge, what is considered actionable knowledge, and who is in control remain uncontested. This observation, which emerged from the body of qualitative studies (both directly and as an analytic interpretation), represents both a barrier to working together and a perceived harm of preparedness efforts (Andrulis et al., 2011; Cordasco et al., 2007; Gin et al., 2016; Hipper et al., 2015; Kamau et al., 2017; Laborde et al., 2011; Messias et al., 2012; Schoch-Spana et al., 2013; Stajura et al., 2012).

Negative experiences from past collaborative relationships may pose barriers to future engagement efforts if potential members think that collaborations do not result in constructive relationships or seldom produce desired results (Stajura et al., 2012). Past failures may be attributed to poor cultural sensitivity within collaborations or conflicts over decision-making principles (notably hierarchical versus consensus approaches) (Andrulis et al., 2011; Ingham and Redshaw, 2017). CBPs may perceive that certain members tend to experience more recognition than others (Laborde et al., 2011; Stajura et al., 2012) or do not provide evidence-based, honest, or reliable information (Andrulis et al., 2011; Charania and Tsuji, 2012); exhibit "egos" and form "gangs" (Cha et al., 2016; Stajura et al., 2012); or are not trustworthy (Cha et al., 2016). Also noted as a concern is the potential for engagement efforts to be token rather than substantive when collaboration is mandated by external government standards or funders (Gin et al., 2016).

Collaborative partners may express frustration when they perceive a short-term rather than sustained focus on emergency preparedness. It needs to be acknowledged that collaboration building is usually a slow process, one complicated by ongoing personnel changes (and resulting loss of institutional memory) within CBPs (Cha et al., 2016; Gin et al., 2016; Hipper et al., 2015; Ingham and Redshaw, 2017; Peterson et al., 2019; Schoch-Spana et al., 2013). Although Charania and Tsuji (2012) observe that collaborative work is not always a long-term endeavor, in most instances, the often limited and short-term funding provided for this work impedes building and sustaining collaborations, and may result in unintended consequences and harms such as collaboration fatigue, which may also exacerbate trust and confidence issues (Gin et al., 2016, 2018; Peterson et al., 2019; Schoch-Spana et al., 2013).

Specifically with regard to training, when there are no opportunities to deliberatively practice learning obtained through training, training becomes an isolated event with no transfer to the workplace, whether for routine or emergency operations (Cuervo et al., 2017). These factors not only create barriers to assessing the effectiveness of training and knowledge transfer, but likely cause harm by potentially creating disenchantment with the usefulness of any training.

Case Report Evidence Synthesis

While case reports included in this review address only benefits of engaging CBPs, unintended consequences may have occurred but not been known or described. Overall, however, case report findings indicate positive impacts of engaging partners, many of which align with the findings on benefits from other evidence types. These reported benefits include the development of new partnerships, enhanced coordination, the potential for surge staffing during an emergency, and improved preparedness and readiness to serve at-risk populations. In support of the qualitative evidence synthesis findings, case reports suggest that engagement and training of direct service personnel, FBOs, and other community partners also present opportunities for leveraging the distinctive capabilities of each, as well as for capacity development. In Philadelphia, an outreach model that included training, education, bidirectional communication via dissemination of quarterly health bulletins to CBOs serving vulnerable populations, and inclusion of evaluation practices was found to increase preparedness and local capacity to prepare for and respond to the needs of vulnerable populations during an emergency (Klaiman et al., 2010). Another case report describes how a statewide tribal public health emergency preparedness network was perceived to have been strengthened as the result of a training collaboration among statewide tribal partners; the Arizona Department of Health Services; and the College of Public Health at the University of Arizona (Peate and Mullins, 2008), which tailored trainings to the unique public health concerns of the tribal communities.

Case reports suggest further that new and strengthened partnerships with CBPs developed through engagement and training efforts can support increased reach to underserved communities before and during a public health emergency. For example, targeted outreach to key community leaders aimed at increasing H1N1 vaccination of African Americans in Los Angeles County resulted in new partnerships with CBPs that were well positioned to extend the reach of public health messaging within the African American community and expanded locations willing to allow on-site vaccinations (Plough et al., 2011). Los Angeles County's experience indicates that integration of public health preparedness within routine prevention messages and community engagement strategies can maximize both effectiveness and efficiency, as well as build trust prior to a public health emergency.

Another benefit of engaging CBPs is improved cultural competency and alignment with the needs of underserved populations. Review findings suggest that including underserved populations in emergency planning, training, and exercises can increase understanding of the needs and expectations of these populations (Chandra et al., 2015; Cripps et al., 2016; Howard et al., 2006; Klaiman et al., 2010; Levin et al., 2014; McCabe et al., 2011; Peate and Mullins, 2008). Case reports also describe improved trust resulting from ongoing engagement. Several case reports emphasize the importance of building trust with CBPs prior to emergencies, as they are often the trusted sources of information for underserved communities (Klaiman et al., 2010; Wells et al., 2013). Some communities may have an underlying historical mistrust of government services, necessitating more rigorous outreach efforts (Plough et al., 2011, 2013).

Including vulnerable populations in planning processes can raise the level of respect for, trust in, and acceptance of emergency plans among underserved communities. Trust may also be built by developing connections with populations that are not formally served by an agency or provider. Such connections can result from reaching out to neighborhood and grassroots groups, including FBOs and limited-English-speaking communities (Klaiman et al., 2010). Trusted leadership and organizational relationships can also be built by providing safe and supportive environments for bidirectional learning (Kiser and Lovelace, 2019). This is important as the lack of preexisting or fully functional relationships among emergency preparedness agencies, CBOs, and vulnerable communities hinders effective engagement in emergency situations (Cripps et al., 2016; Gebbie et al., 2009; McCabe et al., 2011; Plough et al., 2013). Moreover, a lack of strong relationships may lead to confusion around the roles of CBPs, which can serve as an additional barrier to effective engagement (Koh et al., 2006). Case reports also mention opportunities for shared learning and dissemination of best practices through the development of multilevel networks of learning communities, collaborative exercises, and the establishment of trusted relationships that may allow for more rigorous evaluation methodologies and quality improvement (Chandra et al., 2015; Kiser and Lovelace, 2019; Klaiman et al., 2010). Finally, outcomes may be improved by engaging trusted local networks that share a commitment to eliminating health disparities; using a framework of strengths and assets; and providing a safe, supportive, multilevel learning community (Kiser and Lovelace, 2019; McCabe et al., 2011, 2013).

3. Acceptability and Preferences

Qualitative Evidence Synthesis

The body of qualitative studies indicated that CBPs were generally supportive of community preparedness goals and strategies for engagement and training, valuing both representation (inclusion) and involvement (shared ownership). Pushback was most often attributable to issues of nonparticipatory approaches or capacity. CBPs emphasized their everyday roles in serving at-risk individuals and stated that they would continue providing those services during emergencies (Messias et al., 2012). Accordingly, they stressed the need to be involved in planning and preparedness for emergencies at the community level—which also would help with coordination efforts—and the need to identify and strengthen services that could be leveraged during emergency responses (Andrulis et al., 2011; Bromley et al., 2017; Cha et al., 2016; Charania and Tsuji, 2012; Cordasco et al., 2007; Cuervo et al., 2017; Eisenman et al., 2009; Gin et al., 2016; Hipper et al., 2015; Ingham and Redshaw, 2017; Kamau et al., 2017; Miller et al., 2015; Peterson et al., 2019; Rowel et al., 2012; Schoch-Spana et al., 2013; Stajura et al., 2012).

Leadership support has been found to influence acceptability. Leaders are crucial to establishing the importance of preparedness and commitment to participation in preparedness efforts (Cuervo et al., 2017). Four qualitative studies (Bromley et al., 2017; Gagnon et al., 2016; Hipper et al., 2015; Schoch-Spana et al., 2013) indicate that *collaborations are more likely to be effective when CBPs have their leaders' support for cooperative engagement* (moderate confidence in the evidence). Two qualitative studies (Hipper et al., 2015; Laborde et al., 2011) similarly support a finding that *when participating in training, CBP employees and volunteers are more likely to engage when they have the unambiguous support of their leadership and organizational culture* (moderate confidence in the evidence).

Case Report Evidence Synthesis

None of the case reports reviewed for this report addresses in detail acceptability and preferences related to engagement strategies. As with the evidence from qualitative studies, the case report evidence suggests that participatory, collaborative approaches for ensuring the participation of key stakeholders early on in planning processes may facilitate effective engagement. For instance, stakeholder engagement in the development of accessible culturally appropriate emergency preparedness messages has been noted as an important facilitator of effective engagement (Bouye et al., 2009; Cripps et al., 2016; Klaiman et al., 2010; Levin et al., 2014; McCabe et al., 2013; Peate and Mullins, 2008; Wells et al., 2013). A commitment to transparency can also help build the trust needed for effective engagement (Kiser and Lovelace, 2019; Wells et al., 2013).

Case reports address as well the role of organizational culture in facilitating effective engagement (Plough et al., 2013; Wells et al., 2013). For instance, public health departments may need to undergo an internal culture change to both embrace and align with a community-partnered approach. Additionally, emergency preparedness staff may need to develop new skill sets that go beyond traditional individual- and family-focused preparedness efforts to better encompass community coordination, neighborhood planning, and integration with nonemergency community-based activities. Reframing public health emergency preparedness practices to include a commitment to leveraging existing community health activities, along with a strong emphasis on health equity in all activities, can facilitate this organizational shift toward collaborative strategies and community preparedness (Plough et al., 2013).

Descriptive Survey Study Evidence

Two descriptive surveys support the finding from the qualitative evidence synthesis that CBPs generally are supportive of engagement in PHEPR activities and are willing to collaborate with public health, although social desirability bias may influence their reported willingness to collaborate. Baezconde-Garbanati and colleagues (2006) report that 70 percent of surveyed CBOs and nongovernmental organizations serving the Hispanic community across 12 U.S. states were willing to provide services to their community during a large-scale emergency, and most were willing to establish linkages with other organizations to help them become better integrated into emergency planning and management at the local level (74 percent preferred to link with public health agencies), given proper coordination and resources. Agencies were also willing, contingent on funding, to offer additional services to help prepare for an emergency, including the dissemination of information to Hispanic communities through formal and informal channels, which the majority believed public health departments could not accomplish adequately because of a lack of cultural proficiency and language resources. Ablah and colleagues (2010) surveyed local health departments (LHDs) and community health centers (CHCs) in 23 states and found that roughly 97 percent of respondents were willing to collaborate with their neighboring LHD or CHC in emergency preparedness or response activities.

Three descriptive surveys support the findings from the qualitative evidence synthesis that leadership support is an important facilitator for the acceptability of PHEPR-related engagement and training. Wineman and colleagues (2007) found that 22 percent of CHCs cited lack of strong leadership and poor coordination of efforts among stakeholders as barriers to their integration into community preparedness activities. Chi and colleagues (2015) report that 11 percent of Los Angeles County Department of Public Health staff cited lack of leadership support as a challenge to building partnerships with community partners, and 10 percent indicated that partnership building did not align with a program priority. Although not specific to CBP engagement, a national survey of LHDs found that higher-intensity community engagement in PHEPR more broadly was associated with having a formal community engagement policy, funds being allocated for community engagement, receiving strong support from CBOs, and having a coordinator with prior community engagement experience (Schoch-Spana et al., 2015).

4. Feasibility and PHEPR System Considerations

Qualitative Evidence Synthesis

The body of qualitative studies suggests that participatory collaborations and targeted, tailored training are feasible. Although collaborations and trainings can in fact alleviate capacity concerns in some cases, there remain perceived capacity limits, likely to be exacerbated in an emergency (Hipper et al., 2015; Stajura et al., 2012), that serve as a barrier to engagement.

In qualitative studies, CBPs often reported capacity concerns with respect to the delivery of routine services. Nearly all worried about emergencies because such events would increase needs, with concomitant increases in demand for services, and stated that an emergency would stress already stretched human and nonhuman resource capacities (Andrulis et al., 2011; Gin et al., 2016, 2018; Hipper et al., 2015). The more poorly funded a community partner was, the sooner and more deeply these constraints would be felt (Gagnon et al., 2016; Gin et al., 2016; Ingham and Redshaw, 2017). Because it is the less well-funded community partners (often those that are more grassroots, faith based, volunteer based, and emergent) that often serve the most vulnerable populations, they may be the first to experience overwhelmed capacities (Andrulis et al., 2011; Gin et al., 2018; Laborde et al., 2011; Schoch-Spana et al., 2013).

The move toward increasing collaborations frequently runs up against CBPs' concerns over competing priorities (routine versus emergency) and overextended capacities (Cha et al., 2016; Gin et al., 2016; Hipper et al., 2015; Shih et al., 2018). Moreover, large collaborative efforts may be considered too expensive, as well as labor intensive (Charania and Tsuji, 2012). Staff turnover, funding limits, and unrealistic expectations for quick successes compound these challenges (Cha et al., 2016; Gin et al., 2016; Ingham and Redshaw, 2017; Peterson et al., 2019; Schoch-Spana et al., 2013). However, a few studies found that collaborations served as a forum for identifying strategic opportunities. When collaboration members improved their understanding of other CBPs' services, leveraging and coordination of services could expand rather than stress capacities (Cuervo et al., 2017; Gagnon et al., 2016;

Ingham and Redshaw, 2017; Laborde et al., 2011). *Collaborations may expand capacities through coordination, and may help identify new funding and new opportunities, such as working with emergent groups* (high confidence in the evidence). This finding is supported by seven qualitative studies (Bromley et al., 2017; Cuervo et al., 2017; Gagnon et al., 2016; Ingham and Redshaw, 2017; Messias et al., 2012; Miller et al., 2015; Peterson et al., 2019).

Specifically with regard to training, when possible, sponsorship of trainings and provision of monetary incentives may encourage participation and engagement in training activities while minimizing accessibility barriers due to affordability issues (Bromley et al., 2017; Cha et al., 2016; Cuervo et al., 2017; Gin et al., 2016; Hipper et al., 2015; Kamau, 2017; Laborde et al., 2011, 2013).

Case Report Evidence Synthesis

Few case reports address the feasibility of their engagement strategies, although two cite the successful recruitment of CBPs and their willingness to participate in collaborations as evidence of the feasibility of engagement and training initiatives (McCabe et al., 2011, 2013). Still, many note that limited capacity, time, and resources of CBOs, such as CHCs and tribal organizations, can impede engagement because of issues of understaffing, employee turnover, and competing priorities (Chandra et al., 2015; Gebbie et al., 2009; Klaiman et al., 2010; Koh et al., 2006; Levin et al., 2014; Peate and Mullins, 2008). With regard to leveraging FBOs, legal issues regarding separation of church and state are also noted as a potential area for concern (Kiser and Lovelace, 2019; McCabe et al., 2013; Plough et al., 2011). Guidelines in accordance with the U.S. and state constitutions that include non-discriminatory requirements, separation of public health services and religious activities, and no furthering of religious activities may be helpful in addressing this issue (Kiser and Lovelace, 2019).

Descriptive Survey Study Evidence

Five descriptive surveys support the finding from the qualitative evidence synthesis regarding capacity constraints (e.g., human resources, funding) as a commonly cited barrier to engagement and training (raised by both the CBPs and public health agencies). Baezconde-Garbanati and colleagues (2006) report that among Hispanic-serving CBOs that had recently participated in an emergency response, 50 percent said their resources and capabilities had been exceeded when responding, and 96 percent of those surveyed indicated they received little or no funding for public health emergency preparedness. Regarding commonly experienced barriers to integration into community preparedness activities, a national sample of CHCs cited a number of resource and capacity limitations, including staff limitations and time constraints (70 percent), lack of funding for training and equipment (59 percent), and lack of reimbursement (20 percent), as well as the perception that the role of the CHC is not understood by community emergency planners (57 percent) (Wineman et al., 2007).

Adams and colleagues (2018) surveyed LHD preparedness directors nationally and used a multiple linear regression model to identify characteristics of LHDs that enhance collaborations with CBOs and FBOs for emergency preparedness and response. The survey results highlight the importance of LHD staff capacity. Bevc and colleagues (2014) found that with regard to barriers to establishing and maintaining partnerships, 60 percent of LHD respondents reported lack of resources to train community partners, 41 percent cited concerns about high staff turnover, and 37 percent reported lack of skilled and/or experienced staff. When identifying challenges to partnership building with CBPs, staff of the Los Angeles County Department of Public Health cited lack of training on engagement (23 percent), burden of maintaining relationships (12 percent), capacity limitations of CBPs (15 percent), perception of lack of trust by CBPs (5 percent), and lack of interest from the community (10 percent) or the public health staff (14 percent) (Chi et al., 2015).

5. Resource and Economic Considerations

Qualitative Evidence Synthesis

As discussed above, CBPs may perceive participation in collaborations and training related to PHEPR as doing more with no concomitant increase in resources or funding (Cha et al., 2016). This dynamic often discourages collaboration and, to a lesser degree, participation in trainings. It is therefore important to leverage current practices and frame preparedness efforts as an adaptation of existing activities rather than as additional services (Schoch-Spana et al., 2013; Stajura et al., 2012).

Importantly, the qualitative studies included in this review indicate that building and maintaining collaborations requires long-term investment (Cha et al., 2016; Schoch-Spana et al., 2013; Stajura et al., 2012). If federal policy makers decide to embrace and promote collaborations and training, they will need to do so with an understanding of the need for longitudinal funding and appropriate outcome evaluations (Gin et al., 2016; Peterson et al., 2019; Stajura et al., 2012), which also require dedicated financial support (Kamau et al., 2017).

Case Report Evidence Synthesis

Few case reports address resource and economic considerations, but those that do point to resource constraints impeding the ability to attend trainings (e.g., lack of travel funds) or competing needs faced by underfunded tribal health programs (Peate and Mullins, 2008). Issues of staff turnover, inadequate staffing, and competing priorities are also considerations for CBPs with limited resources. The case report evidence thus supports the critical need for policy makers and funders to recognize the time required to establish and maintain authentic partnerships and make continued investments to facilitate effective long-term engagement of CBPs (Wells et al., 2013).

6. Equity

Qualitative Evidence Synthesis

When CBPs and the at-risk populations they serve see themselves represented in community preparedness initiatives, they are more likely to engage in such efforts (Charania and Tsuji, 2012; Peterson et al., 2019). Messias and colleagues (2012) report that inclusion helps combat feelings of being discounted. Equally important, inclusion helps mitigate ongoing histories of distrust and mistrust associated with government or government-supported initiatives (Eisenman et al., 2009). Gin and colleagues (2016) and Stajura and colleagues (2012) discuss how some CBPs see local health departments as focused on "the visible, recognized, or active CBOs and FBOs" to the exclusion of others, which reinforces feelings of marginalization (Cordasco et al., 2007; Gin et al., 2016; Rowel et al., 2012). This marginalization occurs in collaborations and in trainings that target and are tailored for some CBPs to the exclusion of others (Laborde et al., 2011, 2013). If such concerns are not addressed in future collaboration initiatives, many CBPs will continue to be underrepresented, with continued marginalization of the at-risk populations with which they work.

Case Report Evidence Synthesis

None of the case reports assess equitable outcomes; however, some do note historical context and an inadequate focus on addressing the unique needs of underserved populations as defined by such factors as race, access and functional needs, and income (Wells et al., 2013). The CBPR model promotes two-way knowledge exchange across diverse stakeholders, with a focus on equal power and authority of community and academic partners to develop and evaluate programs while building community capacity to use the research findings. Implementing such models may help promote equitable outcomes, mutual respect, and inclusive participation.

For some case reports, it is unclear the extent to which their participants are representative of the populations intended to be served. For instance, FBOs are described mainly as churches (McCabe et al., 2013). Thus, it is possible that people belonging to smaller faith-based communities were overlooked in planning processes and that the case report findings may not be generalizable to other communities. To further promote equitable distribution of resources and improved outcomes, public health agencies need to focus intentionally on issues of equity and social justice when engaging CBPs.

7. Ethical Considerations[4]

The section on equity above notes several ways in which engaging communities, when done well, can promote the ethical principles of justice, or fairness, and equity. The earlier section on balancing benefits and harms also describes some ways in which poorly designed or implemented engagement efforts, even when intended to promote principles of transparency and accountability, can generate mistrust, frustration, or alienation. Overall, these observations suggest that engaging communities is ethically justified if it achieves harm reduction/benefit promotion for relevant stakeholders. Similarly, if engaging communities in preparedness activities is an efficient means of achieving better preparedness, it is supported by the principle of stewardship, which is often considered to be of special importance in public health emergencies when resources can be very limited. Still, it is important to bear in mind that community engagement, like all human relationships, also can hold intrinsic value. That is, building open and trusting relationships is important because it reflects the value placed by society on respect for persons and communities. The principle of respect for persons and communities posits that one has a fundamental obligation to engage people in decisions that might affect their well-being and the well-being of those they care about, and this holds true even if doing so does not change ultimate decisions.

[4] Ethical considerations included in this section were generated through committee discussions, drawing on the ethical principles laid out in Box 3-4 in Chapter 3 and key ethics and policy texts, including the 2009 Institute of Medicine letter report on crisis standards of care (IOM, 2009), the 2008 Centers for Disease Control and Prevention white paper "Ethical Guidance for Public Health Emergency Preparedness and Response: Highlighting Ethics and Values in a Vital Public Health Service" (Jennings and Arras, 2008), *Emergency Ethics: Public Health Preparedness and Response* (Jennings et al., 2016), and *The Oxford Handbook of Public Health Ethics* (Mastroianni et al., 2019).

TABLE B1-10 Evidence to Decision Summary Table for Engaging with and Training Community-Based Partners

<table>
<tr><th colspan="2">What is the effectiveness of different strategies for engaging with and training community-based partners to improve the outcomes of at-risk populations after public health emergencies?</th></tr>
<tr><td>Balance of Benefits and Harms

Engagement and training of community-based partners (CBPs) in public health emergency preparedness and response (PHEPR) can benefit communities in multiple ways, particularly when undertaken using a participatory approach and, in the context of multistakeholder collaborations, when inclusive of diverse membership. These benefits can be observed at multiple levels:

• Individual level—increased reach to at-risk populations, many of which are traditionally underserved, which may improve at-risk individuals' PHEPR knowledge and preparedness behaviors, as well as access to critical services following a public health emergency.
• Organizational level—enhanced CBP PHEPR knowledge and preparedness to meet the needs of at-risk individuals; CBP capacity building; improved mutual awareness of existing community and organizational roles and capacities during routine times to better leverage them during an emergency and to identify gaps.
• Community and system level—relationship building that may benefit routine operations, create opportunities for new collaborations, and facilitate coordination of partners during emergencies; enhanced CBP inclusion and shared sense of ownership of community preparedness efforts; greater appreciation of varied community and cultural perspectives and improved cultural competence; opportunities for shared learning; enhanced trust.

There are also a number of potential undesirable effects, including the potential to raise difficult and uncomfortable issues (e.g., implicit bias, marginalization), disenchantment with preparedness-focused collaborations when past collaborations have failed to achieve desired results or members have had negative experiences, disenchantment with preparedness training if there are no opportunities to apply it, and exacerbation of trust and confidence issues if collaborations cannot be sustained because of the often short-term nature of preparedness funding or changing priorities.</td><td>Sources of Evidence

• Synthesis of evidence of effect
• Qualitative evidence synthesis
• Case report evidence synthesis (no assessment of certainty or confidence)</td></tr>
<tr><td>Acceptability and Preferences

CBPs generally value inclusion and shared ownership of community preparedness efforts and are willing to collaborate with public health agencies. Participatory approaches, leadership support, organizational commitment to CBP engagement and training, and transparency are likely to be important facilitators of acceptability. Some public health departments may require an internal culture change to embrace and align with a community partnering approach. Reframing public health emergency preparedness activities to include a commitment to leveraging existing community health activities, along with a strong emphasis on health equity in all activities, can facilitate this organizational shift toward collaborative strategies and community preparedness.</td><td>Sources of Evidence

• Qualitative evidence synthesis
• Case report evidence synthesis (no assessment of certainty or confidence)
• Descriptive survey study evidence (no synthesis)</td></tr>
<tr><td>Feasibility and PHEPR System Considerations

Engaging with and training CBPs to improve the outcomes of at-risk populations may be time and resource intensive, with intensity varying depending on the specific strategy. Capacity challenges (e.g., human and nonhuman resource limitations, policy impediments) and competing priorities, for both public health organizations and CBPs, are likely to be common barriers. Feasibility may be improved by working strategically to reduce capacity-related barriers through financial support and by leveraging opportunities to expand capacity, for example, through coordination. Studies note legal issues regarding separation of church and state as a potential area for consideration when engaging faith-based organizations. Guidelines in accordance with the U.S. and state constitutions that include nondiscriminatory requirements, separation of public health services and religious activities, and no furthering of religious activities may be helpful in addressing this issue.</td><td>Sources of Evidence

• Qualitative evidence synthesis
• Case report evidence synthesis (no assessment of certainty or confidence)
• Descriptive survey study evidence (no synthesis)</td></tr>
</table>

TABLE B1-10 Continued

Resource and Economic Considerations	Sources of Evidence
Community preparedness efforts may be perceived as having to do more with no concomitant increase in resources. Framing preparedness efforts as an adaptation of existing activities rather than as additional services may reduce concerns regarding resource requirements. Many CBPs and public health agencies are already facing challenges in sustaining underfunded programs while dealing with high staff turnover, which may discourage engagement efforts and impede the ability of CBP representatives to attend trainings. Competing priorities for limited resources may necessitate prioritization of engagement and training initiatives, but identifying opportunities to leverage existing resources and programs can help address financial constraints. Collaboration building and maintenance require a long-term investment. Such activities need to be undertaken with an understanding of the importance of longitudinal funding and appropriate outcome evaluations. Failure to sustain partnerships and lack of clear outcomes from engagement and training initiatives may contribute to disenchantment with preparedness-related engagement efforts.	• Qualitative evidence synthesis • Case report evidence synthesis (no assessment of certainty or confidence)
Equity	**Sources of Evidence**
Although none of the studies included in this review assess the potential effects on equity outcomes, engagement and training of CBPs is presumed to yield equity-related benefits by mitigating the often disproportionate effects of disasters on at-risk populations, many of which have been marginalized historically. The body of qualitative studies suggests that representation and meaningful participation in community preparedness efforts may help counteract feelings of being discounted and mitigate mistrust associated with government initiatives in some populations. In the absence of an inclusive approach to engagement and training, however, many CBPs will continue to be underrepresented, with continued marginalization of the at-risk populations with whom they work. Such models as community-based participatory research that promote two-way knowledge exchange, equal power in the development and evaluation of programs, and building of community capacity to apply findings may help promote equitable outcomes, mutual respect, and inclusive participation, but this is an important research gap. Equity outcomes need to be measured in future studies to better capture the opportunities to embrace a health equity framing and community asset approach to CBP engagement and preparedness training. Careful attention is needed to ensure that participants in CBP engagement and training efforts are representative of the populations intended to be served.	• Qualitative evidence synthesis • Case report evidence synthesis (no assessment of certainty or confidence)
Ethical Considerations	**Source of Evidence**
Engaging communities, when done well, can promote the ethical principles of justice, or fairness, and equity. However, poorly designed or implemented engagement efforts, even when intended to promote principles of transparency and accountability, can generate mistrust, frustration, or alienation. Overall, these observations suggest that engaging communities is ethically justified if it achieves harm reduction/benefit promotion for relevant stakeholders. Similarly, if engaging communities in preparedness activities is an efficient means of achieving better preparedness, it is supported by the principle of stewardship, which is often considered to be of special importance in public health emergencies when resources can be very limited. Still, it is important to bear in mind that community engagement, like all human relationships, also can hold intrinsic value. That is, building open and trusting relationships is important because it reflects the value placed on respect for persons and communities. The principle of respect for persons and communities posits that one has a fundamental obligation to engage people in decisions that might affect their well-being and the well-being of those they care about, and this holds true even if doing so does not change ultimate decisions.	• Committee discussion drawing on key ethics and policy texts

CONSIDERATIONS FOR IMPLEMENTATION

The following considerations for implementation were drawn from the qualitative evidence synthesis and case report evidence synthesis.

8. Facilitators for CBP Engagement

Qualitative Evidence Synthesis

Twelve qualitative studies (Andrulis et al., 2011; Bromley et al., 2017; Charania and Tsuji, 2012; Cuervo et al., 2017; Gagnon et al., 2016; Gin et al., 2018; Ingham and Redshaw, 2017; Laborde et al., 2013; Miller et al., 2015; Peterson et al., 2019; Rowel et al., 2012; Schoch-Spana et al., 2013) support a finding that *a participatory approach appears to improve engagement and training of CBPs. Involvement in research and programmatic efforts from conceptualization to implementation may correspond to more effective engagement and training through enhanced inclusion, cultural acceptability, shared ownership, and capacity building of community members* (high confidence in the evidence). Moreover, *collaborations are more likely to be effective in improving the outcomes of at-risk populations when CBP membership is diverse and inclusive. This means ensuring the inclusion of CBPs traditionally ignored or marginalized, some of which may have strong ties to at-risk populations and experiences that may increase the incorporation of diverse cultural perspectives* (high confidence in the evidence). This finding is supported by 15 qualitative studies (Andrulis et al., 2011; Bromley et al., 2017; Cha et al., 2016; Charania and Tsuji, 2012; Cordasco et al., 2007; Cuervo et al., 2017; Gagnon et al., 2016; Gin et al., 2016, 2018; Ingham and Redshaw, 2017; Laborde et al., 2011; Miller et al., 2015; Peterson et al., 2019; Rowel et al., 2012; Stajura et al., 2012).

Ten qualitative studies (Andrulis et al., 2011; Bromley et al., 2017; Charania and Tsuji, 2012; Gagnon et al., 2016; Hipper et al., 2015; Ingham and Redshaw, 2017; Miller et al., 2015; Peterson et al., 2019; Schoch-Spana et al., 2013; Stajura et al., 2012) indicate that *the effectiveness of collaborations will likely be improved when there is shared understanding and acceptance of operating aspects* (high confidence in the evidence). Four studies (Gin et al., 2016; Peterson et al., 2019; Schoch-Spana et al., 2013; Shih et al., 2018) support a need to ensure *clarity of a collaboration's purpose and goals* (moderate confidence in the evidence). A clearly articulated purpose may help invited members determine the value of their engagement in the collaboration (Gagnon et al., 2016; Shih et al., 2018). Attention also is necessary to building a shared language (rather than elevating or marginalizing a particular sector's vocabulary) to foster constructive and productive relationships (Bromley et al., 2017; Ingham and Redshaw, 2017; Schoch-Spana et al., 2013). Eight qualitative studies (Bromley et al., 2017; Cha et al., 2016; Gin et al., 2016, 2018; Hipper et al., 2015; Ingham and Redshaw, 2017; Shih et al., 2018; Stajura et al., 2012) show that *collaborations are more likely to be effective when they operate with a shared language, whereas an imposed language is likely to be off-putting and perceived by many to carry biases that privilege some members over others* (moderate confidence in the evidence). The qualitative evidence also provides some indication that resiliency and response resonate better than planning, preparedness, recovery, and response as guiding concepts, and therefore facilitate discussions and actions related to emergency and routine operations (Bromley et al., 2017; Cha et al., 2016; Cuervo et al., 2017; Shih et al., 2018).

Collaborations likely include members accustomed to specific decision-making principles. Notably, some studies suggest a divide in principles between emergency managers and CBPs. Emergency managers typically rely on hierarchical rather than horizontal (or consensus) decision-making principles, a perspective that contrasts with the principles utilized by many CBPs. Collaborations will likely be more effective if they bridge these divides proactively (Cha et al., 2016; Cuervo et al., 2017; Ingham and Redshaw, 2017; Peterson et al., 2019; Stajura et al., 2012). Collaborations likely also will be more effective given shared ownership and the absence of perceived abuses or unacceptable differences in power (Cha et al., 2016; Gagnon et al., 2016; Stajura et al., 2012). A sense of ownership usually elevates the priority of coalitions and partnerships and improves outcomes.

Written agreements to manage membership expectations and responsibilities may facilitate CBP engagement. Nine qualitative studies (Bromley et al., 2017; Cha et al., 2016; Charania and Tsuji, 2012; Hipper et al., 2015; Ingham and Redshaw, 2017; Miller et al., 2015; Peterson et al., 2019; Schoch-Spana et al., 2013, Stajura et al., 2012) support a finding that *agreements may help formalize the nature of membership roles and responsibilities in collaborations (including definition of what constitutes participation and engagement), which in turn may minimize conflicts over inequitable participation. It is important for collaborations to retain flexibility and attempt to accommodate different CBP realities* (high confidence in the evidence). Important elements of such agreements include expectations of attendance, participation, engagement, roles of individual members within the coalition, and organizational commitment, among others (Cha et al., 2016; Gin et al., 2016, 2018; Hipper et al., 2015; Ingham and Redshaw, 2017; Rowel et al., 2012). Stajura and colleagues (2012) report on the concerns of smaller and rural CBPs about contractual agreements. Such concerns may be mitigated by openly addressing how perceived barriers and harms from past experiences will be minimized (Bromley et al., 2017; Cha et al., 2016; Charania and Tsuji, 2012; Hipper et al., 2015; Ingham and Redshaw, 2017; Peterson et al., 2019; Schoch-Spana et al., 2013, Stajura et al., 2012).

In addition to formalized agreements, a coalition and partnership coordinator may help protect CBP members from unmanageable workloads, maintain the focus of the coalition, mitigate problems associated with competing priorities, and minimize perceptions of uneven power dynamics among the coalition members (Bromley et al., 2017; Cha et al., 2016; Gagnon et al., 2016; Miller et al., 2015). A coordinator position may merit a full-time position, so it is ill advised to add those responsibilities to the work of an already overburdened employee (Hipper et al., 2015; Stajura et al., 2012). Gagnon and colleagues (2016) report an example in which two coalition members could perform the leadership roles effectively, an approach that may alleviate the burden for any one member.

Case Report Evidence Synthesis

The case report evidence shows that effective engagement of CBPs is tied to efforts to maintain culturally competent trainings and services aligned with the needs of the target audience, which, although time consuming, is important (McCabe et al., 2011; Peate and Mullins, 2008; Wells et al., 2013). The ability to bridge language differences among collaboration members can facilitate alignment of efforts by public health agencies and FBOs as well (Kiser and Lovelace, 2019). Communication mechanisms may also help foster more effective engagement. For instance, bidirectional communication via a free and accessible quarterly health newsletter to CBOs serving vulnerable populations was found to enable greater trust and buy-in prior to an emergency, which could then be leveraged during an emergency (Klaiman et al., 2010). In addition, engaging umbrella organizations may serve to connect local public health departments with smaller, local CBOs to which they would otherwise lack access (Klaiman et al., 2010). Trust may also be built by developing connections with populations that are not formally served by an agency or provider through outreach to neighborhood and grassroots groups, including FBOs and limited-English-speaking communities (Klaiman et al., 2010).

During public health emergencies, leveraging information technology, such as a community-based resource database, may facilitate timely engagement of CBPs and link at-risk populations with needed services. A pilot study in Georgia involved implementing such a database through collaboration with local American Red Cross chapters and public and private community organizations. The Metropolitan Atlanta Chapter of Red Cross in Georgia used this database to better serve clients displaced by Hurricane Katrina with accurate information and locations for referrals (Troy et al., 2008). Another potential facilitator is the use of data already collected by agencies serving vulnerable populations, which could be centrally managed in a shared database and stripped of any identifying or confidential information (Klaiman et al., 2010).

9. Facilitators for CBP Training

Qualitative Evidence Synthesis

Eleven qualitative studies (Ablah et al., 2008; Bromley et al., 2017; Cha et al., 2016; Gin et al., 2016, 2018; Hipper et al., 2015; Kamau et al., 2017; Laborde et al., 2011; Rowel et al., 2012; Schoch-Spana et al., 2013; Stajura et al., 2012) show that *targeting specific learners and learning needs is likely to improve the effectiveness of trainings for CBPs* (high confidence in the evidence). Targeting the specific needs of CBPs helps with recruiting and engaging trainees and facilitates the translation of learning into practice (Schoch-Spana et al., 2013). Additionally, *tailoring with multifaceted strategies is likely to improve the effectiveness of training for CBPs* (high confidence in the evidence), a finding supported by 11 qualitative studies (Ablah et al., 2008; Andrulis et al., 2011; Bromley et al., 2017; Cuervo et al., 2017; Eisenman et al., 2009; Gin et al., 2016; Hipper et al., 2015; Kamau et al., 2017; Laborde et al., 2011, 2013; Rowel et al., 2012). Such strategies may include the following:

- Customize the curriculum to identified needs and specified learning outcomes (Ablah et al., 2008; Bromley et al., 2017; Cuervo et al., 2017; Gin et al., 2016; Kamau et al., 2017; Laborde et al., 2011, 2013; Rowel et al., 2012).
- Create and adapt training and utilized resources so that they are culturally sensitive and appropriate (Ablah et al., 2008; Bromley et al., 2017; Cuervo et al., 2017; Eisenman et al., 2009; Laborde et al., 2011, 2013; Rowel et al., 2012).
- Identify capable, credible, and trusted trainers from the learners' perspective. Potential trainers may include *promatoras* and trainers developed through train-the-trainer models (Bromley et al., 2017; Cuervo et al., 2017; Eisenman et al., 2009; Ingham and Redshaw, 2017; Kamau et al., 2017; Laborde et al., 2011, 2013; Rowel et al., 2012).
- Determine and utilize learner preferences for training methods, such as collaborative learning, tabletop exercises, hands-on experiences, interactive games, and small-group discussions. Multiple methods may be used within a training session (Ablah et al., 2008; Bromley et al., 2017; Eisenman et al., 2009; Ingham and Redshaw, 2017; Laborde et al., 2011, 2013).
- Adjust the length of any training session to accommodate learners' attention spans and time availability (Ablah et al., 2008; Laborde et al., 2011).
- Customize training channels to learners' preferences, and possibly to align with behaviors during emergencies. Channels that have been described include face-to-face and virtual modes of learning, among others. Trainings may also use multiple channels (Ablah et al., 2008; Bromley et al., 2017; Kamau et al., 2017; Laborde et al., 2011, 2013).
- Facilitate bidirectional discussion, interaction, and feedback loops in training activities (Ablah et al., 2008; Bromley et al., 2017; Kamau et al., 2017; Laborde et al., 2011, 2013).

- Consider the timing of training. Most training for preparedness will take place before an emergency, yet just-in-time training may facilitate the transfer of learned knowledge to actual response (Bromley et al., 2017; Hipper et al., 2015).
- Consider the location of training, whether physical or virtual, and its accessibility to learners (Bromley et al., 2017; Eisenman et al., 2009; Hipper et al., 2015; Laborde et al., 2011).
- Provide affordable training (Gin et al., 2016; Kamau et al., 2017; Laborde et al., 2011, 2013).
- Evaluate training and facilitate opportunities for deliberate practice (Ablah et al., 2008; Cuervo et al., 2017; Kamau et al., 2017; Laborde et al., 2013).

Case Report Evidence Synthesis

As noted above, effective engagement of CBPs has been found to be tied to efforts to maintain culturally competent trainings and services aligned with the needs of the target audience (McCabe et al., 2011; Peate and Mullins, 2008; Wells et al., 2013). Integrating evaluation of program materials, training content, and message dissemination mechanisms via focus groups, surveys, and stakeholder feedback can also help ensure the quality of materials and promote stakeholder buy-in (Bouye et al., 2009; Klaiman et al., 2010). It is important to note as well that providers serving vulnerable populations may themselves be directly impacted by an emergency as community members. Thus, the issue of personal preparedness and self-care needs to be stressed during trainings for CBPs, as it can play a role in promoting buy-in for their role as promoters of client preparedness and may enable them to serve those in need more effectively (Levin et al., 2014; Wells et al., 2013).

REFERENCES FOR ARTICLES INCLUDED IN THE MIXED-METHOD REVIEW

Quantitative Comparative Studies

Bromley, E., D. P. Eisenman, A. Magana, M. Williams, B. Kim, M. McCreary, A. Chandra, and K. B. Wells. 2017. How do communities use a participatory public health approach to build resilience? The Los Angeles County Community Disaster Resilience Project. *International Journal of Environmental Research and Public Health* 14(10).

Coady, M. H., S. Galea, S. Blaney, D. C. Ompad, S. Sisco, D. Vlahov, and Project Viva Intervention Working Group. 2008. Project Viva: A multilevel community-based intervention to increase influenza vaccination rates among hard-to-reach populations in New York City. *American Journal of Public Health* 98(7):1314–1321.

Eisenman, D. P., D. Glik, L. Gonzalez, R. Maranon, Q. Zhou, C. H. Tseng, and S. M. Asch. 2009. Improving Latino disaster preparedness using social networks. *American Journal of Preventive Medicine* 37(6):512–517.

Eisenman, D. P., A. Bazzano, D. Koniak-Griffin, C. H. Tseng, M. A. Lewis, K. Lamb, and D. Lehrer. 2014. Peer-mentored preparedness (PM-PREP): A new disaster preparedness program for adults living independently in the community. *Intellectual and Developmental Disabilities* 52(1):49–59.

Hites, L. S., B. S. Granillo, E. R. Garrison, A. D. Cimetta, V. J. Serafin, R. F. Renger, J. F. Wakelee, and J. L. Burgess. 2012. Emergency preparedness training of tribal community health representatives. *Journal of Immigrant & Minority Health* 14(2):323–329.

McCabe, O. L., N. L. Semon, C. B. Thompson, J. M. Lating, G. S. Everly, Jr., C. J. Perry, S. S. Moore, A. M. Mosley, and J. M. Links. 2014a. Building a national model of public mental health preparedness and community resilience: Validation of a dual-intervention, systems-based approach. *Disaster Medicine and Public Health Preparedness* 8(6):511–526.

McCabe, O. L., N. L. Semon, J. M. Lating, G. S. Everly, Jr., C. J. Perry, S. S. Moore, A. M. Mosley, C. B. Thompson, and J. M. Links. 2014b. An academic-government-faith partnership to build disaster mental health preparedness and community resilience. *Public Health Reports* 129(Suppl 4):96–106.

Montgomery County Department of Health and Human Services. 2008. *Emergency preparedness education for the Latino community conducted by health promoters: A mini pilot project.* http://www.cidrap.umn.edu/sites/default/files/public/php/347/347_report.pdf (accessed April 1, 2020).

Williams, M. V., A. Chandra, A. Spears, D. Varda, K. B. Wells, A. L. Plough, and D. P. Eisenman. 2018. Evaluating community partnerships addressing community resilience in Los Angeles, California. *International Journal of Environmental Research and Public Health* 15(4).

Quantitative Noncomparative Studies

Laborde, D. J., K. Magruder, J. Caye, and T. Parrish. 2013. Feasibility of disaster mental health preparedness training for black communities. *Disaster Medicine and Public Health Preparedness* 7(3):302–312.

McCabe, O. L., A. M. Mosley, H. S. Gwon, G. S. Everly, Jr., J. M. Lating, J. M. Links, and M. J. Kaminsky. 2008. The tower of ivory meets the house of worship: Psychological first aid training for the faith community. *International Journal of Emergency Mental Health and Human Resilience* 9(3):171–180.

McCabe, O. L., C. Perry, M. Azur, H. G. Taylor, M. Bailey, and J. M. Links. 2011. Psychological first-aid training for paraprofessionals: A systems-based model for enhancing capacity of rural emergency responses. *Prehospital and Disaster Medicine* 26(4):251–258.

McCabe, O. L., C. Perry, M. Azur, H. G. Taylor, H. Gwon, A. Mosley, N. Semon, and J. M. Links. 2013. Guided preparedness planning with lay communities: Enhancing capacity of rural emergency response through a systems-based partnership. *Prehospital and Disaster Medicine* 28(1):8–15.

Qualitative Studies

Ablah, E., A. M. Tinius, L. Horn, C. Williams, and K. M. Gebbie. 2008. Community health centers and emergency preparedness: An assessment of competencies and training needs. *Journal of Community Health* 33(4):241–247.

Andrulis, D. P., N. J. Siddiqui, and J. P. Purtle. 2011. Integrating racially and ethnically diverse communities into planning for disasters: The California experience. *Disaster Medicine and Public Health Preparedness* 5(3):227–234.

Bromley, E., D. P. Eisenman, A. Magana, M. Williams, B. Kim, M. McCreary, A. Chandra, and K. B. Wells. 2017. How do communities use a participatory public health approach to build resilience? The Los Angeles County Community Disaster Resilience Project. *International Journal of Environmental Research and Public Health* 14(10).

Cha, B. S., R. I. Lawrence, J. C. Bliss, K. B. Wells, A. Chandra, and D. P. Eisenman. 2016. The road to resilience: Insights on training community coalitions in the Los Angeles County Community Disaster Resilience Project. *Disaster Medicine and Public Health Preparedness* 10(6):812–821.

Charania, N. A., and L. J. Tsuji. 2012. A community-based participatory approach and engagement process creates culturally appropriate and community informed pandemic plans after the 2009 H1N1 influenza pandemic: Remote and isolated First Nations communities of sub-arctic Ontario, Canada. *BMC Public Health* 12:268.

Cordasco, K. M. E., D. P. Eisenmann, D. C. Glik, J. F. Golden, and S. M. Asch. 2007. "They blew the levee": Distrust of authorities among Hurricane Katrina evacuees. *Journal of Healthcare for the Poor and Underserved* 18(2):277–282.

Cuervo, I., L. Leopold, and S. Baron. 2017. Promoting community preparedness and resilience: A Latino immigrant community-driven project following Hurricane Sandy. *American Journal of Public Health* 107(S2):S161–S164.

Eisenman, D. P., D. Glik, R. Maranon, L. Gonzales, and S. Asch. 2009. Developing a disaster preparedness campaign targeting low-income Latino immigrants: Focus group results for project PREP. *Journal of Health Care for the Poor and Underserved* 20(2):330–345.

Gagnon, E., T. O'Sullivan, D. E. Lane, and N. Pare. 2016. Exploring partnership functioning within a community-based participatory intervention to improve disaster resilience. *Journal of Higher Education Outreach and Engagement* 20(2):25–52.

Gin, J. L., R. Saia, A. Dobalian, and D. Kranke. 2016. Disaster preparedness in homeless residential organizations in Los Angeles County: Identifying needs, assessing gaps. *Natural Hazards Review* 17(1).

Gin, J. L., R. K. Eisner, C. Der-Martirosian, D. Kranke, and A. Dobalian. 2018. Preparedness is a marathon, not a sprint: A tiered maturity model for assessing preparedness in homeless residential organizations in Los Angeles. *Natural Hazards Review* 19(1).

Hipper, T. J., A. Orr, and E. Chernak. 2015. Are human service agencies ready for disasters? Findings from a mixed-methods needs assessment and planning project. *Health Security* 13(2):106–114.

Ingham, V., and S. Redshaw. 2017. Connecting community organisations for disaster preparedness. *International Journal of Safety and Security Engineering* 7(1):52–64.

Kamau, P. W., S. L. Ivey, S. E. Griese, and S. H. Qari. 2017. Preparedness training programs for working with deaf and hard of hearing communities and older adults: Lessons learned from key informants and literature assessments. *Disaster Medicine and Public Health Preparedness* 12(5):606–614.
Laborde, D. J., K. Brannock, and T. Parrish. 2011. Assessment of training needs for disaster mental health preparedness in black communities. *Journal of the National Medical Association* 103(7):624–634.
Laborde, D. J., K. Magruder, J. Caye, and T. Parrish. 2013. Feasibility of disaster mental health preparedness training for black communities. *Disaster Medicine and Public Health Preparedness* 7(3):302–312.
Messias, D. K. H., C. Barrington, and E. Lacy. 2012. Latino social network dynamics and the Hurricane Katrina disaster. *Disasters* 36(1):101–121.
Miller, A., P. D. Massey, J. Judd, J. Kelly, D. N. Durrheim, A. R. Clough, R. Speare, and S. Saggers. 2015. Using a participatory action research framework to listen to aboriginal and Torres Strait islander people in Australia about pandemic influenza. *Rural & Remote Health* 15(3):2923.
Peterson, P., P. McNabb, S. R. Maddali, J. Heath, and S. Santibanez. 2019. Engaging communities to reach immigrant and minority populations: The Minnesota Immunization Networking Initiative (MINI), 2006–2017. *Public Health Reports* 134(3):241–248.
Rowel, R., P. Sheikhattari, T. M. Barber, and M. Evans-Holland. 2012. Introduction of a guide to enhance risk communication among low-income and minority populations: A grassroots community engagement approach. *Health Promotion Practice* 13(1):124–132.
Schoch-Spana, M., T. K. Sell, and R. Morhard. 2013. Local health department capacity for community engagement and its implications for disaster resilience. *Biosecurity and Bioterrorism* 11(2):118–129.
Shih, R. A., J. D. Acosta, E. K. Chen, E. G. Carbone, L. Xenakis, D. M. Adamson, and A. Chandra. 2018. *Improving disaster resilience among older adults: Insights from public health departments and aging-in-place efforts.* Santa Monica, CA. https://pdfs.semanticscholar.org/1c8d/f1f242c17beed8f6884a3b7887da0a41bc60.pdf?_ga=2.206505498.82203835.1585740408-540380720.1583341124 (accessed April 1, 2020).
Stajura, M., D. Glik, D. Eisenman, M. Prelip, A. Martel, and J. Sammartinova. 2012. Perspectives of community- and faith-based organizations about partnering with local health departments for disasters. *International Journal of Environmental Research and Public Health* 9(7):2293–2311.

Descriptive Survey Studies

Ablah, E., K. S. Konda, K. Konda, M. Melbourne, J. N. Ingoglia, and K. M. Gebbie. 2010. Emergency preparedness training and response among community health centers and local health departments: Results from a multistate survey. *Journal of Community Health* 35(3):285–293.
Adams, R. M., M. L. Prelip, D. C. Glik, I. Donatello, and D. P. Eisenman. 2018. Facilitating partnerships with community- and faith-based organizations for disaster preparedness and response: Results of a national survey of public health departments. *Disaster Medicine and Public Health Preparedness* 12(1):57–66.
Baezconde-Garbanati, L., J. Unger, C. Portugal, J. L. Delgado, A. Falcon, and M. Gaitan. 2006. Maximizing participation of Hispanic community-based/non-governmental organizations (NGOs) in emergency preparedness. *International Quarterly of Community Health Education* 24(4):289–317.
Bevc, C. A., M. C. Simon, T. A. Montoya, and J. A. Horney. 2014. Institutional facilitators and barriers to local public health preparedness planning for vulnerable and at-risk populations. *Public Health Reports* 129(Suppl 4):35–41.
Chi, G. C., M. Williams, A. Chandra, A. Plough, and D. Eisenman. 2015. Partnerships for community resilience: Perspectives from the Los Angeles County Community Disaster Resilience Project. *Public Health.* http://www.escholarship.org/uc/item/30f4f1kf (accessed February 5, 2020).
Schoch-Spana, M., F. W. Selck, and L. A. Goldberg. 2015. A national survey on health department capacity for community engagement in emergency preparedness. *Journal of Public Health Management and Practice* 21(2):196–207.
Wineman, N. V., B. I. Braun, J. A. Barbera, and J. M. Loeb. 2007. Assessing the integration of health center and community emergency preparedness and response planning. *Disaster Medicine and Public Health Preparedness* 1(2):96–105.

Case Reports

Bouye, K., B. I. Truman, S. Hutchins, R. Richard, C. Brown, J. A. Guillory, and J. Rashid. 2009. Pandemic influenza preparedness and response among public-housing residents, single-parent families, and low-income populations. *American Journal of Public Health* 99(Suppl 2):S287–S293.

Chandra, A., M. V. Williams, C. Lopez, J. Tang, D. Eisenman, and A. Magana. 2015. Developing a tabletop exercise to test community resilience: Lessons from the Los Angeles County Community Disaster Resilience Project. *Disaster Medicine and Public Health Preparedness* 9(5):484–488.

Cripps, J. H., S. B. Cooper, and E. N. Austin. 2016. Emergency preparedness with people who sign: Toward the whole community approach. *Journal of Emergency Management* 14(2):101–111.

Gebbie, K. M., L. Horn, M. McCollum, and K. O Hara. 2009. Building a system for preparedness: The NYCEPCE NEST experience. *Journal of Public Health Management and Practice* 15(2 Suppl):S3–S7.

Howard, K. K., C. S. Amie, B. Janette, B. Jon, D. B. Paul, M. S. Crowther, A. S. Richard, R. C. Bradley, A. N. Gilbert, C. L. Mary, M. J. Christine, H. C. Paul, H. B. Kathryn, and A. John. 2006. Building community-based surge capacity through a public health and academic collaboration: The role of community health centers. *Public Health Reports* 121(2):211–216.

Kiser, M., and K. Lovelace. 2019. A national network of public health and faith-based organizations to increase influenza prevention among hard-to-reach populations. *American Journal of Public Health* 109(3):371–377.

Klaiman, T., D. Knorr, S. Fitzgerald, P. Demara, C. Thomas, G. Heake, and A. Hausman. 2010. Locating and communicating with at-risk populations about emergency preparedness: The vulnerable populations outreach model. *Disaster Medicine and Public Health Preparedness* 4(3):246–251.

Koh, H. K., C. S. Amie, B. Janette, B. Jon, D. B. Paul, M. S. Crowther, A. S. Richard, R. C. Bradley, A. N. Gilbert, C. L. Mary, M. J. Christine, H. C. Paul, H. B. Kathryn, and A. John. 2006. Building community-based surge capacity through a public health and academic collaboration: The role of community health centers. *Public Health Reports* 121(2):211–216.

Levin, K. L., M. Berliner, and A. Merdjanoff. 2014. Disaster planning for vulnerable populations: Leveraging community human service organizations direct service delivery personnel. *Journal of Public Health Management and Practice* 20(Suppl 5):S79–S82.

McCabe, O. L., C. Perry, M. J. Azur, H. G. Taylor, M. J. Bailey, and J. M. Links. 2011. Psychological first-aid training for paraprofessionals: A systems-based model for enhancing capacity of rural emergency responses. *Prehospital and Disaster Medicine* 26(4):251–258.

McCabe, O. L., C. Perry, M. Azur, H. G. Taylor, H. Gwon, A. Mosley, and J. M. Links. 2013. Guided preparedness planning with lay communities: Enhancing capacity of rural emergency response through a systems-based partnership. *Prehospital and Disaster Medicine* 28(1):8–15.

NIH (National Institutes of Health), CDC (Centers for Disease Control and Prevention), and ATSDR (Agency for Toxic Substances and Disease Registry). 2011. *Principles of community engagement.* https://www.atsdr.cdc.gov/communityengagement/pdf/PCE_Report_508_FINAL.pdf (accessed May 23, 2020).

Peate, W. F., and J. Mullins. 2008. Disaster preparedness training for tribal leaders. *Journal of Occupational Medicine and Toxicology* 3(1).

Plough, A., B. Bristow, J. Fielding, S. Caldwell, and S. Khan. 2011. Pandemics and health equity: Lessons learned from the H1N1 response in Los Angeles county. *Journal of Public Health Management and Practice* 17(1):20–27.

Plough, A., J. E. Fielding, A. Chandra, M. Williams, D. Eisenman, K. B. Wells, G. Y. Law, S. Fogleman, and A. Magaña. 2013. Building community disaster resilience: Perspectives from a large urban county department of public health. *American Journal of Public Health* 103(7):1190–1197.

Troy, D. A., A. Carson, J. Vanderbeek, and A. Hutton. 2008. Enhancing community-based disaster preparedness with information technology. *Disasters* 32(1):149–165.

Wells, K. B., B. F. Springgate, E. Lizaola, F. Jones, and A. Plough. 2013. Community engagement in disaster preparedness and recovery: A tale of two cities—Los Angeles and New Orleans. *The Psychiatric Clinics of North America* 36(3):451–466.

Parallel Evidence Systematic Reviews

Butler, M., E. McCreedy, N. Schwer, D. Burgess, K. Call, J. Przedworski, S. Rosser, S. Larson, M. Allen, S. Fu, and R. L. Kane. 2016. Improving cultural competence to reduce health disparities. *Comparative Effectiveness Review* 170. https://www.ncbi.nlm.nih.gov/books/NBK361126/pdf/Bookshelf_NBK361126.pdf (accessed April 1, 2020).

Cyril, S., B. J. Smith, A. Possamai-Inesedy, and A. M. Renzaho. 2015. Exploring the role of community engagement in improving the health of disadvantaged populations: A systematic review. *Global Health Action* 8:29842.

DeRose, K. P., and C. Rodriguez. 2019. A systematic review of church-based health interventions among Latinos. *Journal of Immigrant & Minority Health.* https://doi.org/10.1007/s10903-019-00941-2.

Florez, K. R., D. D. Payan, K. Palar, M. V. Williams, B. Katic, and K. P. Derose. 2019. Church-based interventions to address obesity among African Americans and Latinos in the United States: A systematic review. *Nutrition Reviews* 78(4):304–322. https://doi.org/10.1093/nutrit/nuz046.

Kim, K., J. S. Choi, E. Choi, C. L. Nieman, J. H. Joo, F. R. Lin, L. N. Gitlin, and H. R. Han. 2016. Effects of community-based health worker interventions to improve chronic disease management and care among vulnerable populations: A systematic review. *American Journal of Public Health* 106(4):e3–e28.

McCall, T., C. S. Bolton III, R. McCall, and S. Khairat. 2019. The use of culturally-tailored telehealth interventions in managing anxiety and depression in African American adults: A systematic review. *Studies in Health Technology & Informatics* 264:1728–1729.

McCallum, G. B., P. S. Morris, N. Brown, and A. B. Chang. 2017. Culture-specific programs for children and adults from minority groups who have asthma. *Cochrane Database of Systematic Reviews* 8:CD006580.

McCurley, J. L., A. P. Gutierrez, and L. C. Gallo. 2017. Diabetes prevention in U.S. Hispanic adults: A systematic review of culturally tailored interventions. *American Journal of Preventive Medicine* 52(4):519–529.

Nasir, B. F., L. Hides, S. Kisely, G. Ranmuthugala, G. C. Nicholson, E. Black, N. Gill, S. Kondalsamy-Chennakesavan, and M. Toombs. 2016. The need for a culturally tailored gatekeeper training intervention program in preventing suicide among indigenous peoples: A systematic review. *BMC Psychiatry* 16(1):357.

O'Mara-Eves, A., G. Brunton, S. Oliver, J. Kavanagh, F. Jamal, and J. Thomas. 2015. The effectiveness of community engagement in public health interventions for disadvantaged groups: A meta-analysis. *BMC Public Health* 15:129.

Schroeder, K., R. McCormick, A. Perez, and T. H. Lipman. 2018. The role and impact of community health workers in childhood obesity interventions: A systematic review and meta-analysis. *Obesity Reviews* 19(10):1371–1384.

Shommu, N. S., S. Ahmed, N. Rumana, G. R. Barron, K. A. McBrien, and T. C. Turin. 2016. What is the scope of improving immigrant and ethnic minority healthcare using community navigators: A systematic scoping review. *International Journal for Equity in Health* 15:6.

Viswanathan, M., A. Ammerman, E. Eng, G. Garlehner, K. Lohr, D. Griffith, S. Rhodes, C. Samuel-Hodge, S. Maty, L. Lux, L. Webb, S. Sutton, T. Swinson, A. Jackman, and L. Whitener. 2004. *Community-based participatory research: Assessing the evidence.* Rockville, MD: Agency for Healthcare Research and Quality.

Ethics and Policy Text

IOM (Institute of Medicine). 2009. *Guidance for establishing crisis standards of care for use in disaster situations: A letter report.* Washington, DC: The National Academies Press.

Jennings, B., and J. Arras. 2008. *Ethical guidance for public health emergency preparedness and response: Highlighting ethics and values in a vital public health service.* Atlanta, GA: Centers for Disease Control and Prevention. https://www.cdc.gov/od/science/integrity/phethics/docs/white_paper_final_for_website_2012_4_6_12_final_for_web_508_compliant.pdf (accessed February 23, 2020).

Jennings, B., J. D. Arras, D. H. Barrett, and B. A. Ellis. 2016. *Emergency ethics: Public health preparedness and response.* New York: Oxford University Press.

Mastroianni, A. C., J. P. Kahn, and N. E. Kass, eds. 2019. *The Oxford handbook of public health ethics.* New York: Oxford University Press. https://www.oxfordhandbooks.com/view/10.1093/oxfordhb/9780190245191.001.0001/oxfordhb-9780190245191 (accessed June 3, 2020).

B2 Mixed-Method Review of Activating a Public Health Emergency Operations Center

This appendix provides a detailed description of the methods for and the evidence from the mixed-method review examining the activation of a public health emergency operations center, which is summarized in Chapter 5.[1]

KEY REVIEW QUESTIONS AND ANALYTIC FRAMEWORK

Activating a public health emergency operations center (PHEOC) is a common and standard practice in response to a public health emergency. The primary question posed by the committee in this review is: "In what circumstances is activating public health emergency operations appropriate?" To further identify evidence of interest, the committee explored several sub-questions related to activation, separate public health emergency operations, changes in response, benefits and harms, and the factors that create barriers and facilitators (see Box B2-1).

For the purposes of this review, the committee developed an analytic framework to present the causal pathway and interactions between public health emergency operations and its components, populations, and outcomes of interest (see Figure B2-1). The underlying theory is that activating a PHEOC facilitates the coordination of resources and information flow, thereby improving response efforts by increasing the efficiency and timeliness of response (see Figure B2-1).

EVIDENCE SUPPORTING THE PRACTICE RECOMMENDATION

This section summarizes the evidence from the mixed-method review examining PHEOC activation. It begins with a description of the results of the literature search and then sum-

[1] This section draws heavily on two reports commissioned by the committee: "Public Health Emergency Operations Coordination: Qualitative Research Evidence Synthesis" by Pradeep Sopory and Julie Novak; and "Public Health Emergency Operations Coordination: Findings from After Action Reports and Case Reports" by Sneha Patel (see Appendix C).

BOX B2-1 KEY REVIEW QUESTIONS

In what circumstances is activating public health emergency operations appropriate?

- What factors (e.g., type and scale of event, type of command, complexity, past experience, mutual aid requests, policy) are useful for determining when to activate public health emergency operations?
- In what circumstances should public health agencies activate a separate public health emergency operations center (EOC), lead a multiagency EOC, or play a supporting role in a multiagency EOC based on identified or potential public health consequences?
- How does the response change following the activation of public health emergency operations?
- What benefits and harms (desirable and/or undesirable impacts) of activation of public health emergency operations have been described or measured?
- What are the barriers to and facilitators of successful public health emergency operations using an incident command center?

marizes the evidence of effectiveness. The committee considered evidence beyond effectiveness, which was compiled using an Evidence to Decision (EtD) framework encompassing balance of benefits and harms, acceptability and preferences, feasibility and public health emergency preparedness and response (PHEPR) system considerations, resource and economic considerations, equity, and ethical considerations. The evidence from each methodological stream applicable to each of the EtD criteria is discussed; a synthesis is provided in Table B2-2 later in this appendix and in Chapter 5. Graded finding statements from evidence syntheses are italicized in the narrative below.

Full details about the study eligibility criteria, search strategy, and processes for data extraction and individual study quality assessment are available in Appendix A. Appendix C links to all of the commissioned analyses informing this review.

Results of the Literature Search

The searches of bibliographic databases (including a separate targeted search conducted through SCOPUS to identify literature in the military, first responder, and transportation disciplines) identified a total of 5,332 potentially relevant citations (deduplicated) for the mixed-method review of PHEOC activation. A search of the gray literature, reference mining, a call for reports, and a search of the Homeland Security Digital Library for after action reports (AARs) contributed an additional 609 articles. All 5,941 citations were imported into EndNote and were included in title and abstract screening. During screening, 5,708 articles were excluded because their abstracts did not appear to answer any of the key questions or they indicated that the articles were commentaries, editorials, or opinion pieces. After the abstracts had been reviewed, 233 full-text articles were reviewed and assessed for eligibility for inclusion in the mixed-method review. The committee considered 106 articles for data extraction and ultimately included 87 articles in the mixed-method review. Figure B2-2

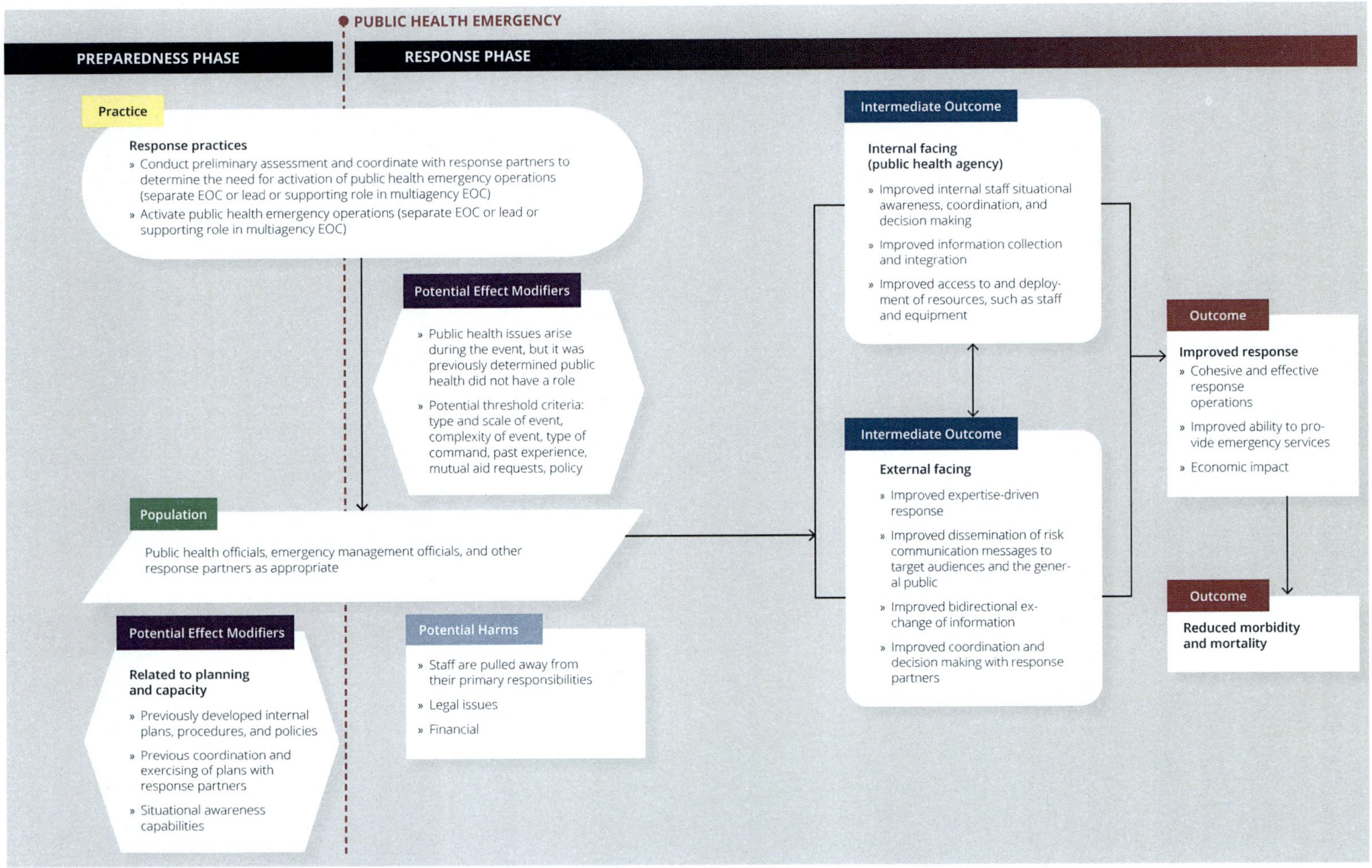

FIGURE B2-1 Analytic framework for public health emergency operations.
NOTES: Arrows in the framework indicate hypothesized causal pathways between interventions and outcomes. Double-headed arrows indicate feedback loops. EOC = emergency operations center.

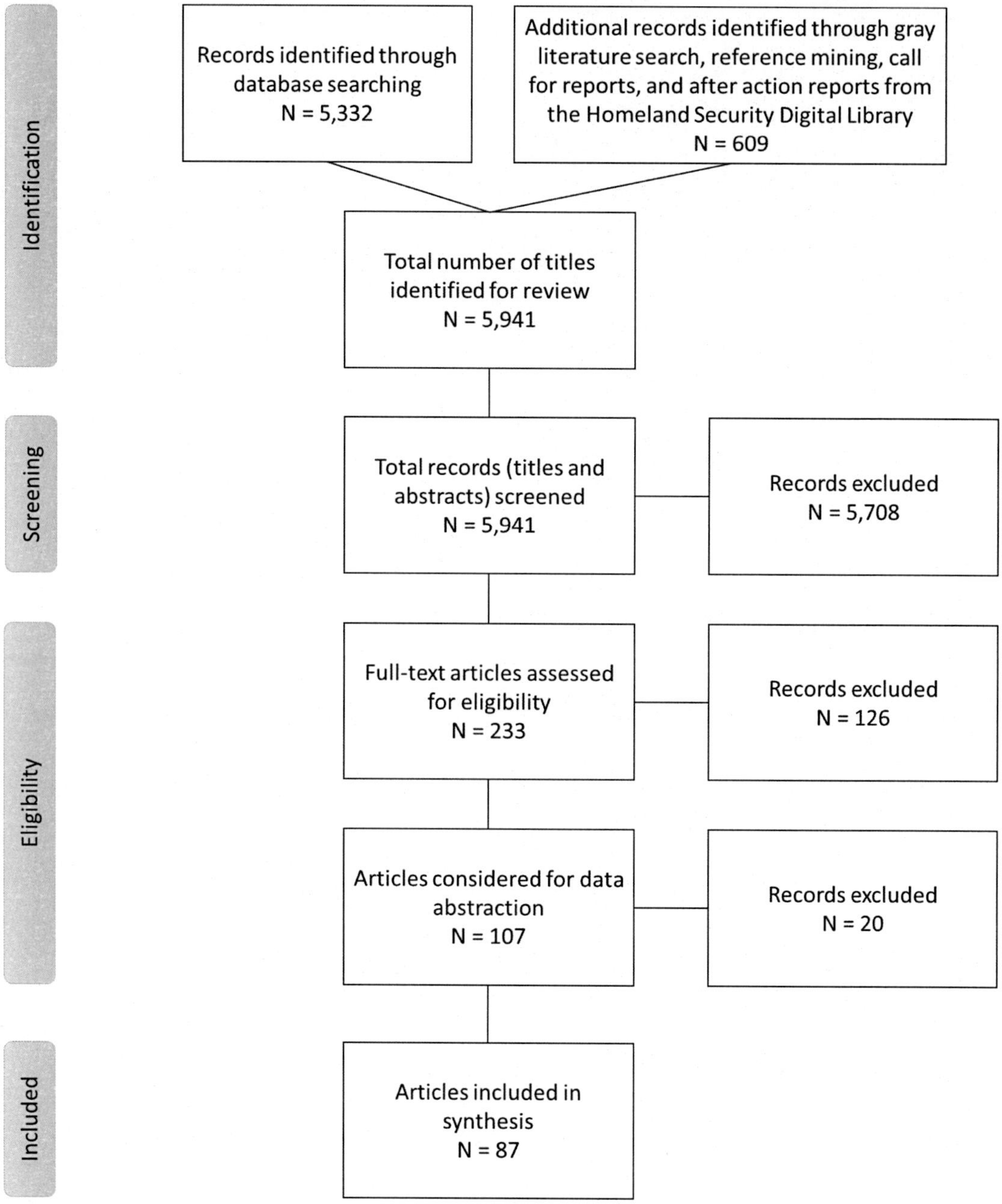

FIGURE B2-2 Preferred Reporting Items for Systematic Reviews and Meta-Analyses diagram for the mixed-method review of activating public health emergency operations.

TABLE B2-1 Evidence Types Included in the Mixed-Method Review of Activating Public Health Emergency Operations

Evidence Type[a]	Number of Studies (as applicable)[b]
Quantitative comparative	0
Quantitative noncomparative (postintervention measure only)	0
Qualitative	21
Modeling	0
Descriptive surveys	1
Case reports	29[c]
After action reports	35[c]
Mechanistic	N/A
Parallel (systematic reviews)	N/A

[a] Evidence types are defined in Chapter 3.
[b] Note that sibling articles (different results from the same study published in separate articles) are counted as one study in this table. Mixed-method studies may be counted in more than one category.
[c] A sample of case reports and after action reports were prioritized for inclusion in this review based on relevance to the key questions, as described in Chapter 3.

depicts the literature flow, indicating the number of articles included and excluded at each screening stage. Table B2-1 indicates the types of evidence included in this review.

1. Determining Evidence of Effect

The review identified no quantitative comparative or noncomparative studies or modeling studies eligible for inclusion, but information gleaned from the qualitative evidence synthesis and the case report and AAR evidence synthesis contributed to understanding in what circumstances activating public health emergency operations is appropriate. This is a difficult evidentiary situation; the lack of quantitative studies, in particular, speaks to the committee's high-level finding that more and improved research is needed in this field. Still, the committee's overriding goal was to distill the available evidence to give practitioners the best possible guidance. Therefore, the evidence gleaned was used to construct a high-level view of what happened and what appeared to work.

2. Balance of Benefits and Harms

As stated above, no research on the effectiveness of PHEOCs was identified. Therefore, findings from the qualitative evidence synthesis and the case reports and AARs evidence synthesis contributed to an understanding of the benefits and harms and undesirable effects of activating a PHEOC.

Qualitative Evidence Synthesis

Several qualitative studies found that staff with experience from responding to prior emergency events made faster and better decisions (presumably relative to staff without such experience), implying that this benefit becomes visible only over time in responses to future events (Bigley and Roberts 2001; Buck et al., 2006; Militello et al., 2007). Similarly, some qualitative studies found that the development of social relations and associated trust across organizations from response to a previous event became manifest in the current event in the form of smoother interorganizational coordination (Buck et al., 2006; Freedman et al., 2013).

Eight qualitative studies examined undesirable impacts associated with PHEOC activation (Bigley and Roberts 2001; Freedman et al., 2013; McMaster and Baber, 2012; Militello et al., 2007; Moynihan, 2008; Reeder and Turner, 2011; Rimstad and Sollid, 2015; Sisco et al., 2019). The qualitative evidence indicates that *activation of public health emergency operations may lead to several undesirable effects, the salient of which are related to staffing deployment, staff stress and burnout, and adaptation-generated interorganizational distrust and chain-of-command disruption* (high confidence in the evidence).

With regard to the benefits and harms of PHEOC activation relative to population health, the qualitative evidence generally reflects an assumption, not explicitly stated, as to the benefits of preventing morbidity and mortality in an emergency event. Qualitative studies found two sets of undesirable effects of PHEOC activation on human health: disruption of routine services that may still be needed in an emergency event (Freedman et al., 2013; Reeder and Turner, 2011), which has the potential to negatively impact public health; and negative effects on staff, such as burnout and stress (Militello et al., 2007; Moynihan, 2008; Rimstad and Sollid, 2015). Undesirable effects of PHEOC activation on the public health system, such as staff stress and burnout, turnover among professionals, uneven distribution of staff workload, and adaptation-generated interorganizational distrust and chain-of-command disruption, were likely to be present only during the span of an event. There may, however, be situations in which these undesirable effects became embedded in the system and carry over from event to event.

Case Report and AAR Evidence Synthesis

Evidence from the case reports and AARs aligns with the qualitative evidence synthesis findings. Case reports and AARs examined in this review suggest that the efficiency of response improved following PHEOC activation. Situational awareness, interagency coordination, and information sharing were strengthened (Minnesota Department of Health, 2014; Texas Department of State Health Services, 2018; Williams et al., 2014). The timeliness of activities also improved as the result of increased availability of resources and/or capabilities for extended, expanded, or emergent responses (Williams et al., 2014). For instance, PHEOC activation during a 2002 response to West Nile virus in Arkansas led to the initiation of a public hotline to answer questions about the virus and the development of a specially designed website to provide instructions for submitting diagnostic specimens (Fleischauer et al., 2003). Findings from the Centers for Disease Control and Prevention's (CDC's) early response to Middle East respiratory syndrome coronavirus (MERS-CoV) show that activating the PHEOC relieved some administrative demands, which meant that the technical staff members could turn their attention to pressing public health issues (CDC, 2013).

Activation has also enabled greater access to subject-matter experts during responses with potential public health implications. During the 2010 *Deepwater Horizon* response, a public health unit coordinated response efforts across a multistate area of operations. The AAR states that the "formation of this unit allowed for the sharing of public health concerns, needs and requests, and thus more efficient and effective coordination of efforts" (Florida Department of Health, 2010). An unintended consequence of activation, however, was staff fatigue due to overreliance on a few key personnel or insufficient staffing depth to meet response needs.

With respect to the benefits and harms of PHEOC activation relative to system-level changes, the evidence from case reports and AARs indicates that following the decision to activate, response operations typically became more efficient and capable of responding to emergent needs with greater flexibility because activation can result in standardized structure, greater clarity of roles, improved coordination, and sustained staffing (Boston Public Health Commission, 2013; Branum et al., 2010; CDC, 2013; Governor's Office of Homeland Security and Emergency Preparedness, 2012; Iskander et al., 2017; Massachusetts Emergency Management et al., 2014; Timm and Gneuhs, 2011). Other benefits include the practical experience gained by staff under urgent and emergent conditions (Quinn et al., 2018).

3. Acceptability and Preferences

Qualitative Evidence Synthesis

While the set of studies included in the qualitative evidence synthesis does not directly, or even indirectly, address the issue of acceptability and preferences, none of the articles reviewed mention any reluctance on the part of any agency to join emergency response operations for a real event or a preparedness training exercise.

Case Report and AAR Evidence Synthesis

Findings from case reports and AARs suggest that overall, the public health agency workforce values and prefers to use an incident command system (ICS) when a PHEOC is activated. Although some tension is noted with regard to shifting from day-to-day responsibilities or balancing them with response needs, public health agencies appeared to value the use of an ICS to coordinate response operations. This was evident in examples of jurisdictions that previously had not used an ICS but preferred to do so in future responses because of the structure it provides (Adams et al., 2010; Contra Costa Health Services, 2012; New Hampshire Department of Health and Human Services and Department of Safety, 2010). Findings from a case report examining CDC's use of the ICS model during the 2009 influenza pandemic indicate that the agency preferred to modify the traditional model by including a policy unit to "guide the interpretation, coordination, and adjudication of policy during the response" (Ansell and Keller, 2014). While this is not a standard element of the ICS model, CDC found it better suited the operational context. Public health agencies could consider similar adaptations with the potential to improve public health response operations.

Descriptive Survey Study Evidence

Jensen and Youngs (Jensen, 2011; Jensen and Youngs, 2015) surveyed county emergency managers so as to describe and explain their implementation behavior with respect to the National Incident Management System (NIMS). They found that not all counties considerd NIMS to be well suited to their jurisdiction, and that those views influenced counties that modified the system and failed to implement it as designed. Likewise, Jensen and Youngs (Jensen, 2011; Jensen and Youngs, 2015) found it was critical that counties believed NIMS had the potential to solve real problems, that they perceived it to be clear and specific, that incentives and sanctions were not only provided but likely, and that capacity-building resources were provided.

4. Feasibility and PHEPR System Considerations

Qualitative Evidence Synthesis

Seventeen qualitative studies examined challenges to effective PHEOC activation (Bigley and Roberts, 2001; Buck et al., 2006; Freedman et al., 2013; Gryth et al., 2010; Klima et al., 2012; Lis and Resnick, 2018; Mase et al., 2017; McMaster and Baber, 2012; Militello et al., 2007; Moynihan, 2008; Obaid et al., 2017; Reeder and Turner, 2011; Rimstad and Sollid, 2015; Shipp Hilts et al., 2016; Sisco et al., 2019; Thomas et al., 2005; Yanson et al., 2017). Many of these challenges relate to general management practices, and it is important to keep in mind that typically, the opposite or absence of a barrier is a facilitator for effective operations. *Challenges to effective public health emergency operations are many. Some of the most salient relate to interorganizational awareness, interorganizational relationships, interorganizational cultural differences, differences in team members' knowledge and experience, communication technology, rules and regulations, volume of information, and lack of training* (high confidence in the evidence).

Lack of interorganizational awareness—members of an operations team from an agency not being aware of other agencies (e.g., public health agencies at different levels and outside the traditional public health domain) or sometimes of other teams within their agency—was a major impediment to an effective PHEOC. This lack of awareness took the form of lack of mutual awareness of operations; lack of shared understanding of an event, particularly between organizations not familiar with each other's domains of expertise and work practices; lack of understanding of role differences; and no common understanding of standard operating procedures among all responding organizations (Buck et al., 2006; Freedman et al., 2013; McMaster and Baber, 2012; Militello et al., 2007). Challenges involving the relationships among team members from different organizations included core members of a team from one or two organizations not interacting with other team members from different organizations; team members from one organization without prior relationships formed during training sessions with members from other organizations working independently; new members added later than others not forming relationships; mistrust between agencies and disagreement over which was in charge; a wide variety of response organizations; and different interpretations of an emergency event (Freedman et al., 2013; Lis and Resnick, 2018; McMaster and Baber, 2012; Militello et al., 2007; Moynihan, 2008; Thomas et al., 2005). Another challenge was cultural differences in organizational values of individual team members, cultures of the organizations, or organizational priorities (Bigley and Roberts, 2001; Moynihan, 2008).

Communication technology also presented challenges to effective PHEOC activation. These challenges included incompatible communication systems, especially those of civil and military organizations; new technologies for emergency events that were different from those used for routine operations and therefore unfamiliar to users; system and equipment noise in communication channels; inadequate numbers of shared electronic displays; lacking or forgotten knowledge of the use of communication systems; outdated email and phone lists; problems with data entry systems and ticket and request software for interagency assistance; and radio traffic overload and lack of radio discipline (Gryth et al., 2010; Klima et al., 2012; Mase et al., 2017; McMaster and Baber, 2012; Militello et al., 2007; Reeder and Turner, 2011; Yanson et al., 2017). Also challenging was the increased volume of information to be processed and integrated resulting from a surge in phone calls, teleconferences, and emails; new, evolving issues generating new information; conflicting information and attempts to resolve it; new guidance and related information; multiple public health roles requiring different streams of information gathering and dissemination; the long duration of an emergency event and the response; and information flow in the entire network (Chandler et al., 2016; Freedman et al., 2013; Gryth et al., 2010; Mase et al., 2017; Reeder and Turner, 2011; Rimstad and Sollid, 2015; Sisco et al., 2019).

Rules and regulations required for routine public health operations were also found to pose challenges for emergency operations. These included rules leading to bottlenecks during surge at public health laboratories; Health Insurance Portability and Accountability Act rules prohibiting access to non–public health staff or secured shared data repositories on individual computers; unclear rules about overtime compensation and working at nonroutine locations; and lack of clarity of rules for information sharing, including with the media and the public (Freedman et al., 2013; Shipps Hilts et al., 2016; Sisco et al., 2019; Yanson et al., 2017).

Differences in team members' knowledge and experience presented a further challenge to an effective PHEOC. These differences were seen in members' willingness to enter affected areas, training in command-control environments, level of facility with tools and systems, knowledge of roles and functions, knowledge of medical procedures and equipment, and emergency operations plans (Freedman et al., 2013; Klima et al., 2012; Militello et al., 2007; Rimstad and Sollid, 2015).

Case Report and AAR Evidence Synthesis

Many AARs examined for this evidence review focus on the barriers to and facilitators of successful PHEOC activation, likely because jurisdictions often use these reports to evaluate their capabilities so as to improve their response processes. Evidence from the case reports and AARs supports the above qualitative evidence with respect to barriers related to interagency relationships and coordination (Ansell and Keller, 2014; Boston Public Health Commission, 2013; Massachusetts Emergency Management et al., 2014; Moynihan, 2007; Oklahoma Department of Emergency Management, 2013; Phillips and Williamson, 2005; San Francisco Department of Public Health, 2010; Shipp Hilts et al., 2016; Texas Department of State Health Services, 2018; Wiesman et al., 2011; Williams et al., 2014); appropriate and reliable communication technology (Beatty et al., 2006; Boston Public Health Comission, 2013; Buffalo Hospital and Wright County Public Health, 2013; Chicago Department of Public Health et al., 2011; Delaware Division of Public Health, 2010; DuPage County Health Department, 2009; Governor's Office of Homeland Security and Emergency Preparedness, 2012; Kilianski et al., 2014; Moynihan, 2007; Multnomah County Health Department, 2010; Redd and Frieden, 2017); lack of prior staff knowledge and experience with ICS and larger-scale disasters (Logan County Health District, 2015; Moynihan, 2007); lack of clarity with respect to roles and responsibilities (Capitol Region Council of Governments, 2016; Multnomah County Health Department, 2009; New Hampshire Department of Safety and Department of Health and Human Services, 2009a,b); lack of training on NIMS, ICS, partner roles, and job-specific roles (Augustine and Shottmer, 2005; Becker County Community Health, 2013; Boston Public Health Comission, 2013; Chicago Department of Public Health et al., 2011; Fishbane et al., 2012; Florida Department of Health, 2017; Minnesota Department of Health, 2013; Oklahoma Department of Emergency Management, 2013; Williams et al., 2014); and inadequate staffing (Boston Public Health Comission, 2013; Buehler et al., 2017; City of Nashua Department of Emergency Management, 2012; Delaware Division of Public Health, 2010; Klein et al., 2005; Multnomah County Health Department, 2009, 2010; New Hampshire Department of Health and Human Services and Department of Safety, 2010; Posid et al., 2005; Texas Department of State Health Services, 2010; Tri-County Health Department, 2017, n.d.; Wood County Health District, 2017).

Descriptive Survey Study Evidence

Further supporting the above evidence are the findings of a survey of county emergency managers conducted by Jensen and Youngs (Jensen, 2011; Jensen and Youngs, 2015) regarding the implementation of NIMS, which indicated that if interorganizational characteristics are not conducive to the implementation of emergency operations, then regardless of what jurisdictions intend, their actual implementation behavior can be negatively impacted. Additionally, when a county thought it had insufficient personnel to implement all of the components, structures, and processes of the response system, they tended to have weaker implementation intent and behavior, and vice versa.

5. Resource and Economic Considerations

Qualitative Evidence Synthesis

The resource, cost, and logistical constraints of PHEOC activation are important considerations for those making the decision to activate. Fourteen qualitative studies examined the types of resources that can facilitate effective public health emergency operations (Freedman et al., 2013; Glick and Barbara, 2013; Gryth et al., 2010; Hambridge et al., 2017; Klima et al., 2012; Lis and Resnick, 2018; Lis et al., 2017; Mase et al., 2017; McMaster and Baber, 2012; Militello et al., 2007; Obaid et al., 2017; Reeder and Turner, 2011; Sisco et al., 2019; Thomas et al., 2005). These studies found that resources for PHEOCs served as facilitators for effective response. They also found that the need for different types of resources and their amounts changed throughout an emergency event (Sisco et al., 2019); for example, resource needs tended to be greater in the earlier phases of an event when there was a demand surge relative to the later phases. *Resources that can facilitate the effectiveness of public health emergency operations can be many. Some of the salient resources include training, databases, supplies, mechanisms for communicating with the public and media, and having a liaison or point-of-contact position. The need for various resources often changes over the course of an event* (high confidence in the evidence).

Case Report and AAR Evidence Synthesis

Although the case reports and AARs reviewed do not address resources in detail, some note that activating and sustaining a response to a major public health event required large numbers of staff at various locations (Posid et al., 2005). One jurisdiction dealt with this need by formally communicating the expectation that all divisions within the public health agency were required to provide staffing resources for response efforts (Tri-County Health Department, 2013). In terms of nonhuman resources, AAR findings suggest that jurisdictions should maintain an alternative PHEOC location with the necessary communication infrastructure (Capitol Region Council of Governments, 2017). Significant resources also are required for trainings and exercises to prepare agencies for a public health emergency response. Reports reviewed indicate that such trainings and exercises were worth the time commitment and were an asset in subsequent response operations (Redd and Frieden, 2017; Wisconsin Division of Public Health, 2010). Some reports emphasize the need for continuous federal investment in public health preparedness capacity as that investment has been shown to help state and local agencies achieve federal benchmarks, carry out capacity-building activities, and develop functional capabilities (Davis et al., 2007; Wiedrich et al., 2013). The reviewed reports indicate further that risk assessments were found to be a useful means of weighing the potential public health impacts of a resource-intensive activation against the cost implications (Quinn et al., 2018).

6. Equity

Qualitative Evidence Synthesis

Two qualitative studies examined the needs of at-risk populations in the context of emergency operations (Chandler et al., 2016; Sisco et al., 2019). The response to vulnerable populations is an important aspect of an effective PHEOC. Yet, pre-event planning for these operations may not always explicitly include consideration of the needs of such groups. Pre-event establishment of an interagency task force that includes community organizations to plan specifically for meeting those needs can greatly facilitate such responses (Sisco et al., 2019). Such a task force, among other things, can ensure the creation of needed databases; the provision of care in shelters, as well as staff availability for specialized services; the availability of medical equipment and medications; alternative sources of power during outages and refueling for such sources; and the availability of regular and specialized transportation (Chandler et al., 2016, Sisco et al., 2019). *The response of public health emergency operations to the needs of at-risk populations can be facilitated by interagency planning that, among other things, addresses establishing a task force, creating needed databases, providing care in shelters, ensuring access to medications, dealing with power outages, and meeting transportation needs* (low confidence in the evidence).

Case Report and AAR Evidence Synthesis

Few case reports and AARs address equity issues associated with PHEOC activation. Recommendations in AARs, however, suggest some consideration of equity during the planning and response phases. For instance, one report notes the inclusion of interpreters and on-site physician consultants during a mass influenza clinic (Phillips and Williamson, 2005). The inclusion of interpreters helped ensure that language barriers would not impede the provision of services. Findings from the response to the Boston Marathon bombing indicate that creating demographic profiles of health care organizations can help in understanding the unique challenges associated with particular neighborhoods and populations (Boston Public Health Commission, 2013).

Another approach highlighted in this evidence stream is including community representatives in the PHEOC for joint decision making (Wiesman et al., 2011), although it is important to ensure that these representatives are well trained in response operations. Also important is considering equity issues internal to the PHEOC. One case report briefly touches on the need to avoid gender bias in training, "given the fact that there is a much greater proportion of women within emergency relevant organizations than in emergency mission organizations" (Lutz and Lindell, 2008). Additional research is needed to better understand how biases or inequities internal to a PHEOC relate to equitable response outcomes.

7. Ethical Considerations[2]

The section on equity above addresses ethical considerations in PHEOC operations related to the principle of justice or fairness. In addition, the primary ethical principle underlying the initiation of a PHEOC is that of stewardship of limited resources. This principle, often framed as a duty to produce the greatest good for the greatest number of people as efficiently as possible, is seen as particularly important during public health emergencies, when resources typically are limited and need to be allocated with care. As a result, ethical concerns with respect to implementing a PHEOC are centered primarily on the pragmatic benefits and harms of doing so—namely, the possibility that implementing a PHEOC will waste resources and generate harms through the neglect of other programs while team members are reassigned to PHEOC operations. Some of the procedural principles in play can include transparency, which is supported when a PHEOC improves communication; and proportionality (acting only in proportion to need, or using the least restrictive means to achieve a desired outcome), which is supported when having an activated PHEOC improves situational awareness and therefore averts unnecessary implementation of interventions.

TABLE B2-2 Evidence to Decision Summary Table for Activation of Public Health Emergency Operations

In what circumstances is activating public health emergency operations appropriate?	
Balance of Benefits and Harms	**Sources of Evidence**
No quantitative research on the effectiveness of public health emergency operations center (PHEOC) activation was identified. The evidence from qualitative studies and from case reports and after action reports (AARs) indicates that activation generally results in more efficient response operations and improved ability to respond to emergent needs with greater flexibility, and as a result may have implicit benefits in relation to improving population health during a public health emergency. The timeliness of response activities also improves because of the increased availability of resources and/or capabilities. Moreover, activation may enable greater access to subject-matter experts during responses with potential public health implications. A long-term benefit of activation is the accumulation of institutional knowledge of what does and does not work (i.e., practical experience) gained by the public health agency under urgent or emergent conditions. Important factors in deciding whether activating a PHEOC will lead to any harms include the potential need for more intensive staffing due to long hours and the need to continue routine public health services, as well as the potential for adaptation-generated interorganizational distrust and chain-of-command disruption. These harms are likely to be present only during an event and not to persist postevent for any appreciable length of time. In some cases, however, such harms may become embedded in the public health system and carry over from event to event (e.g., if a negative interpersonal relationship forms that creates barriers to future successful collaboration). Simply activating a PHEOC is not a comprehensive solution; public health agencies must be ready to manage them effectively, and without that readiness, more harms may be experienced.	• Qualitative evidence synthesis • Case report and AAR evidence synthesis (no assessment of certainty or confidence)

[2] Ethical considerations included in this section were generated through committee discussions, drawing on the ethical principles laid out in Box 3-4 in Chapter 3 and key ethics and policy texts, including the 2009 Institute of Medicine letter report on crisis standards of care (IOM, 2009), the 2008 CDC white paper "Ethical Guidance for Public Health Emergency Preparedness and Response: Highlighting Ethics and Values in a Vital Public Health Service" (Jennings and Arras, 2008), *Emergency Ethics: Public Health Preparedness and Response* (Jennings et al., 2016), and *The Oxford Handbook of Public Health Ethics* (Mastroianni et al., 2019).

TABLE B2-2 Continued

Acceptability and Preferences	**Sources of Evidence**
Public health emergency preparedness and response (PHEPR) practitioners generally find their roles in participating in emergency operations acceptable and are amenable to the resulting changes in work patterns. PHEPR practitioners prefer to use an incident command system (ICS) but appreciate the ability to modify the structure to better suit their operational context and jurisdiction. Furthermore, to facilitate the implementation of public health emergency operations, practitioners must believe that implementation of the National Incident Management System (NIMS)/ICS has the potential to solve real problems and is clear and specific, that incentives and sanctions are not only provided but likely, and that capacity-building resources are being provided. Ongoing support for meaningful work is important, and PHEOCs that provide this support are therefore likely to be more successful.	• Case report and AAR evidence synthesis (no assessment of certainty or confidence) • Descriptive survey study evidence (no synthesis)
Feasibility and PHEPR System Considerations	**Sources of Evidence**
Many barriers impact the feasibility of successful PHEOC activation, and these barriers are often related to challenges involving general management practices. These challenges include interorganizational awareness, relationships, and cultural differences; differences in team members' knowledge and experience; adequate staffing to implement the activation with all of its components, structures, and processes; communication technology; rules and regulations; the volume of information; and a lack of training in NIMS/ICS, partner roles, and job-specific roles. If these interorganizational characteristics are not conducive to implementation, actual implementation behavior can be negatively impacted regardless of what jurisdictions intend.	• Qualitative evidence synthesis • Case report and AAR evidence synthesis (no assessment of certainty or confidence) • Descriptive survey study evidence (no synthesis)
Resource and Economic Considerations	**Sources of Evidence**
The resource, cost, and logistical constraints of PHEOC activation are important considerations in deciding whether to activate. These considerations often change over the course of an event and may be sizable depending on the scope of the event. Salient resources include training; databases; supplies; and mechanism(s) for communicating with the public and media, among which is the creation of liaison or point-of-contact positions. These resource needs may dictate the level at which the public health emergency operations should be coordinated (e.g., local, regional, state, and/or national). Baseline PHEOC operations require an infusion of resources beyond normal operations, in general, and public health agencies need to be prepared to manage those costs, ideally with support from other levels of government.	• Qualitative evidence synthesis • Case report and AAR evidence synthesis (no assessment of certainty or confidence)
Equity	**Sources of Evidence**
Inequities in the implementation of public health emergency operations for different populations due to variability in the availability of resources, infrastructure, and funding likely exist among state, local, tribal, and territorial public health agencies (and are also related to the resource and economic considerations discussed above). Activating a PHEOC can help ensure that the needs of particular at-risk populations are addressed during the response to an event. Accomplishing this requires interagency planning based within the PHEOC that entails establishing a task force to help these population(s), creating a database to collect relevant risk information, providing targeted care in shelters, ensuring access to medications, and addressing specific medical needs caused by power outages and unique transportation requirements. Another approach involves welcoming community representatives into the PHEOC for more inclusive decision making. Additional research is needed to better understand how biases or inequities internal to a PHEOC relate to equitable response outcomes. PHEOCs likely reflect the implicit biases of their decision makers and will support equity more or less well based on the perspective of those individuals.	• Qualitative evidence synthesis • Case report and AAR evidence synthesis (no assessment of certainty or confidence)

continued

TABLE B2-2 Continued

Ethical Considerations	Source of Evidence
The section on equity above addresses ethical considerations in a PHEOC related to the principle of justice or fairness. In addition, the primary ethical principle underlying the initiation of a PHEOC is that of stewardship of limited resources. This principle, often framed as a duty to produce the greatest good for the greatest number of people as efficiently as possible, is frequently seen as particularly important during public health emergencies, since resources in emergencies are typically limited and need to be allocated with care. As a result, ethical concerns related to implementing a PHEOC are centered primarily on the pragmatic benefits and harms of doing so: namely, the possibility that implementing a PHEOC will waste resources and generate harms due to the neglect of other programs while team members are reassigned to PHEOC operations. Some of the procedural principles in play can include transparency, which is supported when a PHEOC improves communication, and proportionality (acting only in proportion to need, or using the least restrictive means to achieve a desired outcome), which is supported when having an activated PHEOC improves situational awareness and therefore averts unnecessary implementation of interventions.	• Committee discussion drawing on key ethics and policy texts

CONSIDERATIONS FOR IMPLEMENTATION

The following considerations for implementation were drawn from the synthesis of qualitative research studies, the synthesis of case reports and AARs, and descriptive surveys.

8. Factors in Determining When to Activate a PHEOC

Qualitative Evidence Synthesis

Seven qualitative studies report on factors in determining when to activate a PHEOC (Freedman et al., 2013; Glick and Barbara, 2013; Lis and Resnick, 2018; Lis et al., 2017; Obaid et al., 2017; Sisco et al., 2019; Yanson et al., 2017). The qualitative evidence indicates that *public health emergency operations are fully activated, as support or lead, when an emergency event is large in size and complex in scope, or when the hazards it poses impact primarily or only human health as opposed to natural or built environments, as is the case, for example, with disease outbreaks. The activation may also include activation of a liaison officer and may precede the onset of an event through advance activation of interagency protocols and memorandums of understanding. Overall aspects of activation include determination of specific thresholds for activation and time to the activation decision* (moderate confidence in the evidence).

As noted above, the scope of an emergency event is associated with the activation of a PHEOC. Measures of scope include the depletion of resources and the imposition of a high burden on operations, used to create a threshold for determining whether public health emergency operations should be activated. Determination of the critical point or specific threshold that elicits an activation decision is thus an essential aspect of activation. Findings from health care settings are informative in this regard. For example, an emergency event can lead to a surge in demand for health care services. Standards of care fall on a continuum ranging from conventional to contingency to crisis care. The triggers and indicators that signal the need to transition to crisis standards of care are characterized by insufficient resources to meet the increased demand for care during an emergency event (Lis et al., 2017). Five factors have been found to influence the time taken to activate a PHEOC: previous knowledge and experience; the degree to which an emergency event is atypical; the amount, speed, and quality of situation data available; integration of the data to build a picture of the situation; and the perception of urgency to make a decision (Glick and Barbara, 2013).

Case Report and AAR Evidence Synthesis

Findings from the case reports and AARs reviewed support the above qualitative evidence, suggesting that it was helpful to activate for more complex and multijurisdictional responses that presented threats to public health and to do so early, even if the event's size and scope were initially unknown (Cruz et al., 2015). There was often a period of initial uncertainty as to the need to activate, particularly regarding exposure to infectious and novel diseases (Cole et al., 2015). New Hampshire was able to respond successfully to a 2012 Nor'easter, for example, because the state activated an ICS ahead of the storm and prepared to respond to a winter weather emergency even though it was predicted to be an average snowstorm. The advance decision to activate allowed for rapid escalation of response operations when needed (City of Nashua Department of Emergency Management, 2012). Other case reports and AARs show that as the demands of an incident extended beyond the capacity of existing resources, activating an ICS enabled an effective surge in capacity (County of San Diego, 2018; Wiedrich et al., 2013; Williams et al., 2014). A typical example is a 2017 hepatitis A outbreak in San Diego during which the number of cases continued to rise, leading to the need for additional vaccination, sanitation, and education measures (County of San Diego, 2018).

The case reports and AARs also reveal that activation triggers were useful in determining when to activate, reactivate, or deactivate response operations. During disease outbreaks, use of the number of cases as a trigger informed the decision to activate and the level at which to do so (Williams et al., 2014). It is important to note that while triggers have been defined in advance of an event, novel diseases have required the development of new triggers, as was the case when CDC developed new triggers for activating a PHEOC for MERS-CoV given the uncertainty of the epidemiology of the disease. Findings from the case reports and AARs indicate further that it is best for predefined triggers to remain flexible, as the adequacy of resources to meet response needs at a given time also plays an important role in the decision to activate. It may be useful as well to consider having flexible triggers at the local level that do not necessarily rely on a state's declaration of an emergency, as response needs can overburden local resources even in the absence of a formal state emergency declaration. Additionally, as was learned from New Hampshire's 2009 H1N1 response, it can be helpful to define standardized triggers among response agencies for physical activation of a regional multiagency coordinating entity (MACE) location (New Hampshire Department of Health and Human Services and Department of Safety, 2009a). Some regions had physically opened a MACE, whereas others simply had one person answering phone calls and sending emails for activation, resulting in a disconnect between state and local expectations for the response.

Findings from the case reports and AARs indicate that local public health agencies activated and benefited from activating PHEOCs to lead local responses to a public health emergency (Branum et al., 2010; Porter et al., 2011). Activation allowed local jurisdictions to keep pace with the response and improved interagency coordination if other agencies were involved (Capitol Region Council of Governments, 2016; New Hampshire Department of Health and Human Services and Department of Safety, 2010). Activation at the local level was also found to be beneficial in support of reponse to state-level public health threats (New Hampshire Department of Health and Human Services and Department of Safety, 2010). A recurring issue raised in AARs is the need to clarify the role of state versus local

PHEOCs (New Hampshire Department of Health and Human Services and Department of Safety, 2009b, 2010; Ohio Department of Health, 2010; Texas Department of State Health Services, 2010, 2018). Noted as particularly important is ensuring clear chains of command and decision-making authority during a response. Regardless of the structure established, public health agencies across levels could thereby better integrate their functions.

Public health agencies led multiagency EOCs in response to public health threats (e.g., infectious disease outbreaks) when coordination and information sharing among response agencies were critical to meeting objectives, a finding that supports those from the qualitative evidence synthesis. Activation helped clarify roles among the supporting response agencies (e.g., emergency management, police, fire, school officials). Numerous AARs and case reports also describe the benefits of public health support functions during planned events or incidents with potential for public health implications (Boston Public Health Commission, 2013; Buehler et al., 2017; Capitol Region Council of Governments, 2016, 2017; Contra Costa Health Services, 2012; Fleischauer et al., 2003; Florida Department of Health, 2010; Hunter et al., 2012; Massachusetts Emergency Management Agency et al., 2014; Wisconsin Division of Public Health, 2010). During the 2013 Boston Marathon bombing, for instance, public health agencies helped facilitate family reunification (Boston Public Health Commission, 2013). During a 2011 tsunami threat in California, public health agencies "activated surveillance and epidemiology, environmental health and mental health and psychological support functions" (Hunter et al., 2012). Public health agencies also participated in mass care and the management and distribution of medical supplies. AARs on environmental disasters with the potential for short- and/or long-term public health impacts (e.g., oil spills, refinery fires) likewise note the importance of including public health in multiagency activations.

9. Other Implementation Considerations

The following conceptual findings inform the perspectives and approaches one should consider when implementing a PHEOC.

Leverage Strong, Decisive Leadership and Create Shared Understanding in Response

Qualitative evidence synthesis Nine qualitative studies examined the use of mental models in public health emergency operations (Bigley and Roberts, 2001; Glick and Barbara, 2013; Gryth et al., 2010; Lis et al., 2017; McMaster and Baber, 2012; Militello et al., 2007; Moynihan, 2008; Rimstad and Sollid, 2015; Sisco et al., 2019). According to these studies, knowledge of different aspects of public health emergency operations, including situational awareness of an event, is cognitively represented through mental models, and building this knowledge base, especially the situational awareness of an event, is critical to emergency operations. When leaders and staff of public health and other agencies undergo preparedness training for an emergency event or act as "eyes and ears" for monitoring of an ongoing event, they are, in fact, creating cognitive representations of the event in the form of mental models. The full representation of all aspects of an event may be within the mind of one leader, although more often, understanding of the different aspects of an event is distributed across multiple leaders and staff (Bigley and Roberts, 2001; McMaster and Baber, 2012; Moynihan, 2008; Rimstad and Sollid, 2015). These mental models evolve, and for some people, they may initially be incorrect (Bigley and Roberts, 2001; Gryth et al., 2010). Therefore, one way to think about coordination among members of a group involved in emergency operations is to view it as coordination of the varying mental models held by staff and leaders within and across agencies. Mental models may serve as the basis for activation decisions. Leaders and commanders rarely have all available information about an ongoing event, but experienced personnel often make rapid decisions based on their mental models of prior events (Glick and Barbara, 2013; Rimstad and Sollid, 2015). Effective coordination of emergency operations depends to some extent on the degree to which accurate mental models are shared among members of the groups involved, leading to a shared understanding of an emergency event, as well as of interagency functions (Bigley and Roberts, 2001; McMaster and Baber, 2012; Militello et al., 2007; Moynihan, 2008; Sisco et al., 2019). *Knowledge of different aspects of public health emergency operations, and especially situational awareness of ongoing events, can be seen as cognitively constituted through mental models that are distributed across leaders and staff and that may be based on less-than-complete information. Viewing shared understanding of public health emergency operations overall in terms of mental models can help in understanding the functioning of activation and coordination activities* (moderate confidence in the evidence).

Case report and AAR evidence synthesis Case reports and AARs implicitly highlight the need for strong leadership willing to be decisive despite uncertainties inherent in emergencies. Leaders need to have the ability to receive new, sometimes unexpected information and to revise objectives as necessary (Redd and Frieden, 2017). Leaders also need to work to promote trust by creating a shared sense of purpose and recognizing the contributions of different network members (Moynihan, 2007).

Ensure Simultaneous Rigidity and Flexibility in a PHEOC

Qualitative evidence synthesis Seven qualitative studies examined simultaneously ensuring rigidity and flexibility in a PHEOC (Bigley and Roberts, 2001; Buck et al., 2006; Chandler et al., 2016; Freedman et al., 2013; Hambridge et al., 2017; McMaster and Baber, 2012; Moynihan, 2008). PHEOCs may be characterized only in terms of their rigid command and control structures, with the potential flexibility of the operations being downplayed. A more accurate overall conceptualization, however, is that these operations entail both command and control functions and preplanned adjustments and ad hoc improvisations (Chandler et al., 2016; Freedman et al., 2013; Hambridge et al., 2017; McMaster and Baber, 2012; Moynihan, 2008). The often changing, complex, and dynamic environment of an emergency event generates unique demands to which available command and control procedures do not fully apply, necessitating the emergence of new organizational structures and responses (Buck et al., 2006; Chandler et al., 2016; Freedman et al., 2013). Formal structures may be reconfigured through such strategies as structure elaboration, role switching, and authority migration so as to enhance organizational flexibility and thus reliability (Bigley and Roberts, 2001; McMaster and Baber, 2012). Similarly, professionals, especially those with experience, may not follow established procedures strictly, but make adjustments and use creative problem solving as required to respond to an evolving event (Bigley and Roberts, 2001; Freedman et al., 2013; McMaster and Baber, 2012; Rimstad and Sollid, 2015). *Emergency operations can be conceptualized and operationalized not just as rigid command and control functions but also as flexible adaptations and improvisations. Taking both perspectives on public health emergency operations can help in designing effective activation and coordination activities* (high confidence in the evidence).

Case report and AAR evidence synthesis While indicating that flexibility is crucial, case reports and AARs also stress the importance of adhering to basic principles. While jurisdictions acknowledged the value of an ICS, lack of adherence to basic principles also led to inefficiencies in some instances. For example, the lack of incident action plans (IAPs), response objectives, and routine briefings was reported to hinder response operations (Florida Department of Health, 2010, 2017; Metropolitan Medical Response System, 2016; New Hampshire Department of Health and Human Services and Department of Safety, 2009b; Ohio Department of Health, 2010). Likewise, the absence of routine updates to the incident commander inhibited well-informed and timely decision making (Logan County Health District, 2015), and an ongoing lack of communication through the chain of command led to delayed emergency notification and mutual aid and impeded timely resource requests (Lyons et al., 2009). Conversely, the inclusion of operations briefings, debriefs, situational reports (SitReps) and IAPs with response objectives, and job action sheets contributed to the success of response (Boston Public Health Comission, 2013; Capitol Region Council of Governments, 2016; Florida Department of Health, 2017; Logan County Health District, 2015; New Hampshire Department of Health and Human Services and Department of Safety, 2009b; San Francisco Department of Public Health, 2010).

View Public Health Emergency Operations Teams as Social Groups

Qualitative evidence synthesis Seven qualitative studies examined viewing public health emergency operations teams as social groups (Bigley and Roberts, 2001; Buck et al., 2006; Freedman et al., 2013; McMaster and Baber, 2012; Militello et al., 2007; Moynihan, 2008; Rimstad and Sollid, 2015). To take this view is to acknowledge that these teams are likely to face issues of differing values, power struggles, and political machinations (Bigley and Roberts, 2001). Also recognized are cultural differences among staff from different organizational cultures, such as those that are strictly hierarchical versus those that value judgment and discretion (Moynihan, 2008), as well as preexisting social power differentials and economic and political interests in the impacted communities during the response and recovery phases of an emergency event (Buck et al., 2006). Recognized as well are issues of affect and emotion, such as fear and concern about personal safety among staff members. Once these intensely social phenomena have been acknowledged, they can be dealt with productively, thereby improving the functioning of emergency operations (Buck et al., 2006; Rimstad and Sollid, 2015). Seeing work teams as social groups improves their functioning in other ways as well. Pre-event training across agencies creates informal relationships and a sense of social closeness and collegiality, which in turn fosters creativity and adaptation in response activities, trust, cohesion, and shared goals linked inextricably to the development of social relations and group formation (Buck et al., 2006; Freedman et al., 2013; McMaster and Baber, 2012; Militello et al., 2007). *Public health emergency operations teams, especially those involving multiple agencies, can be viewed as social groups in their functioning. A history of informal social relationships through prior training leads to familiarity and trust across differences in organizational cultures that can reduce power struggles and political maneuvering and enhance cooperation and coordination* (moderate confidence in the evidence).

Understand How Response Changes Following PHEOC Activation

Qualitative evidence synthesis Five qualitative studies examined how response changes following PHEOC activation (Chandler et al., 2016; Lis et al., 2017; McMaster and Baber, 2012; Rimstad and Sollid, 2015; Sisco et al., 2019). Studies considered several typologies for understanding these changes, but the changes are best described in terms of the Dynes typology, which can be used to classify responses into four categories: established organized response (regular old-task structural arrangements), expanding organized response (regular new-task structural arrangements), extending organized response (nonregular old-task structural arrangements), and emergent organized response (nonregular new-task structural arrangements) (Chandler et al., 2016; Dynes, 1993, 1994). This typology helps clarify how public health agencies navigate their responses by carrying out both regular and irregular tasks while also functioning within both old and new structural arrangements. Response changes can be judged in terms of their adaptation to the emergency event as a deviation from the planned, established responses. At a minimum, response changes can be seen as exhibiting no, some, or a great deal of adaptation, depending on the phase of the emergency event, with a great deal of adaptation being most likely in the event's earliest phases (McMaster and Baber, 2012; Rimstad and Sollid, 2015; Sisco et al., 2019). *Response changes following activation of public health emergency operations can be seen in terms of the degree of adaptation (none, some, a great deal) of established responses. The type of response change may depend on the phase of the emergency event* (high confidence in the evidence).

Leverage Staff with Past Response Experiences

Case report and AAR evidence synthesis Case reports and AARs indicate that lessons learned from decisions not to activate a PHEOC during previous events influenced decisions to activate during subsequent public health emergencies (Adams et al., 2010; Wiedrich et al., 2013). In 1999, for instance, Nassau County, New York, decided not to activate in response to West Nile virus, a new disease of unknown magnitude (Adams et al., 2010). In 2008, however, when the threat reemerged, the decision to activate was made, given the complexities involved and the recognized need for resources. Thus, looking to past experience can be a practical means of determining whether to activate.

Furthermore, staff's level of familiarity with the ICS model represented either a barrier to or facilitator of successful response operations. Numerous AARs indicate that the previous knowledge and experience of staff enabled positive outcomes (Moynihan, 2007; Quinn et al., 2018; San Francisco Department of Public Health, 2010; Wisconsin Division of Public Health, 2010), whereas a lack of familiarity with ICS or limited experience with larger-scale disasters was a barrier to effective response operations (Logan County Health District, 2015; Moynihan, 2007). In some instances, the use of experienced staff and subject-matter experts early on in the response to a novel outbreak is recommended (Multnomah County Health Department, 2010), although overreliance on a few key personnel can lead to staff fatigue (Delaware Division of Public Health, 2010).

REFERENCES FOR ARTICLES INCLUDED IN THE MIXED-METHOD REVIEW

Qualitative Studies

Bigley, G. A., and K. H. Roberts. 2001. The incident command system: High-reliability organizing for complex and volatile task environments. *Academy of Management Journal* 44(6):1281–1299.

Buck, D. A., J. E. Trainor, and B. E. Aguirre. 2006. A critical evaluation of the incident command system and NIMS. *Journal of Homeland Security and Emergency Management* 3(3).

Chandler, T., D. M. Abramson, B. Panigrahi, J. Schlegelmilch, and N. Frye. 2016. Crisis decision-making during Hurricane Sandy: An analysis of established and emergent disaster response behaviors in the New York Metro Area. *Disaster Medicine and Public Health Preparedness* 10(3):436–442.

Freedman, A. M., M. Mindlin, C. Morley, M. Griffin, W. Wooten, and K. Miner. 2013. Addressing the gap between public health emergency planning and incident response lessons learned from the 2009 H1N1 outbreak in San Diego County. *Disaster Health* 1(1):13–20.

Glick, J. A., and J. A. Barbara. 2013. Moving from situational awareness to decisions during disaster response: Transition to decision making. *Journal of Emergency Management* 11(6):423–432.
Gryth, D., M. Radestad, H. Nilsson, O. Nerf, L. Svensson, M. Castren, and A. Ruter. 2010. Evaluation of medical command and control using performance indicators in a full-scale, major aircraft accident exercise. *Prehospital & Disaster Medicine* 25(2):118–123.
Hambridge, N. B., A. M. Howitt, and D. W. Giles. 2017. Coordination in crises: Implementation of the national incident management system by surface transportation agencies. *Homeland Security Affairs* 13.
Klima, D. A., S. H. Seiler, J. B. Peterson, A. B. Christmas, J. M. Green, G. Fleming, M. H. Thomason, and R. F. Sing. 2012. Full-scale regional exercises: Closing the gaps in disaster preparedness. *The Journal of Trauma and Acute Care Surgery* 73(3):592–597; discussion 597–598.
Lis, R., and A. T. Resnick. 2018. Coordinated communications and decision making to support a regional severe infectious disease response. *Health Security* 16(3):158–164.
Lis, R., V. Sakata, and O. Lien. 2017. How to choose? Using the Delphi method to develop consensus triggers and indicators for disaster response. *Disaster Medicine and Public Health Preparedness* 11(4):467–472.
Mase, W. A., B. Bickford, C. L. Thomas, S. D. Jones, and M. Bisesi. 2017. After-action review of the 2009-10 H1N1 influenza outbreak response: Ohio's public health system's performance. *Journal of Emergency Management* 15(5):325–334.
McMaster, R., and C. Baber. 2012. Multi-agency operations: Cooperation during flooding. *Applied Ergonomics* 43(1):38–47.
Militello, L. G., E. S. Patterson, L. Bowman, and R. Wears. 2007. Information flow during crisis management: Challenges to coordination in the emergency operations center. *Cognition, Technology and Work* 9(1):25–31.
Moynihan, D. P. 2008. Combining structural forms in the search for policy tools: Incident command systems in U.S. crisis management. *Governance* 21(2):205–229.
Obaid, J. M., G. Bailey, H. Wheeler, L. Meyers, S. J. Medcalf, K. F. Hansen, K. K. Sanger, and J. J. Lowe. 2017. Utilization of functional exercises to build regional emergency preparedness among rural health organizations in the U.S. *Prehospital & Disaster Medicine* 32(2):224–230.
Reeder, B., and A. M. Turner. 2011. Scenario-based design: A method for connecting information system design with public health operations and emergency management. *Journal of Biomedical Informatics* 44(6):978–988.
Rimstad, R., and S. J. M. Sollid. 2015. A retrospective observational study of medical incident command and decision-making in the 2011 Oslo bombing. *International Journal of Emergency Medicine* 8(1):1–10.
Shipp Hilts, A., S. Mack, M. Eidson, T. Nguyen, and G. S. Birkhead. 2016. New York State public health system response to Hurricane Sandy: Lessons from the field. *Disaster Medicine and Public Health Preparedness* 10(3):443–453.
Sisco, S., E. M. A. Jones, E. K. Giebelhaus, T. Hadi, I. Gonzalez, and F. Lee Kahn. 2019. The role and function of the liaison officer: Lessons learned and applied after Superstorm Sandy. *Health Security* 17(2):109–116.
Thomas, T. L., E. B. Hsu, H. K. Kim, S. Colli, G. Arana, and G. B. Green. 2005. The incident command system in disasters: Evaluation methods for a hospital-based exercise. *Prehospital & Disaster Medicine* 20(1):14–23.
Yanson, A., A. S. Hilts, S. Mack, M. Eidson, T. Nguyen, and G. Birkhead. 2017. Superstorm Sandy: Emergency management staff perceptions of impact and recommendations for future preparedness, New York State. *Journal of Emergency Management* 15(4):209–218.

Descriptive Survey Studies

Jensen, J. 2011. The current NIMS implementation behavior of United States counties. *Journal of Homeland Security and Emergency Management* 8.
Jensen, J., and G. Youngs. 2015. Explaining implementation behaviour of the National Incident Management System (NIMS). *Disasters* 39(2):362–388.

Case Reports

Adams, E. H., E. Scanlon, J. J. Callahan, 3rd, and M. T. Carney. 2010. Utilization of an incident command system for a public health threat: West Nile virus in Nassau County, New York, 2008. *Journal of Public Health Management and Practice* 16(4):309–315.
Ansell, C., and A. Keller. 2014. *Adapting the incident command model for knowledge-based crises: The case of the Centers for Disease Control and Prevention.* Washington, DC: IBM Center for the Business of Government.
Augustine, J., and J. T. Schoettmer. 2005. Evacuation of a rural community hospital: Lessons learned from an unplanned event. *Disaster Management & Response* 3(3):68–72.

Beatty, M. E., S. Phelps, M. C. Rohner, and M. I. Weisfuse. 2006. Blackout of 2003: Public health effects and emergency response. *Public Health Reports* 121(1):36–44.

Branum, A., J. E. Dietz, and D. R. Black. 2010. An evaluation of local incident command system personnel in a pandemic influenza. *Journal of Emergency Management.* https://doi.org/10.5055/jem.2010.0031.

Buehler, J. W., J. Caum, and S. J. Alles. 2017. Public health and the Pope's visit to Philadelphia, 2015. *Health Security* 15(5):548–558.

CDC (Centers for Disease Control and Prevention). 2013. CDC's emergency management program activities—Worldwide, 2003–2012. *Morbidity and Mortality Weekly Report* 62(35):709–713.

Cole, D., M. Peninger, S. Singh, J. Tucker, C. Douglas, and S. Kiernan. 2015. Measles emergency response: Lessons learned from a measles exposure in an 800-bed facility. *American Journal of Infection Control* 43(6 Suppl 1):S14–S15.

Cruz, M. A., N. M. Hawk, C. Poulet, J. Rovira, and E. N. Rouse. 2015. Public health incident management: Logistical and operational aspects of the 2009 initial outbreak of H1N1 influenza in Mexico. *American Journal of Disaster Medicine* 10(4):347–353.

Davis, M. V., P. D. MacDonald, J. S. Cline, and E. L. Baker. 2007. Evaluation of public health response to hurricanes finds North Carolina better prepared for public health emergencies. *Public Health Reports* 122(1):17–26.

Fishbane, M., A. Kist, and R. A. Schieber. 2012. Use of the emergency incident command system for school-located mass influenza vaccination clinics. *Pediatrics* 129(Suppl 2):S101–S106.

Fleischauer, A. T., S. Williams, D. R. O'Leary, T. McChesney, W. Mason, S. Falk, L. Gladden, S. Snow, F. L. Clark, P. Terebuh, and F. W. Boozman. 2003. The West Nile virus epidemic in Arkansas, 2002: The Arkansas Department of Health Response. *Journal of the Arkansas Medical Society* 100(3):94–99.

Hunter, J. C., A. W. Crawley, M. Petrie, J. E. Yang, and T. J. Aragón. 2012. Local public health system response to the tsunami threat in coastal California following the Tohoku earthquake. *PLOS Currents* 2012(4). http://doi.org/10.1371/4f7f57285b804.

Iskander, J., D. A. Rose, and N. D. Ghiya. 2017. Science in emergency response at CDC: Structure and functions. *American Journal of Public Health* 107(S2):S122–S125.

Kilianski, A., A. T. O'Rourke, C. L. Carlson, S. M. Parikh, and F. Shipman-Amuwo. 2014. The planning, execution, and evaluation of a mass prophylaxis full-scale exercise in Cook County, IL. *Biosecurity & Bioterrorism* 12(2):106–116.

Klein, K. R., M. S. Rosenthal, and H. A. Klausner. 2005. Blackout 2003: Preparedness and lessons learned from the perspectives of four hospitals. *Prehospital & Disaster Medicine* 20(5):343–349.

Lutz, L. D., and M. K. Lindell. 2008. Incident command system as a response model within emergency operation centers during Hurricane Rita. *Journal of Contingencies and Crisis Management* 16(3):122–134.

Lyons, W. H., F. M. Burkle, Jr., D. L. Roepke, and J. E. Bertz. 2009. An influenza pandemic exercise in a major urban setting, part I: Hospital health systems lessons learned and implications for future planning. *American Journal of Disaster Medicine* 4(2):120–128.

Moynihan, D. P. 2007. *From forest fires to Hurricane Katrina: Case studies of incident command systems.* Washington, DC: IBM Center for the Business of Government.

Phillips, F. B., and J. P. Williamson. 2005. Local health department applies incident management system for successful mass influenza clinics. *Journal of Public Health Management & Practice* 11(4):269–273.

Porter, D., M. Hall, B. Hartl, C. Raevsky, R. Peacock, D. Kraker, S. Walls, and G. Brink. 2011. Local health department 2009 H1N1 influenza vaccination clinics—CDC staffing model comparison and other best practices. *Journal of Public Health Management & Practice* 17(6):530–533.

Posid, J. M., S. M. Bruce, J. T. Guarnizo, M. L. Taylor, and B. W. Garza. 2005. SARS: Mobilizing and maintaining a public health emergency response. *Journal of Public Health Management and Practice* 11(3):208–215.

Quinn, E., T. Johnstone, Z. Najjar, T. Cains, G. Tan, E. Huhtinen, S. Nilsson, S. Burgess, M. Dunn, and L. Gupta. 2018. Lessons learned from implementing an incident command system during a local multiagency response to a legionnaires' disease cluster in Sydney, NSW. *Disaster Medicine and Public Health Preparedness* 12(4):539–542.

Redd, S. C., and T. R. Frieden. 2017. CDC's evolving approach to emergency response. *Health Security* 15(1):41–52.

Shipp Hilts, A., S. Mack, M. Eidson, T. Nguyen, and G. S. Birkhead. 2016. New York State public health system response to Hurricane Sandy: An analysis of emergency reports. *Disaster Medicine & Public Health Preparedness* 10(3):308–313.

Timm, N. L., and M. Gneuhs. 2011. The pediatric hospital incident command system: An innovative approach to hospital emergency management. *Journal of Trauma—Injury, Infection and Critical Care* 71(5 Suppl 2):S549–S554.

Wiedrich, T. W., J. L. Sickler, B. L. Vossler, and S. P. Pickard. 2013. Critical systems for public health management of floods, North Dakota. *Journal of Public Health Management & Practice* 19(3):259–265.

Wiesman, J., A. Melnick, J. Bright, C. Carreon, K. Richards, J. Sherrill, and J. Vines. 2011. Lessons learned from a policy decision to coordinate a multijurisdiction H1N1 response with a single incident management team. *Journal of Public Health Management & Practice* 17(1):28–35.

Williams, H. A., R. L. Dunville, S. I. Gerber, D. D. Erdman, N. Pesik, D. Kuhar, et al. 2014. CDC's early response to a novel viral disease, middle east respiratory syndrome coronavirus (MERS-CoV), September 2012–May 2014. *Public Health Reports* 130(4):307–317.

AARs[3]

Becker County Community Health. 2013. *People & Stuff 2013—HSEM Region 3 logistics exercise after action report/improvement plan.* Becker County, MN. December 6, 2013.

Boston Public Health Commission. 2013. *2013 Boston Marathon emergency support function F8 (ESF-8) public health and medical planning, response, and recovery operations (April 15–April 16).* https://delvalle.bphc.org/mod/wiki/view.php?pageid=63 (accessed April 3, 2020).

Buffalo Hospital and Wright County Public Health. 2013. *Buffalo hospital closed pod after-action report/improvement plan.* Buffalo, NY. November 21, 2013.

Capitol Region Council of Governments. 2016. *Ebola virus disease functional exercise after action report.* Hartford, CT. May 18, 2016.

Capitol Region Council of Governments. 2017. *Ebola Virus Disease Full Scale Exercise After Action Report.* Hartford, CT. May 19, 2017.

Chicago Department of Public Health, Illinois Department of Public Health, and Metropolitan Chicago Healthcare Council. 2011. *Illinois hospitals pediatric full-scale exercise after action report.* Chicago, IL. May 21, 2011.

City of Nashua Department of Emergency Management. 2012. *October Nor'easter after action report.* Nashua, NH. March 2, 2012.

Contra Costa Health Services. 2012. *Chevron Richmond refinery fire of August 6, 2012: After action report based on medical/health debriefing.* Martinez, CA. December 6, 2012.

County of San Diego. 2018. *Hepatitis A outbreak after action report.* May 2018. San Diego, CA. https://www.sandiegocounty.gov/content/dam/sdc/cosd/SanDiegoHepatitisAOutbreak-2017-18-AfterActionReport.pdf (accessed January 23, 2020).

Delaware Division of Public Health. 2010. *Novel H1N1 influenza Delaware response April 2009 to March 2010: After action report/improvement plan.* Dover, DE. June 1, 2010. https://dhss.delaware.gov/DHSS/DPH/php/files/h1n1aar.pdf (accessed January 23, 2020).

DuPage County Health Department. 2009. 00.10 *H1N1 after action report (AAR)—improvement plan (IP).* Wheaton, IL. April 26, 2009–May 11, 2009.

Florida Department of Health. 2010. *2010* Deepwater Horizon *oil spill response: ESF 8 after action report and improvement plan.* Tallahassee, FL. April 30, 2011. http://www.floridahealth.gov/programs-and-services/emergency-preparedness-and-response/training-exercise/_documents/deepwater-aar.pdf (accessed January 23, 2020).

Florida Department of Health. 2017. *2017 statewide hurricane full scale exercise.* Tallahassee, FL. September 19, 2017. http://www.floridahealth.gov/programs-and-services/emergency-preparedness-and-response/training-exercise/_documents/2017-statewide-hurricane-fse.pdf (accessed January 23, 2020).

Governor's Office of Homeland Security & Emergency Preparedness. 2012. *Hurricane Isaac after action report & improvement plan.* Baton Rouge, LA. December 31, 2012.

Logan County Health District. 2015. *Logan County Health District 2015 full scale exercise.* Bellefontaine, OH. June 9–10, 2015. http://loganhealth.org/documents/2015LCHDAARfinaldraft_06_24_2015.pdf (accessed January 23, 2020).

Massachusetts Emergency Management Agency, Massachusetts Department of Public Health, City of Boston, City of Cambridge, Town of Watertown, Massachusetts Bay Transportation Authority Transit Police Department, and M. S. P. Massachusetts National Guard. 2014. *After action report for the response to the 2013 Boston Marathon bombings.* https://www.policefoundation.org/wp content/uploads/2015/05/after-action-report-for-the-response-to-the-2013-boston-marathon-bombings_0.pdf (accessed January 23, 2020).

Metropolitan Medical Response System. 2016. *CT region 3 ESF-8 Ebola preparedness & response: After action report.* Falls Church, VA. October 29, 2015.

Minnesota Department of Health. 2013. *Operation Loon Call 2013: After-action report/improvement plan.* St. Paul, MN. June 11, 2013.

[3] These AARs were retrieved from the Homeland Security Digital Library at https://www.hsdl.org/c (accessed June 10, 2020); they may be accessed and downloaded there.

Minnesota Department of Health. 2014. *DOC FE flash floods 2014: After-action report/improvement plan 2014.* St. Paul, MN. May 29, 2014.

Multnomah County Health Department. 2009. *"Swine flu Multco" Spring 2009 H1N1 response of April 27–May 12, 2009: After action report/improvement plan.* Portland, OR. December 28, 2009.

Multnomah County Health Department. 2010. *H1N1 Fall 2009–Multco Aug 4–5, 2009–December 8, 2009: After action report/improvement plan.* Portland, OR. May 4, 2010.

New Hampshire Department of Health and Human Services and New Hampshire Department of Safety. 2009a. *2009 spring H1N1 response: After action report/improvement plan.* Concord, NH. September 22, 2009.

New Hampshire Department of Health and Human Services and New Hampshire Department of Safety. 2009b. *Cities ready initiative operation rapid RX full-scale exercise: After action report.* Concord, NH. October 16, 17, 24, 2009.

New Hampshire Department of Health and Human Services and New Hampshire Department of Safety. 2010. *New Hampshire July 1, 2009–March 30, 2010 H1N1 response: After action report/improvement plan.* Concord, NH.

Ohio Department of Health. 2010. *Fall 2009 H1N1 response: ICS operations conducted through September 21, 2009–Febuary 4, 2010: After action report—Improvement plan.* Columbus, OH. June 29, 2010.

Oklahoma Department of Emergency Management. 2013. *Earth, wind, and fire 2013: After-action report/corrective action plan.* Oklahoma City, OK. November 14, 2013.

San Francisco Department of Public Health. 2010. *Fall/winter 2009–2010 H1N1 swine flu response: San Francisco, California: September 28, 2009–March 9,2010: After action report/improvement plan.* August 20, 2010. https://www.sfcdcp.org/wp-content/uploads/2018/01/H1N1-AAR-Executive-Summary.Fall-Winter-2009-2010-id639.pdf (accessed January 23, 2020).

Texas Department of State Health Services. 2010. *Texas Department of State Health Services response to the novel H1N1 pandemic influenza (2009 and 2010): After action report.* The Litaker Group LLC. Austin, TX. August 30, 2010.

Texas Department of State Health Services. 2018. *Hurricane Harvey response: After-action report.* Austin, TX. May 30, 2018.

Tri-County Health Department. 2013. *PHIMT NACCHO model practice award application.* Greenwood Village, CO.

Tri-County Health Department. 2017. *Public health emergency dispensing exercise (PHEDX) after action report and improvement plan.* Greenwood Village, CO. June 15–17, 2017.

Tri-County Health Department. n.d. *Public health incident management team (PHIMT).* Greenwood Village, CO.

Wisconsin Division of Public Health. 2010. *2009 H1N1 influenza response after action report and improvement plan.* Madison, WI. July 2010.

Wisconsin Hospital Emergency Preparedness Program. 2010. *After action report (AAR) for H1N1 influenza.* Madison, WI. April 24, 2009–Spring 2010.

Wood County Health District. 2017. *2017 regional functional/full-scale exercise: After-action report/improvement plan.* Bowling Green, OH. June 12, 2017.

Ethics and Policy Text

IOM (Institute of Medicine). 2009. *Guidance for establishing crisis standards of care for use in disaster situations: A letter report.* Washington, DC: The National Academies Press

Jennings, B. and J. Arras. 2008. *Ethical guidance for public health emergency preparedness and response: Highlighting ethics and values in a vital public health service.* https://www.cdc.gov/od/science/integrity/phethics/docs/white_paper_final_for_website_2012_4_6_12_final_for_web_508_compliant.pdf (accessed February 23, 2020).

Jennings, B., J. D. Arras, D. H. Barrett, and B. A. Ellis. 2016. *Emergency ethics: Public health preparedness and response.* New York: Oxford University Press.

Mastroianni, A. C., J. P. Kahn, and N. E. Kass, eds. 2019. *The Oxford handbook of public health ethics.* New York: Oxford University Press. https://www.oxfordhandbooks.com/view/10.1093/oxfordhb/9780190245191.001.0001/oxfordhb-9780190245191 (accessed June 3, 2020).

ARTICLES NOT FORMALLY INCLUDED IN THE MIXED-METHOD REVIEW

Dynes, R. R. 1993. Disaster reduction: The importance of adequate assumptions about social organization. *Sociological Spectrum* 13:175–192.

Dynes, R. R. 1994. Community emergency planning: False assumptions and inappropriate analogies. *International Journal of Mass Emergencies and Disasters* 12:141–158.

B3 Mixed-Method Review of Channels for Communicating Public Health Alerts and Guidance with Technical Audiences During a Public Health Emergency

This appendix provides a detailed description of the methods for and the evidence from the mixed-method review of channels for communicating public health alerts and guidance with technical audiences during a public health emergency, which is summarized in Chapter 6.[1]

KEY REVIEW QUESTIONS AND ANALYTIC FRAMEWORK

The overarching question that guided this review addresses the effectiveness of different channels for communicating public health alerts and guidance with technical audiences during a public health emergency. To answer this overarching question, the committee sought evidence on several sub-questions related to documented benefits and harms associated with the channels themselves, as well as the engagement of technical audiences in the development of communication plans and channels. The committee also examined the evidence on the factors that create barriers to and facilitators of effective communication with technical audiences (see Box B3-1).

Effective communication channels provide a conduit for information to be transmitted from public health authorities to recipient technical audiences (and in some cases, allow for bidirectional exchange). The objective of this public health emergency preparedness and response (PHEPR) practice is to ensure that technical audiences are aware of and understand up-to-date information about a particular public health threat. As depicted in the analytic framework in Figure B3-1, awareness of current alerts and guidance may influence the behaviors of information recipients (e.g., changes in diagnostic testing protocols, use of

[1] This appendix draws heavily on three reports commissioned by the committee: "Data Extraction and Quality Assessment: Methodology and Evidence Tables" by the Brown University Center for Evidence Synthesis in Health; "Communicating Public Health Alerts and Guidance with Technical Audiences: Qualitative Research Evidence Synthesis" by Julie Novak and Pradeep Sopory; and "Information Sharing with Technical Audiences: Findings from After Action Reports and Case Reports" by Sneha Patel (see Appendix C).

BOX B3-1 KEY REVIEW QUESTIONS

What is the effectiveness of different channels for communicating public health alerts and guidance with technical audiences during a public health emergency (e.g., Health Alert Network, conference calls, bidirectional text-based messaging/SMS, provider access line, email, website, written guidance documents)?

- What are the benefits and harms of engaging technical audiences in the development of communication plans, protocols, and channels?
- What benefits and harms (desirable and/or undesirable impacts) of different communication channels have been described or measured?
- What are the barriers to and facilitators of effective communication with technical audiences?

personal protective equipment, case reporting), which may in turn improve the response to a public health threat (e.g., through improved situational awareness and coordination of response partners) and reduce associated morbidity and mortality (e.g., by reducing or better managing infections).

EVIDENCE SUPPORTING THE PRACTICE RECOMMENDATION

This section summarizes the evidence from the mixed-method review examining different channels for communicating public health alerts and guidance with technical audiences during a public health emergency. It begins with a description of the results of the literature search and then summarizes the evidence of effectiveness. In formulating its practice recommendation, the committee considered evidence beyond effectiveness, which was compiled using an Evidence to Decision (EtD) framework encompassing balance of benefits and harms, acceptability and preferences, feasibility and PHEPR system considerations, resource and economic considerations, equity, and ethical considerations. The evidence from each methodological stream applicable to each of the EtD criteria is discussed; a synthesis is provided in Table B3-4 later in this appendix and in Chapter 6. Graded finding statements from evidence syntheses are italicized in the narrative below.

Full details about the study eligibility criteria, search strategy, and processes for data extraction and individual study quality assessment are available in Appendix A. Appendix C links to all of the commissioned analyses informing this review.

Results of the Literature Search

The searches of bibliographic databases identified a total of 5,853 potentially relevant citations (deduplicated) for the mixed-method review of channels for communicating public health alerts and guidance with technical audiences during a public health emergency. A search of the gray literature, reference mining, and a call for papers contributed an additional 599 articles. All 6,452 citations were imported into EndNote and were included in title and abstract screening. During screening, 6,279 articles were excluded because their abstracts did not appear to answer any of the key questions or they indicated that the articles were

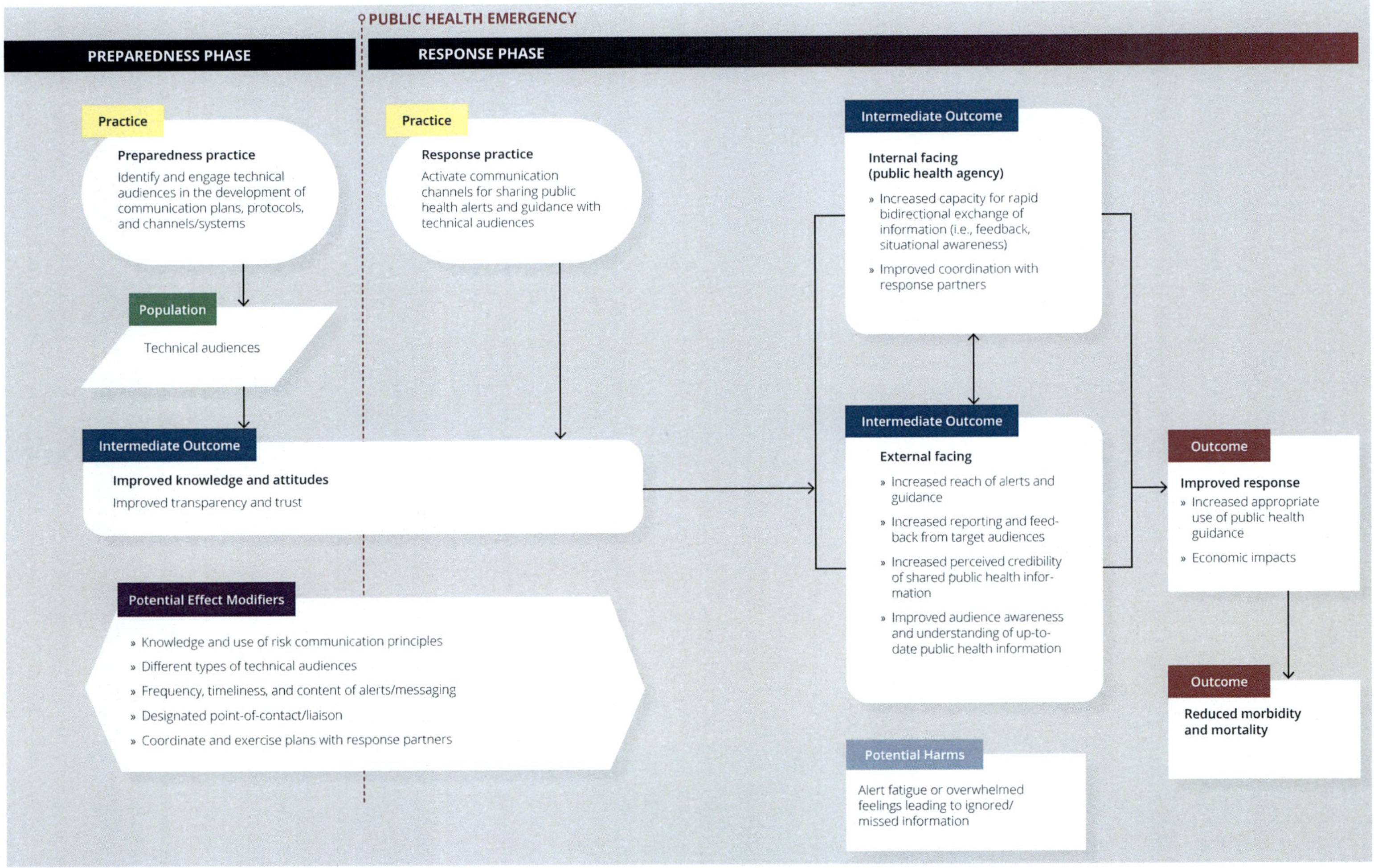

FIGURE B3-1 Analytic framework for communicating public health alerts and guidance with technical audiences during a public health emergency.
NOTES: Arrows in the framework indicate hypothesized causal pathways between interventions and outcomes. Double-headed arrows indicate feedback loops.

commentaries, editorials, or opinion pieces. After the abstracts had been reviewed, 173 full-text articles were reviewed and assessed for eligibility for inclusion in the mixed-method review. The committee considered 79 articles for data extraction and ultimately included 61 articles in the mixed-method review. Figure B3-2 depicts the literature flow, indicating the number of articles included and excluded at each screening stage. Table B3-1 indicates the types of evidence included in this review.

1. Determining Evidence of Effect

Two quantitative comparative studies directly addressed the overarching key question regarding the effectiveness of different channels for communicating public health alerts and guidance with technical audiences during a public health emergency. Both studies evaluated types of electronic messaging systems (e.g., email, fax, text messaging) that are used to push information out to target audiences (rather than relying on target audiences to pull information down). A meta-analysis of the evidence for the effectiveness of these communication channels was not feasible, so the committee conducted a synthesis without meta-analysis (as described in Chapter 3).

Consistent with the methods described in Chapter 3, in making its final judgment on the evidence of effectiveness for electronic messaging channels for communicating public health alerts and guidance with technical audiences during a public health emergency, the committee considered other types of evidence that could inform a determination of what works for whom and in which contexts, ultimately reaching consensus on the certainty of the evidence (COE) for each outcome. Including forms of evidence beyond quantitative comparative studies is particularly important when assessing evidence in settings where controlled studies are challenging to conduct and/or other forms of quantitative comparative data are difficult to obtain. As discussed in Chapter 3, descriptive evidence from real-world implementation of practices offers the potential to corroborate research findings or explain differences in outcomes in practice settings, even if it has lesser value for causal inference. Moreover, qualitative studies can complement quantitative studies by providing additional useful evidence to guide real-world decision making, because well-conducted qualitative studies produce deep and rich understandings of how interventions are implemented, delivered, and experienced. Other forms of evidence considered for evaluation of effectiveness included quantitative data reported in descriptive surveys, case reports, and after action reports (AARs) that involved a real disaster or public health emergency.

Of note, some surveys, case reports, and AARs report on passive electronic messaging systems that rely on the information-seeking behavior of the target audience (e.g., websites) and communication channels other than electronic messaging systems (e.g., telephone conferencing, hotlines). In the absence of comparative data from which conclusions regarding effectiveness could be drawn, however, these other communication channels were not included in the committee's synthesis of quantitative evidence. While it is clear that channels other than electronic messaging systems are being used in practice to communicate public health alerts and guidance with technical audiences, the effectiveness of these channels has not yet been rigorously studied in the PHEPR context.

Evidence from Quantitative Research Studies

Two quantitative comparative research studies examined the effectiveness of different channels for communicating public health alerts and guidance with technical audiences. A randomized controlled trial conducted by Baseman and colleagues (2016) from 2009

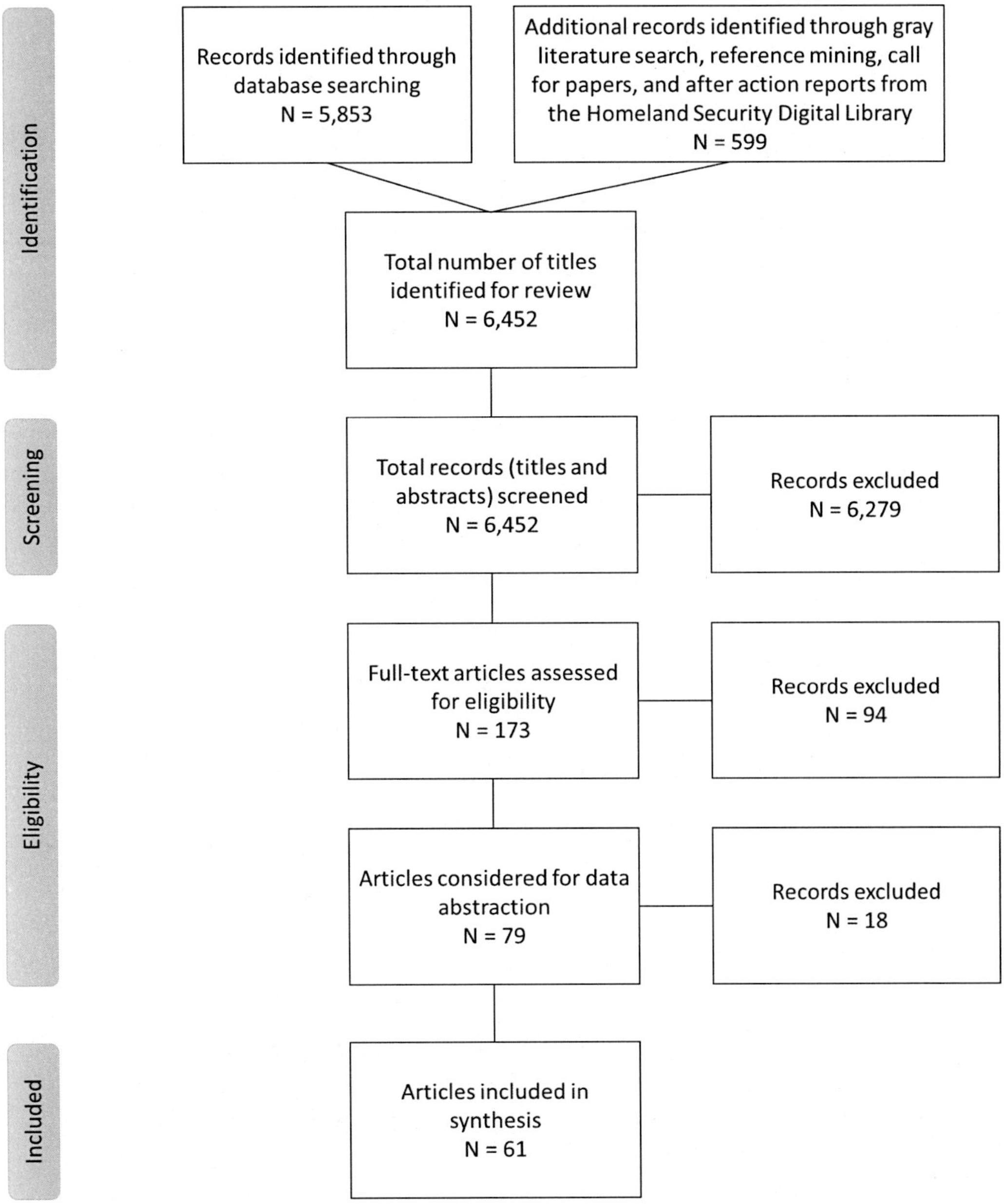

FIGURE B3-2 Preferred Reporting Items for Systematic Reviews and Meta-Analyses diagram for the mixed-method review of channels for communicating public health alerts and guidance with technical audiences during a public health emergency.

TABLE B3-1 Evidence Types Included in the Mixed-Method Review of Channels for Communicating Public Health Alerts and Guidance with Technical Audiences During a Public Health Emergency

Evidence Type[a]	Number of Studies (as applicable)[b]
Quantitative comparative	2
Quantitative noncomparative (postintervention measure only)	0
Qualitative	8[c]
Modeling	0
Descriptive surveys	8
Case reports	12[d]
After action reports	29[d]
Mechanistic	N/A
Parallel (systematic reviews)	N/A

[a] Evidence types are defined in Chapter 3.
[b] Note that sibling articles (different results from the same study published in separate articles) are counted as one study in this table. Mixed-method studies may be counted in more than one category.
[c] Two surveys containing a qualitative analysis of free-text responses were included in the qualitative evidence synthesis. The two studies were not classified as qualitative research studies and are not included in the qualitative study count for this table. As described in Chapter 3, the findings from these sources were extracted and considered separately in the qualitative evidence synthesis to affirm or question those findings from the more complete qualitative studies.
[d] A sample of case reports and after action reports was prioritized for inclusion in this review based on relevance to the key questions, as described in Chapter 3.

to 2012 (the REACH trial) compared what then were considered "traditional" and new (mobile) communication strategies for use by public health agencies to transmit time-sensitive health information to health care providers in Washington State and Montana over a 6- to 12-month period. The trial compared email, fax, SMS (text messaging), and no messaging. The investigators assessed 846 providers' recall of message topics, correcting for the possibility of false recall. All messaging methods were more successful with respect to recall of message topics than no (active) messaging. Email was statistically significantly more effective than either fax or text (45 percent message topic recall versus 38 percent and 37 percent for fax and text, respectively, $p < 0.05$) (Baseman et al., 2016). Accessing available hyperlinks (available through all messaging methods) was associated with greater recall (odds ratio [OR] = 3.9; $p < 0.001$). Text messaging resulted in a statistically significantly greater likelihood of accessing hyperlinks relative to either phone or fax messages ($p \leq 0.001$). A substudy of the REACH trial ($N = 528$) showed that increases in the number of messages sent to a provider were associated with a decreased likelihood of correct recall of message content. Every increase of one public health message per week resulted in a statistically significant 41.2 percent decrease ($p < 0.01$) in the odds of recalling the study message content, a finding suggestive of alert fatigue (Baseman et al., 2013). The committee was concerned that the comparisons made in this study are outdated and potentially not relevant (in part because simultaneous messages via multiple modalities are common practice today). Also important is that although study messages were time sensitive, they were not real emergency alerts. These concerns were not incorporated into the assessment of risk of bias and methodological quality for this study as they were not considered to be issues of bias or methodological quality. The trial had no serious methodological limitations, and overall, the study (and each outcome) was deemed to be of good methodological quality.

A retrospective, nonrandomized comparative study by van Woerden and colleagues (2007) evaluated data from 2001 and 2002 to determine whether the number of patients tested for Q fever was affected by sending faxes to primary care physicians about a Q fever outbreak in Wales that occurred in 2002. After the Q fever outbreak was identified at an urban factory, the National Public Health Service used a fax cascade system to alert primary care practices. Physicians were asked to submit serum samples on any patient meeting a clinical case definition of Q fever and having an association with the area where the outbreak appeared to be occurring. The researchers compared the number of Q fever diagnostic tests ordered during the same 2-month period in 2001 and 2002, which included the dates of the fax cascade in mid-September 2002, as well as the preceding 2 weeks. Approximately 565,000 people lived in the analyzed community. The number of requests for Q fever tests during the 2-month period in 2002 was three times higher than the number of requests during the corresponding time period of the preceding year, and the difference in the proportion of the population tested in 2001 and 2002 was statistically significant ($p < 0.001$). The researchers found an association between the timing of the faxes and the significant increase in the number of requests for Q fever tests, in contrast with similar numbers of test requests in the prior 2 weeks in both analyzed years. This study had major limitations related to lack of adjustment for differences between the two analyzed years, as well as poor power. In addition, the researchers did not attempt to account for other factors (such as the local press) that may have impacted the number of tests ordered. Overall, the study (and each outcome) was deemed to be of poor methodological quality.

Other Evidence That May Inform Effectiveness

The results of one survey support the above findings from quantitative comparative studies regarding the effectiveness of electronic messaging systems.[2] Argonne National Laboratory surveyed stakeholders of the Illinois Department of Public Health (IDPH) representing a mix of health and nonhealth (e.g., schools, businesses) sectors regarding strengths and weaknesses of IDPH information-sharing practices during the response to the H1N1 outbreak. Only 24 percent of respondents reported fax to be an effective means of communication during such a disease outbreak, while 64 percent reported that the IDPH website provided timely and useful information. Fewer than half of respondents identified the hospital Health Alert Network (H-HAN) as a "useful" communication tool during a disease outbreak, although 72 percent of hospital respondents did so (most other stakeholders lacked access to the H-HAN) (Walsh et al., 2010).

The committee reviewed six case reports containing quantitative data related to electronic messaging systems used for communicating public health alerts and guidance with technical audiences during public health emergencies. One supportive case report, published in a 2013 *Morbidity and Mortality Weekly Report,* describes how the Iowa Department of Public Health's multipronged communication strategy featuring multiple electronic messaging channels (HAN, electronic newsletter, website, Twitter) resulted in increased test-

[2] As described in Chapter 3, the committee reviewed other evidence that informed the COE (e.g., mechanistic evidence, experiential evidence from case reports and AARs, qualitative evidence) for coherence with the findings from the quantitative research studies and classified that evidence as very supportive, supportive, inconclusive (no conclusion can be drawn on coherence, either because results are mixed or the data are insufficient), or unsupportive (discordant with the findings). The distinction between supportive and very supportive is based on the magnitude of the reported effect and the directness of the evidence to the question of interest.

ing (as compared with the month prior to the alerts) for an infectious agent presumed to be causing an outbreak of cyclosporiasis. One health care provider ordered *Cyclospora* testing for a patient with undiagnosed and recurring vomiting and diarrhea after reading the electronic newsletter alert, which resulted in appropriate treatment for that patient (CDC, 2013).

A second supportive case report, published by Nagykaldi and colleagues (2006), describes a web-based alerting and surveillance system for influenza-like illness (ILI) in Oklahoma (OKAlert-ILI). The Oklahoma State Department of Health used this system to send a weekly message containing surveillance data for influenza and other infectious diseases to members of the Oklahoma practice-based research network and to collect ILI reports from users. OKAlert-ILI sentinel reports were correlated with culture-positive laboratory influenza test results (Pearson correlation coefficient = 0.827), but there was a 7-day lag for laboratory test results (i.e., the bidirectional ILI system resulted in more timely case reporting).

A third, very supportive case report, published by Lurio and colleagues (2010), describes an alerting system whereby HAN alerts sent from the public health department are received by leadership at the Institute for Family Health (a network of community health centers) and may, if appropriate, be translated into a best practice advisory (BPA) that alerts clinicians and provides diagnostic/treatment guidance through a popup in the electronic health record (EHR). HAN notifications that were translated into BPAs resulted in orders for diagnostic tests:

- In a case of a *Legionella* outbreak, a BPA was triggered for 142 patients, and orders were activated in 5 instances (3.5 percent). Two orders were submitted for *Legionella* urine antigen, a test that had not been ordered in the 5 years prior to the alert.
- During an *E. coli* O157:H7 outbreak, a BPA was triggered for 287 patients and orders for diagnostic tests were activated 65 times (22.6 percent), but no instance of *E. coli* O157:H7 was identified.
- During a measles outbreak, a BPA was triggered for 198 patients and orders were activated on four occasions (2 percent). Specimens from a potential case identified through the system were sent to the Department of Health but were not confirmed as measles.

The remaining three case reports with quantitative data (Daniel et al., 2005; Gamache et al., 2010; Gotham et al., 2007) are inconclusive with respect to the effectiveness of the communication channels discussed.

Few AARs addressing the use of communication channels report quantitative data, and among those that do, the findings regarding the effectiveness of electronic messaging channels are mixed. Two of the AARs in the sample collected for this mixed-method review report survey results regarding the perceived "effectiveness" of or satisfaction with electronic communication channels used during a public health emergency. In a survey of registered vaccine providers in New Hampshire during the H1N1 outbreak (N = 141), 92 percent of respondents agreed or strongly agreed that the HAN is "an effective vehicle for communicating information to [their] organization" (New Hampshire Department of Health and Human Services and New Hampshire Department of Safety, 2010). In contrast, another AAR from the H1N1 response reports that only 38 percent of survey respondents were satisfied or very satisfied with the HAN, but 93 percent were satisfied or very satisfied with H1N1 information provided by webcasts, while ~90 percent were satisfied or very satisfied with such information provided though the state government website (Wisconsin Division of Public Health, 2010).

Some AARs include information on the number or proportion of individuals who received electronic alerts. For example, a poll launched during a hospital exercise showed that only

70 percent of participating hospitals reported receiving the HAN alert (Chicago Department of Public Health et al., 2011). This and other AARs raise concerns regarding the distribution of electronic alerts, such as messages not being sent to the full recipient list, delays in receipt due to the passive nature of communication (i.e., intended recipients were not actively monitoring for messages), and failure by initial recipients to ensure that the HAN alert is passed along to other stakeholders. Thus, AARs raise the potential of an undesirable effect whereby reliance on electronic messaging methods could interfere with other, traditional modalities and delay responses.

Summary of the Evidence: Technical Audience Awareness

The committee concluded that *there is moderate COE that electronic messaging systems such as email, fax, and text messaging are effective communication channels for increasing technical audiences' awareness of public health alerts and guidance during a public health emergency.* Two quantitative comparative studies (Baseman et al., 2016; van Woerden et al., 2007) provide moderate COE regarding the effects of electronic messaging systems on technical audiences' awareness of public health alerts and guidance during a public health emergency (see Table B3-2). Other forms of evidence, which include one supportive survey, two supportive and one very supportive case reports, and mixed AAR evidence that raises questions about potential undesirable effects (although providing no conclusive data on harms) were insufficient to upgrade the COE but also did not warrant downgrading.

TABLE B3-2 Effect of Electronic Messaging System Channels (Email, Text, and Fax) on Improved Technical Audiences' Awareness of Public Health Alerts and Guidance During a Public Health Emergency

Quality Assessment	Number of Studies	2
	Study Infomation	Baseman et al., 2016 Randomized controlled trial (RCT), good methodological quality (▲) van Woerden et al., 2007 Nonrandomized comparative study (NRCS), retrospective, poor methodological quality (▲)
	Risk of Bias	Not serious
	Inconsistency	Not serious
	Indirectness	Serious (Baseman et al., 2016, study not conducted during a public health emergency)
	Imprecision	Not serious
	Publication Bias	Unlikely
	Upgrade for Large Effect, Dose Response, Plausible Confounding	No
Summary of Findings	Initial Certainty of the Evidence (COE)	Moderate
	Other Evidence	One supportive survey, case report evidence (two supportive and one very supportive), mixed after action report (AAR) evidence that raises concerns about undesirable effects
	COE	Moderate (improves technical audiences' awareness)

NOTE: Effect direction: upward arrow (▲) = improvement/beneficial effect; downward arrow (▼) = harm/negative effect; sideways arrows (◄►) = no effect; up and down arrows (▲▼) = mixed effect/conflicting findings.

Summary of the Evidence: Technical Audience Use of Guidance

The committee concluded that *there is very low COE that electronic messaging systems are effective communication channels for increasing technical audiences' use of current public health guidance during a public health emergency.* One quantitative comparative study (van Woerden et al., 2007) provides very low COE regarding the effects of electronic messaging systems on technical audiences' use of current public health guidance during a public health emergency (see Table B3-3). Other forms of evidence, which include a supportive survey, two supportive and one very supportive case reports, and mixed AAR evidence that raises questions about potential undesirable effects (although providing no conclusive data on harms) were insufficient to upgrade the COE but also did not warrant downgrading.

TABLE B3-3 Effect of Electronic Messaging System Channels (Email, Text, and Fax) on Improved Technical Audiences' Use of Public Health Guidance During a Public Health Emergency

Quality Assessment	Number of Studies	1
	Study Infomation	van Woerden et al., 2007 Nonrandomized comparative study (NRCS), retrospective, poor methodological quality (▲)
	Risk of Bias	Very serious
	Inconsistency	Not applicable
	Indirectness	Not serious
	Imprecision	Serious
	Publication Bias	Unlikely
	Upgrade for Large Effect, Dose Response, Plausible Confounding	No
Summary of Findings	Initial Certainty of the Evidence (COE)	Very low
	Other Evidence	One supportive survey, case report evidence (two supportive and one very supportive), mixed after action report (AAR) evidence that raises concerns about undesirable effects
	COE	Very low (improves technical audiences' use of guidance)

NOTE: Effect direction: upward arrow (▲) = improvement/beneficial effect; downward arrow (▼) = harm/negative effect; sideways arrows (◄►) = no effect; up and down arrows (▲▼) = mixed effect/conflicting findings.

Based on the evidence described above, the committee concludes that there is evidence of differential impact of different technologies employed as electronic messaging systems for communicating public health alerts and guidance with technical audiences during a public health emergency to increase awareness and appropriate use. However, data are insufficient to conclude what technology is best for which audiences in which scenarios.

2. Balance of Benefits and Harms

Synthesis of Evidence of Effect

As discussed in the section on effectiveness above, electronic messaging communication channels may have beneficial effects on technical audiences' awareness of public health alerts and guidance (moderate COE). However, these effects may be dampened by alert fatigue arising from excessive message volume.

Qualitative Evidence Synthesis

The 10 studies included in the body of qualitative evidence include very little discussion of the benefits and harms per se of communication channels. Instead, the studies largely considered how different channels corresponded to facilitators of and barriers to communication with technical audiences, after incorporating contextual factors. Participants reported what did and did not work well and offered suggestions for consideration. Notably, however, clear benefits were observed when public health officials engaged in thoughtful and inclusive deliberations with stakeholders about providing guidance. Such deliberations not only facilitated effective communication but also built relationships with health care providers and other stakeholders that were characterized by trust, respect, responsiveness, transparency, and flexibility (Khan et al., 2017; Lis and Resnick, 2018).

Although not specific to particular channels, technical audiences reported undesirable impacts related to the approach taken to communication of alerts and guidance. For example, although some duplication across different channels could be helpful, the volume of messages could quickly pose a burden and discourage rather than encourage the use of arriving guidance (Khan et al., 2017; Markiewicz et al., 2012; Staes et al., 2011). In addition, some important technical audiences could be excluded from existing communication channels. Leung and colleagues (2008) report that some smaller agencies and community-based partners were not included in prepared email listservs or other directories specifying recipients for public health guidance, and therefore received information through other pathways and relationships. Filice and colleagues (2013) point to a notable harm that manifests when no guidance is received or when guidance is incongruent with practice in public health emergencies. Such instances can lead to poor implementation of guidance, as health care providers may adhere to routine practices and institutionally determined adaptations. Additionally, when past experience and lessons learned fail to lead to changes in protocols and practices, disillusionment with future, coordinated efforts for preparedness may result.

Case Report and AAR Evidence Synthesis

Case reports and AARs included in this review do not specifically assess the benefits or unintended consequences of specific modes of communication. However, a few attributes improved timeliness to specific communication mechanisms. For instance, Cavey and colleagues (2009) assert that the use of telephone reporting through a shelter hotline improved timeliness, reporting compliance, accuracy, and staff satisfaction and knowledge. Gamache and colleagues (2010) also identify timeliness as a benefit of sending public health alerts through Health Information Exchange platforms. Similarly, Nagykaldi and colleagues' (2006) findings from an evaluation of the OKAlert-ILI system discussed earlier indicate more timely and accurate responses to ILI cases. Reports suggest that in-person meetings, teleconferences, and webcasts also improve timeliness by providing for real-time feedback (Delaware Division of Public Health, 2010; Wisconsin Division of Public Health, 2010).

One noted harm relates to the potential for important stakeholders to be omitted from those channels that require enrollment (New Hampshire Department of Health and Human Services and New Hampshire Department of Safety, 2009b). For example, while the HAN is cited as an important direct communication link to technical audiences, several reports point to the need to expand its reach, as not all technical audiences (e.g., first responders, individual providers, emergency medical departments, medical practices, local boards of health) are enrolled in that network (Boston Public Health Commission, 2013; Daniel et al., 2005; Delaware Division of Public Health, 2010; Gamache et al., 2010; Gursky et al., 2003; Massachusetts Emergency Management Agency et al., 2014; New Hampshire Department of Health and Human Services and New Hampshire Department of Safety, 2009b; Ohio Department of Health, 2010).

Although the evidence from case reports and AARs indicates that hotlines can facilitate bidirectional information sharing, hotline staff may experience excess fatigue as a result of stress associated with response efforts (Boston Public Health Commission, 2013). Additionally, Lurio and colleagues (2010) discuss the potential for alert fatigue if alerts are not targeted and tailored to specific provider types. "Paralysis by analysis" can also result from an overwhelming amount of information being shared in a short time without clear guidance (Metropolitan Medical Response System, 2016). Furthermore, the Delaware Division of Public Health (2010) reports experiencing a loss of "credibility of the public health community" due to frequent and delayed Centers for Disease Control and Prevention (CDC) modifications to recommendations on vaccine distribution resulting from a temporary vaccine shortage.

Descriptive Survey Study Evidence

Results of one survey support the above findings from the syntheses of qualitative and case report and AAR evidence regarding the potential for information overload. Staes and colleagues (2011) surveyed primary care physicians in Utah and found that they often received emails with information on H1N1 from multiple sources, which could result in an excessive amount of email and information overload. One survey also supports the finding that stakeholders may miss public health alerts and guidance as a result of not being enrolled in communication systems. An Argonne National Laboratory (Walsh et al., 2010) survey found that many stakeholders of the IDPH lacked awareness of or access to some communication channels (e.g., conference calls, H-HAN) used to communicate public health information during the H1N1 outbreak.

3. Acceptability and Preferences

Quantitative Study Evidence

Baseman and colleagues (2016) report on health care providers' preferences regarding channels used by public health authorities to transmit time-sensitive alerts and advisories as part of the REACH trial described earlier in this appendix. Email was the preferred communication channel, while SMS (text messaging) was preferred over fax for alerts but not advisories. There were differences in preferred channels based on age, gender, provider type, and whether the provider read emails on the phone or a computer.

Qualitative Evidence Synthesis

The body of qualitative evidence shows that technical audiences prefer email and fax as channels for communicating public health alerts and guidance (Khan et al., 2017; Ockers, 2011; Revere et al., 2015). Such audiences also stress the importance of and preference for just-in-time dissemination of guidance (Janssen et al., 2006; Leung et al., 2008).

An inclusive, collaborative, and dynamic process of engaging technical audiences in discussions on communication channels and processes for the generation of public health guidance before and during a public health event may improve providers' acceptance of and implementation fidelity to that guidance (Filice et al., 2013). Another factor that may affect the acceptability of communication strategies is the potential for bidirectional exchange of information between public health agencies and their stakeholders. To this end, public health agencies can share results generated from information submitted by technical audiences to demonstrate its utility and value, thus ensuring that these results can be utilized by those audiences in carrying out their own work and by public health agencies in improving the community's health (Revere et al., 2015).

Case Report and AAR Evidence Synthesis

The vast majority of case reports and AARs reviewed do not address the acceptability of communication channels or preferences of technical audiences with regard to information sharing, indicating a need for further research on the acceptability and feasibility of specific communication channels to determine how to best improve traditional channels and whether reported innovations (e.g., OKAlert-ILI, shelter hotlines) are replicable. However, it is evident that technical audiences prefer timely, accurate, consistent information that is easy to navigate and bidirectional (i.e., the ability to both send and receive information). Alerts and guidance tailored to specific audiences are also preferred to facilitate translating the information into appropriate action. Additionally, some audiences desire flexibility in their application of the guidance provided. According to the Delaware Division of Public Health (2010), for example, during the 2009 H1N1 response in that state, physicians looked to public health to determine appropriate priority groups for treatment and prophylaxis, but they also wanted the flexibility to reevaluate priority groups based on the data available from the state as the crisis progressed. The AAR suggests further that physicians preferred direct communication from a credible source and that the majority looked to the department of health or their medical society for leadership. Multiple AARs point to an appreciation of webcasts and a direct line of communication to experts (by phone or in person) (County of San Diego, 2018; Minnesota Department of Health, 2013a; Ohio Department of Health, 2010; Wisconsin Division of Public Health, 2010; Wisconsin Hospital Emergency Preparedness Program, 2010).

Descriptive Survey Study Evidence

Six surveys asked about the preferences of technical audiences (mainly health care providers) for communication channels and sources of alerts and guidance during a public health emergency. This survey evidence supports the finding from other evidence streams that email is the preferred channel for communicating this information. Few surveys addressed text messaging and social media, but when queried on these communication channels, technical audiences did not appear to prefer them. Ockers (2011) found that email and fax blast were the most preferred communication channels for vaccine providers in California, Louisiana, Oregon, and Washington, while text messages and social media were least preferred, as many providers reported they could not receive messages by these latter channels. Surveyed health care providers in New York City during the city's Zika response indicated a preference for receiving alerts and guidance through email (77 percent of respondents), while fewer than 10 percent preferred hard-copy mailings, in-person presentations, online webinars, or conference calls (Quinn et al., 2018). Seidl and colleagues (2010) report that approximately 94 percent of survey respondents found emails from the health incident controller to be somewhat or very useful as sources of information on H1N1, and nearly 90 percent found local health information bulletins useful (Seidl et al., 2010). In a survey of infectious disease physicians, 91 percent reported that emailed and faxed health alerts were useful, versus 43 percent for mailed notifications, 22 percent for social media, and 46 percent for smartphone applications (Santibanez et al., 2016). According to an Argonne National Laboratory report on surveys sent to various public health stakeholders to solicit feedback on the IDPH's communication during the H1N1 outbreak, survey respondents indicated a preference for receiving information via email and the health department's websites versus conference calls (Walsh et al., 2010).

Survey evidence also supports findings from the synthesis of case report and AAR evidence regarding public health authorities and medical societies being trusted information sources, although one survey found that primary care providers in Utah preferred institutional sources (73 percent) over public health sources for information and guidance (Staes et al., 2011). Seidl and colleagues (2010) report that during the H1N1 response, communications from the local health authority were favored as a source of updated information. Santibanez and colleagues (2016) report that physicians generally preferred information from professional authorities, including CDC (98 percent of respondents), professional societies (92 percent), and online medical resources such as ProMed mail (23 percent), over public websites (22 percent) and social media (5 percent). Ockers (2011) notes that surveyed vaccine providers most frequently relied on state and local health departments for timely, accurate information about outbreaks and other public health threats, with less reliance on federal agencies, professional societies, and the news media. Among surveyed health care providers in New York City, the HAN was the preferred local source of information for providers (73 percent) (Quinn et al., 2018). Among nonlocal sources, information from CDC (64 percent) was preferred over that from the state health department (47 percent), followed by roughly similar levels of preference (30–35 percent) for public websites, medical journals and other online or point-of-care resources, and professional societies and associations. The majority of respondents to the Argonne National Laboratory (Walsh et al., 2010) survey mentioned above expressed the view that local health departments, but not the state health department, should customize CDC messages and updates to incorporate local information.

4. Feasibility and PHEPR System Considerations

Qualitative Evidence Synthesis

The body of qualitative evidence included in the review suggests that some communication channels are presently more feasible than others. Use of EHRs remains somewhat limited although EHRs are highly pertinent to the delivery of alerts and guidance at the point of individual care. Text-based messages/SMS are already in use. Advances in information technology often push the public health system to examine and adopt new channels (Janssen et al., 2006; Revere et al., 2015). Doing so, however, may raise concerns about compounding the burdens of message volume and availability of resources, such as personal or work devices and technical support. It appears important to weigh the strengths and limitations of any technology as a channel for communication during a public health emergency in context.

Case Report and AAR Evidence Synthesis

Findings on feasibility and PHEPR system considerations from case reports and AARs are discussed in the above section on this evidence stream relative to acceptability and preferences.

5. Resource and Economic Considerations

Qualitative Evidence Synthesis

All communication channels incur ongoing costs. However, as emphasized in one qualitative study, the indirect costs of new technologies related to training and technical support need to be added to their direct cost (Revere et al., 2015).

Case Report and AAR Evidence Synthesis

Adequate resources—from such resources as phones, radios, computers, servers, software platforms, and notification systems to human resources for hotline management, message development, message delivery, bidirectional communication, and many other functions—are critical for successful information sharing with technical audiences. Gamache and colleagues (2010) report that providing public health alerts through community health information exchanges yielded a cost savings to public health agencies relative to the traditional mail-based alerts. The estimated total cost savings was $3,638 for each set of alerts, based on sending 3,085 alerts to providers. Given advancements in technology, however, it may be more relevant to consider cost savings from this channel relative to other electronic channels. The OKAlert-ILI system was funded by a $50,000 health department contract, and has been made available to participating clinicians at no cost (Nagykaldi et al., 2006). The New York State Hospital Emergency Response Data System (HERDS), developed in 2001 by the New York State Department of Health in partnership with health care and public health agencies, reduced costs by implementing the application within an existing infrastructure used by response partner communities and leveraging existing multimillion-dollar investments (Gotham et al., 2007). Costs included development ($130,000) and the system's annual recurring cost ($200,000).

Beyond the necessary technologies, findings from case reports and AARs suggest that successful information sharing depends on the availability of critical staff, such as liaison officers and subject-matter experts (Minnesota Department of Health, 2014; New Hampshire Department of Health and Human Services and New Hampshire Department of Safety, 2009a). Mathur and Beckermann (2010) discuss the frequent need to adjust communication strategies during Canada's H1N1 response. Additional management support was brought in, the frequency of teleconferences was increased, target audiences were expanded, and on-site expert support was provided. This ability to adapt based on need was made possible by a strong, adequately resourced and supported team with vaccine expertise. Conversely, reliance on a handful of liaison officers during a full-scale exercise testing information sharing in the context of a novel respiratory illness was shown to be ineffective (Tri-County Health Department, 2017). Staff were overwhelmed by the sheer volume of calls and unable to meet the demand for information. Many partners were unable to get in touch, further highlighting the need for sufficient human resources to support effective information sharing.

6. Equity

Qualitative Evidence Synthesis

The qualitative evidence included in this review provides some indication that small jurisdictions and rural areas are less able to adapt to changes in technology and communication channels relative to other areas (Revere et al., 2015).

Case Report and AAR Evidence Synthesis

Overall, the body of case reports and AARs does not address equity issues associated with different channels for communicating public health alerts and guidance with technical audiences, highlighting an important evaluation gap. The AAR from the 2009 H1N1 response in Washington's Seattle & King County identifies an opportunity for "improved relationships with smaller and ethnic pharmacies to expand outreach to ethnic and vulnerable populations" (Public Health—Seattle & King County, 2009). Although this opportunity is not directly related to sharing information with pharmacies, improving relationships with technical audiences serving underserved populations may lead to more targeted and tailored information sharing during a public health emergency.

Wynn and Moore (2012) are the only authors to mention equity explicitly, stating, "especially during a public health emergency, the health care system must show sensitivity to socioeconomic circumstance and use an understanding of the determinants of health when developing emergency mitigation strategies." The authors go on to describe the bidirectional role of family health teams during the 2009 H1N1 response in Ontario. These teams were able to relay patient needs to public health agencies through communication with primary care providers. The United States may be able to apply similar approaches when developing communication channels for technical audiences to promote greater equity.

7. Ethical Considerations[3]

In addition to the equity concerns noted above, which are often considered as reflecting ethical values, the primary value of communication using appropriate channels is often considered to be *instrumental,* meaning that it is important because using appropriate channels to convey information presumably leads to better information delivery, which can facilitate better decision making. In the language of ethical principles, communication using appropriate channels is important because it promotes the principle of harm reduction/benefit promotion. But problems of overcommunication (such as information overload or alert fatigue) are also possible when appropriate communication channels are used, which can lead to worse or delayed decisions. In addition, communication using appropriate channels also has intrinsic value; that is, setting aside whether decision making is improved by better information delivery, communicating with individuals and communities in ways that are most effective for them is important to achieve transparency, which reflects the principle of respect for persons and communities. As in considering the instrumental value of using more effective channels for communication, one should remember that while communication using ineffective channels is obviously disrespectful, overloading effective communication channels is also disrespectful during crises, when recipients have limited time and bandwidth. In sum, selecting appropriate communication channels is ethically important, and so is careful selection of the information to be delivered over those channels.

[3] Ethical considerations included in this section were generated through committee discussions, drawing on the ethical principles laid out in Box 3-4 in Chapter 3 and key ethics and policy texts, including the 2009 Institute of Medicine letter report on crisis standards of care (IOM, 2009), the 2008 CDC white paper "Ethical Guidance for Public Health Emergency Preparedness and Response: Highlighting Ethics and Values in a Vital Public Health Service" (Jennings and Arras, 2008), *Emergency Ethics: Public Health Preparedness and Response* (Jennings et al., 2016), and *The Oxford Handbook of Public Health Ethics* (Mastroianni et al., 2019).

TABLE B3-4 Evidence to Decision Summary Table for Channels Used to Communicate Public Health Alerts and Guidance with Technical Audiences During a Public Health Emergency

What is the effectiveness of different channels for communicating public health alerts and guidance with technical audiences during a public health emergency?	
Balance of Benefits and Harms Although only two quantitative comparative research studies evaluate the effectiveness or benefits of specific channels for communicating public health alerts and guidance, case reports and after action reports (AARs) also cite improved audience awareness and the timeliness of messaging as benefits for some communication channels, such as electronic messaging systems (e.g., fax, email, web-based alerting and surveillance systems), teleconferences, and hotlines. Reported harms and undesirable impacts rarely relate to a specific communication channel but arise as a result of how communication is implemented. For example, several evidence sources note the potential for important stakeholders to be left out of the loop if excluded from the systems used to distribute messages (e.g., the Health Alert Network, teleconferences) and/or if contact information is not kept up to date. Also commonly reported as undesirable impacts of public health messaging are alert fatigue and information overload (particularly when guidance is constantly changing), with potential downstream effects of loss of credibility for the public health agency and disillusionment with future preparedness and response efforts. Finally, one study notes that when guidance does not align with what can feasibly be carried out in practice, it may be ignored.	**Sources of Evidence** • Synthesis of the evidence of effect • Qualitative evidence synthesis • Case report and AAR evidence synthesis (no assessment of certainty or confidence) • Descriptive survey study evidence (no synthesis)
Acceptability and Preferences Email and fax have consistently been reported as preferred channels for communicating public health alerts and guidance, although published technology preferences may be outdated given the rapid pace of technology development and adoption. Recent AARs may be useful sources of more current information on preferred communication channels (e.g., webcasts, social media). Technical audiences generally prefer information from local sources (public health or health care institutional sources) or such national authorities as the Centers for Disease Control and Prevention and medical societies. Engaging technical audiences in communication strategies, providing a direct line of communication, offering opportunities for bidirectional exchange, and ensuring information reciprocity (i.e., returning results generated from information submitted by stakeholders to demonstrate the utility and value of the shared information) may improve the acceptability of and responsiveness to messaging. Tailoring guidance to specific audiences, sending just-in-time guidance, and ensuring that guidance is congruent with practice and allows sufficient flexibility in implementation may help enable the translation of information to appropriate action.	**Sources of Evidence** • Quantitative study evidence • Qualitative evidence synthesis • Case report and AAR evidence synthesis (no assessment of certainty or confidence) • Descriptive survey study evidence (no synthesis)
Feasibility and PHEPR System Considerations Some communication channels are more feasible than others for public health agencies and technical audiences to implement. The widespread use of traditional channels (e.g., email, fax, phone calls) indicates their feasibility, but further research is needed on the acceptability and feasibility of newer channels (e.g., health information exchange– and electronic health record–based alerting, purpose-built bidirectional surveillance and alert systems). For example, while advances in information technology may lead the public health system to examine and adopt new communication channels, the adoption of these new channels may raise concerns about adding to the burden of message volume and about the availability of needed resources, such as personal or work devices, and technical support.	**Sources of Evidence** • Qualitative evidence synthesis • Case report and AAR evidence synthesis (no assessment of certainty or confidence)
Resource and Economic Considerations Resource requirements for communicating public health alerts and guidance with technical audiences include both technology costs (e.g., phones, radios, computers, servers, software platforms) and human resources. Little research has examined the cost-effectiveness of different communication channels. Many public health agencies and technical audiences already have the technology necessary for traditional communication methods, such as email and conference calls. The initial costs for some purpose-built systems may exceed tens or even hundreds of thousands of dollars, which does not include ongoing maintenance costs. However, such systems often have multiple functions of value to public health agencies, including situational awareness and surveillance. Moreover, the indirect costs of new technologies related to training and technical support need to be added to the direct costs. Designated liaisons and communication networks may help amplify messaging and build or maintain trusted relationships, but the human resource costs of these strategies need to be considered.	**Sources of Evidence** • Qualitative evidence synthesis • Case report and AAR evidence synthesis (no assessment of certainty or confidence)

TABLE B3-4 Continued

Equity	**Sources of Evidence**
Equity issues associated with different channels for communicating public health alerts and guidance with technical audiences are rarely raised in research studies and evaluations (e.g., AARs), and represent an important evaluation gap. One such issue is access to technology, which may be a consideration with respect to rural and underserved populations. Improving relationships with technical audiences that serve disadvantaged populations could lead to more targeted and tailored information sharing during a public health emergency, which in turn could help address equity issues.	• Qualitative evidence synthesis • Case report and AAR evidence synthesis (no assessment of certainty or confidence)
Ethical Considerations	**Source of Evidence**
The primary value of communication using appropriate channels is often considered to be instrumental, meaning that it is important because using appropriate channels to convey information presumably leads to better information delivery, which can facilitate better decision making. In the language of ethical principles, communication using appropriate channels is important because it promotes the principle of harm reduction/benefit promotion. But problems of overcommunication (such as information overload or alert fatigue) are also possible when appropriate communication channels are used, which can lead to worse or delayed decisions. In addition, communication using appropriate channels also has intrinsic value; that is, setting aside whether decision making is improved by better information delivery, communicating with individuals and communities in ways that are most effective for them is important to achieve transparency, which reflects the principle of respect for persons and communities. As in considering the instrumental value of using more effective channels for communication, one should remember that while communication using ineffective channels is obviously disrespectful, overloading effective communication channels is also disrespectful during crises, when recipients have limited time and bandwidth. In sum, selecting appropriate communication channels is ethically important, and so is careful selection of the information to be delivered over those channels.	• Committee discussion drawing on key ethics and policy texts

CONSIDERATIONS FOR IMPLEMENTATION

The following considerations for implementation are drawn from the qualitative evidence synthesis, the case report and AAR evidence synthesis, and evidence from descriptive surveys.

8. Engaging Technical Audiences in the Development of Communication Plans, Protocols, and Channels

Qualitative Evidence Synthesis

Six qualitative studies (Filice et al., 2013; Janssen et al., 2006; Khan et al., 2017; Leung et al., 2008; Lis and Resnick, 2018; Markiewicz et al., 2012) support a finding that *engaging technical audiences in the development of communication plans, protocols, and channels appears to help in the dissemination of guidance* (moderate confidence in the evidence). Additionally, three qualitative studies (Filice et al., 2013; Khan et al., 2017; Lis and Resnick, 2018) indicate that such engagement efforts *also improve the usefulness of guidance, especially through prior attention to how the guidance is translated into actionable knowledge* (moderate confidence in the evidence). The act and process of engaging technical audiences prior to public health emergencies facilitates relationship building (also coalition building and the identification of liaisons and points of contact), which may in turn improve emergency response by enhancing understanding of institutional needs, sharing of expertise, dissemination and implementation of guidance, and situational awareness (Filice et al., 2013; Leung et al., 2008; Markiewicz et al., 2012). Health care stakeholders value strong (and especially preexisting) relationships with local public health and other health care entities, and report those relationships as being beneficial to response scenarios. They similarly report the value of partnerships and coalitions as strategies for effective communication (Filice et al., 2013; Khan et al., 2017). Additionally, when technical audiences are engaged in the development of communication channels, plans, and processes, they can foresee the resulting improvements in interdisciplinary coordination during response (Filice et al., 2013; Khan et al., 2017; Lis and Resnick, 2018). Likewise, there is some indication that engaging technical audiences may facilitate the incorporation of lessons learned from past experience into revised plans and protocols (Filice et al., 2013; Lis and Resnick, 2018).

Case Report and AAR Evidence Synthesis

Although few of the case reports and AARs examined in this review address whether technical audiences were engaged in the development of communication plans, protocols, or channels, several AARs point out the need for better stakeholder engagement in the future (Blue Earth County Public Health, 2014; Capitol Region Council of Governments, 2016; Delaware Division of Public Health, 2010; Metropolitan Medical Response System, 2016; Minnesota Department of Health, 2013b; Ohio Department of Public Health, 2010; Public Health—Seattle & King County, 2009; Wisconsin Hospital Emergency Preparedness Program, 2010). Lessons learned from both exercises and real events suggest that insufficient engagement of partners in planning processes may impede effective communication during responses as a result of planning gaps and unclear communication channels and vetting processes.

Because of staffing gaps resulting from a hiring freeze during Delaware's 2009 response to the H1N1 outbreak, for example, hospitals and the medical community were not engaged earlier in the planning process (Delaware Division of Public Health, 2010). Following the response, the state's Division of Public Health recognized the need to further engage partners in the planning and decision-making processes because of confusion around the vaccine ordering process. Blast faxes did not reach physicians, decisions made during meetings sometimes changed based on vaccine allocations, and changes were not well communicated to all parties. The Division subsequently proposed establishing a hotline for medical providers to address this issue, using a stakeholder-engaged process. Wisconsin experienced similar challenges during its 2009 H1N1 response (Wisconsin Hospital Emergency Preparedness Program, 2010). Given how quickly information changed, it was difficult for physicians and employees to keep pace with the information, and some questioned the credibility of the guidelines being provided because of the frequent changes. The public health department recommended engaging the Wisconsin Medical Society to issue a mandate or advisory and establish a point of contact at each hospital to whom emails and communications would be directed. Overall, then, engaging appropriate partners during the planning process in anticipation of a dynamic environment may enhance the credibility and effectiveness of messaging.

Evidence suggests that the public health field is moving toward a more inclusive planning approach. However, the effectiveness of communication channels warrants further study (Boston Public Health Commission, 2013; Cavey et al., 2009; Gamache et al., 2010; Gotham et al., 2007; Massachusetts Emergency Management Agency et al., 2014; McKenna et al., 2003). Some jurisdictions have developed new channels based on direct feedback from stakeholders. For instance, Mississippi developed and tested an infectious disease hotline with surveillance and education capabilities in the aftermath of Hurricane Katrina in response to requests made by shelter staff for "both a reporting system and infectious disease education" (Cavey et al., 2009). The hotline enabled direct verbal communication between shelter staff and hotline managers, allowing for immediate feedback and education for staff unfamiliar with diseases and reporting processes. A satisfaction survey confirmed immediate positive feedback from the system's users. This example illustrates a truly stakeholder-driven approach based on an identified need.

Gamache and colleagues (2010) highlight the importance of evaluating end-user acceptance of a new data-sharing mechanism designed to deliver public health alerts to Iowa providers by leveraging an existing electronic clinical messaging system within the context of a health information exchange. Although they do not present findings from their evaluation, they emphasize the value of engaging both clinical and public health stakeholders as a means of building trust and establishing infrastructure for a more complex public health decision support process. Similarly, the HERDS, discussed earlier, serves as the infrastructure for linking and exchanging health preparedness and response information in the state (Gotham et al., 2007). A key lesson learned in developing this system was the need for a bottom-up approach to system requirements that cut across jurisdictions and knowledge domains.

Descriptive Survey Study Evidence

Seidl and colleagues (2010) report on a survey-based real-time quality improvement mechanism that enabled public health authorities to tailor communications and better meet stakeholders' information needs.

9. Considerations for Selection of Communication Channels

Qualitative Evidence Synthesis

Table B3-5 summarizes considerations that can inform the use of the various channels for communicating public health alerts and guidance with technical audiences that are discussed in the qualitative studies included in this review. Both public health and health care stakeholders describe using judgment to select the optimal communication channel depending on the context at hand, such as the level of uncertainty or urgency (Khan et al., 2017; Staes et al., 2011).

Multiple channels facilitate effective communication by attending differentially to contextual dynamics while avoiding message overload. Contextual dynamics include such priorities as access, accuracy, coordination, dissemination, reciprocity, and timeliness (moderate confidence in the evidence). This finding is supported by seven qualitative studies (Garrett et al., 2011; Janssen et al., 2006; Khan et al., 2017; Leung et al., 2008; Ockers, 2011; Revere et al., 2015; Staes et al., 2011). A decision as to which among multiple communication strategies should be utilized needs to balance message content (emergency versus routine communications), delivery (one- versus two-way), and channel (e.g., text, email) with stakeholder preferences and technical capabilities, all the while mitigating the risk of incurring message overload and overlooking important information (Janssen et al., 2006). Participants in one study described utilizing multipronged approaches, first using one method, followed up with another (Khan et al., 2017). Specifically mentioned was following up on email with a phone call for something urgent.

As discussed earlier, some channels allow for bidirectional communication. The decision to use bidirectional messaging strategies is complex, and public health agencies need to manage concerns about and barriers to such strategies to ensure benefits for all parties

TABLE B3-5 Considerations for Selection of Communication Channels

Face to Face	Direct contact through in-person meetings is synchronous (i.e., allows real-time exchange of information), which allows for degrees of nuance and flexibility related to the uptake and understanding of public health guidance (Khan et al., 2017). In-person meetings between public health personnel and clinicians are useful, especially when there is perceived anxiety or discomfort about particular guidance (Khan et al., 2017).
Phone Calls	Direct contact through phone calls and teleconferences is synchronous, which allows for degrees of nuance and flexibility related to the uptake and understanding of public health guidance. Such contact is also helpful for very urgent communication (Khan et al., 2017). In one example, public health epidemiologists, in their role as liaisons, participated in weekly phone calls with the state public health department (Markiewicz et al., 2012). In another example, the use of two-tiered conference calls (a triage call followed by a coordination call) expedited specific decision making for coordinated patient care decisions (Lis and Resnick, 2018). Such two-tiered calls allow for collaborative, cross-agency decision making.
Email	Regardless of situational context (emergency versus nonurgent) and message recipients (target audience[s]), email is a favored modality for receiving public health messages (Revere et al., 2015). Email is a push-type channel, generally used in the one-way delivery of alerts and guidance to target audiences. Despite its limitations (see below), email was cited as the preferred channel for communication of public health guidance to frontline staff by emergency department clinician administrators, who judged it the fastest way of presenting information to clinicians (Khan et al., 2017). Email dissemination relies on an established listserv, prepared in advance. This may be seen as a limitation, as some key people may not be on the list, and/or the list may require constant maintenance to be kept up to date (Khan et al., 2017; Leung et al., 2008).
Fax	Fax is often used in tandem with email (Ockers, 2011; Revere et al., 2015). Faxes still may arrive when phone calls cannot connect.
Internet/Websites/ Social Media	One study showed that providers were as likely to seek information from Google as from the Centers for Disease Control and Prevention (Janssen et al., 2006). Revere and colleagues (2015) note that some health care providers and community-based organizations are currently using social media as a communication channel to some degree; however, this is less so for public health agencies. Evident in the body of studies included in this review is the lag time of research related to emerging technologies.
Text Messaging/ SMS	Text messaging/SMS provides rapid, in-the-field short messages, probably helpful in emergencies but not for mass communications. When information is lengthy, email appears to be better suited and preferred (Revere et al., 2015). Both public health agencies and their stakeholders have noted multiple values and uses as well as concerns regarding two-way public health text messaging (Revere et al., 2015). For example, this channel can readily provide "eyes on the ground" reports, short polls, and postdisaster check-in on status and availability, and is an alternative when phone lines are out of service. Conversely, there are concerns with this channel, including receipt of text messages on personal phones, restrictive screen space, ease of ignoring messages, limited cell coverage, security, and the inability to forward messages. Whether mobile phones are sufficiently made available or supported by workplaces appears to be understudied (Revere et al., 2015).
Electronic Health Records	Enabling guidance to arrive directly at the point of individual care and monitoring, electronic health records have the potential to serve as a channel for communicating public health alerts and guidance with health care audiences. However, many issues related to technology, resources, and compatibility with emergency guidance would need to be considered and managed before effective implementation of this channel could occur (Garrett et al., 2011).

(Revere et al., 2015). Public health participants in some studies discussed using direct contact and bidirectional communication practices to follow up and facilitate closing the communication loop (Khan et al., 2017; Leung et al., 2008; Markiewicz et al., 2012). In another study, community-based partners expressed wanting the option to reply to a message, whether they would actually do so or not (Revere et al., 2015). Yet, despite the benefits of bidirectional communication channels (e.g., ability to receive confirmation of message receipt and information from stakeholders for purposes of surveillance or surge capacity awareness), concerns have been raised regarding burden; management; technology requirements; privacy, security, and Health Insurance Portability and Accountability Act[4] considerations; information utility; and the potential for misunderstanding replies. Other concerns include the funding for new technologies, whether the technology is supported by the workplace, and the need to learn how to utilize a new system (Revere et al., 2015).

It should be noted that there is a time lag between the adoption of new communication technologies in the field and evaluation studies. Although text messaging and some Internet-based technologies have existed as communication channels for at least a couple of decades and are being used to some degree for PHEPR messaging, relatively little research has investigated their use or effectiveness for this purpose. Thus, there is an urgent need for more research in this area.

10. Barriers to and Facilitators of Communicating Alerts and Guidance During a Public Health Emergency

Qualitative Evidence Synthesis

Target audiences have noted the difficulties that they experience when there are multiple sources of guidance—international, national, state, and local public health agencies, as well as institutional sources—and often inconsistencies in guidance information resulting from uncoordinated messaging (Filice et al., 2013; Khan et al., 2017; Leung et al., 2008; Staes et al., 2011). In one study, a clinician commented that if "medical office emails duplicated health department ones, reading both to find discrepancies was too time consuming," and "if [health care institution] recommendations are different than the CDC's then this difference should be explicitly noted and explained" (Staes et al., 2011, p. 6). Compounding this barrier to accurate and quality guidance is the rapidly changing nature of information during a response and, in turn, the need for rapid dissemination of updated guidance (Filice et al., 2013; Khan et al., 2017; Leung et al., 2008). Additionally, some study participants have identified inconsistencies in channel use as a challenge; they have come to expect certain sources to use certain channels, and when those expectations are not met, timely access may be hindered. Inconsistencies in channel use or differences in channel preferences across institutions and jurisdictions also are frustrating challenges for health care providers (Khan et al., 2017; Staes et al., 2011). Overall, six qualitative studies (Filice et al., 2013; Janssen et al., 2006; Khan et al., 2017; Leung et al., 2008; Markiewicz et al., 2012; Staes et al., 2011) support a finding that *source and channel inconsistencies, excessive message volume, guidance and practice incongruences, and poor coordination within and between agencies work against effective communication during emergencies* (moderate confidence in the evidence).

Liaisons and institutional points of contact may facilitate message dissemination, congruence between guidance and practice, and coordination efforts during emergencies (moderate

[4] Health Insurance Portability and Accountability Act, HR 3103. Public Law 104-901, 104th Cong. (August 21, 1996).

confidence in the evidence), a finding supported by seven qualitative studies (Filice et al., 2013; Janssen et al., 2006; Khan et al., 2017; Leung et al., 2008; Lis and Resnick, 2018; Markiewicz et al., 2012; Staes et al., 2011). Liaisons and institutional points of contact can increase the speed of dissemination of public health messages (Markiewicz et al., 2012), but beyond amplifying message dissemination, they can have additional influences on the communication process. The institutional knowledge afforded by their roles appears to aid in reaching target audiences within organizations, and by identifying key contacts within public health agencies, they gain an advance understanding of the public health bureaucracy during response (Filice et al., 2013; Khan et al., 2017; Leung et al., 2008; Markiewicz et al., 2012). Additionally, they have facilitated reciprocity by promptly meeting needs for bidirectional information sharing between institutions and public health agencies and adapting as needed to changing dynamics (Markiewicz et al., 2012). Hospitals and other health care entities appear to readily designate these individuals as team leaders for preparedness efforts, protocol development and revision, and integration of institutional learning (Filice et al., 2013; Khan et al., 2017; Markiewicz et al., 2012).

In addition to liaisons and points of contact, coalitions, through developed relationships and networks, have facilitated improvements in interdisciplinary communication and coordination during responses. Khan and colleagues (2017) found that a regional coalition helped with challenges related to the coordination of communication across institutions and jurisdictions and differences in work environments across sectors. Another study found that a coalition helped with developing consistent use of communication channels (e.g., teleconferences) and collaborative decision making (Lis and Resnick, 2018). At the same time, two studies found that coalitions can be very time intensive to maintain. Such challenges may be felt most acutely by smaller agencies (Leung et al., 2008; Lis and Resnick, 2018).

Case Report and AAR Evidence Synthesis

Given the often dynamic nature of public health emergencies, the ability to maintain consistent messaging remains a substantial challenge (ASTHO, n.d.; Capitol Region Council of Governments, 2017; Chicago Department of Public Health et al., 2011; Multnomah County Health Department, 2010; New Hampshire Department of Health and Human Services and New Hampshire Department of Safety, 2009b; Texas Department of State Health Services, 2010; Wisconsin Hospital Emergency Preparedness Program, 2010). Consistent with the findings from the qualitative evidence synthesis, several AARs mention how lack of coordination among partners led to conflicting or inconsistent messaging, resulting in confusion and frustration among technical audiences. During the H1N1 outbreak, guidance sometimes changed several times a day, with multiple guidance documents, forms, and instructions being distributed, some remaining valid while others were superseded (New Hampshire Department of Health and Human Services and New Hampshire Department of Safety, 2009b). Providers with clinics in bordering states often received conflicting messages (Wisconsin Hospital Emergency Preparedness Program, 2010). Regions that established joint information centers struggled to avoid conflicting recommendations from states (Multnomah County Health Department, 2010). More coordinated messaging can help prevent information overload, duplication of effort, and conflicting recommendations (ASTHO, n.d.). Some AARs point to other simple solutions for addressing the challenges of a dynamic information environment, solutions that require minimal resources, such as posting of webinar highlights on relevant websites, sharing of meeting notes after conference calls, and color coding of new information in frequently changing guidance documents (Maine Center for Disease Control and Prevention, 2010; Texas Department of State Health Services, 2018).

Amplification of public health guidance through media (including social media) has been shown to help facilitate the dissemination of technical guidance (CDC, 2013; Maine Center for Disease Control and Prevention, 2010), as has engaging medical societies (County of San Diego, 2018; Delaware Division of Public Health, 2010; Wisconsin Division of Public Health, 2010). Delaware's joint health department and Medical Society of Delaware communication to Delaware physicians during the state's H1N1 response, for example, was considered an effective strategy for crisis management as "physicians were more likely to use professional channels for getting technical information during a crisis" (Delaware Division of Public Health, 2010).

A commonly cited barrier to access to and the reach and timeliness of public health guidance during an emergency is the lack of preexisting or up-to-date distribution lists (ASTHO, n.d.; Buffalo Hospital and Wright County Public Health, 2013; Texas Department of State Health Services, 2018). For example, many hospitals' points of contact participating in a 2011 pediatric full-scale mass casualty incident exercise in Chicago did not report receiving the HAN or State of Illinois Rapid Electronic Notification alert (Chicago Department of Public Health et al., 2011). Additionally, it is often unclear just who is on alert distribution lists, especially when there are multiple channels with various permission rights to each (e.g., WebEOC, agency email, Everbridge) (Boston Public Health Commission, 2013). A lesson learned from Hurricane Harvey was the need to develop and maintain standard distribution lists for health care providers, local health departments, executive leadership, and response managers; to predetermine routine communications to be sent to each recipient based on need; and to develop an automated system (e.g., RedSky) to ensure that all necessary recipients receive the appropriate information (Texas Department of State Health Services, 2018). Maintaining these lists and systems as a routine preparedness activity can save valuable time during responses. It is also important to keep in mind that communication systems can fail as a result of technical issues or power outages (Chicago Department of Public Health et al., 2011; Gursky et al., 2003; McKenna et al., 2003; Montana Department of Public Health and Human Services, 2014; Ramsey County Public Health, 2014). Therefore, redundant individual contact information (e.g., cell phone, email, pager) and redundant systems are critical to ensure that technical audiences receive alerts and guidance in a timely manner.

Another similar barrier mentioned in AARs is the lack of access to such platforms as WebEOC across the local, state, and regional levels (Capitol Region Council of Governments, 2016, 2017). Establishing this linkage would enhance information sharing between levels. Additionally, even when use of WebEOC is limited to a specific locality, ensuring that passwords are updated routinely is important to maintaining accessibility (Boston Public Health Commission, 2013).

Unclear vetting processes, roles and responsibilities, and communication channels can also hinder the effectiveness of communication (Florida Department of Health, 2010). During San Francisco's 2009 H1N1 response, the lack of protocols led to confusion over how reports should be reviewed, who should review them prior to release, and the appropriate target audiences (San Francisco Department of Public Health, 2009). Similarly, during the potential Ebola threat in Connecticut, Regional Emergency Support Function (ESF) #8's role in the development and vetting process was unclear (Metropolitan Medical Response System, 2016). In the absence of guidance from the health department, ESF #8 developed recommendations based on the information available, which concerned the health department because it had not vetted the guidance before it was disseminated. Vetting processes therefore need to be formally documented and shared to minimize confusion over roles (Boston Public Health Commission, 2013). Furthermore, overly complex processes can hinder the timeliness of alerts and guidance. Findings suggest that simplified review protocols and easily customizable alerting frameworks are essential for providing timely decision support to technical audiences (Lurio et al., 2010).

Descriptive Survey Study Evidence

Survey findings align with several of the barriers identified in the qualitative and case report and AAR syntheses. Santibanez and colleagues (2016), for example, surveyed infectious disease physicians and found that problems related to not knowing whom to contact at the public health department and the connection to automated answering services impeded communication. Physicians wanted phone numbers for designated points of contact. They also suggested that building trust relationships in advance (e.g., through online joint rounds or in-person updates at periodic meetings) would help overcome these barriers. In addition, Staes and colleagues (2011) found that changing public health guidance was associated with reduced awareness of current guidance.

Surveys also were sources of strategies (often suggested by representatives of technical audiences) for facilitating communication with technical audiences. Note that the following compilation of these strategies, although potentially of use to public health stakeholders, should not be viewed as an exhaustive list and that additional evidence is needed before these strategies can be recommended as evidence-based practices:

- Given the need for increased coordination of messaging, public health authorities should consider routing notifications regarding alerts and guidance through preferred institutional communication channels (Staes et al., 2011).
- As messages received from public health authorities are often communicated to the full clinic staff in person, public health agencies should consider disseminating talking points as an attachment to their notifications (Ockers, 2011).
- When communicating text message alerts, inclusion of the following information should be considered: topic, recommendations, geographic location, signs and symptoms, population affected, and a hyperlink to additional information (Revere et al., 2014).
- When communicating changing information and guidance, including executive summaries at the beginning of informational emails can help quickly highlight new, important information for technical audiences (Seidl et al., 2010).
- Having a public information officer and a pandemic influenza plan was associated with greater odds of health care stakeholders receiving H1N1 information from the local health department, suggesting that these strategies may facilitate the sharing of information with technical audiences (Howard et al., 2012).

REFERENCES FOR ARTICLES INCLUDED IN THE MIXED-METHOD REVIEW

Quantitative Comparative Studies

Baseman, J. G., D. Revere, I. Painter, M. Toyoji, H. Thiede, and J. Duchin. 2013. Public health communications and alert fatigue. *BMC Health Services Research* 13:295.

Baseman, J., D. Revere, I. Painter, M. Oberle, J. Duchin, H. Thiede, R. Nett, D. MacEachern, and A. Stergachis. 2016. A randomized controlled trial of the effectiveness of traditional and mobile public health communications with health care providers. *Disaster Medicine and Public Health Preparedness* 10(1):98–107.

Revere, D., I. Painter, M. Oberle, and J. Baseman. 2014. Health-care provider preferences for time-sensitive communications from public health agencies. *Public Health Reports* 129(6 Suppl 4):67–76.

van Woerden, H. C., M. R. Evans, B. W. Mason, and L. Nehaul. 2007. Using facsimile cascade to assist case searching during a Q fever outbreak. *Epidemiology & Infection* 135(5):798–801.

Qualitative Studies

References marked with an asterisk (*) are surveys containing a qualitative analysis of free-text responses.

Filice, C. E., F. E. Vaca, L. Curry, S. Platis, N. Lurie, S. Bogucki, and M. N. Shah. 2013. Pandemic planning and response in academic pediatric emergency departments during the 2009 H1N1 influenza pandemic. *Academic Emergency Medicine* 20(1):54–62. http://doi.org/10.1111/acem.12061.

Garrett, N. Y., N. Mishra, B. Nichols, C. J. Staes, C. Akin, and C. Safran. 2011. Characterization of public health alerts and their suitability for alerting in electronic health record systems. *Journal of Public Health Management & Practice* 17(1):77–83.

Janssen, A. P., R. R. Tardif, S. R. Landry, and J. E. Warner. 2006. "Why tell me now?" The public and healthcare providers weigh in on pandemic influenza messages. *Journal of Public Health Management & Practice* 12(4):388–394.

Khan, Y., S. Sanford, D. Sider, K. Moore, G. Garber, E. de Villa, and B. Schwartz. 2017. Effective communication of public health guidance to emergency department clinicians in the setting of emerging incidents: A qualitative study and framework. *BMC Health Services Research* 17(1).

Leung, C. S., M. M. Ho, A. Kiss, A. V. Gundlapalli, and S. W. Hwang. 2008. Homelessness and the response to emerging infectious disease outbreaks: Lessons from SARS. *Journal of Urban Health* 85(3):402–410.

Lis, R., and A. T. Resnick. 2018. Coordinated communications and decision making to support a regional severe infectious disease response. *Health Security* 16(3):158–164.

Markiewicz, M., C. A. Bevc, J. Hegle, J. A. Horney, M. Davies, and P. D. MacDonald. 2012. Linking public health agencies and hospitals for improved emergency preparedness: North Carolina's public health epidemiologist program. *BMC Public Health* 12:141.

*Ockers, S. 2011. *Communication preferences of health care providers during an emergency: Data from four state surveys conducted before and after the H1N1 influenza mass vaccination campaigns.* (Master's thesis—joint program MPH/PA). Atlanta, GA: Rollins School of Public Health, Emory University.

Revere, D., R. Calhoun, J. Baseman, and M. Oberle. 2015. Exploring bi-directional and SMS messaging for communications between public health agencies and their stakeholders: A qualitative study. *BMC Public Health* 15:621.

*Staes, C. J., A. Wuthrich, P. Gesteland, M. A. Allison, M. Leecaster, J. H. Shakib, M. E. Carter, B. M. Mallin, S. Mottice, R. Rolfs, A. T. Pavia, B. Wallace, A. V. Gundlapalli, M. Samore, and C. L. Byington. 2011. Public health communication with frontline clinicians during the first wave of the 2009 influenza pandemic. *Journal of Public Health Management & Practice* 17(1):36–44.

Descriptive Survey Studies

Howard, A. F., H. M. Bush, R. M. Shapiro, and A. Dearinger. 2012. Characteristics of Kentucky local health departments that influence public health communication during times of crisis: Information dissemination associated with H1N1 novel influenza. *Journal of Public Health Management & Practice* 18(2):169–174.

Ockers, S. 2011. *Communication preferences of health care providers during an emergency: Data from four state surveys conducted before and after the H1N1 influenza mass vaccination campaigns.* (Master's thesis—joint program MPH/PA). Atlanta, GA: Rollins School of Public Health, Emory University.

Quinn, C., E. Poirot, A. Sanders Kim, A. L. Viswanath, S. N. Patel, D. M. Abramson, and R. Piltch-Loeb. 2018. Variations in healthcare provider use of public health and other information sources by provider type and practice setting during New York City's response to the emerging threat of Zika virus disease, 2016. *Health Security* 16(4):252–261.

Revere, D., M. R. Schwartz, and J. Baseman. 2014. How 2 txt: An exploration of crafting public health messages in SMS. *BMC Research Notes* 7:514.

Santibanez, S., P. M. Polgreen, S. E. Beekmann, C. Cairns, G. A. Filice, M. Layton, and J. M. Hughes. 2016. Communication between infectious disease physicians and U.S. state and local public health agencies: Strengths, challenges, and opportunities. *Public Health Reports* 131(5):666–670.

Seidl, I. A., A. J. Johnson, P. Mantel, and P. Aitken. 2010. A strategy for real time improvement (RTI) in communication during the H1N1 emergency response. *Australian Health Review* 34(4):493–498.

Staes, C. J., A. Wuthrich, P. Gesteland, M. A. Allison, M. Leecaster, J. H. Shakib, M. E. Carter, B. M. Mallin, S. Mottice, R. Rolfs, A. T. Pavia, B. Wallace, A. V. Gundlapalli, M. Samore, and C. L. Byington. 2011. Public health communication with frontline clinicians during the first wave of the 2009 influenza pandemic. *Journal of Public Health Management & Practice* 17(1):36–44.

Walsh, D., M. Barry, and K. Overly. 2010. Illinois Department of Public Health 2009 H1N1 influenza A: Pandemic communications evaluation survey. Argonne, IL: Argonne National Laboratory. https://digital.library.unt.edu/ark:/67531/metadc1013467/m2/1/high_res_d/990518.pdf (accessed April 9, 2020).

Case Reports

ASTHO (Association of State and Territorial Health Officals). n.d. *Addressing communication challenges during an infectious disease emergency response: State experiences from the H1N1 pandemic.* https://www.astho.org/Programs/Infectious-Disease/Addressing-Communication-Challenges-During-an-Infectious-Disease-Emergency-Response (accessed April 9, 2020).

Cavey, A. M., J. M. Spector, D. Ehrhardt, T. Kittle, M. McNeill, P. G. Greenough, and T. D. Kirsch. 2009. Mississippi's infectious disease hotline: A surveillance and education model for future disasters. *Prehospital & Disaster Medicine* 24(1):11–17.

CDC (Centers for Disease Control and Prevention). 2013. Notes from the field: Use of electronic messaging and the news media to increase case finding during a cyclospora outbreak—Iowa, July 2013. *Morbidity & Mortality Weekly Report* 62(30):613–614.

Daniel, J. B., D. Heisey-Grove, P. Gadam, W. Yih, K. Mandl, A. Demaria, Jr., and R. Platt. 2005. Connecting health departments and providers: Syndromic surveillance's last mile. *Morbidity and Mortality Weekly Report* 54:147–150.

Gamache, R., K. C. Stevens, R. Merriwether, B. E. Dixon, and S. Grannis. 2010. Development and assessment of a public health alert delivered through a community health information exchange. *Online Journal of Public Health Informatics* 2(2).

Gotham, I. J., D. L. Sottolano, M. E. Hennessy, J. P. Napoli, G. Dobkins, L. H. Le, R. L. Burhans, and B. I. Fage. 2007. An integrated information system for all-hazards health preparedness and response: New York State health emergency response data system. *Journal of Public Health Management and Practice* 13(5).

Gursky, E., T. V. Inglesby, and T. O'Toole. 2003. Anthrax 2001: Observations on the medical and public health response. *Biosecurity and Bioterrorism* 1(2):97–110.

Lurio, J., F. P. Morrison, M. Pichardo, R. Berg, M. D. Buck, W. Wu, K. Kitson, F. Mostashari, and N. Calman. 2010. Using electronic health record alerts to provide public health situational awareness to clinicians. *Journal of the American Medical Informatics Association* 17(2):217–219.

Mathur, A., and K. Beckermann. 2010. Moving up, moving down: Communications flow to and from mass immunization clinics. *Canadian Journal of Infectious Diseases and Medical Microbiology* 21(4):209.

McKenna, V. B., J. E. Gunn, J. Auerbach, K. H. Brinsfield, K. S. Dyer, and M. A. Barry. 2003. Local collaborations: Development and implementation of Boston's bioterrorism surveillance system. *Journal of Public Health Management and Practice* 9(5):384–393.

Nagykaldi, Z., J. W. Mold, K. K. Bradley, and J. E. Bos. 2006. Bridging the gap between public and private healthcare: Influenza-like illness surveillance in a practice-based research network. *Journal of Public Health Management and Practice* 12(4):356–364.

Wynn, A., and K. M. Moore. 2012. Integration of primary health care and public health during a public health emergency. *American Journal of Public Health* 102(11):e9–e12.

AARs[5]

Blue Earth County Public Health. 2014. *Information sharing or TB contact investigation after action report/improvement plan.* Mankato, MN. June 20, 2014.

Boston Public Health Commission. 2013. *2013 Boston Marathon emergency support function 8 (ESF-8) public health and medical planning, response, and recovery operations (April 15–April 26): Final after-action report/improvement plan.* Boston, MA. December 20, 2013. https://delvalle.bphc.org/mod/wiki/view.php?pageid=63 (accessed April 9, 2020).

[5] These AARs were retrieved from the Homeland Security Digital Library at https://www.hsdl.org/c (accessed June 10, 2020). They may be accessed and downloaded there.

Buffalo Hospital and Wright County Public Health. 2013. *Buffalo Hospital closed pod after-action report/improvement plan.* Buffalo, NY. November 21, 2013.

Capitol Region Council of Governments. 2016. *Ebola virus disease functional exercise after action report.* Hartford, CT. May 18, 2016.

Capitol Region Council of Governments. 2017. *Ebola virus disease full scale exercise after action report.* http://woodcountyhealth.org/ep/documents/2017%20WCHD%20Functional_Full-Scale%20Exercise%20AAR_IP.pdf (accessed April 9, 2020).

Chicago Department of Public Health, Illinois Department of Public Health, and Metropolitan Chicago Healthcare Council. 2011. *Illinois hospitals' pediatric full-scale exercise after action report.* Chicago, IL. May 21, 2011.

County of San Diego. 2018. *Hepatitis A outbreak after action report.* May 2018. San Diego, California. https://www.sandiegocounty.gov/content/dam/sdc/cosd/SanDiegoHepatitisAOutbreak-2017-18-AfterActionReport.pdf (accessed January 23, 2020).

Delaware Division of Public Health. 2010. *Novel H1N1 influenza Delaware response April 2009 to March 2010: After action report/improvement plan.* Dover, DE. June 1, 2010. https://dhss.delaware.gov/DHSS/DPH/php/files/h1n1aar.pdf (accessed January 23, 2020).

Florida Department of Health. 2010. *2010* Deepwater Horizon *oil spill response: ESF 8 after action report and improvement plan.* Tallahassee, FL. April 30, 2011. http://www.floridahealth.gov/programs-and-services/emergency-preparedness-and-response/training-exercise/_documents/deepwater-aar.pdf (accessed January 23, 2020).

Maine Center for Disease Control and Prevention. (2010). *Maine CDC 2009 H1N1 Influenza Pandemic After Action Summary. https://www.maine.gov/dhhs/mecdc/infectious-disease/epi/influenza/maineflu/documents/piop/AAR%20MECDC%202009%20H1N1%20Pandemic%202.11.pdf* (accessed May 23, 2020).

Massachusetts Emergency Management Agency, Massachusetts Department of Public Health, City of Boston, City of Cambridge, Town of Watertown, Massachusetts Bay Transportation Authority Transit Police Department, Massachusetts National Guard, and Massachusetts State Police. 2014. *After action report for the response to the 2013 Boston Marathon bombings.* https://www.policefoundation.org/wp-content/uploads/2015/05/after-action-report-for-the-response-to-the-2013-boston-marathon-bombings_0.pdf (accessed January 23, 2020).

Metropolitan Medical Response System. 2016. *CT Region 3 ESF-8 Ebola preparedness and response: After action report.* Falls Church, VA. October 29, 2015.

Minnesota Department of Health. 2013a. *Operation Loon Call 2013: After-action report/improvement plan.* St. Paul, MN. June 11, 2013.

Minnesota Department of Health. 2013b. *White powder incident November 2013 after action report/improvement plan.* St. Paul, MN. February 2014.

Minnesota Department of Health. 2014. *DOC FE flash floods 2014. After-action report/improvement plan 2014.* St. Paul, MN. May 29, 2014.

Montana Department of Public Health and Human Services. 2014. *Big Sky Push II: Medical supplies management and distribution full scale exercise March 21—April 11, 2014.* Great Falls, MT. May 22, 2014.

Multnomah County Health Department. 2010. *H1N1 Fall 2009–Multco Aug 4–5, 2009–December 8, 2009: After action report/improvement plan.* Portland, OR. May 4, 2010.

New Hampshire Department of Health and Human Services and New Hampshire Department of Safety. 2009a. *Cities ready initiative operation rapid RX full-scale exercise: After action report.* Concord, NH. October 16, 17, 24, 2009.

New Hampshire Department of Health and Human Services and New Hampshire Department of Safety. 2009b. *2009 Spring H1N1 response: After action report/improvement plan.* Concord, NH. September 22, 2009.

New Hampshire Department of Health and Human Services and New Hampshire Department of Safety. 2010. *New Hampshire July 1, 2009–March 30, 2010 H1N1 response: After action report/improvement plan.* Concord, NH.

Ohio Department of Health. 2010. *Fall 2009 H1N1 response. ICS operations conducted through September 21, 2009–February 4, 2010. After action report/improvement plan.* Columbus, OH. June 29, 2010.

Public Health—Seattle & King County and King County Healthcare Coalition. 2009. *H1N1 influenza (swine flu) 2009. King County ESF-8 after action report.* April 26, 2009–May 15, 2009.

Ramsey County Public Health. 2014. *Operation: Communication woes: After-action report/improvement plan.* St. Paul, MN. May 5, 2014.

San Francisco Department of Public Health. 2009. *Fall/Winter 2009–2010 H1N1 swine flu response: San Francisco, California. September 28, 2009–March 9, 2010: After action report/improvement plan.* August 20, 2010. https://www.sfcdcp.org/wp-content/uploads/2018/01/H1N1-AAR-Executive-Summary.Fall-Winter-2009-2010-id639.pdf (accessed January 23, 2020).

Texas Department of State Health Services. 2010. *Texas Department of State Health Services response to the novel H1N1 pandemic influenza (2009 and 2010): After action report.* The Litaker Group, LLC. Austin, TX. August 30, 2010.

Texas Department of State Health Services. 2018. *Hurricane Harvey response: After-action report.* Austin, TX. May 30, 2018.

Tri-County Health Department. 2017. *Public health emergency dispensing exercise (PHEDEX) after action report and improvement plan.* Greenwood Village, CO. June 15–17, 2017.

Wisconsin Division of Public Health. 2010. *2009 H1N1 influenza response after action report and improvement plan.* Madison, WI. July 2010.

Wisconsin Hospital Emergency Preparedness Program. 2010. *After action report (AAR) for H1N1 influenza.* Madison, WI. April 24, 2009–Spring 2010.

Ethics and Policy Text

IOM (Institute of Medicine). 2009. *Guidance for establishing crisis standards of care for use in disaster situations: A letter report.* Washington, DC: The National Academies Press.

Jennings, B., and J. Arras. 2008. *Ethical guidance for public health emergency preparedness and response: Highlighting ethics and values in a vital public health service.* https://www.cdc.gov/od/science/integrity/phethics/docs/white_paper_final_for_website_2012_4_6_12_final_for_web_508_compliant.pdf (accessed February 23, 2020).

Jennings, B., J. D. Arras, D. H. Barrett, and B. A. Ellis. 2016. *Emergency ethics: Public health preparedness and response.* New York: Oxford University Press.

Mastroianni, A. C., J. P. Kahn, and N. E. Kass, eds. 2019. *The Oxford handbook of public health ethics.* New York: Oxford University Press. https://www.oxfordhandbooks.com/view/10.1093/oxfordhb/9780190245191.001.0001/oxfordhb-9780190245191 (accessed June 3, 2020).

B4

Mixed-Method Review of Implementing Quarantine to Reduce or Stop the Spread of a Contagious Disease

This appendix provides a detailed description of the methods for and the evidence from the mixed-method review examining the implementation of quarantine to reduce the spread of a contagious disease, which is summarized in Chapter 7.[1]

KEY REVIEW QUESTIONS AND ANALYTIC FRAMEWORK

Theoretically, the perceived benefit of quarantine is effective curbing of the spread of contagious diseases by not allowing person-to-person transmission. Therefore, the primary question posed by the committee in this review is: "In what circumstances (e.g., based on biologic factors, risks, resource availability, legal authorities, social context) is quarantine effective in reducing or stopping the spread of a contagious disease?" To answer this primary question, the committee sought evidence on several sub-questions related to evidence on the pros and cons of specific adherence strategies, the documented benefits and harms of implementing quarantine, and the factors that create barriers to and facilitators of its implementation (see Box B4-1).

For the purposes of this review, the committee developed an analytic framework to present the causal pathway and interactions between quarantine and its components, populations, and outcomes of interest (see Figure B4-1). The mechanism by which quarantine can ultimately reduce or stop the spread of contagious disease is well established and noncontroversial: there is a period of time (the incubation period) between when a person is exposed to a contagious illness and when that person, if infected, becomes contagious to others; and if individuals who are exposed and become infected are not in contact with anyone else at the time they become contagious, they cannot spread the infection (Drews, 2013).

[1] This appendix draws heavily on four reports commissioned by the committee: "Data Extraction and Quality Assessment: Methodology and Evidence Tables" by the Brown University Center for Evidence Synthesis in Health; "Quarantine as a Non-Pharmaceutical Intervention: Qualitative Research Evidence Synthesis" by Pradeep Sopory and Julie Novak; "Use of Quarantine as a Non-Pharmaceutical Intervention for Public Health Emergencies: Findings from Case Reports" by Sneha Patel; and "In What Situations Do Modeling Studies Suggest Quarantine is More Versus Less Effective to Control Infectious Disease Outbreaks?" by Jeremy Goldhaber-Fiebert (see Appendix C).

BOX B4-1 KEY REVIEW QUESTIONS

In what circumstances (e.g., based on biologic factors, risks, resource availability, legal authorities, social context) is quarantine effective at reducing or stopping the spread of a contagious disease?

- What strategies affect adherence to quarantine?
- What benefits and harms (desirable and/or undesirable impacts) of quarantine have been described or measured?
- What are the barriers to and facilitators of effective quarantine?

EVIDENCE SUPPORTING THE PRACTICE RECOMMENDATION

This section summarizes the evidence from the mixed-method review examining implementing quarantine to reduce or stop the spread of a contagious disease. It begins with a description of the results of the literature search and then summarizes the evidence of effectiveness. In formulating its practice recommendation, the committee considered evidence beyond effectiveness, which was compiled using an Evidence to Decision (EtD) framework encompassing balance of benefits and harms, acceptability and preferences, feasibility and public health emergency preparedness and response (PHEPR) system considerations, resource and economic considerations, equity, and ethical considerations. The evidence from each methodological stream applicable to each of the EtD criteria is discussed; a synthesis is provided in Table B4-10 later in this appendix and in Chapter 7. Graded finding statements from evidence syntheses are italicized in the narrative below.

Full details about the study eligibility criteria, search strategy, and processes for data extraction and individual study quality assessment are available in Appendix A. Appendix C links to all the commissioned analyses informing this review.

Results of the Literature Search

The searches of bibliographic databases identified a total of 1,588 potentially relevant citations (deduplicated) for the mixed-method review of implementing quarantine to reduce or stop the spread of a contagious disease. A search of the gray literature, reference mining, and a call for reports contributed an additional 224 articles. All 1,812 citations were imported into EndNote and were included in title and abstract screening. During screening, 1,528 articles were excluded because their abstracts did not appear to answer any of the key questions or they indicated that the articles were commentaries, editorials, or opinion pieces. After the abstracts had been reviewed, 284 full-text articles were reviewed and assessed for eligibility for inclusion in the mixed-method review. The committee considered 136 articles for data extraction and ultimately included 88 articles in the mixed-method review. Figure B4-2 depicts the literature flow, indicating the number of articles included and excluded at each screening stage. Table B4-1 indicates the types of evidence included in this review.

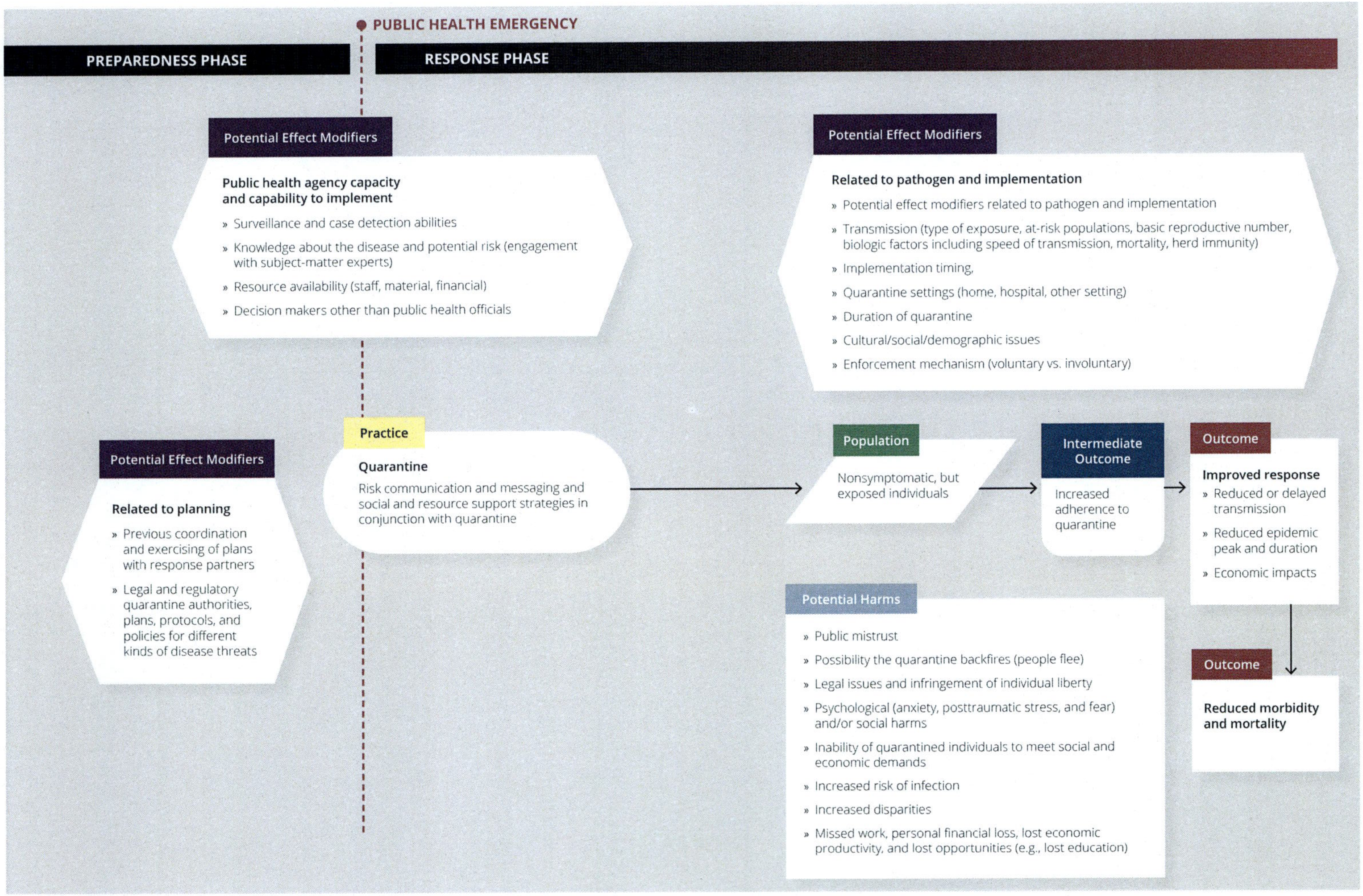

FIGURE B4-1 Analytic framework for implementing quarantine during a public health emergency.
NOTE: Arrows in the framework indicate hypothesized causal pathways between interventions and outcomes.

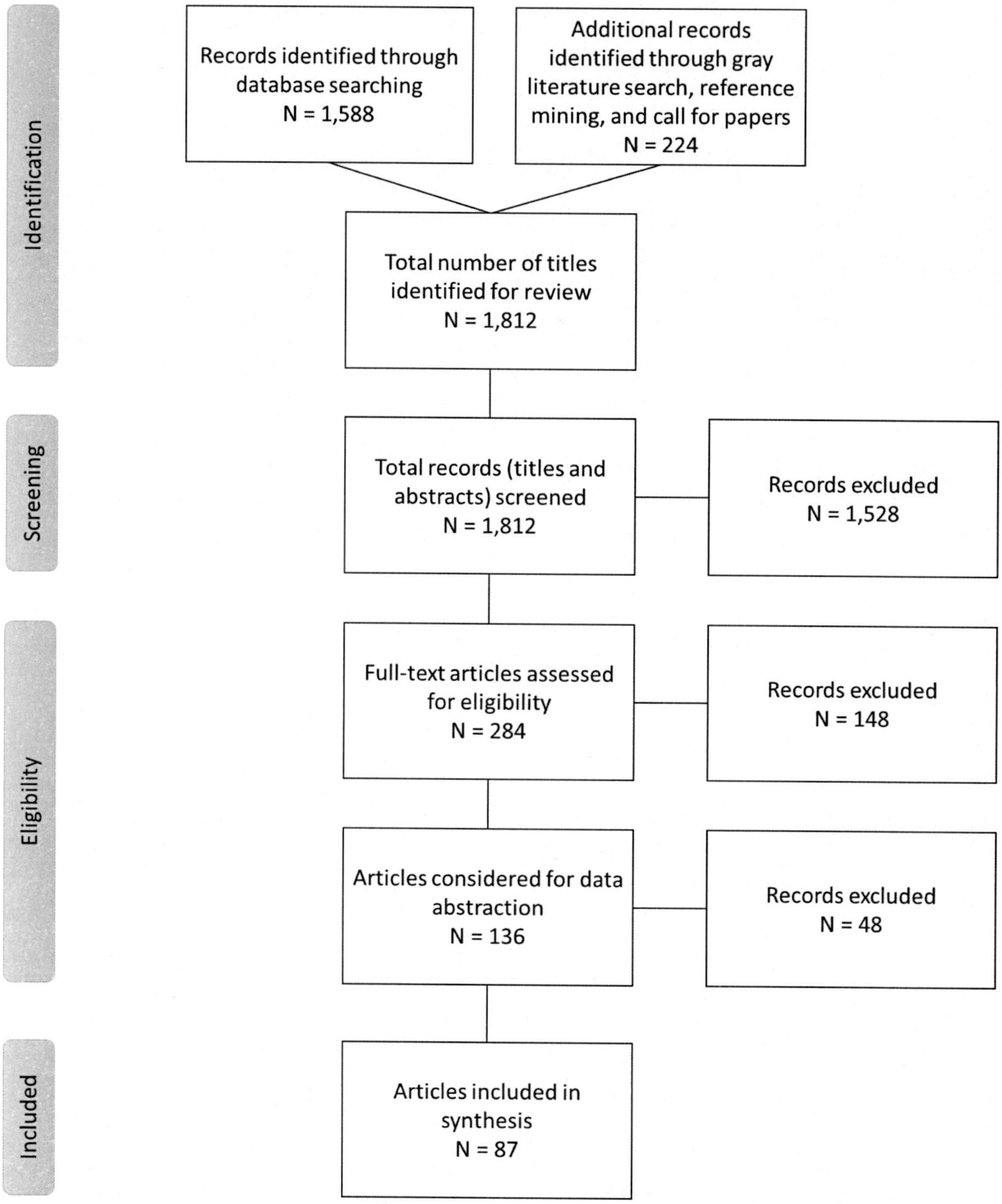

FIGURE B4-2 Preferred Reporting Items for Systematic Reviews and Meta-Analyses diagram for the mixed-method review of implementing quarantine to reduce or stop the spread of a contagious disease.

TABLE B4-1 Evidence Types Included in the Mixed-Method Review of Implementing Quarantine to Reduce or Stop the Spread of a Contagious Disease

Evidence Type[a]	Number of Studies (as applicable)[b]
Quantitative comparative	9
Quantitative noncomparative (postintervention measure only)	4
Qualitative	16
Modeling	12[c]
Descriptive surveys	13
Case reports	28
After action reports	N/A
Mechanistic[d]	Yes
Parallel (systematic reviews)	N/A

[a] Evidence types are defined in Chapter 3.
[b] Note that sibling articles (different results from the same study published in separate articles) are counted as one study in this table. Mixed-method studies may be counted in more than one category.
[c] The committee chose a sample of 12 studies out of 47 modeling studies for detailed review based on an assessment of their methodologic approach, data sources, relevance to the key questions for this practice, potential implications for public health practice, and disease condition studied. Given the time and resources available, the committee had to exclude a number of well-conducted modeling studies. Studies were excluded from detailed review if they reported major limitations to their model conclusions due to such factors as excessive uncertainty about modeling parameter values.
[d] For the purposes of this report, the committee defined mechanistic evidence as relationships for which causality has been established—generally from other scientific fields, such as chemistry, biology, economics, and physics (e.g., the accelerating effect of the gravitational attraction of Earth and the slowing effect of air resistance)—which can reasonably be applied to the PHEPR context through mechanistic reasoning. Mechanistic evidence is further discussed in Chapter 3.

1. Determining Evidence of Effect

Three quantitative comparative studies addressed the overarching key question regarding in what circumstances quarantine is effective at reducing or stopping the spread of a contagious disease in the community. These three studies examined whether quarantine reduced disease transmission in response to three different contagious diseases: H1N1 pandemic influenza, severe acute respiratory syndrome (SARS), and measles. Another six quantitative comparative studies and four quantitative noncomparative studies examined other potential benefits and harms of quarantine, as well as strategies that may be effective at improving adherence to quarantine.

A meta-analysis of the evidence for the effectiveness of quarantine was not feasible, so the committee conducted a synthesis without meta-analysis (as described in Chapter 3). Consistent with the methods described in Chapter 3, in making its final judgment on the evidence of effectiveness for quarantine, the committee considered other types of evidence that could inform a determination of what works for whom and in which contexts, ultimately reaching consensus on the certainty of the evidence (COE) for each outcome. Including forms of evidence beyond quantitative comparative studies is particularly important when assessing evidence in settings where controlled studies and/or other forms of quantitative comparative data are difficult to obtain, as is the case with studying quarantine. As discussed in Chapter 3, descriptive evidence from real-world implementation of practices offers the potential to corroborate research findings or explain differences in outcomes in practice settings, even if it has lesser value for causal inference. Moreover, qualitative studies can complement quantitative studies by providing additional useful evidence to guide real-world decision making, because well-conducted qualitative studies produce deep and rich understandings of how interventions are implemented, delivered, and experienced. Other forms of evidence considered for effectiveness included mechanistic evidence, evidence from modeling studies, and quantitative data reported in case reports of real disasters or public health emergencies.

Benefit: Reduced Overall Disease Transmission in the Community

Evidence from quantitative research studies Three quantitative comparative studies examined whether the use of quarantine can reduce disease transmission in the community. First, a "quasi-cluster randomized" controlled trial conducted by Miyaki and colleagues (2011) evaluated quarantine as an intervention in Japanese workplaces during the H1N1 influenza pandemic in 2009–2010. Employees of one of two randomly selected automobile factories were assigned to follow a home quarantine protocol, while employees at the other automobile factory were assigned to follow their company's standard operating procedures. At the factory implementing quarantine (N = 6,634), employees who developed influenza-like illness were ordered to stay home with pay (i.e., they were placed in non-state-enforced home quarantine), and employees whose cohabiting family members developed influenza-like illness were asked to stay home under quarantine. The factory's health management department managed implementation of the quarantine protocol. In the control factory (N = 8,500), employees reported to work or stayed home when ill per their normal practice. The researchers found a statistically significant 20 percent lower odds of employees testing positive for H1N1 influenza in the factory implementing quarantine compared with the control factory (hazard ratio 0.799; 95% confidence interval [CI] 0.658–0.970; $p = 0.023$). No one died of H1N1 influenza. The study was limited because outcome measurement was inadequate (use of a rapid test and clinical diagnosis may have greatly underestimated influenza infections), the study did not adjust for baseline differences between groups, and the study was underpowered for death. The study was deemed to be of moderate methodological quality for the analysis of overall H1N1 infection rates.

Second, Bondy and colleagues (2009) conducted a retrospective nonrandomized comparative study on quarantine using data from the 2003 SARS outbreak in Toronto, Canada. The authors made quantitative estimates of the reduction in secondary cases attributable to quarantine, based on information from 8,498 people who were quarantined. They estimated that the "secondary case count difference" (the average transmissions per case, similar to a risk difference) was −0.133 (95% CI −0.213, −0.053) transmitted cases for quarantined versus nonquarantined cases, which translated to a "number needed to quarantine" of 7.51 (95% CI 4.68, 18.9). That is, for every 7.51 people quarantined after exposure to SARS, one additional case of SARS was prevented. The adjusted secondary case count ratio (similar to the incident rate ratio) was 0.352 (95% CI 0.127, 0.981). The authors note that their study was underpowered, and to estimate statistical significance, they used multiple analyses that did not all agree. The article addresses measurement errors, but it is unclear whether this was a major concern with respect to the conclusions drawn. Overall, the study (and each outcome) was deemed to be of moderate methodological quality.

Finally, a retrospective nonrandomized comparative study conducted by Delaporte and colleagues (2013) evaluated 73 people exposed to measles who were quarantined and 173 people who were exposed to measles but not quarantined during a measles epidemic in Geneva, Switzerland, in 2011. The quarantined group represented all of those who met quarantine criteria and were quarantined; the nonquarantined group represented an undescribed sample of those who met quarantine criteria but were not quarantined. Those who were quarantined were half as likely to transmit measles within their household compared with those who were not quarantined and did not transmit any cases outside the household. Overall, quarantine reduced the risk of measles transmission by nearly 75 percent ($p = 0.002$). In this study, every case of transmission outside the household was connected to a nonquarantined person. The authors of this study defined their analyzed samples poorly, and the characteristics of the two samples were not compared or adjusted for. Overall, the study (and each outcome) was deemed to be of poor methodological quality.

Other evidence that may inform effectiveness The committee considered mechanistic evidence, modeling evidence, and quantitative data from case reports for the primary outcome of interest—reducing or stopping disease transmission. Relevant mechanistic evidence was identified from published historical reviews, and as noted earlier, there is little dispute that properly applied quarantine can reduce disease transmission rates (Drews, 2013; Tognotti, 2013). Indeed, the practice of quarantine was an effective response to disease outbreaks before the underlying causes of contagious diseases were understood. For centuries, quarantine has been the cornerstone of a coordinated outbreak-control strategy, which also has included isolation, sanitary cordons, bills of health issued to ships, fumigation, disinfection, and regulation of persons believed to be responsible for spreading illness. The advent of the germ theory of disease in the 1800s brought a new and powerful scientific underpinning to support modern quarantine. The idea that microscopic "germs" could lead to disease and that these germs could be passed from one person to another led to notions of exposure, infection, latent infection, incubation periods, and more (Drews, 2013). Thus, the mechanistic evidence behind quarantine as a means of reducing disease transmission, given the right circumstances, is very solid: quarantine aims to interrupt the chain of contagious disease transmission by separating individuals at risk of becoming contagious from susceptible populations.

The committee identified relevant modeling evidence from a detailed synthesis of 12 selected modeling studies. Across these 12 modeling studies, quarantine was found to be more effective for pathogens with certain specific characteristics (see the section on findings from modeling studies later in this appendix, and specifically Table B4-9). In addition, quarantine was more likely to be effective in several specific types of populations and settings. In summary, quarantine was found to drive the effective reproductive number (R_e)[2] <1 for Ebola; hepatitis A; Middle East respiratory syndrome (MERS); and possibly pandemic influenza, SARS, smallpox, and measles. It was not found to drive $R_e <1$ for pertussis. Given that a number of assumptions in these studies tend to lead to overestimation of the potential effectiveness of quarantine, it is likely prudent to assume that quarantine's effectiveness is somewhat lower than what is estimated and predicted by the modeling studies.

Across the remaining 35 modeling studies (those that were not examined in detail), 24 models considered the effectiveness of quarantine per se, and all 24 models found it to be effective in at least some circumstances. However, in nine of these studies, quarantine was inextricably linked with co-strategies such as safe burial practices (as are typical of real-world practice).

Finally, the committee identified relevant evidence on this question from case reports that also include some epidemiological quantitative data. Specifically, the committee exam-

---

[2] Effective reproductive number (R_e): Note that the pathogen's basic reproductive number (R_0) changes over time as the result of interventions and as the infection establishes immunity. The R_e (in this case in the presence of quarantine) is conceptually related to the ability of an infection to have persistent or growing prevalence in a population (when the R_e is above 1, the disease will have growing prevalence; below 1, prevalence will decline).

ined case reports that report on the number of individuals who eventually developed confirmed or probable illness during the time they were under quarantine. The rationale for examining such data is that a quarantine protocol that ended up placing only healthy people into quarantine was, by definition, ineffective at reducing the spread of a disease since those healthy people never posed a risk to the larger population. By contrast, a quarantine protocol that placed people in quarantine who eventually did end up being infected has a definable probability of having prevented one or more subsequent infections (as suggested by the three quantitative studies summarized above). The committee found 12 case reports that provide information on whether any individuals in quarantine developed illness. In five of these studies, none of those quarantined had confirmed or probable illness (CDC, 2004; Collier et al., 2013; Ehlkes et al., 2017; Grigg et al., 2015; Plipat et al., 2017); in the other seven, at least one quarantined person developed confirmed or probable illness during the quarantine period (CDC, 2003a,b; Chen et al., 2005; Pang et al., 2003; Reaves et al., 2014; Svoboda et al., 2004; Ward et al., 2010).

Summary of the evidence The committee concluded that *there is high COE that quarantine can be effective at reducing overall disease transmission in the community in certain circumstances.* Three quantitative comparative studies (Bondy et al., 2009; Delaporte et al., 2013; Miyaki et al., 2011) provide low COE regarding the effect of quarantine on reduced overall disease transmission (see Table B4-2). As for other forms of evidence,[3] taken together, the weight of the evidence is sufficient to upgrade the COE to high. Mechanistic data support the practice, as do modeling data, although effectiveness varies with characteristics of the pathogen. In addition, seven case reports may be seen as supportive, as there were illnesses in the quarantine groups that could have been transmitted; an additional five case reports with no illnesses in the quarantine groups have an equivocal impact on the COE. There are no discordant studies.

[3] As described in Chapter 3, the committee reviewed other evidence that informed the COE (e.g., mechanistic evidence, experiential evidence from case reports and after action reports, qualitative evidence) for coherence with the findings from the quantitative research studies and classified that evidence as very supportive, supportive, inconclusive (no conclusion can be drawn on coherence, either because results are mixed or the data are insufficient), or unsupportive (discordant with the findings from the quantitative research studies). The distinction between supportive and very supportive is based on the magnitude of the reported effect and the directness of the evidence to the question of interest.

TABLE B4-2 Effect of Quarantine on Reduced Overall Disease Transmission in the Community in Certain Circumstances

Quality Assessment	Number of Studies	3
	Study Infomation	Miyaki et al., 2011 Quasi-cluster randomized controlled trial, moderate methodological quality (▲) Bondy et al., 2009 Retrospective nonrandomized comparative study (NRCS), moderate methodological quality (▲) Delaporte et al., 2013 Retrospective NRCS, poor methodological quality (▲)
	Risk of Bias	Serious
	Inconsistency	Not serious
	Indirectness	Serious (Miyaki et al., 2011, study was conducted in an occupational health setting)
	Imprecision	Not serious
	Publication Bias	Unlikely
	Upgrade for Large Effect, Dose Response, Plausible Confounding	No
Summary of Findings	Initial Certainty of the Evidence (COE)	Low
	Other Evidence	Supportive mechanistic evidence, supportive modeling evidence, supportive case report evidence, and no discordant studies
	COE	High (reduces overall disease transmission)

NOTE: Effect direction: upward arrow (▲) = improvement/beneficial effect; downward arrow (▼) = harm/negative effect; sideways arrows (◀▶) = no effect; up and down arrows (▲▼) = mixed effect/conflicting findings.

Benefit: Reduced Time from Symptom Onset to Diagnosis

Evidence from quantitative research studies A single retrospective nonrandomized comparative study conducted by Hsieh and colleagues (2005) during the SARS outbreak in Taiwan in 2003 compared quarantined (N = 24) and nonquarantined people (N = 452) with respect to the time from onset of symptoms to diagnosis for those who became ill. Those who were not quarantined had a longer time (2.89 days) from onset of symptoms to clinical diagnosis (and hospital admission) relative to quarantined people (1.20 days) ($p = 0.0061$), but there was no difference in time from clinical diagnosis to final classification (i.e., confirmation of diagnosis of SARS) (7.54 days for nonquarantined people and 7.76 days for quarantined people; $p = 0.7864$). The authors did not adjust for differences between groups, and there was high loss to follow-up for time to classification. Overall, the study (and each outcome) was deemed to be of poor methodological quality.

Other evidence that may inform effectiveness The committee considered mechanistic evidence, modeling evidence, and quantitative data from case reports for the outcome of reduced time from symptom onset to diagnosis. Mechanistically, people in quarantine—

especially hospital quarantine—might also receive very close follow-up care, which could lead to a shorter time from symptom onset to diagnosis. Some modeling studies also assume that quarantine can help accelerate isolation in some circumstances, and may be a more effective option when the process of closely monitoring and then isolating individuals once they become symptomatic is slow or unreliable. One case report also addresses the importance of the difference in time from onset of illness to diagnosis with respect to the diffusion velocity of an epidemic in the early stages of pandemic influenza (Zhang et al., 2012). This case report shows that quarantine of close contacts allowed these high-risk subjects to be monitored closely over a longer period of time, which had important implications in reducing the risk of disease transmission by enabling timely detection of disease in those who had onset of illness.

Summary of the evidence The committee concluded that *there is low COE that quarantine can reduce the time from symptom onset to diagnosis in quarantined individuals.* One quantitative comparative study (Hsieh et al., 2005) provides very low COE regarding the effect of quarantine on this outcome (see Table B4-3). The weight of other forms of evidence, taken together, is sufficient to upgrade the COE to low. There are no discordant studies.

TABLE B4-3 Effect of Quarantine on Reduced Time from Symptom Onset to Diagnosis in Quarantined Individuals

Quality Assessment	Number of Studies	1
	Study Infomation	Hsieh et al., 2005 Retrospective nonrandomized comparative study (NRCS), poor methodological quality (▲)
	Risk of Bias	Very serious
	Inconsistency	Not applicable
	Indirectness	Not serious
	Imprecision	Serious
	Publication Bias	Unlikely
	Upgrade for Large Effect, Dose Response, Plausible Confounding	No
Summary of Findings	Initial Certainty of the Evidence (COE)	Very low
	Other Evidence	Supportive mechanistic evidence, supportive modeling evidence supportive evidence from one case report, and no discordant studies
	COE	Low (reduces time from symptom onset to diagnosis)

NOTE: Effect direction: upward arrow (▲) = improvement/beneficial effect; downward arrow (▼) = harm/negative effect; sideways arrows (◄►) = no effect; up and down arrows (▲▼) = mixed effect/conflicting findings.

Harm: Increased Risk of Infection in Congregate Quarantine Settings

Evidence from quantitative research studies Two quantitative comparative studies examined risk of infection in congregate quarantine settings,[4] both finding an increased risk. The "quasi-cluster randomized" controlled trial conducted by Miyaki and colleagues (2011) was discussed previously. In addition to the findings from this study noted earlier, the researchers found that factory employees with ill family members who were told to quarantine at home (with their ill family members) were twice as likely to develop H1N1 influenza compared with workers with ill family members from the control factory, who were not required to stay home (relative risk 2.17; $p < 0.001$). The second study, a retrospective nonrandomized comparative study conducted by Chu and colleagues (2010) during the pandemic H1N1 influenza season in China in 2009, assigned asymptomatic students who had been exposed to influenza during a train ride (N = 152) to different quarantine dormitory rooming situations for 12 days upon their return to a university. Quarantined students either shared both a room and a toilet with other quarantined students or shared a toilet but had a single room. Students were also categorized based on whether they had (by the end of quarantine) shared either a toilet or a room with another student who became ill. Students were not assigned randomly, but rooming situations were dictated by available rooms without regard for rooming preferences. Among those who shared rooms or toilets, those who shared with virus-positive contacts were more than three times more likely to develop a fever or influenza-like illness ($p = 0.02$, although H1N1 positivity was not generally tested). The rooming situation of those not exposed to virus-positive students during quarantine was not associated with the likelihood of developing a fever or illness. This study had serious methodological limitations related to the way in which students were assigned to rooming situations, inadequate outcome assessment, and lack of adjustment, among other concerns, nor did it directly analyze the effect of the different rooming situations (for all quarantined students). Overall, the study (and each outcome) was deemed to be of poor methodological quality.

Other evidence that may inform effectiveness The committee considered mechanistic evidence for the outcome of increased risk of infection in congregate quarantine settings. The mechanism by which quarantine results in an increased risk of infection in congregate settings is underpinned by the germ theory of disease. Quarantine may increase the contact between symptomatically ill individuals and people who are not ill or infected (i.e., only suspected of being exposed) with whom they come in contact within the quarantine area (mechanistic evidence for quarantine was discussed in prior sections).

Summary of the evidence The committee concluded that *there is high COE that congregate quarantine for influenza and agents with similar transmissibility can increase the risk of infection among those in the shared setting.* Two quantitative comparative studies (Chu et al., 2010; Miyaki et al., 2011) provide moderate COE regarding the effect of congregate quarantine on increased risk of infection among those quarantined together (see Table B4-4). In considering other evidence, the weight of the mechanistic evidence is sufficient to upgrade the COE to high.

---

[4] A congregate quarantine setting is the sharing of the same room or facilities with an infected case. This is applicable mainly to individuals quarantined at home who fall ill and thereby increase the likelihood that another household member will acquire the illness.

TABLE B4-4 Effect of Congregate Quarantine for Influenza and Agents with Similar Transmissibility on Increased Risk of Infection Among Those in the Shared Setting

Quality Assessment	Number of Studies	2
	Study Infomation	Miyaki et al., 2011 Quasi-cluster randomized controlled trial, moderate methodological quality (▼) Chu et al., 2010 Retrospective nonrandomized comparative study (NRCS), poor methodological quality (▼)
	Risk of Bias	Serious
	Inconsistency	Not serious
	Indirectness	Not serious
	Imprecision	Not serious
	Publication Bias	Unlikely
	Upgrade for Large Effect, Dose Response, Plausible Confounding	No
Summary of Findings	Initial Certainty of the Evidence (COE)	Moderate
	Other Evidence	Very supportive mechanistic evidence (no counterfactual)
	COE	High (increases risk of infection among those in the shared setting)

NOTE: Effect direction: upward arrow (▲) = improvement/beneficial effect; downward arrow (▼) = harm/negative effect; sideways arrows (◀▶) = no effect; up and down arrows (▲▼) = mixed effect/conflicting findings.

Harm: Psychological

Evidence from quantitative research studies Three quantitative comparative studies and three noncomparative quantitative studies examined the potential for psychological harms in quarantined individuals. They are briefly summarized below in the order in which they were published, which also corresponds to specific epidemics (SARS and MERS).

A cross-sectional (postintervention) survey conducted by Hawryluck and colleagues (2004) in 2003 examined the experiences of 129 people quarantined during the 2003 Toronto SARS outbreak, "after participants ended their quarantine period." The study found no statistically significant difference in adherence to recommended infection control measures during quarantine (e.g., remaining in residences, wearing masks, temperature monitoring) by health care workers compared with non–health care workers. Symptoms of posttraumatic stress disorder (PTSD) (as measured with the Impact of Event Scale-Revised [IES-R], a measure of levels of psychological distress) and depression (as measured with the Center for Epidemiologic Studies-Depression Scale [CES-D]) were similar among those who underwent home- versus work-based quarantine. Those who experienced ≥10 days of quarantine had statistically significantly worse PTSD symptoms ($p = 0.005$) and had nonsignificantly worse depression symptoms ($p = 0.07$) compared with those who underwent <10 days of quarantine. Those who wore a mask at all times during quarantine (against recommendations, which allowed for masks to be taken off under some circumstances) had statistically significantly higher PTSD and depression symptoms relative to those who followed the recommendations and those who never wore a mask ($p = 0.003$). Worse PTSD and depression symptoms during quarantine were also associated with lower income. According to the study authors, the survey may have preferentially selected those with greater distress. The survey also captured a very small sample of those quarantined (<1 percent). Overall, the study (and each outcome) was deemed to be of poor methodological quality.

Reynolds and colleagues (2008) conducted a similar but much larger cross-sectional (postintervention) survey in 2003, 6 weeks after the Toronto SARS outbreak, among 1,057 quarantined people. Compared with non–health care workers, they found that health care workers had a greater likelihood of severe PTSD symptoms (by IES-R score ≥20; $p < 0.001$) and reported more PTSD symptoms; more avoidance symptoms, intrusion symptoms, and hyperarousal symptoms; and greater loss of income related to being quarantined ($p = 0.001$). The survey underrepresented younger people, and the authors note a high risk of recall bias. Overall, the study (and each outcome) was deemed to be of poor methodological quality.

In a retrospective, nonrandomized comparative study, Marjanovic and colleagues (2007) evaluated the experiences of 333 nurses quarantined during the 2003 Toronto SARS epidemic. In adjusted analyses, quarantine (or longer quarantine time) was associated with higher scores on a then-unvalidated measure of avoidance behavior ($p < 0.001$) and state anger (by the State-Trait Anger Expression Inventory [STAXI] anger subscale) ($p = 0.008$), but not greater emotional exhaustion (as measured by the Maslach Burnout Inventory-General Survey emotional exhaustion subscale) ($p = 0.113$). Overall, the study (and each outcome) was deemed to be of poor methodological quality largely because of a lack of clarity about the comparison that was made.

Wu and colleagues (2008, 2009) and Liu and colleagues (2012) report on a retrospective nonrandomized comparative study of employees at a major Beijing hospital (N = 549) 3 years after that city's SARS outbreak in 2003. Compared with nonquarantined employees, those who were quarantined were found to have been more likely to have had alcohol-related symptoms (questions adapted from the National Household Survey on Drug Abuse), PTSD symptoms (by IES-R) ($p < 0.001$), and depression symptoms (by CES-D) ($p < 0.0001$) during the 3 years after the SARS epidemic. The study authors do not provide a clear definition of quarantine, and it is possible that some of those considered quarantined were actually in isolation and experienced illness with SARS. For PTSD and depression symptoms, the study was deemed to be of moderate methodological quality, and for alcohol-related symptoms, the study was deemed to be of poor methodological quality because of the use of an unvalidated tool.

A cross-sectional (postintervention) survey conducted by Jeong and colleagues (2016) 4 to 6 months after a MERS outbreak in South Korea in 2015 compared psychological and other outcomes between people quarantined for 2 weeks who ended up having MERS (N = 36) and those quarantined who did not (N = 1,656). The study also compared quarantined individuals based on their degree of exposure to individuals with MERS before being placed in quarantine. Quarantined people who developed MERS reported having more medical expenses ($p < 0.001$) and less sufficient food and water, ability to bathe, or access to self-care products ($p < 0.001$) during quarantine compared with quarantined people who did not develop MERS. Individuals with greater prior exposure to people with MERS reported greater anxiety and anger symptoms 4 to 6 months after quarantine. Of note, the study did not compare people quarantined with similarly exposed people who were not quarantined. The study authors report that the anxiety and anger scales used (Generalized Anxiety Disorder Scale and STAXI, respectively) may not be valid in this population, and notably, many angry people refused to participate in the survey. Overall, the study (and each outcome) was deemed to be of poor methodological quality.

Lee and colleagues (2018) conducted a retrospective nonrandomized comparative study (a longitudinal series of surveys) during and following the MERS outbreak of 2015 in South Korea, comparing quarantined and nonquarantined health care personnel at a MERS-affected hospital. In a first survey during the MERS epidemic quarantine period, quarantined and nonquarantined health care personnel (N = 359 total respondents) had similar scores on the IES-R scale. Six weeks later, the authors conducted a follow-up survey (N = 77 total respondents) of just those personnel who had high distress scores on the first survey (scoring in a range that made them "PTSD eligible"). Overall, at 6 weeks, IES-R scores were similar among quarantined and nonquarantined employees. In the follow-up survey of more distressed health care personnel, however, those who had been quarantined were statistically significantly more likely ($p = 0.03$) to have "sleep and numbness" symptoms on the IES-R. For both surveys, the respondents were substantially different from the nonrespondents with respect to their health care roles; response rates varied widely by job description. Nonresponse rates, in particular on the follow-up survey, were high. The authors do not define quarantine. The "sleep and numbness" outcome is inadequately reported and appears to be an ad hoc measure. Outcome results are not fully reported. Overall, the study (and each outcome) was deemed to be of poor methodological quality.

Other evidence that may inform effectiveness The committee considered findings from a qualitative evidence synthesis and quantitative data from case reports for the outcome of psychological harm. Overall, eight qualitative studies examined the psychological harms of quarantine, including social isolation and social stigma (Cava et al., 2005a; Desclaux et al., 2017; DiGiovanni et al., 2004; Lin et al., 2010; Maunder et al., 2003; Pellecchia et al., 2015; Robertson et al., 2004; Schemm Dwyer et al., 2017).

People on whom quarantine is imposed may experience the harm of social isolation (high confidence in the evidence).[5] This harm is documented in four quarantine studies among members of the general public, as well as health care workers placed under quarantine (Cava et al., 2005a; DiGiovanni et al., 2004; Lin et al., 2010; Robertson et al., 2004). Quarantine typically required restriction of physical contact with close others, including spouses, children, and siblings; wearing a mask, which is further distancing; and even home quarantine, all of which resulted in feelings of physical and psychological isolation.

People on whom quarantine is imposed may experience the harm of social stigma (high confidence in the evidence). Unless the quarantine is kept secret, people on whom it is imposed may be publicly labeled as potential carriers of a contagious disease, which may in turn lead others to develop feelings of avoidance, suspicion, mistrust, and fear, and thus stigma, toward the quarantined people. The seven qualitative studies found that when people from already-marginalized communities were quarantined, this stigmatization could exacerbate discrimination and marginalization, a situation that could last well beyond the quarantine period (Cava et al., 2005a; Desclaux et al., 2017; DiGiovanni et al., 2004; Lin et al., 2010; Pellecchia et al., 2015; Robertson et al., 2004; Schemm Dwyer et al., 2017).

People on whom quarantine is imposed may also experience the harm of negative psychological states, including anxiety, fear, worry, stress, and loneliness (high confidence in the evidence). Six qualitative studies found that the sources for these psychological harms

[5] This italicized statement with an associated confidence level is a qualitative evidence finding statement from the commissioned report "Quarantine as a Non-Pharmaceutical Intervention: Qualitative Research Evidence Synthesis" by Pradeep Sopory and Julie Novak (see Appendix C). The Grading of Recommendations Assessment, Development and Evaluation Confidence in the Evidence from Reviews of Qualitative Research (GRADE-CERQual) was used to assess the confidence in synthesized qualitative findings (analytic and some descriptive themes). Additional details on GRADE-CERQual can be found in Chapter 3.

could be the social isolation and stigmatization noted above, as well as the financial stress that can accompany quarantine and worry about the possibility of inflicting harm on others (Cava et al., 2005a; DiGiovanni et al., 2004; Lin et al., 2010; Maunder et al., 2003; Pellecchia et al., 2015; Robertson et al., 2004).

Health care workers on whom quarantine is imposed may experience additional harms (high confidence in the evidence). Three qualitative studies found amplified harms for health care workers (Desclaux et al., 2017; Maunder et al., 2003; Robertson et al., 2004). For example, they experienced stronger negative psychological states such as anxiety, and additional stress from fear, guilt, or shame that they could have infected patients before being quarantined. Health care workers under quarantine also worried about leaving their colleagues understaffed and overworked. In cases of "work quarantine," where essential health care workers must continue to come to work, having contact with patients known to be infected could lead to even greater anxiety. This situation could also lead to resentment and conflict with nonessential coworkers placed in home instead of work quarantine. One case report includes data on the frequency of mental disorders among 6,231 people placed in quarantine for exposure to MERS in South Korea; 1,221 (19.3 percent) showed emotional disturbances such as depression (Yoon et al., 2016).

Summary of the evidence The committee concluded that *there is moderate COE that quarantine can result in psychological harm among quarantined individuals, including PTSD, anxiety, and anger, the risk of which increases with the duration of quarantine.* Three quantitative comparative studies (Lee et al., 2018; Liu et al., 2012; Marjanovic et al., 2007; Wu et al., 2008, 2009) and three quantitative noncomparative studies (Hawryluck et al., 2004; Jeong et al., 2016; Reynolds et al., 2008) provide low COE regarding the effect of quarantine on psychological harms among quarantined individuals (see Table B4-5). The weight of other forms of evidence, taken together, is sufficient to upgrade the COE to moderate. There is very supportive evidence with high certainty from a synthesis of eight qualitative studies and a supportive case report. There are no discordant studies.

TABLE B4-5 Effect of Quarantine on Psychological Harms in Quarantined Individuals

Quality Assessment	Number of Studies	6
	Study Infomation	Lee et al., 2018 Retrospective nonrandomized comparative study (NRCS), poor methodological quality (▼) Liu et al., 2012; Wu et al., 2008, 2009 Retrospective NRCS, moderate methodological quality (▼) Marjanovic et al., 2007 Retrospective NRCS, poor methodological quality (▼) Hawryluck et al., 2004 Cross-sectional (postintervention), poor methodological quality (▼) Jeong et al., 2016 Cross-sectional (postintervention), poor methodological quality (▼) Reynolds et al., 2008 Cross-sectional (postintervention), poor methodological quality (▼)
	Risk of Bias	Serious
	Inconsistency	Not serious
	Indirectness	Not serious
	Imprecision	Not serious
	Publication Bias	Unlikely
	Upgrade for Large Effect, Dose Response, Plausible Confounding	Large effect
Summary of Findings	Initial Certainty of the Evidence (COE)	Low
	Other Evidence	Very supportive qualitative evidence, supportive evidence from one case report, and no discordant studies
	COE	Moderate (increases psychological harm)

NOTE: Effect direction: upward arrow (▲) = improvement/beneficial effect; downward arrow (▼) = harm/negative effect; sideways arrows (◄►) = no effect; up and down arrows (▲▼) = mixed effect/conflicting findings.

Harm: Individual Financial Hardship

Evidence from quantitative research studies Two quantitative noncomparative studies—by Reynolds and colleagues (2008), discussed above, and Kavanagh and colleagues (2012), discussed in a following section—examined whether being placed in quarantine led to financial losses for quarantined individuals. Both found that it did. Kavanagh and colleagues (2012) found that 38 percent of surveyed households lost pay to care for a child in home quarantine, which in 42 percent of cases led to financial difficulties (e.g., unable to pay a bill). Lost pay occurred more frequently in households without access to leave ($p < 0.001$). Reynolds and colleagues (2008) found that health care workers were more likely than non–health care workers to experience a decline in household income during the 2003 SARS outbreak in Toronto ($p < 0.05$).

Other evidence that may inform effectiveness The committee considered mechanistic evidence and findings from a qualitative evidence synthesis for the outcome of individual financial hardship. Mechanistic evidence applies to understanding the process by which quarantine can be associated with financial loss: people who are quarantined are unable to work, which may result in a loss of income.

People on whom quarantine is imposed may experience the harm of financial instability (high confidence in the evidence). Five qualitative studies examined financial losses among quarantined individuals (Baum et al., 2009; Braunack-Mayer et al., 2010; Cava et al., 2005a; Desclaux et al., 2017; DiGiovanni et al., 2004). People were often placed in quarantine with little advance notice, which affected their employment status and resulted in the loss of regular wages and other income without compensation. This situation could be exacerbated for people whose income comes from part-time work, casual work, or self-employment.

Summary of the evidence The committee concluded that *there is high COE that quarantine can be associated with individual financial hardship for people who are quarantined.* Two nonquantitative comparative studies (Kavanagh et al., 2012; Reynolds et al., 2008) provide low COE regarding the effect of quarantine on financial hardship among quarantined individuals (see Table B4-6). The weight of other forms of evidence, taken together, is sufficient to upgrade the COE to high. There is very supportive mechanistic evidence, as well as very supportive evidence with high certainty from a synthesis of five qualitative studies. There are no discordant studies.

TABLE B4-6 Effect of Quarantine on Financial Hardship in Quarantined Individuals

Quality Assessment	Number of Studies	2
	Study Infomation	Kavanagh et al., 2012 Cross-sectional (postintervention), moderate methodological quality (▼) Reynolds et al., 2008 Cross-sectional (postintervention), poor methodological quality (▼)
	Risk of Bias	Serious
	Inconsistency	Not serious
	Indirectness	Not serious
	Imprecision	Not serious
	Publication Bias	Unlikely
	Upgrade for Large Effect, Dose Response, Plausible Confounding	Large effect
Summary of Findings	Initial Certainty of the Evidence (COE)	Low
	Other Evidence	Very supportive mechanistic evidence, very supportive qualitative evidence, and no discordant studies
	COE	High (increases financial hardship)

NOTE: Effect direction: upward arrow (▲) = improvement/beneficial effect; downward arrow (▼) = harm/negative effect; sideways arrows (◄►) = no effect; up and down arrows (▲▼) = mixed effect/conflicting findings.

Strategies for Reducing Harms

Evidence from quantitative research studies A single quantitative noncomparative study examined depression in quarantined individuals and the provision of family support and the promotion and emphasis of health by those leading the outbreak response (i.e., "health-promoting leadership"). Adler and colleagues (2018) published a cross-sectional (postintervention) survey of 501 soldiers on a U.S. military base who had returned from West Africa with possible exposure to Ebola in 2014. The study evaluated the association of family support and health-promoting leadership behaviors by local senior leaders with the soldiers' mental health and attitudes toward the quarantine. Using a regression model, the authors found that health-promoting leadership behaviors were independently associated with fewer depression ($p = 0.04$) and anxiety ($p = 0.008$) symptoms, less functional impairment ($p = 0.03$), and more positive attitudes toward quarantine ($p < 0.001$) and preventive medicine ($p < 0.001$). No statistically significant associations were found with PTSD symptoms or insomnia. Perception of family support was not associated with PTSD, depression, or anxiety symptoms but was associated with fewer insomnia symptoms ($p < 0.001$), less functional impairment ($p = 0.04$), and more positive attitudes toward the quarantine ($p < 0.001$) and the preventive medicine practices enacted during the quarantine ($p < 0.001$). The survey methods and outcomes are not described and were not validated. The predictor "health-promoting leadership behaviors" was based on soldiers' answers to the survey about their leaders; however, it is unclear how this variable (or variables) was entered into the model. Overall, the study (and each outcome) was deemed to be of poor methodological quality.

Summary of the evidence The committee concluded that there is *very low COE that an emphasis on health by those leading the outbreak response (i.e., health-promoting leadership) can reduce depression and anxiety symptoms in quarantined individuals.* One non-quantitative comparative study (Adler et al., 2018) provides very low COE regarding the effect of health-promoting leadership on depression in quarantined individuals (see Table B4-7).

TABLE B4-7 Effect of Health-Promoting Leadership on Reduced Depression and Anxiety Symptoms in Quarantined Individuals

Quality Assessment	Number of Studies	1
	Study Infomation	Adler et al., 2018 Cross-sectional (postintervention), poor methodological quality (▲)
	Risk of Bias	Very serious
	Inconsistency	Not applicable
	Indirectness	Not serious
	Imprecision	Serious
	Publication Bias	Unlikely
	Upgrade for Large Effect, Dose Response, Plausible Confounding	No
Summary of Findings	Initial Certainty of the Evidence (COE)	Very low
	Other Evidence	Not applicable
	COE	Very low (reduces depression and anxiety symptoms)

NOTE: Effect direction: upward arrow (▲) = improvement/beneficial effect; downward arrow (▼) = harm/negative effect; sideways arrows (◄►) = no effect; up and down arrows (▲▼) = mixed effect/conflicting findings.

Strategies for Improving Adherence to Quarantine Measures

Evidence from quantitative research studies A single quantitative noncomparative study examined the implementation of risk communication and messaging and social and resource support strategies as ways of improving adherence to quarantine. Kavanagh and colleagues (2011, 2012) and McVernon and colleagues (2011) conducted this cross-sectional (postintervention) survey about 6 months after a pandemic of H1N1 influenza in Australia in 2009 among 297 households affected by the quarantine of children thought to have been exposed at school. Households that reported understanding what they were meant to do during quarantine were more than twice as likely to comply fully with quarantine recommendations compared with those that did not (odds ratio [OR] 2.27; 95% CI 1.35–3.80) (Kavanagh et al., 2011). Among families in which all resident parents were employed, those with available sick leave were twice as likely to stay home throughout quarantine (OR 2.07; 95% CI 0.82–5.23) (Kavanagh et al., 2012). Those who took time off were more than twice as likely to stay home throughout quarantine (OR 2.47; 95% CI 1.17–5.22; $p = 0.02$), although whether parents took time off from work was not associated with full compliance (OR 1.27; 95% CI 0.61–2.67). Households without access to paid leave were about three times more likely to have lost pay to care for their quarantined child ($p < 0.001$). Households in which the child was not ill were much more likely to have another child visit the household compared with those with ill children ($p < 0.001$) (McVernon et al., 2011). Similarly, households in which no family members were ill were more likely to have another adult visit during quarantine ($p = 0.04$). The authors note a high risk of recall bias, and the response rate may have been low. Overall, the study (and each outcome) was deemed to be of moderate methodological quality.

Other evidence that may inform effectiveness The committee considered findings from a qualitative evidence synthesis for the outcome of improved adherence. Eight qualitative studies examined the importance of risk communication for adherence to quarantine measures (Cava et al., 2005b; DiGiovanni et al., 2004; Lin et al., 2010; Pellecchia et al., 2015; Robertson et al., 2004; Schemm Dwyer et al., 2017; Sell et al., 2018; Smith et al., 2012). This evidence suggests that *agencies can use communication strategically to increase adherence to quarantine during a contagious disease event. This communication is equally important for both the public and the health care staff on whom quarantine has been imposed* (high confidence in the evidence). The findings of these qualitative studies indicate that communication should emphasize persuasion over threat and aim to be bidirectional. They suggest further that communication should take place over the full course of the event and should involve multiple channels, including mass media and interpersonal channels, and multiple sources, including public health and health care staff. The communication should, in particular, provide information about the disease, as well as the need for and instructions for the quarantine; not arouse fear and anxiety; not be stigmatizing; not use terms with confusing meanings; and include clear and consistent information about infection control and coping strategies.

Summary of the evidence The committee concluded that *there is moderate COE that while adherence to quarantine measures can vary by culture, disease, and socioeconomic status, use of various strategies, including risk communication and messaging and access to employment leave, can improve adherence.* One quantitative noncomparative study (Kavanagh et al., 2011, 2012; McVernon et al., 2011) provides low COE regarding the effect of risk communication and messaging and access to employment leave on improved adherence to quarantine measures (see Table B4-8). The weight of other forms of evidence, taken together, is sufficient to upgrade the COE to moderate. There is very supportive evidence with high certainty from a synthesis of eight qualitative studies. There are no discordant studies.

TABLE B4-8 Effect of Risk Communication and Messaging and Employment Leave on Improved Adherence to Quarantine Measures

Quality Assessment	Number of Studies	1
	Study Infomation	Kavanagh et al., 2011, 2012; McVernon et al., 2011 Cross-sectional, moderate methodological quality (▲)
	Risk of Bias	Serious
	Inconsistency	Not applicable
	Indirectness	Not serious
	Imprecision	Serious
	Publication Bias	Unlikely
	Upgrade for Large Effect, Dose Response, Plausible Confounding	Large effect
Summary of Findings	Initial Certainty of the Evidence (COE)	Low
	Other Evidence	Very supportive qualitative evidence and no discordant studies
	COE	Moderate (improves adherence)

NOTE: Effect direction: upward arrow (▲) = improvement/beneficial effect; downward arrow (▼) = harm/negative effect; sideways arrows (◄►) = no effect; up and down arrows (▲▼) = mixed effect/conflicting findings.

2. Findings from a Synthesis of Modeling Studies: Quarantine Is More Effective Under Certain Circumstances

As previously discussed, across the 12 modeling studies considered, quarantine was found to be more or less likely to be effective depending on systematic and consistent factors related both to characteristics of the pathogen and to the population and setting (see Table B4-9).[6] Understanding of these systematic relationships is aided specifically by one of the modeling studies included in this review (Peak et al., 2017), whose authors provide analyses for a range of diseases and attempt to provide answers to this question within a common modeling framework.[7]

Consistent with the findings of Peak and colleagues (2017), as well as the other modeling studies and the drivers of effectiveness their authors identify or imply, quarantine was more likely to be effective at reducing or stopping the spread of a contagious disease in the following circumstances:

- *Moderate basic reproductive number* (R_0)—when the R_0 of a given pathogen is in a range in which quarantine can be expected to reduce transmission importantly. Quarantine may be more effective for a pathogen with a moderate R_0 or for a pathogen with a higher R_0 that has previously produced durable immunity in a population (i.e., the population in question has been exposed previously) such that the effective reproductive number (R_e) in the population even without intervention is relatively lower. If a pathogen has a high R_0, more transmission may occur before quarantine can be implemented, reducing quarantine's effectiveness at limiting the final extent of the outbreak. As a practical matter, for pathogens with a very low R_0 (i.e., <1) disease transmission will not be sustained, making quarantine theoretically effective but perhaps practically unnecessary (see also footnote 2 earlier in this appendix).

- *Shorter incubation period*—when quarantine can reliably separate identified individuals from the general population for durations commensurate with the expected duration of asymptomatic infectiousness. Quarantine may become infeasible or less effective as the result of reduced adherence if its duration must be very long because of a prolonged incubation period (the period between exposure and when infection becomes detectable).
- *Relatively short asymptomatic infectious period*—when the asymptomatic infectious period is short or there is no asymptomatic infectious period. When there is a long period of asymptomatic infectiousness, quarantine of recently infected people must be extremely rapid and comprehensive to prevent transmission by asymptomatic individuals, which may be so logistically challenging as to be practically infeasible. In addition, if the asymptomatic infectious period is long in absolute terms, quarantine may become infeasible or less effective because of reduced adherence (see the previous bullet).
- *Rapid identification*—when exposed individuals can be identified reliably and quickly.
- *Use of quarantine to aid isolation*—when isolation of individuals once they become symptomatic is slow or unreliable without quarantine. In these circumstances, quarantine may reduce transmission through its effects on facilitating more rapid isolation of ill and contagious individuals.

TABLE B4-9 Summary of Findings on the Effectiveness of Quarantine from 12 Modeling Studies

Disease	Quarantine Likely Effective?	Notes
Ebola	Yes	Two studies found that quarantine can drive R_e <1[a] (D'Silva and Eisenberg, 2017; Peak et al., 2017).
Hepatitis A	Yes based on 1 study	One study found that quarantine can drive R_e <1 (Peak et al., 2017).
Influenza A/ H1N1	Maybe	Two studies. One study found that quarantine can drive R_e <1 (Peak et al., 2017). Another study focused on delaying the epidemic peak and indicated that quarantine can possibly be effective depending on the specific features of the pathogen in the population and the level of intervention (An der Heiden et al., 2009).
Middle East respiratory syndrome (MERS)	Yes	Two studies found that quarantine can drive R_e <1 (Ahn et al., 2018; Peak et al., 2017).
Pertussis	No based on 1 study	One study found that quarantine is unlikely to drive R_e <1 (Peak et al., 2017).
Severe acute respiratory syndrome (SARS)	Maybe	Seven studies. Three studies identified situations in which quarantine may not be effective in driving R_e <1, with effectiveness depending on the pathogen's basic reproductive number in a given population (less likely with higher R_0 [b]), the likely effectiveness of isolation of symptomatic individuals as an alternative strategy, the likelihood of there being individuals who are asymptomatic but contagious and the fraction of those individuals, and the ability to quickly identify a large fraction of exposed individuals for quarantine (Day et al., 2006; Hsieh et al., 2007; Peak et al., 2017). Four studies found (or in essence their authors assumed [based on models of past limited outbreaks]) that sufficiently effective, properly scaled and targeted, or potentially dynamic quarantine policies can drive R_e <1 (Feng et al., 2009; Gupta et al., 2005; Mubayi et al., 2010; Podder et al., 2007).
Smallpox	Maybe	Two studies. One study found that quarantine is unlikely to drive R_e <1. Another study found that early initiation of quarantine for a large fraction of exposed cases can likely avoid an epidemic resulting from a smallpox bioterrorism attack (Meltzer et al., 2001; Peak et al., 2017).
Measles	Yes/maybe based on 1 study	One study found that despite measles having a high R_0, if there is a sufficient level of background immunity, it may be possible to use quarantine to end an outbreak quickly. However, with lower levels of background immunity, quarantine is unlikely to drive R_e <1 or to do so quickly (Enanoria et al., 2016).

[a] R_e = effective reproductive number (in this case in the presence of quarantine), which conceptually is related to the ability of an infection to have persistent or growing prevalence in a population (when R_e is above 1, the disease will have growing prevalence; when it is below 1, prevalence will decline).
[b] R_0 = basic reproductive number.

3. Balance of Benefits and Harms

Synthesis of Evidence of Effect

The synthesis of evidence of effect (described above) shows that quarantine can be effective at reducing overall disease transmission in the community in certain circumstances (high COE) and reducing time from symptom onset to diagnosis in quarantined individuals (low COE). The modeling studies reviewed also support these benefits. However, quarantine can result in harms for those quarantined, including increased risk of infection among those quarantined together in congregate quarantine settings (high COE), psychological harm (moderate COE), and individual financial hardship (high COE).

Qualitative Evidence Synthesis

Indirectly, the qualitative studies included in this review found that quarantine is an important response to contagious disease outbreaks that is likely to be effective in lowering morbidity and mortality in the larger population. The 16 qualitative studies in this corpus, however, were focused much more on the process of quarantine than on disease-related outcomes, in particular on understanding the experience of the people on whom quarantine is imposed. The study findings indicate that quarantine has the potential to result in the removal of civil rights protections and, as discussed in the above section on determining evidence of effect, the occurrence of such undesirable impacts as financial instability, social stigma, and compromised psychological well-being. Given these undesirable impacts of quarantine, which can be both short and long term, the balance of benefits and harms is open to debate.

Case Report Evidence Synthesis

As with the qualitative studies, most of the case reports reviewed do not directly address the benefits of quarantine. Those that do so mention potential benefits of reduced risk of transmission and increased public confidence based on experience with SARS in China, Singapore, and Taiwan (CDC, 2003a,b; Ooi et al., 2005). Although acknowledging challenges with careful application of quarantine measures, the Centers for Disease Control and Prevention's (CDC's) *Morbidity and Mortality Weekly Report* indicates that quarantine effectively eliminated the risk for transmission of SARS from quarantined people to community members (CDC, 2003a). Ooi and colleagues (2005) describe how quarantine gave the public in Singapore confidence to continue with their daily activities, given their knowledge of public health safeguards against SARS (Ooi et al., 2005). They conjecture that the public would otherwise have taken actions to avoid public places, resulting in a situation in which the unaffected majority instead of the affected minority would stay at home. Most of the case reports reviewed note the unintended consequences or harms related to quarantine, including the potential for increased transmission and mortality due to its inappropriate application, its impact on emergency and routine services, restrictions on civil liberties, psychological impacts and stigmatization, and lost wages and school absence.

4. Acceptability and Preferences

Qualitative Evidence Synthesis

Nine qualitative studies examined the acceptability of quarantine (Baum et al., 2009; Bell and WHO, 2004; Cava et al., 2005b; Desclaux et al., 2017; DiGiovanni et al., 2004; Leung et al., 2008; Lin et al., 2010; Pellecchia et al., 2015; Robertson et al., 2004). These studies found that the public understood and accepted the general concept of quarantine as one of the mechanisms for slowing the transmission of a contagious disease through a population. Even vulnerable groups, such as the homeless, were not opposed to the idea in general. People had several reasons for this view, including a sense of duty, ethical concerns, and civic-mindedness. Thus, *agencies can facilitate adherence to quarantine by acknowledging that the public in general accepts, and does not resist, the general idea of quarantine as a response to an infectious disease event* (high confidence in the evidence). These qualitative studies also found that the acceptability of and preference for quarantine differed across the various agencies working together to implement quarantine, with some advocating an emphasis on voluntary adherence and others seeking mandatory enforcement, which may include a militaristic response. If community groups are added as stakeholders, which in many instances they should be, the divergence of views on the acceptability of quarantine as a public health intervention may become even wider. Open-ended deliberations among stakeholders could address this divergence and achieve common ground. Furthermore, the implementation of quarantine is unique to contagious disease outbreaks and perhaps to other emergencies in which the health hazard may be communicable through contact. Therefore, capacity building, such as through training, may require a dedicated one-hazard focus, which may not be feasible for an agency to implement on a regular basis.

Case Report Evidence Synthesis

Quarantine may not be acceptable to all communities, given case reports of psychological distress; anxiety; and fear of income loss, stigma, and social isolation. Furthermore, as noted above and as evidenced by findings from a tabletop exercise in San Diego, authorities and public health agencies may have differing preferences with regard to the implementation of quarantine (DiGiovanni et al., 2005).

It is possible that the provision of food, wage compensation, and other financial or in-kind supports can enhance the acceptability of quarantine. Making quarantine voluntary instead of mandatory also could increase its acceptability (CDC, 2003b; Chen et al., 2005; Chung et al., 2015; Ehlkes et al., 2017; Pang et al., 2003; Reaves et al., 2014; Yoon et al., 2016; Zhang et al., 2012). Lessons learned from case reports in Liberia and Ohio indicate that engaging local leaders and involving community members during the planning and implementation phases helped support safe and effective quarantine (Gastañaduy et al., 2016; Nyenswah et al., 2015). Additionally, efforts made to minimize stigmatization of Ebola survivors through education, social mobilization, and reintegration programs may have led to greater adherence to voluntary quarantine because community members did not fear being stigmatized (Reaves et al., 2014). By contrast, a case report of MERS from South Korea indicates that many quarantined individuals were unwilling to provide personal information because of anticipated sigma or negative local perception of MERS (Yoon et al., 2016).

Descriptive Survey Study Evidence

Tracy and colleagues (2009) conducted a survey of the public perceptions of quarantine following a contagious disease outbreak in Canada. Responses revealed a high rate of public acceptance of quarantine as a means of controlling the spread of a contagious disease. The vast majority of respondents expressed strong support for the use of quarantine in a contagious disease outbreak, for legal penalties against absconders, for social supports for those affected, and for public safeguards against potential inappropriate use. A survey conducted by Teh and colleagues (2012) collected information on attitudes toward and understanding of quarantine measures in quarantined households in Australia during the H1N1 outbreak in that country. Most respondents said that they considered quarantine useful and that the quarantine measures imposed were justified; the proportion of respondents who expressed the latter view increased when the survey asked about a scenario of more serious pandemic influenza. A survey examining the public's reaction to the use of quarantine in Hong Kong, Singapore, Taiwan, and the United States found strong majorities favor quarantining in each country (Blendon et al., 2006). In general, Americans were less supportive of more restrictive monitoring methods (e.g., use of electronic bracelets or guards) than were people living in other regions and strongly preferred home quarantine. Kelly and colleagues (2015) assessed perceptions and beliefs about possible Ebola-related policies, such as mandatory quarantine, in the United States. A majority of respondents said that all individuals who have been exposed to an Ebola patient should be quarantined for 21 days whether or not they show symptoms. Among respondents to a survey examining trust in government and public attitudes toward mandatory quarantine in the case of a smallpox outbreak in the United States, statistically significant predictors of opposition to mandatory quarantine policy were believing government would abuse power and personal liberties would be violated (Taylor-Clark et al., 2005). Conversely, having children and fears about personally contracting smallpox were significant predictors of support for mandatory quarantine. Overall, more people were opposed to mandatory vaccination than to mandatory quarantine.

5. Feasibility and PHEPR System Considerations

Synthesis of Modeling Studies

Findings from the synthesis of 12 modeling studies indicate the importance of pre-outbreak surveillance. Initiating quarantine in a timely manner requires accurate and granular pre- and intra-outbreak surveillance, as well as linkages to rapid decision making and implementation efforts. Modeling studies that explored the use of quarantine in various localities or focused effects of differential quarantine on locally exposed individuals and travelers entering an area found that the relative value of these efforts depends on the fraction of an epidemic or outbreak that is driven by local transmission versus imported cases. A further finding of modeling studies is that if quarantine is implemented in an uncoordinated manner in multiple areas, the result can be redundancy and the expenditure of excess effort and resources.

Qualitative Evidence Synthesis

The corpus of qualitative studies makes clear that all of the staffing and operational capacities necessary to implement quarantine, such as the ability to initiate a legal order and ensure its enforcement, conduct contact tracing, and monitor adherence to quarantine, currently exist in many agencies and need not be newly created. Some study authors point out that if quarantine will need to be scaled up from a small number of people, to a very large population, shortages of staffing and supplies may occur, but these shortages can be planned for in advance (Sell et al., 2018). However, for implementation of quarantine to be effective in a broader sense and avert restrictions on civil liberties and other harms requires that agencies clearly articulate their overall strategic vision and a corresponding plan for conducting quarantine operations. As noted in the above section on acceptability and preferences, moreover, the unique applicability of quarantine to emergencies in which a health hazard may be communicable through contact may necessitate a dedicated one-hazard focus for capacity building, whose regular implementation may be problematic.

Case Report Evidence Synthesis

Few case reports address the feasibility of quarantine; however, those that do so describe issues related to resources and scale (Grigg et al., 2015; Pang et al., 2003; Reaves et al., 2014). To achieve effective quarantine at a large scale, jurisdictions must have adequate capabilities and resources (Grigg et al., 2015; Reaves et al., 2014). Preexisting organizational frameworks also are necessary to support effective quarantine (Reaves et al., 2014). Pang and colleagues (2003) cite several factors to be considered in deciding who should be quarantined, such as resource availability, the ability to mobilize public health personnel, and social acceptability (Pang et al., 2003). Weighing these factors together is important in developing a feasible plan for quarantine or alternative measures that may be more effective in a given set of circumstances.

6. Resource and Economic Considerations

Qualitative Evidence Synthesis

As noted earlier, the provision of financial compensation, food, and professional social support to people on whom quarantine is imposed can facilitate adherence. The qualitative evidence base does not address the economic considerations associated with providing these resources; however, one can surmise that providing financial compensation for people in quarantine will require a large commitment of financial resources. Some authors (Cava et al., 2005b; DiGiovanni et al., 2004) suggest that the government or employers could assume this responsibility. Assistance with food will also require substantial economic resources, and some authors (Cava et al., 2005b; Desclaux et al., 2017; Pellecchia et al., 2015; Schemm Dwyer et al., 2017) suggest that funding for this purpose could be provided by the government or its agencies. Support may be required in particular for certain populations under quarantine, such as university students (Beaton et al., 2007) or homeless people (Leung et al., 2008). Economic resources will be required as well for the provision of professional support and the creation of organizational mechanisms for interagency deliberations and training. Resources related to the medical care of quarantined individuals include those needed for environmental decontamination, waste management, safe transportation, and availability of sufficient stocks of such supplies as masks and thermometers (Schemm Dwyer et al., 2017; Sell et al., 2018). Whether funding for all of these resources is to be provided by the government or the agencies themselves can be discussed among the agencies.

Case Report Evidence

Some case reports address the need to carefully consider the resources needed for quarantine against the expected benefits (CDC, 2003b; Chung et al., 2015; Collier et al., 2013; Gastañaduy et al., 2016; Nyenswah et al., 2015; Yasuoka, 2009; Zhang et al., 2012). For instance, during a 2011 measles outbreak in Indiana, the state health department incurred costs in the tens of thousands of dollars for public health measures. Although it is unclear how much of this expenditure was allocated to quarantine, findings suggest a greater need to weigh the burden of time and resources associated with quarantine against the desired outcomes (Collier et al., 2013). A further consideration is the provision of food and accommodations for health care workers quarantined in hospitals, as well as wage compensation for those placed on administrative leave (Chung et al., 2015). Still another is payment for quarantined people who are self-employed to compensate for some of their lost income, as well as compensation for small businesses employing 50 or fewer people that were ordered to close temporarily, costs that one case report indicates were funded by the government (Ooi et al., 2005). In another example, the city of Dallas made provisions for food and water for a pet in a household that had potentially been exposed to Ebola, and also requested state assistance to support quarantine-related costs (Spengler et al., 2015). In addition, the ability of agencies to quickly mobilize resource and surge capacity to cope with workloads imposed by quarantine (Binns et al., 2010; Tay et al., 2010; Tsang and Lam, 2003) requires substantial investment in public health personnel and infrastructure, including training and exercises for health care workers and leadership (Nathawad et al., 2013). Finally, as previously mentioned, the implementation of quarantine may be costly not only for public health agencies, hospitals, and local authorities but also for the public. Members of the public may incur both direct and indirect costs, including child care expenses, lost wages due to a lack of employer or government compensation, psychological harm, social stigma, and curtailment of civil liberties.

Descriptive Survey Study Evidence

Porten and colleagues (2006) assessed the amount of extra resources necessary for local public health agencies to implement quarantine and other control measures during the SARS outbreak in Germany. They found that local public health agencies with at least one SARS case under investigation had invested nearly double the working hours of those without a case under investigation. Many local public health agencies may have been hesitant to impose home quarantine on professionally active contacts for extended periods of time because they wished to avoid the need to provide financial compensation. Katz and colleagues (2019) sought to identify key features of preparedness, such as facilities, budget, and legal authority, that affected state and local public health officials' decision to implement social distancing (isolation or quarantine) measures. A majority of public health agencies reported that despite having legal authority to make social distancing decisions, they lacked facilities and a line item in their budget for isolation or quarantine measures.

7. Equity

Synthesis of Evidence of Effect

The committee's synthesis of evidence of effect showed that harms can result for those individuals placed in quarantine, including psychological harm (moderate COE) and individual financial hardship (high COE). As discussed earlier in the section on evidence of effect, quarantined households without access to paid leave from work are more likely to lose pay, and many experience further financial consequences. For low-income households in particular, being forced to take leave from work can exacerbate existing socioeconomic inequalities. Moreover, when people from already-marginalized communities are quarantined, the resulting stigmatization can result in an exacerbation of discrimination and marginalization that can last well beyond the quarantine period (Cava et al., 2005a; Desclaux et al., 2017; DiGiovanni et al., 2004; Lin et al., 2010; Pellecchia et al., 2015; Robertson et al., 2004; Schemm Dwyer et al., 2017). Unless the quarantine is kept confidential, those on whom it is imposed may be publicly labeled as potential carriers of a contagious disease, which may lead others to develop feelings of avoidance, suspicion, mistrust, and fear, and thus stigma, toward them. Thus, *people on whom quarantine is imposed may experience the harm of social stigma* (high confidence in the evidence). Furthermore, health care workers on whom quarantine is imposed may experience several harms—financial, social, and psychological, among others—similar to those experienced by the general public, but sometimes amplified (Desclaux et al., 2017; Maunder et al., 2003; Robertson et al., 2004). Three qualitative studies found that *health care workers on whom quarantine is imposed may experience additional harms beyond those experienced by the general public* (high confidence in the evidence).

Qualitative Evidence Synthesis

Five qualitative studies examined considerations with respect to at-risk populations when implementing quarantine (Baum et al., 2009; Charania and Tsuji, 2013; Desclaux et al., 2017; Leung et al., 2008; Pellecchia et al., 2015). These populations have unique needs that require modified quarantine policies to meet their life needs. In addition, as noted above, the harms of quarantine, such as financial, social, and psychological harms, may be especially pronounced for these groups. Thus, quarantine needs to be applied to at-risk groups with caution and a strong orientation of care. *When imposing quarantine on at-risk populations relative to the general population, agencies should accept a greater need for modifications to standard policies and assume that greater harms will result from the quarantine* (high confidence in the evidence).

Synthesis of Case Report Evidence Synthesis

Case reports note the importance of considering the impact of quarantine on various sub-populations based on demographics, socioeconomic considerations, and access to resources. They observe that potential challenges to quarantine arise when it involves transient populations, such as homeless people, as they may be difficult to locate and monitor (Smith et al., 2015). Residents of homeless shelters who have challenges with continuity of care due to a lack of documentation in health records may pose additional challenges, as was the case with a measles outbreak in Minnesota when the disease was confirmed in a 9-month-old, U.S.-born infant who resided in a homeless shelter and had recently returned from abroad (Gahr et al., 2014). Extra effort is also necessary to support those quarantined in homeless shelters, who may face unique challenges and have access to fewer resources compared with people who self-quarantine in their own homes (CDC, 2003b; Gahr et al., 2014). Insufficient support may lead to ineffective quarantine and increase the risk of transmission in this population. Additionally, members of communities that are hesitant to engage with the public health system may require strategic, culturally tailored outreach to ease their fear and anxiety (Gastañaduy et al., 2016; Smith et al., 2015). As discussed earlier, unintended consequences of quarantine orders may include stigmatization of certain groups if adequate attention is not paid to cultural and social considerations (CDC, 2004; Smith et al., 2015). The Ebola case report from Dallas, for example, describes concerted efforts to minimize stigma by working with organizations and leaders from the local Liberian community (Smith et al., 2015). In addition, schoolchildren were provided with laptops, textbooks, and lesson plans to encourage adherence to quarantine measures. Financial assistance may help ease an otherwise inequitable burden among lower-income communities (Chung et al., 2015; DiGiovanni et al., 2005; Smith et al., 2015).

Descriptive Survey Study Evidence

Seale and colleagues (2009) conducted a survey to determine the community's attitude toward pandemic influenza in Australia, and found that respondents who were self-employed or in casual employment were statistically significantly more likely to view being unable to work during home quarantine as problematic. Blake and colleagues (2010) found that some employment characteristics (inability to work from home, lack of paid sick leave) were statistically significantly associated with working adults' perceived likelihood of financial problems and thus their ability to comply with quarantine recommendations. Respondents who would not be paid if unable to work were almost five times more likely than those who would be paid to say that they would likely lose their job or business as a result of having to stay home from work for 7 to 10 days. Wray and colleagues (2012) assessed individual and community factors likely to facilitate or hinder adherence to public health directives. They found that community demographics (e.g., measures of ethnic homogeneity and poverty) were likely to have the greatest influence on public health directives that last long and require high levels of sacrifice.

8. Ethical Considerations[8]

Because being placed in quarantine represents an infringement of an individual's or group's core liberty rights, it must be justified by an appeal to some equally or more important rights of others that it protects. Specifically, quarantine is almost always justified by the notion that it will protect unexposed people from the harm of being exposed to and contracting a contagious disease, or what is referred to as the harm principle. Given this ethical justification, one could say that any quarantine action that does not in fact reduce or stop the spread of a contagious disease is, by definition, unethical. Of course, the problem with saying this is that one might not know whether quarantine will be effective until it has been tried. In reality, then, the core ethical obligation of those considering whether to implement quarantine is to do the very best they can to determine in advance whether the quarantine will work, and to implement it in ways that will maximize its effectiveness while minimizing the extent to which it infringes on individual or group liberty rights. This latter idea—that if one is required to take actions that will restrict people's liberties, one should do so in the least restrictive way possible that achieves the desired effect—is called the proportionality principle. This principle is widely discussed in public health ethics, as well as written into laws that allow public health authorities to implement quarantine and other measures that restrict people's liberties.

Another ethical consideration is the need to recognize that people in quarantine are giving up their personal freedoms (whether voluntarily or not) in an effort to protect their community, and therefore are deserving of gratitude and respect. This is one justification for ensuring that people in quarantine are well cared for and that they do not suffer stigma later on. The other reason to be as kind as possible to those in quarantine is utilitarian: people who are deathly afraid of being placed in quarantine may flee the area, potentially spreading the contagion farther than it might have spread without a threatened quarantine. This is not an entirely hypothetical concern; there are several real-world examples of quarantines that failed or even backfired when people threatened with quarantine fled the area. With regard to legal justifications, essentially all governments have laws and regulations that allow for the implementation of quarantine in some circumstances. In the United States, these laws are primarily at the state rather than the federal level, which means it is important for public health professionals to be familiar with the specific legal requirements in their locality.

---

[8] Ethical considerations included in this section were generated through committee discussions, drawing on the ethical principles laid out in Box 3-4 in Chapter 3 and key ethics and policy texts, including the 2009 Institute of Medicine letter report on crisis standards of care (IOM, 2009), the 2008 CDC white paper "Ethical Guidance for Public Health Emergency Preparedness and Response: Highlighting Ethics and Values in a Vital Public Health Service" (Jennings and Arras, 2008), *Emergency Ethics: Public Health Preparedness and Response* (Jennings et al., 2016), and *The Oxford Handbook of Public Health Ethics* (Mastroianni et al., 2019).

TABLE B4-10 Evidence to Decision Summary Table for Implementing Quarantine

In what circumstances (e.g., based on biologic factors, risks, resource availability, legal authorities, social context) is quarantine effective?	
Balance of Benefits and Harms Quarantine can be effective at reducing the transmission of contagious disease and has the possible additional benefit of reducing the time to diagnosis for infected patients who are being monitored while under quarantine. However, it also can result in a number of harms. In particular, quarantine has the potential to result in abridging individual or community rights of freedom, movement, and association. In addition, there may be an increased risk of infection among those placed together in congregate quarantine settings. Quarantine can also create financial instability, social stigma, and compromised psychological well-being for quarantined individuals. Given these undesirable effects of quarantine, which can be both short and long term, the balance of benefits and harms is open to debate and should be assessed on a case-by-case basis.	**Sources of Evidence** • Synthesis of evidence of effect • Qualitative evidence synthesis • Case report evidence synthesis (no assessment of certainty or confidence)
Acceptability and Preferences Overall, the public understands and accepts the general concept of quarantine, but this understanding and acceptance is not uniform across all societies, and the acceptability of quarantine can vary depending on levels of social trust in the authorities implementing it. Moreover, fear of harms may make quarantine unacceptable in some communities. The acceptability of and preference for quarantine may differ as well across the multiple individuals and agencies that often must work together to implement quarantine, with some advocating an emphasis on voluntary adherence and others seeking mandatory enforcement, which may include a militaristic response. In general, the evidence suggests that voluntary quarantine is more acceptable, and therefore can be more effective, than mandatory quarantine.	**Sources of Evidence** • Qualitative evidence synthesis • Case report evidence (no assessment of certainty or confidence) • Descriptive survey study evidence (no synthesis)
Feasibility and Public Health Emergency Preparedness and Response System Considerations Quarantine is more effective at reducing or stopping the transmission of a contagious disease when exposed individuals can be identified reliably and quickly. To initiate quarantine in a timely manner requires accurate, up-to-date, and specific pre- and intra-outbreak surveillance, as well as preexisting organizational frameworks and linkages to rapid decision making, including an in-place legal framework. Feasibility is also related to the scale of quarantine; if quarantine is uncoordinated and implemented at an intense level in multiple geographic areas, there is greater potential for redundancy and excess effort and resource expenditures, as well as for flight of individuals beyond designated boundaries. In addition, quarantine may become infeasible or less effective because of reduced adherence when the proposed duration of quarantine is longer. Although staffing and operational capacities to implement quarantine currently exist in many agencies, operational limitations may arise when quarantine is implemented on a large scale. Home quarantine may be more feasible than providing designated facilities for quarantined individuals, but is not without concerns over such harms as increased risk of infection among those housed together and challenges with adherence.	**Sources of Evidence** • Synthesis of modeling studies • Qualitative evidence synthesis • Case report evidence synthesis (no assessment of certainty or confidence)
Resource and Economic Considerations Implementing quarantine is highly resource intensive (e.g., the potential need to provide financial compensation, food, and social support). Therefore, factors that need to be considered when deciding whether to implement quarantine include resource availability, such as the ability to mobilize public health personnel to conduct contact tracing (to identify those who might warrant being placed in quarantine) and regular symptom monitoring of those in quarantine (to detect those who are becoming ill and require isolation and medical care). Resources related to the medical care of quarantined individuals include those needed for environmental decontamination, waste management, safe transportation, and availability of sufficient stocks of such supplies as masks and thermometers. Quarantine may be costly not only for response agencies but also for the individuals placed in quarantine, and has the potential to result in broad social and economic disruption. Quarantined individuals may incur both direct and indirect costs, including child care expenses and lost wages due to a lack of employer or government compensation. Thus, public health agencies need to consider the resources required for quarantine against its expected benefits.	**Sources of Evidence** • Qualitative evidence synthesis • Case report evidence synthesis (no assessment of certainty or confidence) • Descriptive survey study evidence (no synthesis)

continued

TABLE B4-10 Continued

Equity	Sources of Evidence
When considering whether or how to impose quarantine on members of at-risk populations, public health leaders and agencies need to acknowledge that greater harms are likely to result for marginalized populations, creating a stronger obligation to protect them. At-risk populations can have additional needs affecting their ability to adhere to quarantine, and agencies need to consider the impact on various subpopulations based on demographics, socioeconomic considerations, and baseline access to resources. For example, potential challenges to quarantine arise when it involves transient populations such as people that are homeless, as they may be difficult to locate and monitor. Additionally, being forced to miss work can potentially exacerbate preexisting socioeconomic inequalities. The inequitable impacts of quarantine tend to be compounded over time such that the longer a quarantine lasts, the more sacrifice it requires of those being quarantined, and the more likely it is to exacerbate underlying societal, economic, and health care inequities. Finally, health care workers on whom quarantine is imposed may experience financial, social, and psychological harms, similar to those that occur to the general public; however, these harms may be amplified for health care workers for a number of reasons because of their responsibilities.	• Synthesis of evidence of effect • Qualitative evidence synthesis • Case report evidence synthesis (no assessment of certainty or confidence) • Descriptive survey study evidence (no synthesis)
Ethical Considerations	**Source of Evidence**
When implemented correctly and in the proper setting, quarantine is ethically justified by the expectation that it will protect unexposed people from the harm of being exposed to and contracting a contagious disease—a notion that has been called the harm principle. Given this ethical justification (i.e., that quarantine prevents harm), one could say that any quarantine action that does not in fact reduce or stop the spread of a contagious disease is unethical. Of course, the problem with saying this is that one may not know whether a quarantine will be effective until it is tried. In reality, then, the core ethical obligation involved in considering whether to implement quarantine is to do the very best to determine in advance whether the quarantine will work, and to implement it in ways that will maximize its effectiveness while minimizing the extent to which it infringes on individual or group liberties and rights (principle of proportionality). Another ethical consideration for quarantine is the need to recognize that people in quarantine are giving up their personal freedoms (whether voluntarily or not) in an effort to protect their community, and thus deserve gratitude and respect (principle of respect for persons and communities). Indeed, this consideration represents one justification for efforts to ensure that people in quarantine are well cared for and that they do not suffer stigma later on. The other justification for such efforts is utilitarian (principle of harm reduction and benefit promotion): people who fear being placed in quarantine may flee the area, potentially spreading the contagion even farther than it might have spread without a threatened quarantine. This is not an entirely hypothetical concern; there are several real-world examples of quarantines that failed or even backfired when people threatened with quarantine fled the area. With regard to legal justifications, essentially all governments have laws and regulations that allow for the implementation of quarantine in some circumstances. In the United States, these laws are primarily at the state rather than the federal level, which means it is important for public health professionals to be familiar with the specific legal requirements in their locality.	• Committee discussion drawing on key ethics and policy texts

CONSIDERATIONS FOR IMPLEMENTATION

The following considerations for implementation were drawn from the syntheses of quantitative comparative studies, modeling studies, qualitative research studies, and case reports, as well as descriptive surveys.

9. Facilitating Adherence to and Minimizing Harms from Quarantine Measures

Ensure Transparent and Strategic Risk Communication Using Clear Definitions

Synthesis of evidence of effect The committee's synthesis of evidence of effect showed that while adherence to quarantine measures can vary by culture, disease, and socioeconomic status, use of various strategies, including risk communication and messaging and access to leave, can improve adherence (moderate COE).

Case report evidence synthesis Lessons learned from case reports also stress the importance of open, frequent, and transparent communication with the public to ease fear and anxiety (Ehlkes et al., 2017; Tay et al., 2010; Tsang and Lam, 2003; Ward et al., 2010). Useful channels for public communication include daily press briefings, television and radio announcements, Internet bulletins, health talks, and a hotline for public enquiry. During the SARS outbreak in Beijing, the city's Ministry of Health and municipal government also ran education campaigns via billboards, bus advertisements, and traditional banners (Pang et al., 2003). In the U.S. context, during the 2011 measles outbreak in Indiana, the state issued local media releases and used the Indiana Health Alert Network to inform community members and providers about potential exposure to the disease (Collier et al., 2013).

Strategic timing of communication can be an important facilitator of effective quarantine. During the H1N1 pandemic of 2009 in Singapore, a gradual strategic shift from containment to mitigation as part of the risk communication strategy enabled the public to adapt to new measures (Tay et al., 2010). Home visits to provide health education for those quarantined at home may also promote adherence (Ooi et al., 2005). In addition, the public and health care workers need to have a clear understanding of the term "quarantine," which is often misunderstood despite having backing by legal authority (Barbisch et al., 2015), and differences in interpretation may lead to inconsistent application of quarantine laws across jurisdictional boundaries.

Descriptive survey study evidence Eastwood and colleagues (2009, 2010) found that having a basic knowledge of pandemic influenza was statistically associated with willingness to adhere to quarantine measures. Their findings suggest further that discordance between what people state they will do and what they actually do relates to how they perceive risk. Bauerle Bass and colleagues (2010) investigated factors and specific sociodemographic characteristics that may influence an individual's decision to adhere to quarantine measures. Their findings indicate that overall knowledge regarding avian influenza, beliefs about its severity, and the perceived likelihood that the respondent and/or his or her significant other(s) might contract it were predictive of willingness to adhere.

Adapt Policy: Voluntary Versus Legally Enforced Quarantine

Synthesis of modeling studies Some modeling studies found that adherence may be greater with less strict quarantine procedures, making those procedures more effective despite them being less strict.

Qualitative evidence synthesis Seven qualitative studies found a flexible quarantine implementation policy to be important (Bell and WHO, 2004; Cava et al., 2005b; Charania and

Tsuji, 2013; Desclaux et al., 2017; DiGiovanni et al., 2004; Leung et al., 2008; Sell et al., 2018). Findings from these studies suggest that *people on whom quarantine is imposed may find the restrictions acceptable if agencies adapt quarantine policies to suit populations and situations* (moderate confidence in the evidence). Quarantine restrictions may be more acceptable if reasonable modifications of rules and procedures are made to suit the needs of the situation and the people being placed under quarantine. These modifications might include changes to policies related to using tobacco and alcohol in group facilities, leaving quarantine sites to obtain supplies or go to work, and using public transportation to get to work. In this regard, quarantine can be seen as a nuanced measure that is dependent on the situation.

Case report evidence synthesis Several case reports address the use of both voluntary and compulsory quarantine; however, they do not examine whether one of these strategies leads to greater adherence than the other (CDC, 2004; Chen et al., 2005; Chung et al., 2015; Collier et al., 2013; Ehlkes et al., 2017; Ooi et al., 2005; Plipat et al., 2017; Reaves et al., 2014; Tay et al., 2010). Voluntary self-quarantine of health care workers in Dallas during the 2014 cluster of Ebola had high adherence; more than 30 health care workers adhered to the quarantine in the absence of a public health order, as did all but a small subset of additional contacts (Chung et al., 2015). Similarly, during the SARS outbreak in Toronto, only 0.1 percent of contacts requiring quarantine had to be issued an enforceable quarantine order because of initial noncompliance. At the same time, while voluntary quarantine may motivate people to adhere because of a sense of choice, fear of prosecution and hefty fines may encourage even greater adherence. Some case reports cite use of police, sheriffs, and security agencies to enforce quarantine policies, some guarding doors and buildings and others conducting random checks on quarantined individuals (Barbisch et al., 2015; CDC, 2003b; Collier et al., 2013; Ooi et al., 2005; Pang et al., 2003). Yet, while some legally enforceable strategies may be relevant in the U.S. context, more invasive or aggressive measures may face resistance. Therefore, cultural context needs to be carefully considered when strategies are developed. This was the case during a tabletop exercise in San Diego focused on quarantine, when civilian law enforcement officials frequently expressed concerns about carrying out enforcement measures requested by civilian public health authorities (DiGiovanni et al., 2005), instead urging an emphasis on public education to minimize the need for enforcement.

Provide Financial Compensation, Food, and Social and Psychological Support

Synthesis of evidence of effect The committee's synthesis of the evidence of effect showed that an emphasis on health by those leading the outbreak response (i.e., health-promoting leadership, discussed earlier) can reduce depression and anxiety symptoms among quarantined individuals (very low COE). The evidence of effect also indicates that while adherence to quarantine measures can vary by culture, disease, and socioeconomic status, it can be improved through the use of various strategies, including risk communication and messaging and access to employment leave (moderate COE).

Qualitative evidence synthesis Four qualitative studies found providing financial compensation for people subject to quarantine to be important (Baum et al., 2009; Braunack-Mayer et al., 2010; Cava et al., 2005a; Desclaux et al., 2017). This compensation included partial or full income replacement for the duration of the quarantine; assurance of job security and economic recovery following the end of quarantine; and payment for rent, water, electricity, and other utilities. Findings from these studies suggest that *people on whom quarantine is imposed may find the restrictions acceptable depending on the provision of financial compensation by government or other agencies* (high confidence in the evidence).

Six qualitative studies found that providing food for quarantined people is important (Braunack-Mayer et al., 2010; Cava et al., 2005a; Desclaux et al., 2017; DiGiovanni et al., 2004; Leung et al., 2008; Pellecchia et al., 2015). Findings from these studies suggest that government and other agencies can deliver food directly or assist neighbors, friends, and volunteers with its purchase and delivery. Agencies need to keep in mind that any food support provided should match the dietary needs and wishes of the people under quarantine. *People on whom quarantine is imposed may find the restrictions acceptable depending on the provision of food and other basic necessities by government and other agencies* (high confidence in the evidence).

Six qualitative studies found that providing professional social support to quarantined people is important (Braunack-Mayer et al., 2010; Cava et al., 2005a; Desclaux et al., 2017; Lin et al., 2010; Maunder et al., 2003; Schemm Dwyer et al., 2017). Authors of these studies cite the provision of such support in the form of a dedicated new or preexisting general confidential telephone hotline that offers professional counseling and the provision of cell phones to those who do not possess one so they can stay connected to support networks. *People on whom quarantine is imposed may find the quarantine restrictions acceptable depending on the provision of professional social support by government and other agencies* (high confidence in the evidence).

Case report evidence synthesis Several case reports describe provision of food, accommodations, social and psychological support, medical leave, and wage compensation to quarantined people (CDC, 2003b; Chen et al., 2005; Chung et al., 2015; Ehlkes et al., 2017; Pang et al., 2003; Reaves et al., 2014; Yoon et al., 2016; Zhang et al., 2012). During the 2014 Ebola cluster in Dallas, for instance, the hospital where health care workers were quarantined provided food, accommodations, and wage compensation (Chung et al., 2015). Based on Dallas's experience, Smith and colleagues (2015) suggest that public health emergency preparedness for an Ebola outbreak could be enhanced by engaging a wide range of community partners, such as businesses, schools, charitable foundations, community and faith-based organizations, and mental health providers and organizations in readying support resources to meet potential needs of quarantined individuals (Smith et al., 2015). They also cite the importance of providing laptops, textbooks, and school supplies and developing lesson plans that can be completed at home. Although the effectiveness of these measures is not specifically assessed, case reports from Beijing, Liberia, South Korea, and Taiwan also mention the role of social and psychological supports—for example, having community committees mobilize to make such gestures as giving flowers and comforting letters, conducting prayer services, providing social services through local health or civic affairs departments, offering day care, and providing mental health services (CDC, 2003b; Nyenswah et al., 2015; Pang et al., 2003; Yoon et al., 2016). During the 2009 H1N1 outbreak in China, people quarantined in hotels were provided room service, and the government budget supported living expenses (Zhang et al., 2012).

Descriptive survey study evidence Wray and colleagues (2012) assessed individual and community factors that are likely to facilitate or hinder adherence to public health quarantine directives. They found less likelihood of adherence to a 6-day quarantine among individuals anticipating a need for supplies and those finding it difficult to stay home.

Use Culturally and Contextually Relevant Approaches: A Community and Care Orientation

Qualitative evidence synthesis The authors of eight qualitative studies emphasize the importance of considering the community perspective rather than the individual perspective when developing a quarantine strategy (Baum et al., 2009; Braunack-Mayer et al., 2010; Cava et al., 2005b; Charania and Tsuji, 2013; Desclaux et al., 2017; Leung et al., 2008; Pellecchia et al., 2015; Smith et al., 2012). Findings from these studies suggest that *agencies need to understand that the members of a community on whom quarantine is imposed often regard its impact at the community rather than the individual or abstract "common good" level to be more important. Therefore, agencies need to consider the life circumstances of and work cooperatively with the community to increase adherence to quarantine* (high confidence in the evidence). Quarantine is generally conceptualized as restriction of the rights of individuals for the benefit of the abstract "common good," which may be thought of as the larger society. Between these two levels of the individual and the larger society, however, exists the level of the community, which may be understood as a group of individuals with strong social bonds (Smith et al., 2012). When quarantine is imposed on some members of a community, those tight social bonds mean that the life of the whole community is affected as well. Thus, to ensure that individuals on whom quarantine is imposed adhere to its restrictions, agencies need to understand the community's life circumstances, such as economic status, political history, trust of agencies and government, and cultural and religious customs, and work in cooperation with its existing power and leadership social structures.

Two qualitative studies highlight the importance of considering the care rather than the enforcement perspective with respect to those placed in quarantine (Desclaux et al., 2017; Maunder et al., 2003). Findings from these studies suggest that agencies can have an orientation of care, as opposed to an orientation of enforcement, toward the people on whom quarantine is imposed to increase adherence (low confidence in the evidence). Such an orientation means interacting with quarantined people in a way that resembles care, showing concern for their needs, and extending empathetic support rather than emphasizing control and enforcement.

Case report evidence synthesis Given the cultural diversity of the United States, culturally informed strategies may enable more effective quarantine. For instance, during measles outbreaks in a Somali community in Minnesota and an Amish community in Ohio, efforts were made to engage community, religious, and spiritual leaders as advisors because of their strong influence on social networks (Gahr et al., 2014; Gastañaduy et al., 2016). Lessons learned from the Ebola outbreak in Dallas include that "recognizing unique cultural, linguistic, and socioeconomic differences helped ensure contacts' compliance with monitoring, particularly among the community contacts" (Smith et al., 2015). Contact tracers found that because the first Ebola patient was Liberian, many of his contacts were part of the local Liberian community. Therefore, they engaged aid organizations to provide familiar food and clothing in a culturally sensitive manner.

Trust is mentioned as an important factor in facilitating effective quarantine in case reports from Germany, Liberia, and Singapore (Ehlkes et al., 2017; Nyenswah et al., 2015; Tay et al., 2010). During the 2014 Ebola outbreak in Liberia, community trust and confidence in response efforts were found to be challenging at times, as some community members might not have been willing to accept proposed quarantine without first witnessing the devastating effect of the disease on their village (Nyenswah et al., 2015). Trusted local leaders helped facilitate trust and acted as liaisons between community leaders and district health authorities, suggesting that integrating trusted local leaders into response planning and giving them an opportunity to provide feedback before decisions related to public health interventions are made may promote effective quarantine. A case report of the 2009 H1N1 outbreak in Singapore also mentions the importance of building trust in advance of a public health crisis (Tay et al., 2010). Public perception of the quality and credibility of decisions related to control measures and policies reportedly enabled buy-in from health care stakeholders during the response to that outbreak, particularly for policies that were burdensome to implement. The authors recommend regular engagement among stakeholders during "peacetime" as a way of fostering stronger coordination of public health control measures during a crisis. In their case report of the 2016 outbreak of Lassa fever in Germany, Ehlkes and colleagues (2017) describe how contact-tracing interviews can be used as an opportunity to build trust between investigators and interviewees to enhance adherence to quarantine (Ehlkes et al., 2017). Although these findings are based on case reports from abroad, they may be applicable in the United States as well, given that the level of trust between the public and key stakeholders is likely to influence the effectiveness of quarantine, particularly in communities that may have a historical distrust of the U.S. government.

Descriptive survey study evidence Bauerle Bass and colleagues (2010) investigated factors and specific sociodemographic characteristics that may influence an individual's decision to adhere to quarantine measures. The findings of this survey align with the qualitative and case report evidence regarding the importance of understanding the life circumstances of and working in cooperation with the community to increase adherence. Differences were observed among demographic groups in the willingness to comply with quarantine orders, with women and individuals who were not employed being more willing to remain at or to go to a government-designated facility if ordered to do so.

10. Other Implementation Considerations

The following conceptual findings inform the perspectives and approaches public health agencies could consider when implementing quarantine.

Define the Effectiveness of Quarantine More Broadly

Qualitative evidence synthesis Fourteen qualitative studies highlight the potential need for a broader definition of effectiveness for quarantine (Baum et al., 2009; Beaton et al., 2007; Bell and WHO, 2004; Braunack-Mayer et al., 2010; Cava et al., 2005b; Desclaux et al., 2017; DiGiovanni et al., 2004; Lin et al., 2010; Maunder et al., 2003; Pellecchia et al., 2015; Robertson et al., 2004; Schemm Dwyer et al., 2017; Sell et al., 2018; Smith et al., 2012). The results of these studies suggest that *agencies may want to judge the effectiveness of quarantine not only using the metric of medical outcomes but also in terms of the degree of protection of the civil rights of the public on whom quarantine is imposed. Along the same lines, agencies may also want to judge the effectiveness of quarantine in terms of the extent to which the public on whom quarantine is being imposed is protected from harms that result from the quarantine restrictions* (moderate confidence in the evidence). Agencies typically judge the effectiveness of quarantine only from a single utilitarian criterion of reduction of morbidity and mortality in the general population. However, because quarantine almost always is imposed on a group of people without their consent, it may also be important to include two additional criteria—protection of civil rights and protection from harms—when judging the effectiveness of quarantine.

Case report evidence synthesis Barbisch and colleagues (2015) are the only authors who explicitly mention difficulty with determining the effectiveness and equitable application of quarantine policies, particularly given the issues of personal liberties. The authors assert that the restrictive nature of quarantine means it should be evaluated for efficacy. For instance,

> Is the action supported by evidence of improved outcomes?; can it be effectively implemented given the need for balanced [Stuff, Staff, and Structure] surge?; will it lead to unintended negative outcomes?; are other less restrictive public health measures such as monitoring and social distancing equally effective?; and finally, given the impact on civil liberties, is it reasonable, and is it enforceable? (Barbisch et al., 2015)

Develop Options for Different Levels of Quarantine and Plan for Integration with Other Non-Pharmaceutical Interventions

Synthesis of modeling studies The modeling studies reviewed provide a number of other important points regarding the invasiveness of quarantine. Findings from modeling studies that compared quarantine with other, less invasive or intensive interventions, such as symptom monitoring or voluntary reporting, suggest that these alternatives may make it possible to achieve similar levels of effectiveness and control for less transmissible infections that lack asymptomatic infectious periods without incurring the potential harms of social stigma, social and economic disruption, and large-scale use of resources. Results of modeling studies that explored quarantine efforts carried out in various localities or focused differential quarantine efforts on locally exposed individuals and travelers entering an area suggest that the relative value of these control efforts depended on the fraction of an epidemic or outbreak driven by local transmission versus imported cases.

Local quarantine efforts may have both direct and indirect spillover effects, reducing transmission in areas not implementing quarantine. If quarantine is used to help control an outbreak in one area, nearby areas may face fewer imported cases; hence, the need to implement quarantine in these surrounding areas may be reduced (an example of direct spillover). Moreover, chains of such spillovers to areas not directly connected to the original area can occur, which may alter the need for or required level and speed of quarantine in these areas as well (indirect spillovers). As a result, if quarantines are implemented in an uncoordinated manner in multiple areas, redundancy and excess expenditure of effort and resources may result.

Qualitative evidence synthesis Four qualitative studies addressed different levels of quarantine (Bell and WHO, 2004; Charania and Tsuji, 2013; Desclaux et al., 2017; Smith et al., 2012). Findings from these studies suggest that *agencies can enhance the effectiveness of quarantine by developing screening and monitoring criteria that allow for graded quarantine options matched to the characteristics of the infectious disease and its spread* (moderate confidence in the evidence). Different levels of quarantine appropriately depend on the severity and magnitude of the contagious disease situation. Similarly, criteria for placing people in quarantine can differ based on risk of exposure; contacts, such as people exposed to ill family members in close quarters, are at highest risk (aside from health care workers with certain unprotected patient care exposures).

Consider Implementing Quarantine Early, Especially When There Is a Lack of Available Medical Countermeasures

Synthesis of modeling studies Results of modeling studies that explored the timing of initiating quarantine tend to emphasize that it is more effective if implemented closer to when the first case occurs or is equivalently effective but involves quarantining substantially fewer exposed individuals.

Qualitative evidence synthesis Three qualitative studies examined the implementation of quarantine in situations in which medical response infrastructure is lacking (Bell and WHO, 2004; Braunack-Mayer et al., 2010; Charania and Tsuji, 2013). Findings from these studies suggest that *agencies need to recognize that for regions lacking robust medical response infrastructures, non-pharmaceutical interventions such as quarantine may be especially effective* (moderate confidence in the evidence). The international experience shows that at the start of a contagious disease outbreak, countries may lack targeted countermeasures, such as drugs and vaccines. Similarly, there may be regions in a country where the stockpile of drugs and vaccines is limited or where the delivery of such supplies may take time because of remoteness or other logistical obstacles. In these circumstances, non-pharmaceutical interventions have often been the only measures available to combat epidemics, especially at the beginning of an outbreak (Bell and WHO, 2004; Braunack-Mayer, 2010; Charania and Tsuji, 2013).

Case report evidence synthesis A SARS case report from Singapore describes how the decision to undertake quarantine measures was not necessarily based on scientific evidence of the merits of quarantine but on the need to protect the public from a serious new disease with a high case fatality rate (14 percent) (Ooi et al., 2005). The absence of effective vaccination and antiviral treatment strengthened the argument for quarantine management to stop the spread of the disease, given its potentially catastrophic consequences.

Integrate and Coordinate Response at the Systems Level

Qualitative evidence synthesis Four qualitative studies examined the importance of understanding that quarantine requires interagency coordination (Desclaux et al., 2017; DiGiovanni et al., 2004; Schemm Dwyer et al., 2017; Sell et al., 2018). Findings from these studies suggest that *agencies can facilitate adherence to quarantine by understanding that to implement quarantine, multiple agencies and multiple jurisdictions are required to work in concert* (moderate confidence in the evidence). Planning and implementation of quarantine require interagency coordination that includes the legal system. This interagency coordination needs to include plans for the scalability of operations in terms of the number of people placed in quarantine during the course of a contagious disease outbreak.

Case report evidence synthesis Findings from case reports indicate that effective control measures do not work in isolation and require coordination among key stakeholders (Tsang and Lam, 2003). The majority of case reports describe quarantine as one of multiple measures implemented during a response. Integrated responses at the systems level have been found to be essential for a coherent response in fostering a better-coordinated system (Tay et al., 2010). Reliance on preexisting organizational frameworks can also enable efficient redirection of resources (Reaves et al., 2014). In addition, collaborative agreements and coordinated incident command are highlighted as essential for areas with multiple jurisdictions (e.g., civilian, military, federal, tribal) (DiGiovanni et al., 2005). Case reports mention as well the general need for public health surge capacity in light of the threats of emerging diseases and large-scale outbreaks (Binns et al., 2010; Svoboda et al., 2004; Tsang and Lam, 2003). A strong sense of political will and urgency is viewed as facilitating the rapid establishment of command structures aimed at steering action and mobilizing relevant sectors and resources (Tsang and Lam, 2003). Furthermore, the need for flexibility is stressed, as existing plans and predetermined control measures may need to be modified as a public health emergency evolves (Chung et al., 2015; Tay et al., 2010).

REFERENCES FOR ARTICLES INCLUDED IN THE MIXED-METHOD REVIEW

Quantitative Comparative Studies

Adler, A. B., P. Y. Kim, S. J. Thomas, and M. L. Sipos. 2018. Quarantine and the U.S. military response to the Ebola crisis: Soldier health and attitudes. *Public Health* 155:95–98.

Bondy, S. J., M. L. Russell, J. M. Lafleche, and E. Rea. 2009. Quantifying the impact of community quarantine on sars transmission in Ontario: Estimation of secondary case count difference and number needed to quarantine. *BMC Public Health* 9:488.

Chu, C. Y., C. Y. Li, H. Zhang, Y. Wang, D. H. Huo, L. Wen, Z. T. Yin, F. Li, and H. B. Song. 2010. Quarantine methods and prevention of secondary outbreak of pandemic (H1N1) 2009. *Emerging Infectious Diseases* 16(8):1300–1302.

Delaporte, E., C. A. Wyler Lazarevic, A. Iten, and P. Sudre. 2013. Large measles outbreak in Geneva, Switzerland, January to August 2011: Descriptive epidemiology and demonstration of quarantine effectiveness. *European Communicable Disease Bulletin* 18(6):7.

Hawryluck, L., W. L. Gold, S. Robinson, S. Pogorski, S. Galea, and R. Styra. 2004. SARS control and psychological effects of quarantine, Toronto, Canada. *Emerging Infectious Diseases* 10(7):1206–1212.

Hsieh, Y. H., C. C. King, C. W. Chen, M. S. Ho, J. Y. Lee, F. C. Liu, Y. C. Wu, and J. S. JulianWu. 2005. Quarantine for SARS, Taiwan. *Emerging Infectious Diseases* 11(2):278–282.

Jeong, H., H. W. Yim, Y. J. Song, M. Ki, J. A. Min, J. Cho, and J. H. Chae. 2016. Mental health status of people isolated due to Middle East Respiratory Syndrome. *Epidemiology and Health* 38:e2016048.

Kavanagh, A. M., R. J. Bentley, K. E. Mason, J. McVernon, S. Petrony, J. Fielding, A. D. LaMontagne, and D. M. Studdert. 2011. Sources, perceived usefulness and understanding of information disseminated to families who entered home quarantine during the H1N1 pandemic in Victoria, Australia: A cross-sectional study. *BMC Infectious Diseases* 11:2.

Kavanagh, A. M., K. E. Mason, R. J. Bentley, D. M. Studdert, J. McVernon, J. E. Fielding, S. Petrony, L. Gurrin, and A. D. LaMontagne. 2012. Leave entitlements, time off work and the household financial impacts of quarantine compliance during an H1N1 outbreak. *BMC Infectious Diseases* 12:311.

Lee, S. M., W. S. Kang, A. R. Cho, T. Kim, and J. K. Park. 2018. Psychological impact of the 2015 MERS outbreak on hospital workers and quarantined hemodialysis patients. *Comprehensive Psychiatry* 87:123–127.

Liu, X., M. Kakade, C. J. Fuller, B. Fan, Y. Fang, J. Kong, Z. Guan, and P. Wu. 2012. Depression after exposure to stressful events: Lessons learned from the severe acute respiratory syndrome epidemic. *Comprehensive Psychiatry* 53(1):15–23.

Marjanovic, Z., E. R. Greenglass, and S. Coffey. 2007. The relevance of psychosocial variables and working conditions in predicting nurses' coping strategies during the SARS crisis: An online questionnaire survey. *International Journal of Nursing Studies* 44(6):991–998.

McVernon, J., K. Mason, S. Petrony, P. Nathan, A. D. LaMontagne, R. Bentley, J. Fielding, D. M. Studdert, and A. Kavanagh. 2011. Recommendations for and compliance with social restrictions during implementation of school closures in the early phase of the influenza a (H1N1) 2009 outbreak in Melbourne, Australia. *BMC Infectious Diseases* 11:257.

Miyaki, K., H. Sakurazawa, H. Mikurube, M. Nishizaka, H. Ando, Y. Song, and T. Shimbo. 2011. An effective quarantine measure reduced the total incidence of influenza A H1N1 in the workplace: Another way to control the H1N1 flu pandemic. *Journal of Occupational Health* 53(4):287–292.

Reynolds, D. L., J. R. Garay, S. L. Deamond, M. K. Moran, W. Gold, and R. Styra. 2008. Understanding, compliance and psychological impact of the SARS quarantine experience. *Epidemiology and Infection* 136(7):997–1007.

Wu, P., X. Liu, Y. Fang, B. Fan, C. J. Fuller, Z. Guan, Z. Yao, J. Kong, J. Lu, and I. J. Litvak. 2008. Alcohol abuse/dependence symptoms among hospital employees exposed to a SARS outbreak. *Alcohol and Alcoholism* 43(6):706–712.

Wu, P., Y. Fang, Z. Guan, B. Fan, J. Kong, Z. Yao, X. Liu, C. J. Fuller, E. Susser, J. Lu, and C. W. Hoven. 2009. The psychological impact of the SARS epidemic on hospital employees in China: Exposure, risk perception, and altruistic acceptance of risk. *Canadian Journal of Psychiatry* 54(5):302–311.

Modeling Studies

Included in Detailed Analysis

Ahn, I., S. Heo, S. Ji, K. H. Kim, T. Kim, E. J. Lee, J. Park, and K. Sung. 2018. Investigation of nonlinear epidemiological models for analyzing and controlling the MERS outbreak in Korea. *Journal of Theoretical Biology* 437:17–28.

An der Heiden, M., U. Buchholz, G. Krause, G. Kirchner, H. Claus, and W. H. Haas. 2009. Breaking the waves: Modeling the potential impact of public health measures to defer the epidemic peak of novel influenza A/H1N1. *PLOS ONE [Electronic Resource]* 4(12):e8356.

Day, T., A. Park, N. Madras, A. Gumel, and J. Wu. 2006. When is quarantine a useful control strategy for emerging infectious diseases? *American Journal of Epidemiology* 163(5):479–485.

D'Silva, J. P., and M. C. Eisenberg. 2017. Modeling spatial invasion of Ebola in West Africa. *Journal of Theoretical Biology* 428:65–75.

Enanoria, W. T., F. Liu, J. Zipprich, K. Harriman, S. Ackley, S. Blumberg, L. Worden, and T. C. Porco. 2016. The effect of contact investigations and public health interventions in the control and prevention of measles transmission: A simulation study. *PLOS ONE [Electronic Resource]* 11(12):e0167160.

Feng, Z., Y. Yang, D. Xu, P. Zhang, M. M. McCauley, and J. W. Glasser. 2009. Timely identification of optimal control strategies for emerging infectious diseases. *Journal of Theoretical Biology* 259(1):165–171.

Gupta, A. G., C. A. Moyer, and D. T. Stern. 2005. The economic impact of quarantine: SARS in Toronto as a case study. *Journal of Infection* 50(5):386–393.

Hsieh, Y. H., C. C. King, C. W. Chen, M. S. Ho, S. B. Hsu, and Y. C. Wu. 2007. Impact of quarantine on the 2003 SARS outbreak: A retrospective modeling study. *Journal of Theoretical Biology* 244(4):729–736.

Meltzer, M. I., I. Damon, J. W. LeDuc, and J. D. Millar. 2001. Modeling potential responses to smallpox as a bioterrorist weapon. *Emerging Infectious Diseases* 7(6):959–969.

Mubayi, A., C. K. Zaleta, M. Martcheva, and C. Castillo-Chavez. 2010. A cost-based comparison of quarantine strategies for new emerging diseases. *Mathematical Biosciences & Engineering* 7(3):687–717.

Peak, C. M., L. M. Childs, Y. H. Grad, and C. O. Buckee. 2017. Comparing nonpharmaceutical interventions for containing emerging epidemics. *Proceedings of the National Academy of Sciences of the United States of America* 114(15):4023–4028.

Podder, C. N., A. B. Gumel, C. S. Bowman, and R. G. McLeod. 2007. Mathematical study of the impact of quarantine, isolation and vaccination in curtailing an epidemic. *Journal of Biological Systems* 15(2):185–202.

Not Included in Detailed Analysis

Adams, B. 2016. Household demographic determinants of Ebola epidemic risk. *Journal of Theoretical Biology* 392:99–106.

Ahmad, M. D., M. Usman, A. Khan, and M. Imran. 2016. Optimal control analysis of Ebola disease with control strategies of quarantine and vaccination. *Infectious Diseases of Poverty* 5(1):72.

Aldis, G. K., and M. G. Roberts. 2005. An integral equation model for the control of a smallpox outbreak. *Mathematical Biosciences* 195(1):1–22.

Bachinsky, A. G., and L. P. Nizolenko. 2013. A universal model for predicting dynamics of the epidemics caused by special pathogens. *BioMed Research International* 2013:467078.

Barrett, C. L., S. G. Eubank, and J. P. Smith. 2005. If smallpox strikes Portland. *Scientific American* 292(3):42–49.

Blackwood, J. C., and L. M. Childs. 2016. The role of interconnectivity in control of an Ebola epidemic. *Scientific Reports* 6:29262.

Carrat, F., J. Luong, H. Lao, A. V. Salle, C. Lajaunie, and H. Wackernagel. 2006. A "small-world-like" model for comparing interventions aimed at preventing and controlling influenza pandemics. *BMC Medicine* 4:26.

Chau, P. H., and P. S. Yip. 2003. Monitoring the severe acute respiratory syndrome epidemic and assessing effectiveness of interventions in Hong Kong special administrative region. *Journal of Epidemiology and Community Health* 57(10):766–769.

Davey, V. J., R. J. Glass, H. J. Min, W. E. Beyeler, and L. M. Glass. 2008. Effective, robust design of community mitigation for pandemic influenza: A systematic examination of proposed us guidance. *PLOS ONE [Electronic Resource]* 3(7):e2606.

Del Valle, S., H. Hethcote, J. M. Hyman, and C. Castillo-Chavez. 2005. Effects of behavioral changes in a smallpox attack model. *Mathematical Biosciences* 195(2):228–251.

Dénes, A., and A. B. Gumel. 2019. Modeling the impact of quarantine during an outbreak of Ebola virus disease. *Infectious Disease Modelling* 4:12–27.

Ferguson, N. M., D. A. Cummings, S. Cauchemez, C. Fraser, S. Riley, A. Meeyai, S. Iamsirithaworn, and D. S. Burke. 2005. Strategies for containing an emerging influenza pandemic in Southeast Asia. *Nature* 437(7056):209–214.

Gumel, A. B., S. Ruan, T. Day, J. Watmough, F. Brauer, P. van den Driessche, D. Gabrielson, C. Bowman, M. E. Alexander, S. Ardal, J. Wu, and B. M. Sahai. 2004. Modeling strategies for controlling SARS outbreaks. *Proceedings of the Royal Society of London—Series B: Biological Sciences* 271(1554):2223–2232.

Halloran, M. E., N. M. Ferguson, S. Eubank, I. M. Longini, Jr., D. A. Cummings, B. Lewis, S. Xu, C. Fraser, A. Vullikanti, T. C. Germann, D. Wagener, R. Beckman, K. Kadau, C. Barrett, C. A. Macken, D. S. Burke, and P. Cooley. 2008. Modeling targeted layered containment of an influenza pandemic in the United States. *Proceedings of the National Academy of Sciences of the United States of America* 105(12):4639–4644.

Huo, X. 2015. Modeling of contact tracing in epidemic populations structured by disease age. *Discrete and Continuous Dynamical Systems—Series B* 20(6):1685–1713.

Iwami, S., Y. Takeuchi, and X. Liu. 2009. Avian flu pandemic: Can we prevent it? *Journal of Theoretical Biology* 257(1):181–190.

Jung, E., S. Iwami, Y. Takeuchi, and T. C. Jo. 2009. Optimal control strategy for prevention of avian influenza pandemic. *Journal of Theoretical Biology* 260(2):220–229.

Kato, F., K. Tainaka, S. Sone, S. Morita, H. Iida, and J. Yoshimura. 2011. Combined effects of prevention and quarantine on a breakout in SIR model. *Scientific Reports* 1:10.

Lagorio, C., M. Dickison, F. Vazquez, L. A. Braunstein, P. A. Macri, M. V. Migueles, S. Havlin, and H. E. Stanley. 2011. Quarantine-generated phase transition in epidemic spreading. *Physical Review E: Statistical, Nonlinear, & Soft Matter Physics* 83(2 Pt 2):026102.

Li, X., W. Geng, H. Tian, and D. Lai. 2013. Was mandatory quarantine necessary in China for controlling the 2009 H1N1 pandemic? *International Journal of Environmental Research and Public Health [Electronic Resource]* 10(10):4690–4700.

Lipsitch, M., T. Cohen, B. Cooper, J. M. Robins, S. Ma, L. James, G. Gopalakrishna, S. K. Chew, C. C. Tan, M. H. Samore, D. Fisman, and M. Murray. 2003. Transmission dynamics and control of severe acute respiratory syndrome. *Science* 300(5627):1966–1970.

Lloyd-Smith, J. O., A. P. Galvani, and W. M. Getz. 2003. Curtailing transmission of severe acute respiratory syndrome within a community and its hospital. *Proceedings of the Royal Society of London—Series B: Biological Sciences* 270(1528):1979–1989.

Longini, I. M., Jr., A. Nizam, S. Xu, K. Ungchusak, W. Hanshaoworakul, D. A. Cummings, and M. E. Halloran. 2005. Containing pandemic influenza at the source. *Science* 309(5737):1083–1087.

Mesnard, A., and P. Seabright. 2009. Escaping epidemics through migration? Quarantine measures under incomplete information about infection risk. *Journal of Public Economics* 93(7):931–938.

Ngwa, G. A., and M. I. Teboh-Ewungkem. 2016. A mathematical model with quarantine states for the dynamics of Ebola virus disease in human populations. *Computational and Mathematical Methods in Medicine* 2016:9352725.

Nishiura, H., K. Patanarapelert, M. Sriprom, W. Sarakorn, S. Sriyab, and I. Ming Tang. 2004. Modeling potential responses to severe acute respiratory syndrome in Japan: The role of initial attack size, precaution, and quarantine. *Journal of Epidemiology and Community Health* 58(3):186–191.

Pandey, A., K. E. Atkins, J. Medlock, N. Wenzel, J. P. Townsend, J. E. Childs, T. G. Nyenswah, M. L. Ndeffo-Mbah, and A. P. Galvani. 2014. Strategies for containing Ebola in West Africa. *Science* 346(6212):991–995.

Perlroth, D. J., R. J. Glass, V. J. Davey, D. Cannon, A. M. Garber, and D. K. Owens. 2010. Health outcomes and costs of community mitigation strategies for an influenza pandemic in the United States. *Clinical Infectious Diseases* 50(2):165–174.

Roberts, M. G., M. Baker, L. C. Jennings, G. Sertsou, and N. Wilson. 2007. A model for the spread and control of pandemic influenza in an isolated geographical region. *Journal of the Royal Society Interface* 4(13):325–330.

Sang, Z., Z. Qiu, X. Yan, and Y. Zou. 2012. Assessing the effect of non-pharmaceutical interventions on containing an emerging disease. *Mathematical Biosciences and Engineering* 9(1):147–164.

Uribe-Sánchez, A., A. Savachkin, A. Santana, D. Prieto-Santa, and T. K. Das. 2011. A predictive decision-aid methodology for dynamic mitigation of influenza pandemics. *Operations Research Spectrum* 33(3):751–786.

Wu, J. T., S. Riley, C. Fraser, and G. M. Leung. 2006. Reducing the impact of the next influenza pandemic using household-based public health interventions. *PLOS Medicine* 3(9):e361.

Yan, X., Y. Zou, and J. Li. 2007. Optimal quarantine and isolation strategies in epidemics control. *World Journal of Modelling and Simulation* 3(3):202–211.

Yang, Y., P. M. Atkinson, and D. Ettema. 2011. Analysis of CDC social control measures using an agent-based simulation of an influenza epidemic in a city. *BMC Infectious Diseases* 11:199.

Zhang, Q., and D. Wang. 2015. Assessing the role of voluntary self-isolation in the control of pandemic influenza using a household epidemic model. *International Journal of Environmental Research and Public Health [Electronic Resource]* 12(8):9750–9767.

Qualitative Studies

Baum, N. M., P. D. Jacobson, and S. D. Goold. 2009. "Listen to the people": Public deliberation about social distancing measures in a pandemic. *American Journal of Bioethics* 9(11):4–14.

Beaton, R., A. Stergachis, J. Thompson, C. Osaki, C. Johnson, S. J. Charvat, and N. Marsden-Haug. 2007. Pandemic policy and planning considerations for universities: Findings from a tabletop exercise. *Biosecurity and Bioterrorism* 5(4):327–334.

Bell, D. M., and WHO (World Health Organization Working Group on Prevention of International and Community Transmission of SARS). 2004. Public health interventions and SARS spread, 2003. *Emerging Infectious Diseases* 10(11):1900–1906.

Braunack-Mayer, A. J., J. M. Street, W. A. Rogers, R. Givney, J. R. Moss, J. E. Hiller, and Flu Views Team. 2010. Including the public in pandemic planning: A deliberative approach. *BMC Public Health* 10:501.

Cava, M. A., K. E. Fay, H. J. Beanlands, E. A. McCay, and R. Wignall. 2005a. The experience of quarantine for individuals affected by SARS in Toronto. *Public Health Nursing* 22(5):398–406.

Cava, M. A., K. E. Fay, H. J. Beanlands, E. A. McCay, and R. Wignall. 2005b. Risk perception and compliance with quarantine during the SARS outbreak. *Journal of Nursing Scholarship* 37(4):343–347.

Charania, N. A., and L. J. Tsuji. 2013. Assessing the effectiveness and feasibility of implementing mitigation measures for an influenza pandemic in remote and isolated first nations communities: A qualitative community-based participatory research approach. *Rural and Remote Health* 13(4):2566.

Desclaux, A., D. Badji, A. G. Ndione, and K. Sow. 2017. Accepted monitoring or endured quarantine? Ebola contacts' perceptions in Senegal. *Social Science and Medicine* 178:38–45.

DiGiovanni, C., J. Conley, D. Chiu, and J. Zaborski. 2004. Factors influencing compliance with quarantine in Toronto during the 2003 SARS outbreak. *Biosecurity and Bioterrorism* 2(4):265–272.

Leung, C. S., M. M. Ho, A. Kiss, A. V. Gundlapalli, and S. W. Hwang. 2008. Homelessness and the response to emerging infectious disease outbreaks: Lessons from SARS. *Journal of Urban Health* 85(3):402–410.

Lin, E. C., Y. C. Peng, and J. C. Tsai. 2010. Lessons learned from the anti-SARS quarantine experience in a hospital-based fever screening station in Taiwan. *American Journal of Infection Control* 38(4):302–307.

Maunder, R., J. Hunter, L. Vincent, J. Bennett, N. Peladeau, M. Leszcz, J. Sadavoy, L. M. Verhaeghe, R. Steinberg, and T. Mazzulli. 2003. The immediate psychological and occupational impact of the 2003 SARS outbreak in a teaching hospital. *Canadian Medical Association Journal* 168(10):1245–1251.

Pellecchia, U., R. Crestani, T. Decroo, R. Van den Bergh, and Y. Al-Kourdi. 2015. Social consequences of Ebola containment measures in Liberia. *PLOS ONE* 10(12):e0143036.

Robertson, E., K. Hershenfield, S. L. Grace, and D. E. Stewart. 2004. The psychosocial effects of being quarantined following exposure to SARS: A qualitative study of Toronto health care workers. *Canadian Journal of Psychiatry* 49(6):403–407.

Schemm Dwyer, K., H. Misner, S. Chang, and N. Fajardo. 2017. An interim examination of the U.S. public health response to Ebola. *Health Security* 15(5):527–538.

Sell, T. K., M. P. Shearer, D. Meyer, H. Chandler, M. Schoch-Spana, E. Thomas, D. A. Rose, E. G. Carbone, and E. Toner. 2018. Public health resilience checklist for high-consequence infectious diseases—Informed by the domestic Ebola response in the United States. *Journal of Public Health Management and Practice* 24(6):510–518.

Smith, M. J., C. M. Bensimon, D. F. Perez, S. S. Sahni, and R. E. G. Upshur. 2012. Restrictive measures in an influenza pandemic: A qualitative study of public perspectives. *Canadian Journal of Public Health* 103(5):348–352.

Descriptive Survey Studies

Bauerle Bass, S., S. Burt Ruzek, L. Ward, T. F. Gordon, A. Hanlon, A. J. Hausman, and M. Hagen. 2010. If you ask them, will they come? Predictors of quarantine compliance during a hypothetical avian influenza pandemic: Results from a statewide survey. *Disaster Medicine and Public Health Preparedness* 4(2):135–144.

Blake, K. D., R. J. Blendon, and K. Viswanath. 2010. Employment and compliance with pandemic influenza mitigation recommendations. *Emerging Infectious Diseases* 16(2):212–218.

Blendon, R. J., C. M. DesRoches, M. S. Cetron, J. M. Benson, T. Meinhardt, and W. Pollard. 2006. Attitudes toward the use of quarantine in a public health emergency in four countries. *Health Affairs* 25(2):w15–w25.

Eastwood, K., D. Durrheim, J. L. Francis, E. T. d'Espaignet, S. Duncan, F. Islam, and R. Speare. 2009. Knowledge about pandemic influenza and compliance with containment measures among Australians. *Bulletin of the World Health Organization* 87(8):588–594.

Eastwood, K., D. N. Durrheim, M. Butler, and A. Jon. 2010. Responses to pandemic (H1N1) 2009, Australia. *Emerging Infectious Diseases* 16(8):1211–1216.

Katz, R., A. Vaught, and S. J. Simmens. 2019. Local decision making for implementing social distancing in response to outbreaks. *Public Health Reports* 134(2):150–154.

Kelly, B., L. Squiers, C. Bann, A. Stine, H. Hansen, and M. Lynch. 2015. Perceptions and plans for prevention of Ebola: Results from a national survey. *BMC Public Health* 15:1136.

Porten, K., D. Faensen, and G. Krause. 2006. SARS outbreak in Germany 2003: Workload of local health departments and their compliance in quarantine measures—Implications for outbreak modeling and surge capacity? *Journal of Public Health Management and Practice* 12(3):242–247.

Seale, H., M. L. McLaws, A. E. Heywood, K. F. Ward, C. P. Lowbridge, D. Van, J. Gralton, and C. R. MacIntyre. 2009. The community's attitude towards swine flu and pandemic influenza. *Medical Journal of Australia* 191(5):267–269.

Taylor-Clark, K., R. J. Blendon, A. Zaslavsky, and J. Benson. 2005. Confidence in crisis? Understanding trust in government and public attitudes toward mandatory state health powers. *Biosecurity and Bioterrorism* 3(2):138–147.

Teh, B., K. Olsen, J. Black, A. C. Cheng, C. Aboltins, K. Bull, P. D. Johnson, M. L. Grayson, and J. Torresi. 2012. Impact of swine influenza and quarantine measures on patients and households during the H1N1/09 pandemic. *Scandinavian Journal of Infectious Diseases* 44(4):289–296.

Tracy, C. S., E. Rea, and R. E. Upshur. 2009. Public perceptions of quarantine: Community-based telephone survey following an infectious disease outbreak. *BMC Public Health* 9:470.

Wray, R. J., J. K. Harris, K. Jupka, S. Vijaykumar, E. W. Mitchell, W. Pollard, E. Zielinski-Gutierrez, D. Reissman, and K. Lubell. 2012. Individual and community influences on adherence to directives in the ecommmunvent of a plague attack: Survey results. *Disaster Medicine and Public Health Preparedness* 6(3):253–262.

Case Reports

Barbisch, D., K. L. Koenig, and F. Y. Shih. 2015. Is there a case for quarantine? Perspectives from SARS to Ebola. *Disaster Medicine and Public Health Preparedness* 9(5):547–553.

Binns, P. L., V. Sheppeard, and M. P. Staff. 2010. Isolation and quarantine during pandemic (H1N1) 2009 influenza in NSW: The operational experience of public health units. *New South Wales Public Health Bulletin* 21(1–2):10–15.

CDC (Centers for Disease Control and Prevention). 2003a. Efficiency of quarantine during an epidemic of severe acute respiratory syndrome—Beijing, China, 2003. *Morbidity and Mortality Weekly Report* 52(43):1037–1040.

CDC. 2003b. Use of quarantine to prevent transmission of severe acute respiratory syndrome—Taiwan, 2003. *Morbidity and Mortality Weekly Report* 52(29):680–683.

CDC. 2004. Postexposure prophylaxis, isolation, and quarantine to control an import-associated measles outbreak—Iowa, 2004. *Morbidity and Mortality Weekly Report* 53(41):969–971.

Chen, K. T., S. J. Twu, H. L. Chang, Y. C. Wu, C. T. Chen, T. H. Lin, S. J. Olsen, S. F. Dowell, I. J. Su, and S. R. T. Taiwan. 2005. SARS in Taiwan: An overview and lessons learned. *International Journal of Infectious Diseases* 9(2):77–85.

Chung, W. M., J. C. Smith, L. M. Weil, S. M. Hughes, S. N. Joyner, E. M. Hall, J. Ritch, D. Srinath, E. Goodman, M. S. Chevalier, L. Epstein, J. C. Hunter, A. J. Kallen, M. P. Karwowski, D. T. Kuhar, C. Smith, L. R. Petersen, B. E. Mahon, D. L. Lakey, and S. J. Schrag. 2015. Active tracing and monitoring of contacts associated with the first cluster of Ebola in the United States. *Annals of Internal Medicine* 163(3):164–173.

Collier, M. G., A. Cierzniewski, T. Duszynski, C. Munson, M. Wenger, B. Beard, R. Gentry, J. Duwve, P. K. Kutty, and P. Pontones. 2013. Measles outbreak associated with international travel, Indiana, 2011. *Journal of the Pediatric Infectious Diseases Society* 2(2):110–118.

DiGiovanni, C., N. Bowen, M. Ginsberg, and G. Giles. 2005. Quarantine stressing voluntary compliance. *Emerging Infectious Diseases* 11(11):1778–1779.

Ehlkes, L., M. George, G. Samosny, F. Burckhardt, M. Vogt, S. Bent, K. Jahn, and P. Zanger. 2017. Management of a Lassa fever outbreak, Rhineland-Palatinate, Germany, 2016. *European Communicable Disease Bulletin* 22(39).

Gahr, P., A. S. DeVries, G. Wallace, C. Miller, C. Kenyon, K. Sweet, K. Martin, K. White, E. Bagstad, C. Hooker, G. Krawczynski, D. Boxrud, G. Liu, P. Stinchfield, J. LeBlanc, C. Hickman, L. Bahta, A. Barskey, and R. Lynfield. 2014. An outbreak of measles in an undervaccinated community. *Pediatrics* 134(1):e220–e228.

Gastañaduy, P. A., J. Budd, N. Fisher, S. B. Redd, J. Fletcher, J. Miller, D. J. McFadden, 3rd, J. Rota, P. A. Rota, C. Hickman, B. Fowler, L. Tatham, G. S. Wallace, S. de Fijter, A. Parker Fiebelkorn, and M. DiOrio. 2016. A measles outbreak in an underimmunized Amish community in Ohio. *New England Journal of Medicine* 375(14):1343–1354.

Grigg, C., N. E. Waziri, A. T. Olayinka, J. F. Vertefeuille, and Centers for Disease Control and Prevention. 2015. Use of group quarantine in Ebola control—Nigeria, 2014. *Morbidity and Mortality Weekly Report* 64(5):124.

Nathawad, R., P. M. Roblin, D. Pruitt, and B. Arquilla. 2013. Addressing the gaps in preparation for quarantine. *Prehospital and Disaster Medicine* 28(2):132–138.

Nyenswah, T., D. J. Blackley, T. Freeman, K. A. Lindblade, S. K. Arzoaquoi, J. A. Mott, J. N. Williams, C. N. Halldin, F. Kollie, and A. S. Laney. 2015. Community quarantine to interrupt Ebola virus transmission—Mawah Village, Bong County, Liberia, August–October, 2014. *Morbidity and Mortality Weekly Report* 64(7):179–182.

Ooi, P. L., S. Lim, and S. K. Chew. 2005. Use of quarantine in the control of SARS in Singapore. *American Journal of Infection Control* 33(5):252–257.

Pang, X., Z. Zhu, F. Xu, J. Guo, X. Gong, D. Liu, Z. Liu, D. P. Chin, and D. R. Feikin. 2003. Evaluation of control measures implemented in the severe acute respiratory syndrome outbreak in Beijing, 2003. *JAMA* 290(24):3215–3221.

Plipat, T., R. Buathong, S. Wacharapluesadee, P. Siriarayapon, C. Pittayawonganon, C. Sangsajja, T. Kaewpom, S. Petcharat, T. Ponpinit, J. Jumpasri, Y. Joyjinda, A. Rodpan, S. Ghai, A. Jittmittraphap, S. Khongwichit, D. R. Smith, V. M. Corman, C. Drosten, and T. Hemachudha. 2017. Imported case of Middle East respiratory syndrome coronavirus (MERS-CoV) infection from Oman to Thailand, June 2015. *European Communicable Disease Bulletin* 22(33):17.

Reaves, E. J., L. G. Mabande, D. A. Thoroughman, M. A. Arwady, and J. M. Montgomery. 2014. Control of Ebola virus disease—Firestone District, Liberia, 2014. *Morbidity and Mortality Weekly Report* 63(42):959–965.

Smith, C. L., S. M. Hughes, M. P. Karwowski, M. S. Chevalier, E. Hall, S. N. Joyner, J. Ritch, J. C. Smith, L. M. Weil, W. M. Chung, S. Schrag, S. Santibanez, and Centers for Disease Control and Prevention. 2015. Addressing needs of contacts of Ebola patients during an investigation of an Ebola cluster in the United States—Dallas, Texas, 2014. *Morbidity and Mortality Weekly Report* 64(5):121–123.

Spengler, J. R., S. Stonecipher, C. McManus, H. Hughes-Garza, M. Dow, D. L. Zoran, W. Bissett, T. Beckham, D. A. Alves, M. Wolcott, S. Tostenson, B. Dorman, J. Jones, T. J. Sidwa, B. Knust, and C. B. Behravesh. 2015. Management of a pet dog after exposure to a human patient with Ebola virus disease. *Journal of the American Veterinary Medical Association* 247(5):531–538.

Svoboda, T., B. Henry, L. Shulman, E. Kennedy, E. Rea, W. Ng, T. Wallington, B. Yaffe, E. Gournis, E. Vicencio, S. Basrur, and R. H. Glazier. 2004. Public health measures to control the spread of the severe acute respiratory syndrome during the outbreak in Toronto. *New England Journal of Medicine* 350(23):2352–2361.

Tay, J., Y. F. Ng, J. Cutter, and L. James. 2010. Influenza A (H1N1-2009) pandemic in Singapore—Public health control measures implemented and lessons learnt. *Annals of the Academy of Medicine Singapore* 39(4):313–324.

Tsang, T., and T. H. Lam. 2003. SARS: Public health measures in Hong Kong. *Respirology* 8(Suppl):S46–S48.

Ward, K. A., P. Armstrong, J. M. McAnulty, J. M. Iwasenko, and D. E. Dwyer. 2010. Outbreaks of pandemic (H1N1) 2009 and seasonal influenza A (H3N2) on cruise ship. *Emerging Infectious Diseases* 16(11):1731–1737.

Yasuoka, A. 2009. Infection control of the H1N1 influenza in hospitals and local region. *Respirology* 3:A120.

Yoon, M. K., S. Y. Kim, H. S. Ko, and M. S. Lee. 2016. System effectiveness of detection, brief intervention and refer to treatment for the people with post-traumatic emotional distress by MERS: A case report of community-based proactive intervention in South Korea. *International Journal of Mental Health Systems* 10(1):51.

Zhang, Y., P. Yang, S. Liyanage, H. Seale, Y. Deng, X. Pang, L. Tian, B. Liu, L. Zhang, and Q. Wang. 2012. The characteristics of imported cases and the effectiveness of outbreak control strategies of pandemic influenza A (H1N1) in China. *Asia-Pacific Journal of Public Health* 24(6):932–939.

Mechanistic Evidence

Drews, K. 2013. A brief history of quarantine. *The Virginia Tech Undergraduate Historical Review* 2. http://doi.org/10.21061/vtuhr.v2i0.16.

Tognotti, E. 2013. Lessons from the history of quarantine, from plague to influenza A. *Emerging Infectious Diseases* 19(2):254–259. https://dx.doi.org/10.3201/eid1902.120312.

Ethics and Policy Text

IOM (Institute of Medicine). 2009. *Guidance for establishing crisis standards of care for use in disaster situations: A letter report.* Washington, DC: The National Academies Press

Jennings, B., and J. Arras. 2008. *Ethical guidance for public health emergency preparedness and response: Highlighting ethics and values in a vital public health service.* https://www.cdc.gov/od/science/integrity/phethics/docs/white_paper_final_for_website_2012_4_6_12_final_for_web_508_compliant.pdf (accessed February 23, 2020).

Jennings, B., J. D. Arras, D. H. Barrett, and B. A. Ellis. 2016. *Emergency ethics: Public health preparedness and response.* New York: Oxford University Press.

Mastroianni, A. C., J. P. Kahn, and N. E. Kass, eds. 2019. *The Oxford handbook of public health ethics.* New York: Oxford University Press. https://www.oxfordhandbooks.com/view/10.1093/oxfordhb/9780190245191.001.0001/oxfordhb-9780190245191 (accessed June 3, 2020).

C Commissioned Reports That Informed the Four Mixed-Method Reviews

This appendix lists the 10 works commissioned by the committee to inform its mixed-method reviews. These commissioned papers can be found under the Resources tab at http://www.nap.edu/catalog/25650.

- Brown University Center for Evidence Synthesis in Health's commissioned report
  - *Data Extraction and Quality Assessment: Methodology and Evidence Tables*
- Wayne State University's commissioned reports
  - *Engaging with and Training Community-Based Partners for Public Health Emergencies: Qualitative Research Evidence Synthesis*
  - *Public Health Emergency Operations Coordination: Qualitative Research Evidence Synthesis*
  - *Communicating Public Health Alerts and Guidance with Technical Audiences: Qualitative Research Evidence Synthesis*
  - *Quarantine as a Non-Pharmaceutical Intervention: Qualitative Research Evidence Synthesis*
- Sneha Patel's commissioned reports
  - *Engaging with and Training Community-Based Partners to Improve the Outcomes of At-Risk Populations After Public Health Emergencies: Findings from Case Reports*
  - *Public Health Emergency Operations Coordination: Findings from After Action Reports and Case Reports*
  - *Information Sharing with Technical Audiences: Findings from After Action Reports and Case Reports*
  - *Use of Quarantine as a Non-Pharmaceutical Intervention for Public Health Emergencies: Findings from Case Reports*
- Jeremy Goldhaber-Fiebert's commissioned report
  - *In What Situations Do Modeling Studies Suggest Quarantine Is More Versus Less Effective to Control Infectious Disease Outbreaks?*

D

Commissioned Scoping Review and Series of Evidence Maps

The committee sought to understand the extent, range, and nature of public health emergency preparedness and response (PHEPR) research across the 15 Centers for Disease Control and Prevention (CDC) PHEPR Capabilities, with a specific focus on studies evaluating the impact of PHEPR practices, and commissioned an expert group to visualize these findings using high-level evidence maps. This appendix contains excerpts and evidence maps from the group's full paper, "Review and Evidence Mapping of Scholarly Publications Within the CDC's 15 Public Health Emergency Preparedness and Response Capabilities."[1]

A total of 1,692 articles (published 2001–2019), consisting of quantitative (comparative and noncomparative) impact studies, quantitative nonimpact studies, qualitative studies, modeling studies, literature reviews, after action reports and case reports, and commentaries, were initially included in the commissioned scoping review.[2] Ultimately, the committee was most interested in those studies that could potentially provide evidence regarding the 15 PHEPR Capabilities. Therefore, after this initial classification of all study designs, commentaries and literature reviews were excluded from subsequent analyses, resulting in a total of 1,106 articles for final inclusion.[3]

---

[1] The full paper can be found under the Resources tab at http://www.nap.edu/catalog/25650.

[2] The task of finding and classifying the body of research underlying all of the 15 PHEPR Capabilities was challenging because of the broad scope, complexity, and nature of the research topics. The evidence maps prepared for this study certainly do not contain every published study examining PHEPR practices since 2001. The authors of the scoping review did not attempt to capture after action reports that were not published in journals and searchable in bibliographic databases. Future efforts could focus on conducting detailed scoping reviews on specific capabilities or practices.

[3] The 1,106 articles included in the final analysis were described in the commissioned report as "evidentiary studies," which required some form of systematic data collection and analysis that could provide evidence regarding the PHEPR Capabilities. Nonevidentiary studies include opinion, concept, and position papers, as well as literature reviews.

DESCRIPTIVE MAPS OF ARTICLES WITHIN THE 15 PHEPR CAPABILITIES

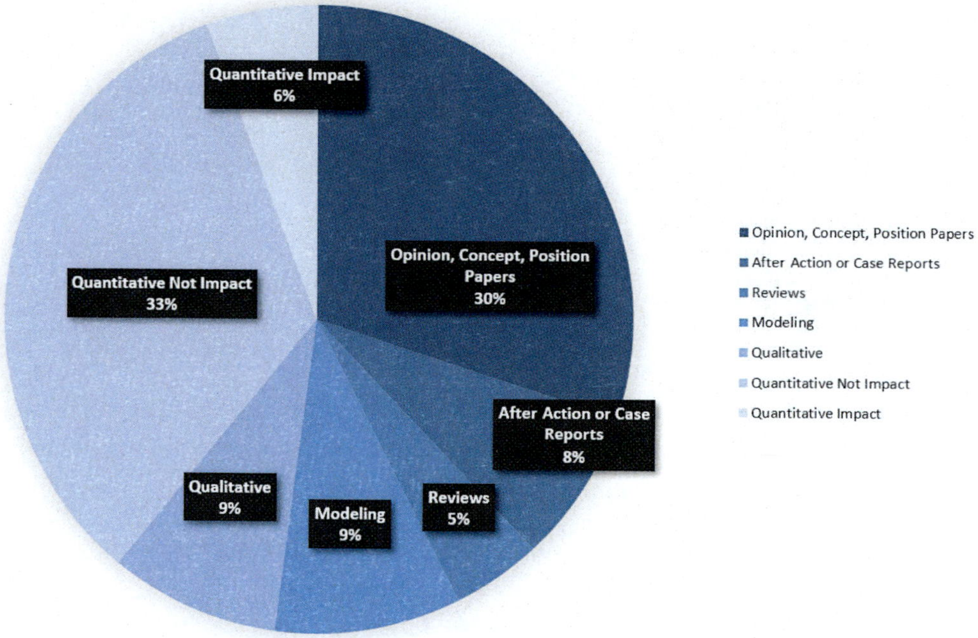

FIGURE D-1 Distribution of all articles by study design (N = 1,692).

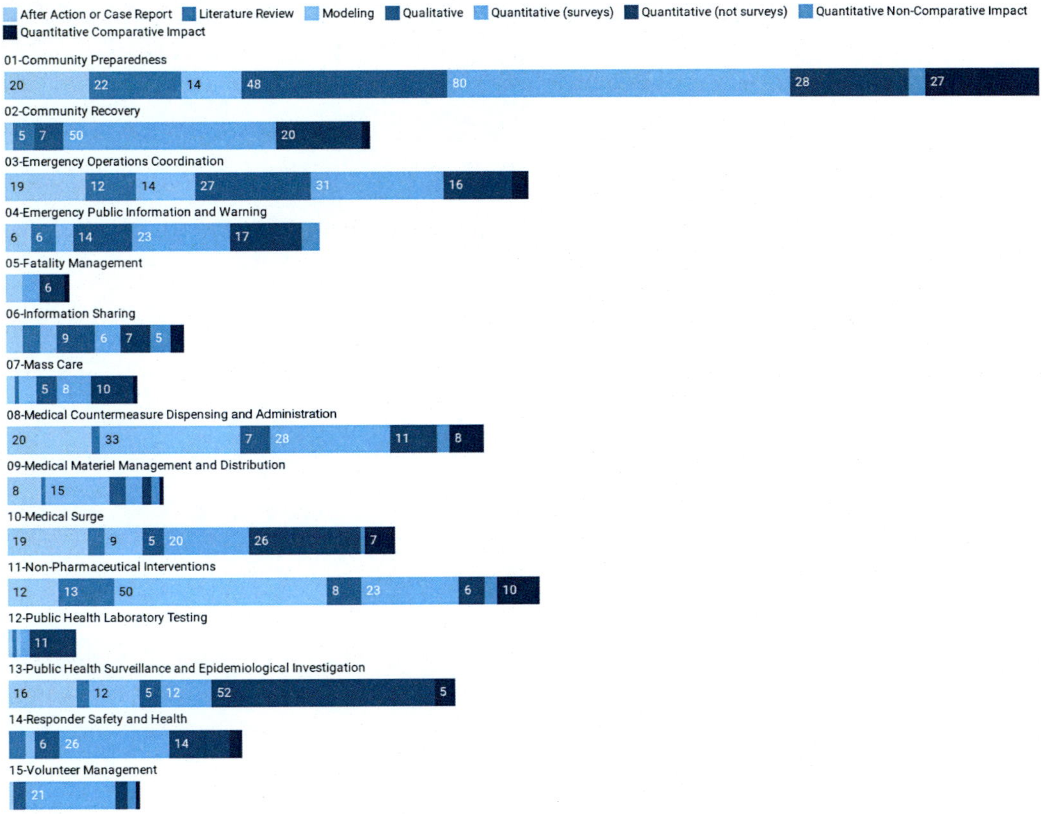

FIGURE D-2 Study design by PHEPR Capability (N = 1,184).

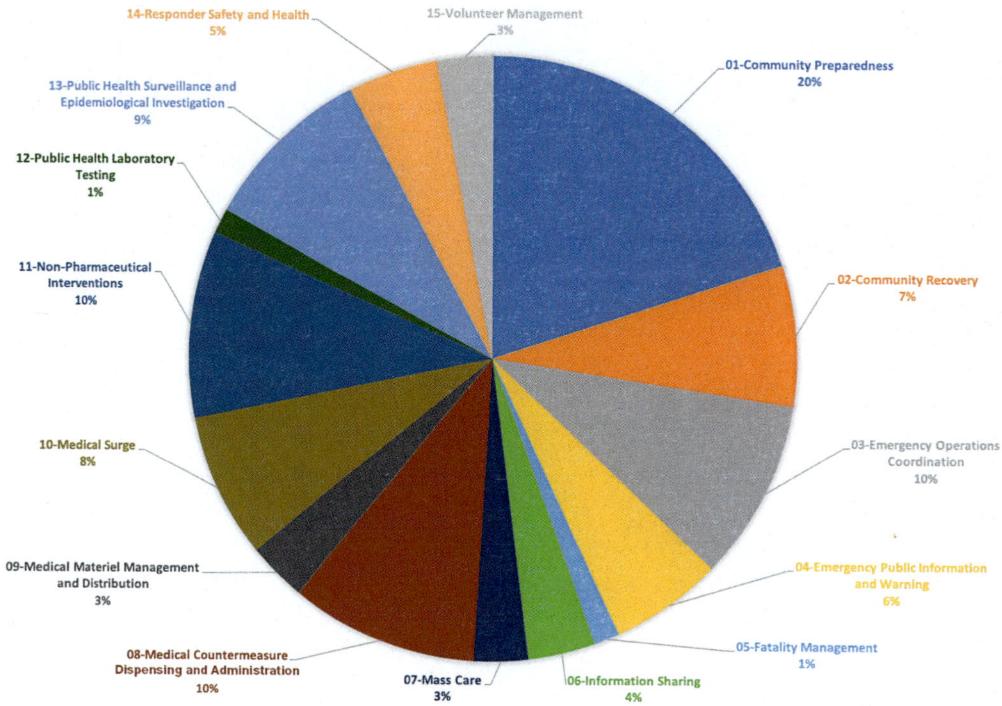

FIGURE D-3 Distribution of evidentiary articles by PHEPR Capability (N = 1,106).

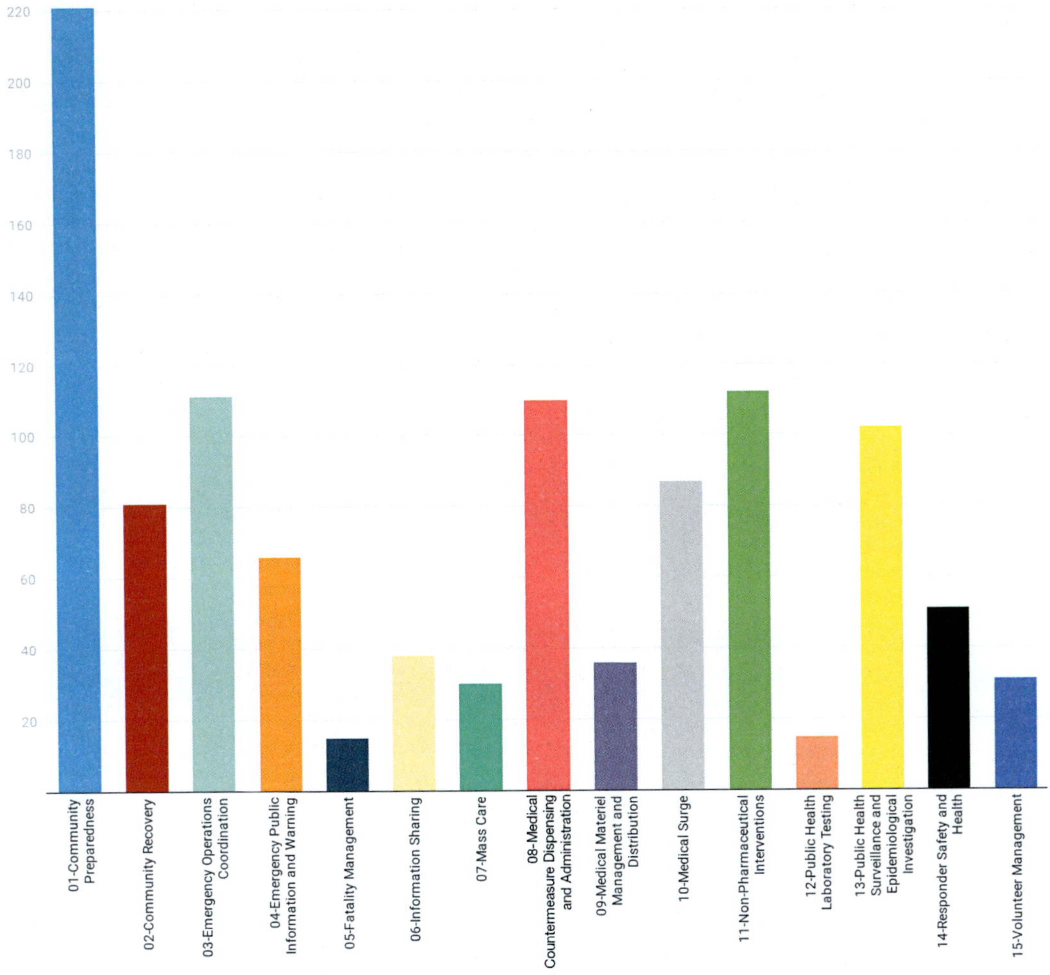

FIGURE D-4 Distribution of evidentiary articles across PHEPR Capabilities (N = 1,106).

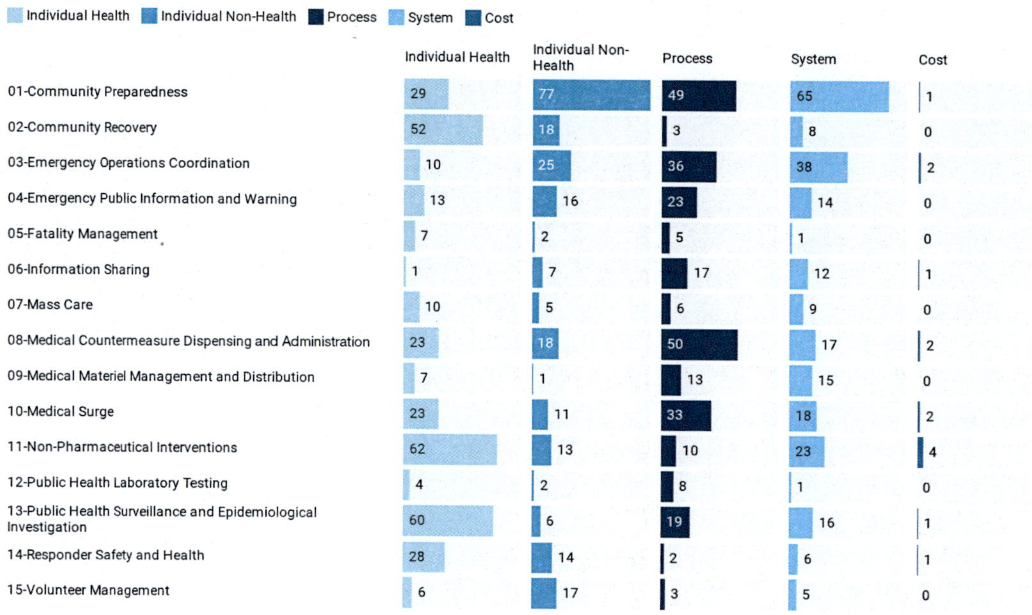

FIGURE D-5 Type of outcome by PHEPR Capability (N = 1,106).

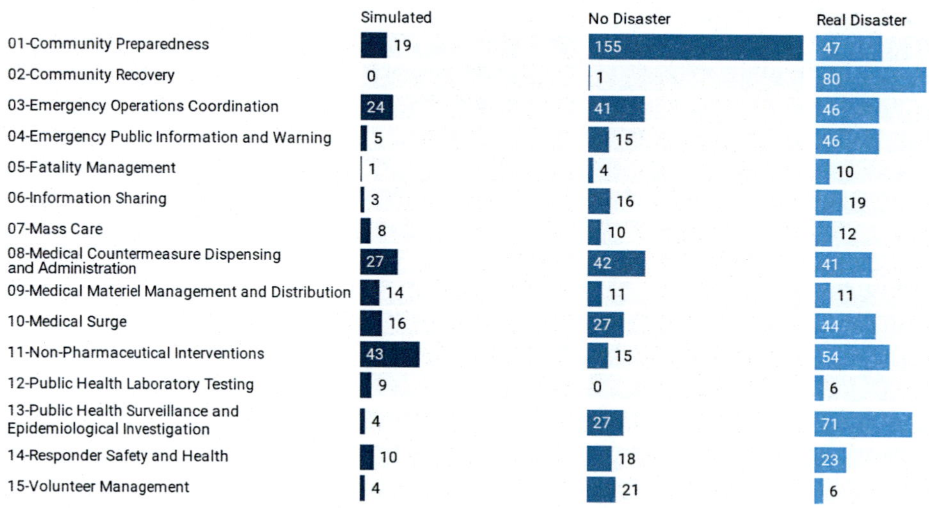

FIGURE D-6 Type of disaster by PHEPR Capability (N = 1,106).

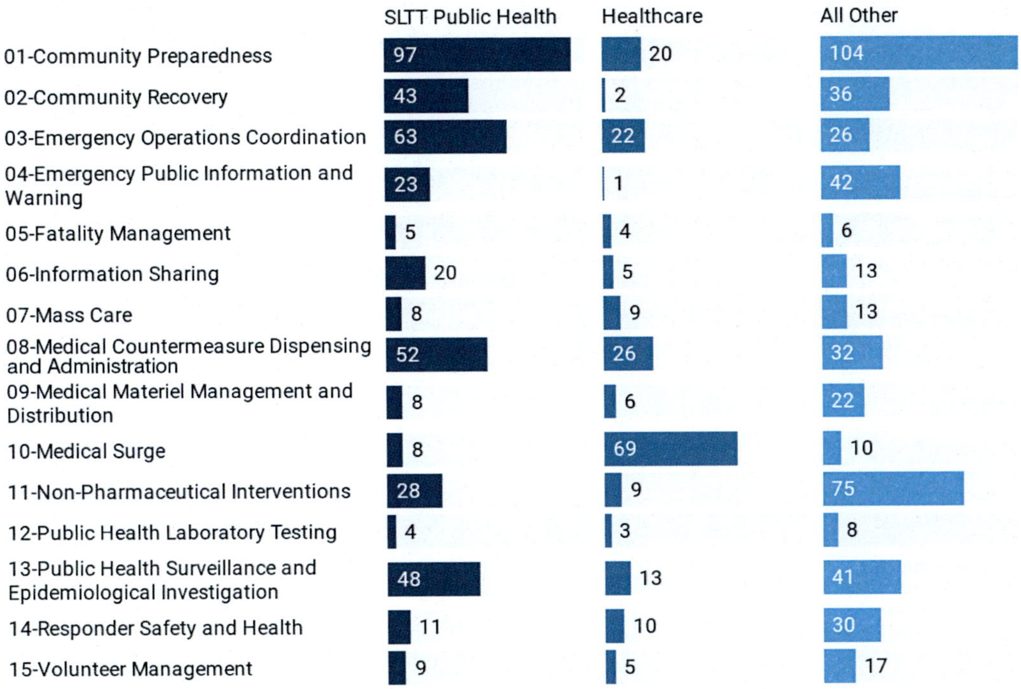

FIGURE D-7 Organization by PHEPR Capability (N = 1,106).

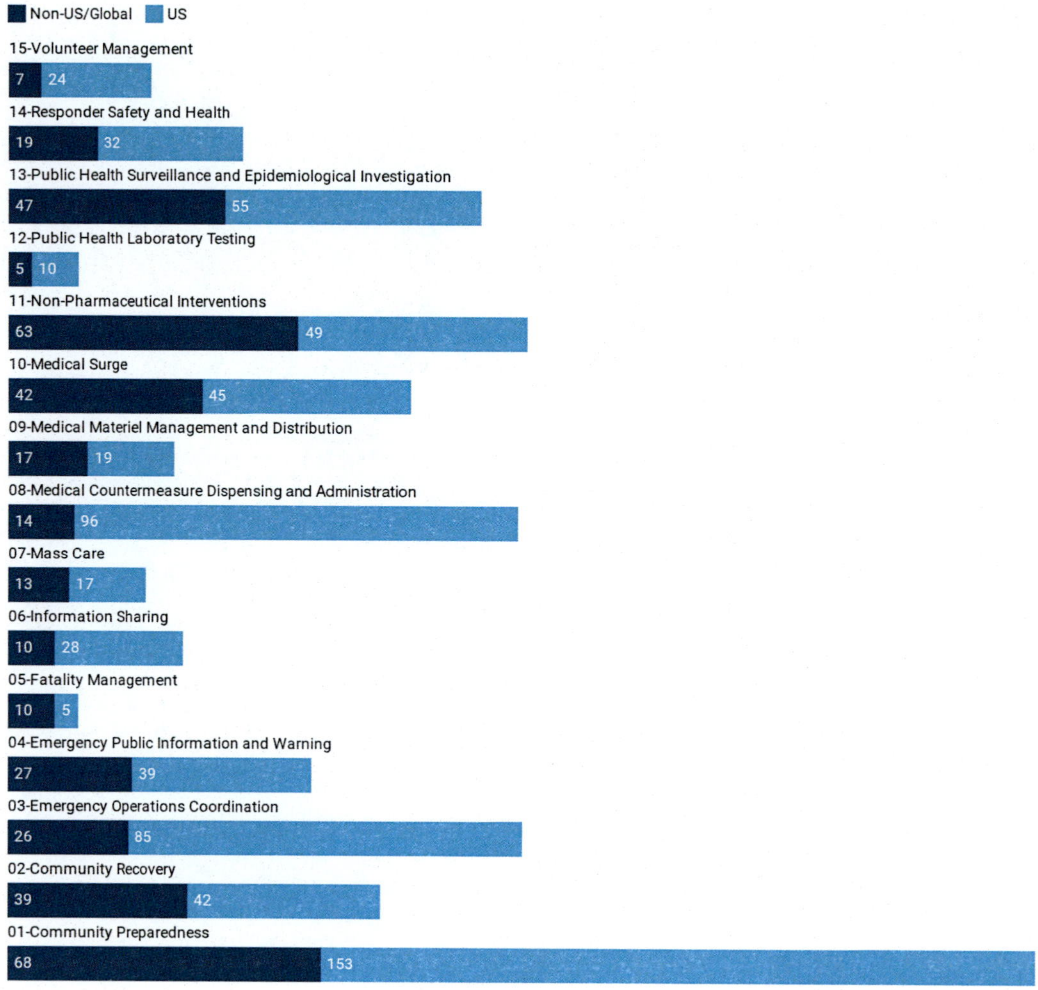

FIGURE D-8 Setting by PHEPR Capability (N = 1,106).

MATRIX EVIDENCE MAPS OF QUANTITATIVE IMPACT STUDIES WITHIN THE 15 PHEPR CAPABILITIES

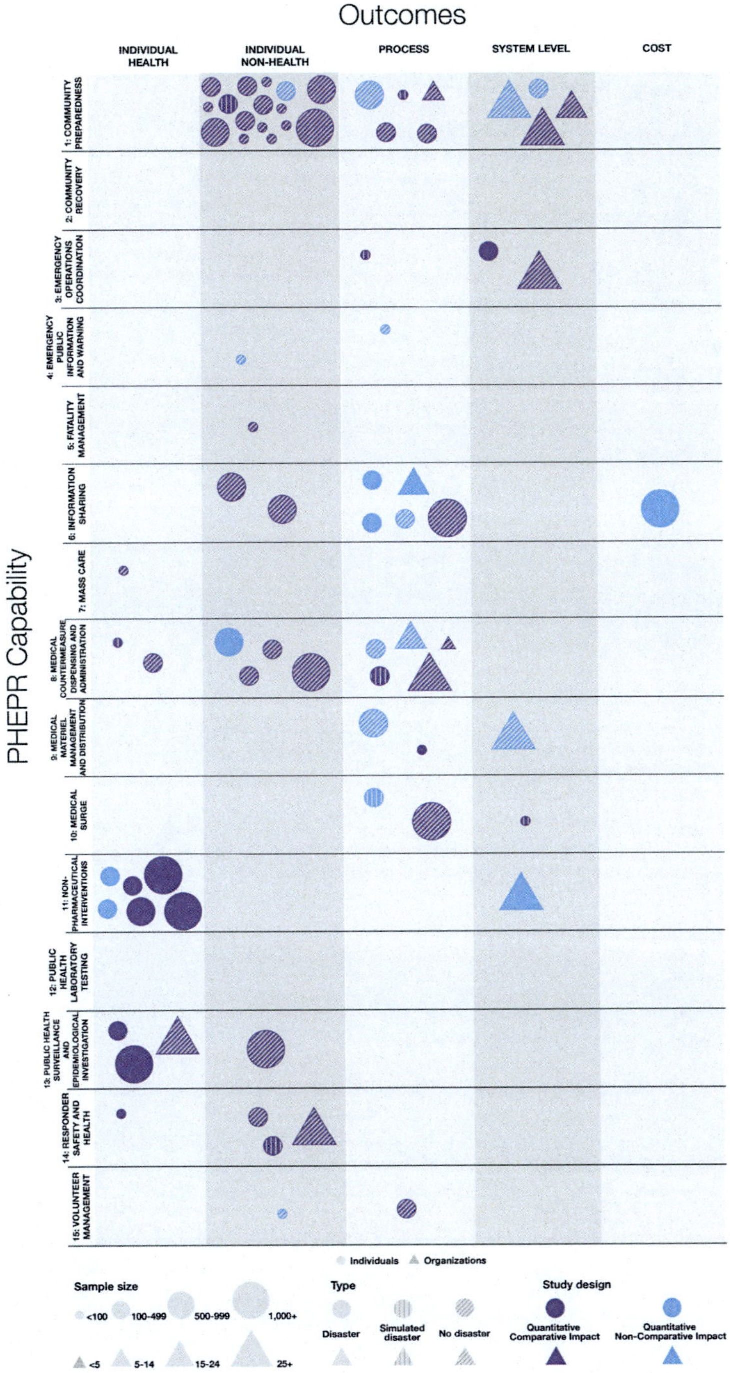

FIGURE D-9 Evidence map: Characteristics of U.S. quantitative impact studies across the PHEPR Capabilities (N = 72).

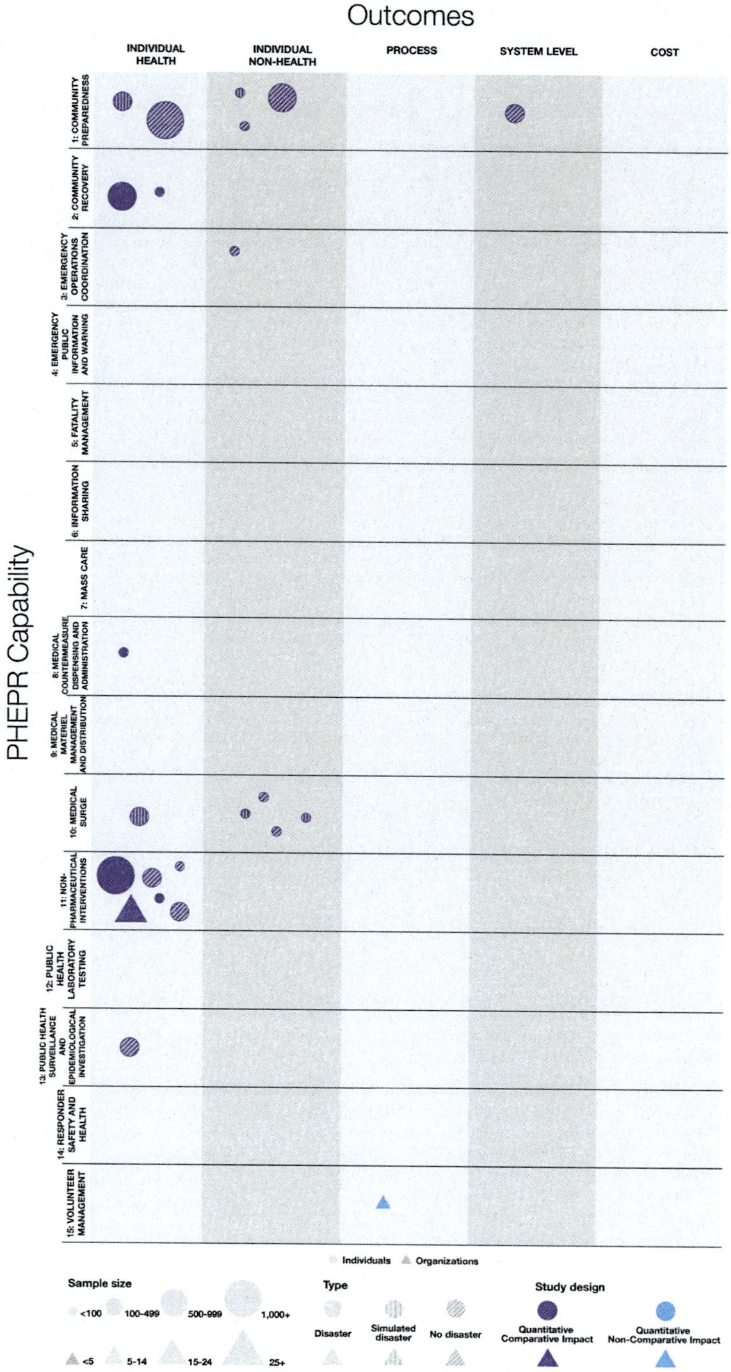

FIGURE D-10 Evidence map: Characteristics of non-U.S. quantitative impact studies across the PHEPR Capabilities (N = 23).

MATRIX EVIDENCE MAPS OF STUDIES WITHIN SPECIFIC PRACTICE AREAS OF THE 15 PHEPR CAPABILITIES

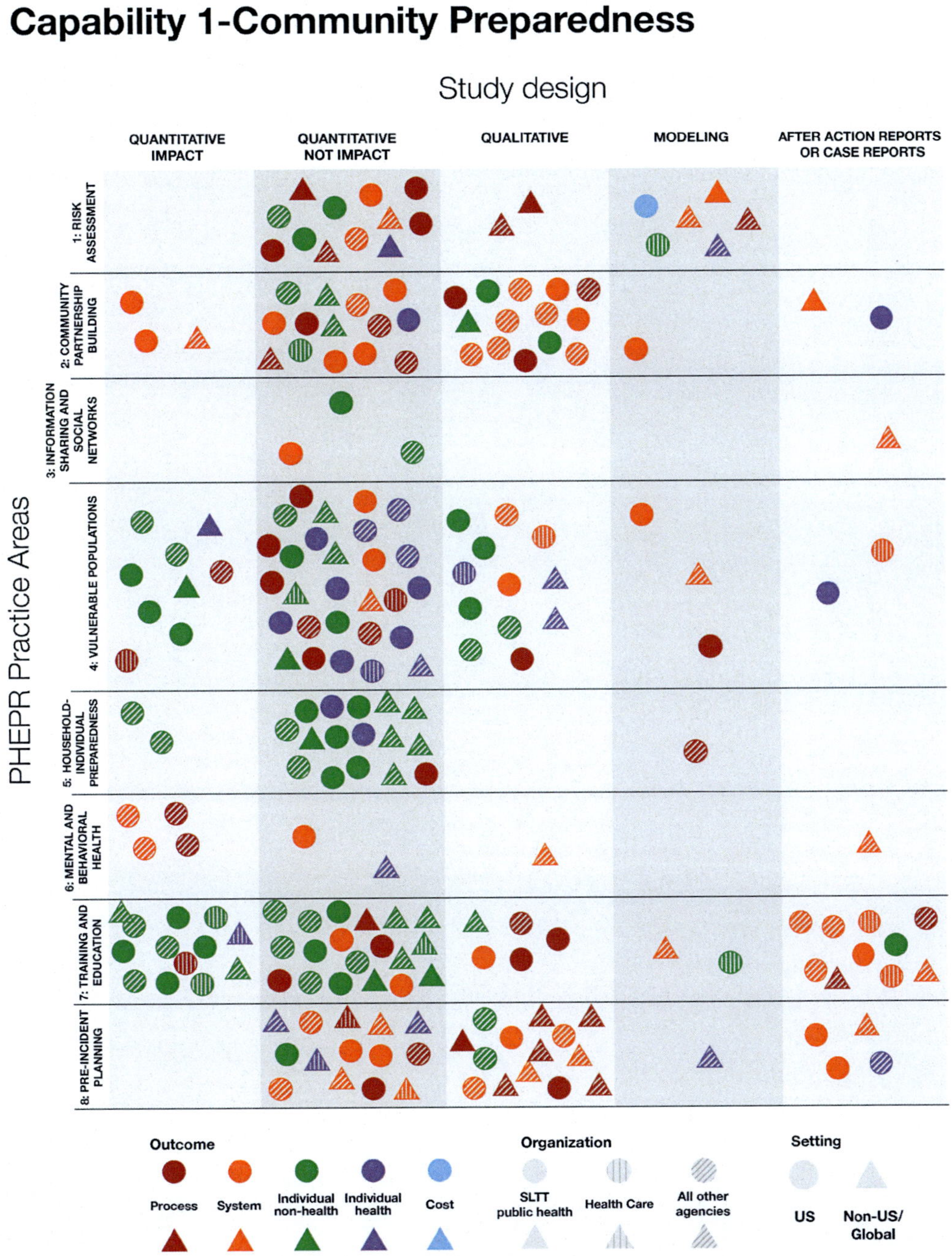

FIGURE D-11 Evidence map: Characteristics of studies for Community Preparedness (N = 221).

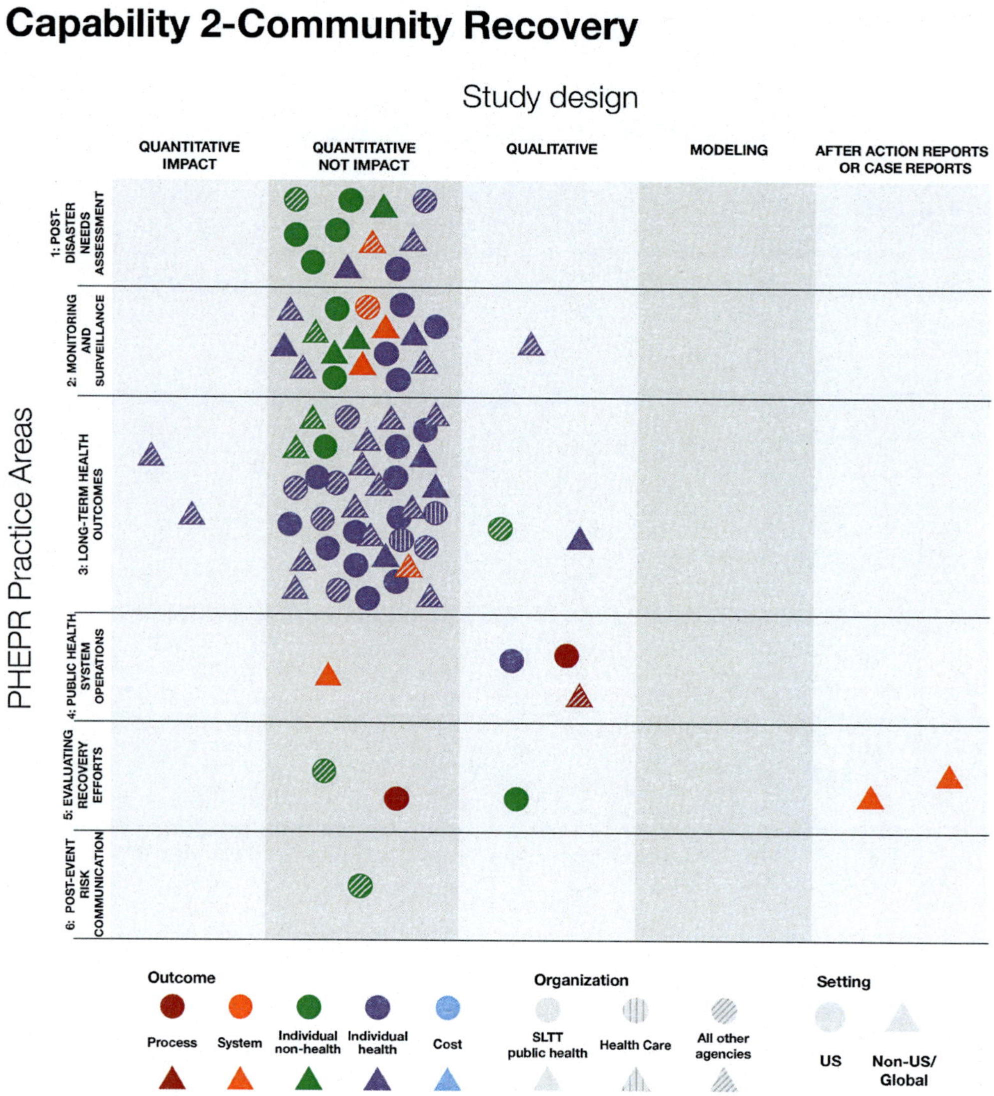

FIGURE D-12 Evidence map: Characteristics of studies for Community Recovery (N = 78).

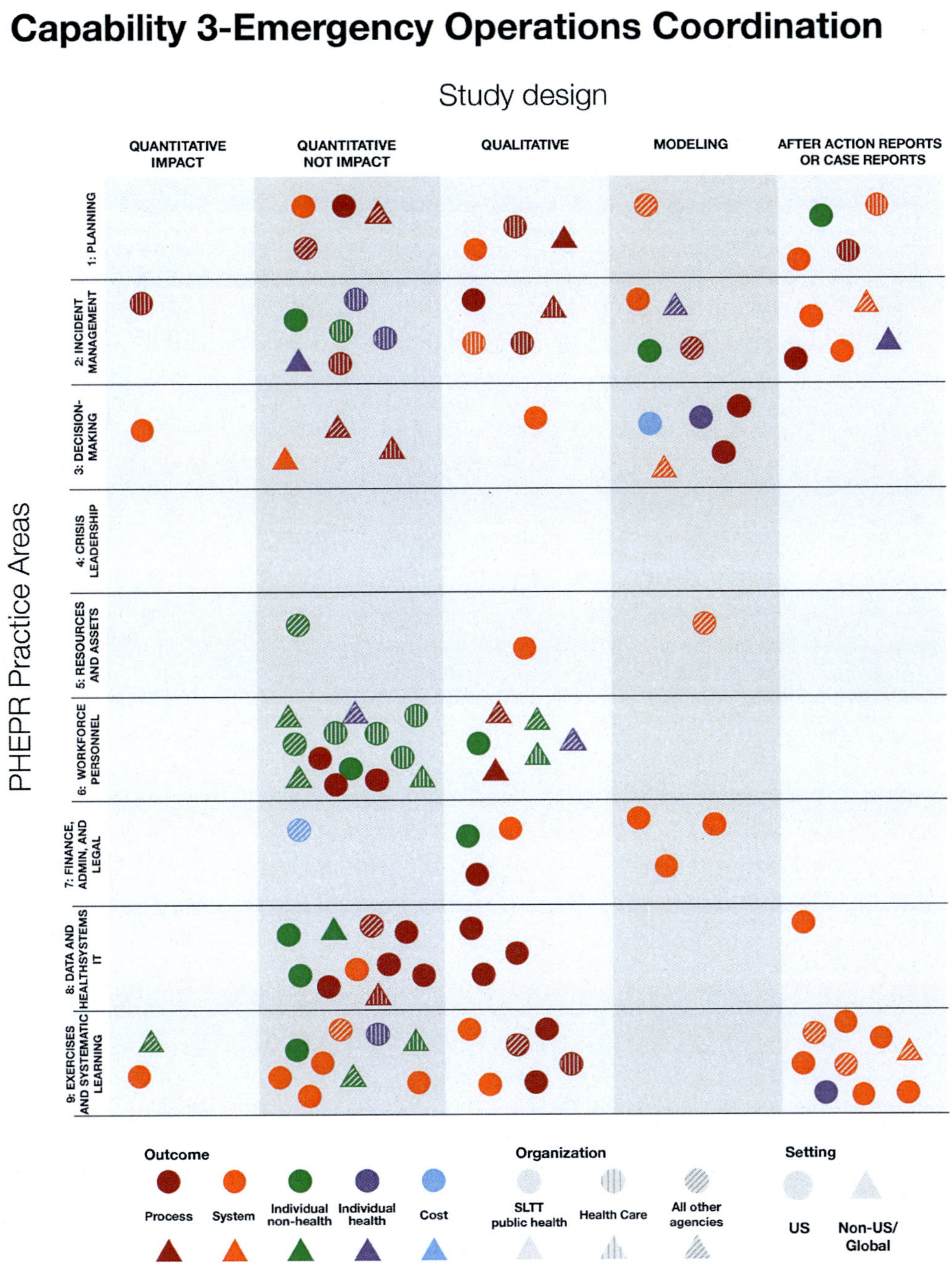

FIGURE D-13 Evidence map: Characteristics of studies for Emergency Operations Coordination (N = 111).

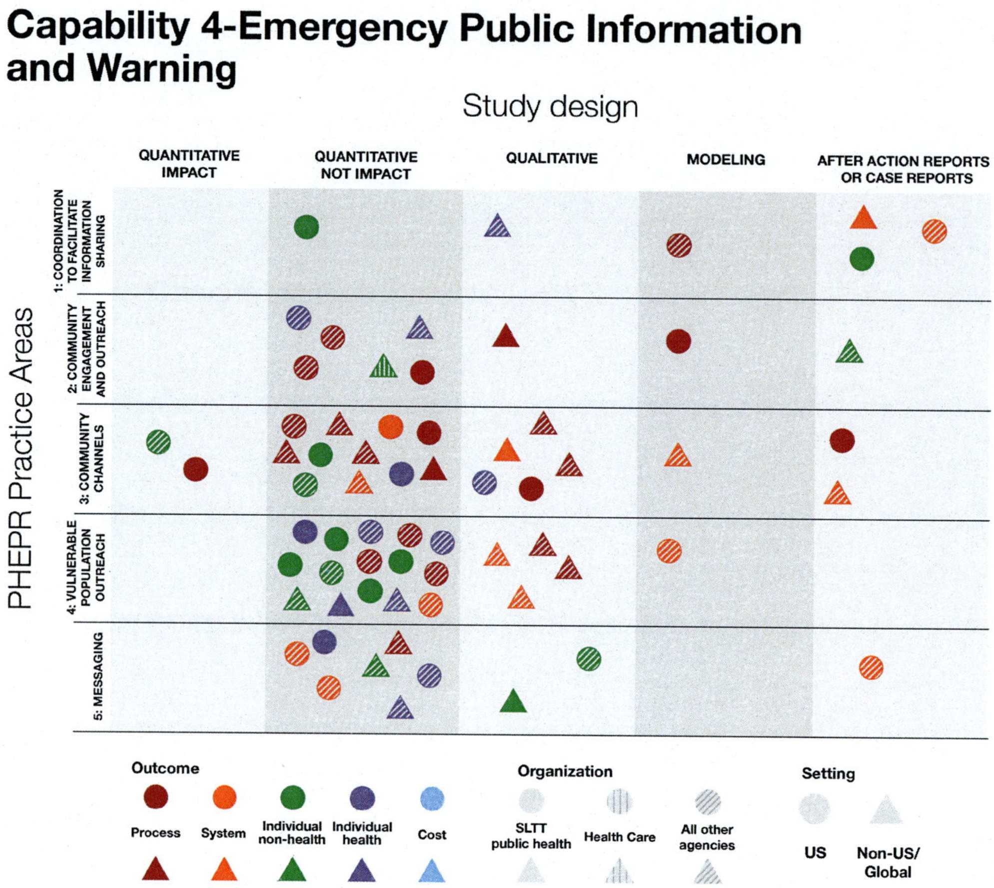

FIGURE D-14 Evidence map: Characteristics of studies for Emergency Public Information and Warning (N = 66).

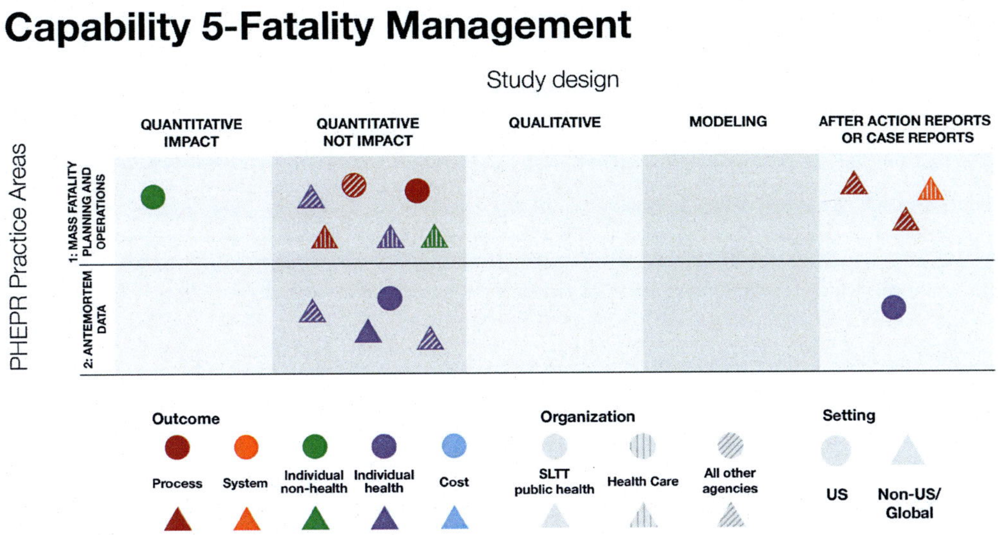

FIGURE D-15 Evidence map: Characteristics of studies for Fatality Management (N = 15).

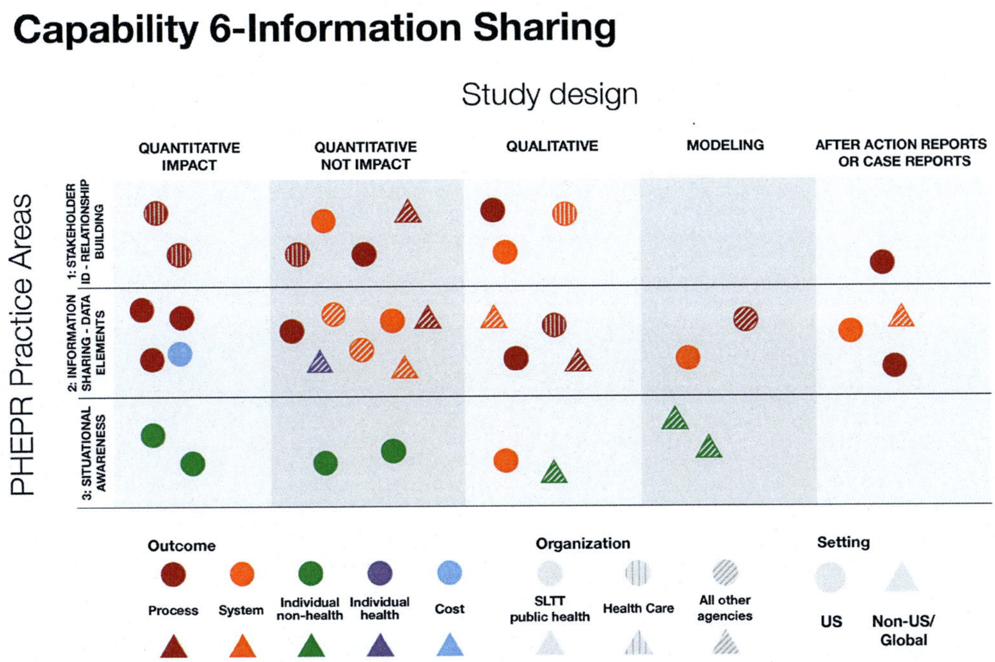

FIGURE D-16 Evidence map: Characteristics of studies for Information Sharing (N = 38).

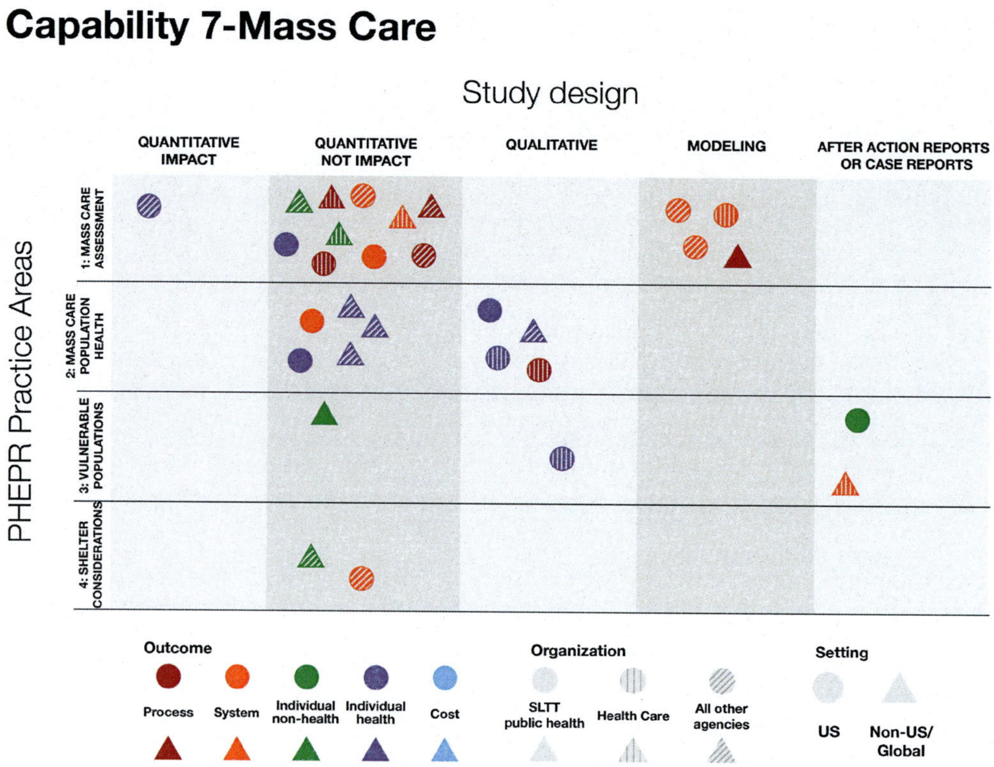

FIGURE D-17 Evidence map: Characteristics of studies for Mass Care (N = 30).

Capability 8-Medical Countermeasure Dispensing and Administration

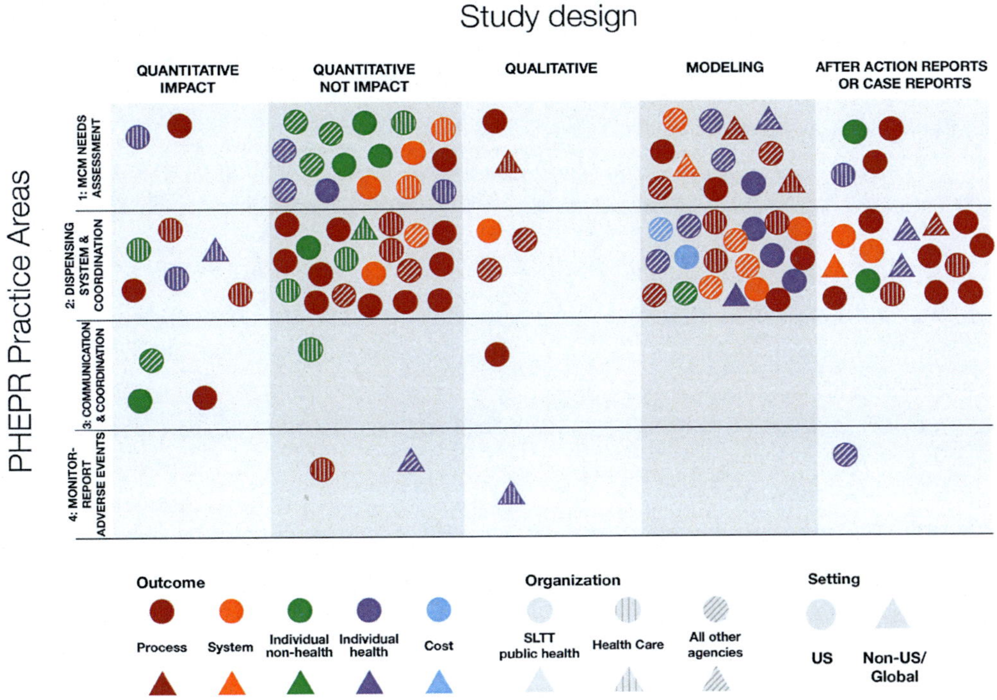

FIGURE D-18 Evidence map: Characteristics of studies for Medical Countermeasure Dispensing and Administration (N = 110).

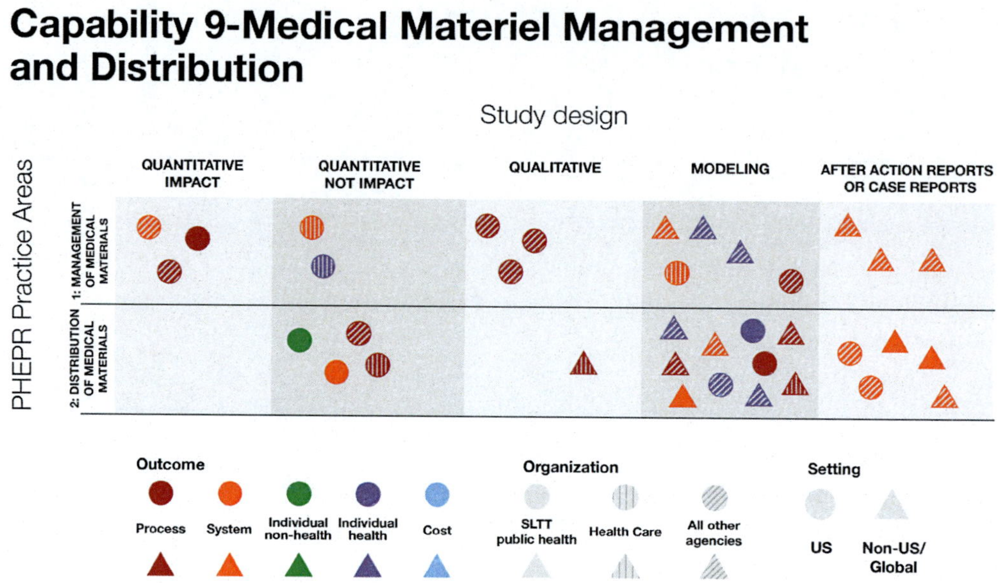

FIGURE D-19 Evidence map: Characteristics of studies for Medical Materiel Management and Distribution (N = 36).

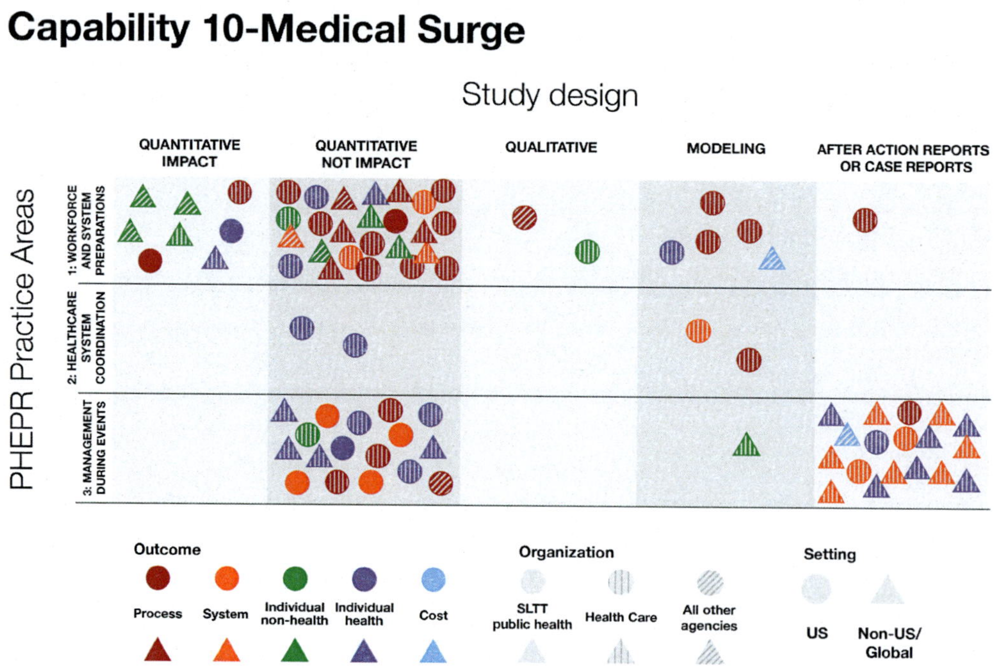

FIGURE D-20 Evidence map: Characteristics of studies for Medical Surge (N = 87).

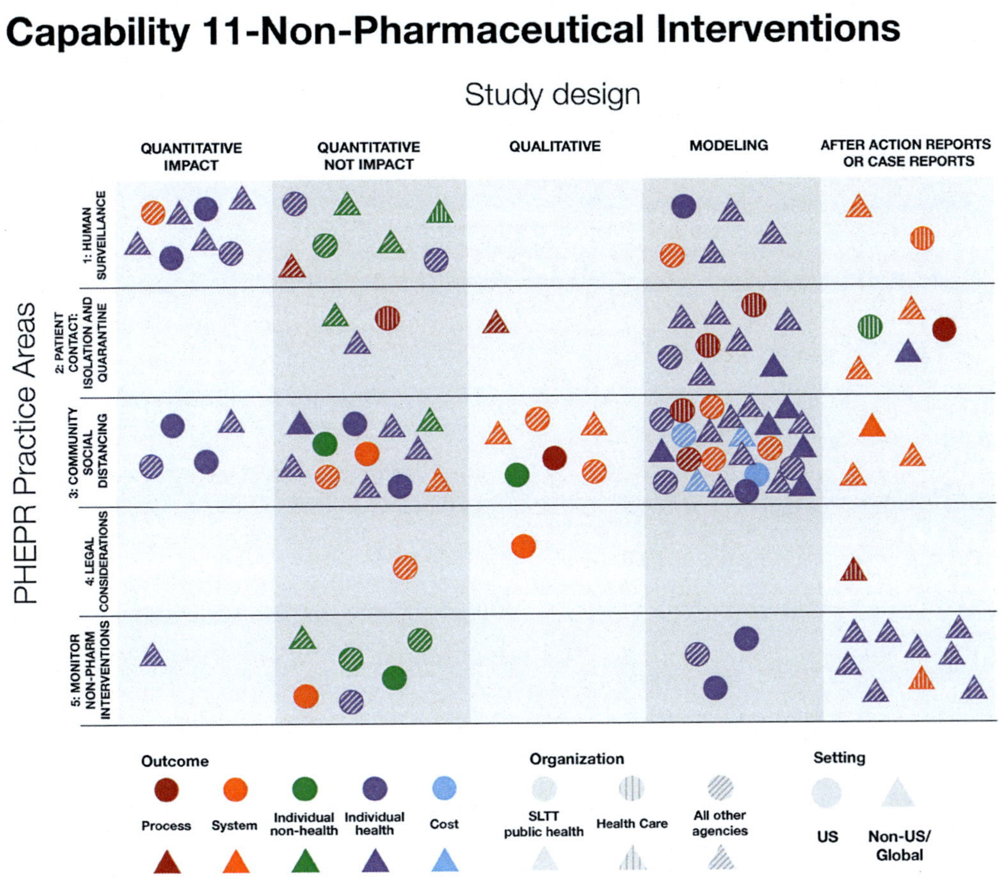

FIGURE D-21 Evidence map: Characteristics of studies for Non-Pharmaceutical Interventions (N = 112).

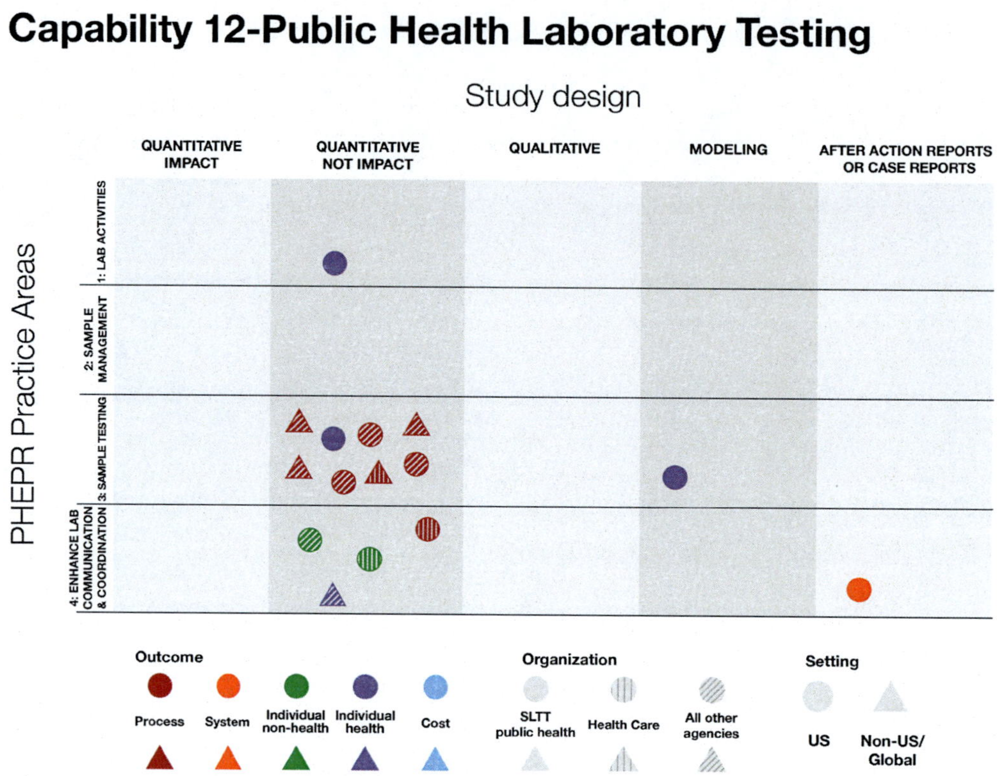

FIGURE D-22 Evidence map: Characteristics of studies for Public Health Laboratory Testing (N = 15).

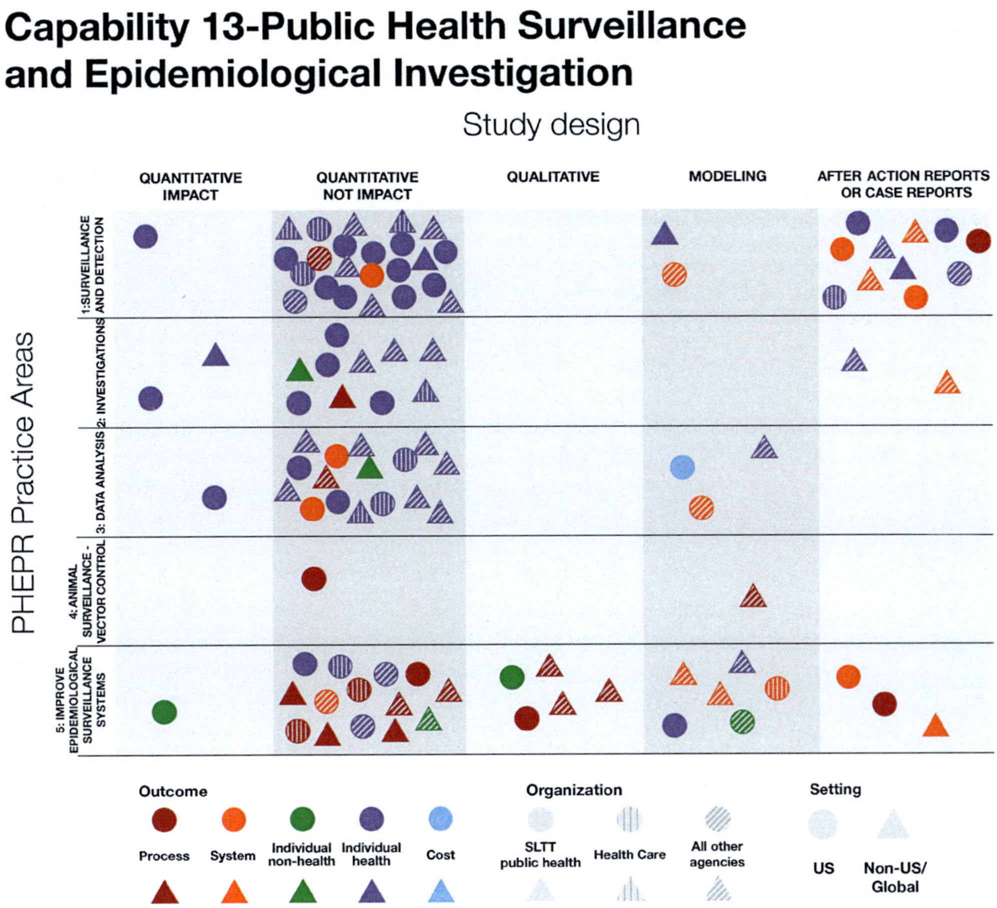

FIGURE D-23 Evidence map: Characteristics of studies for Public Health Surveillance and Epidemiological Investigation (N = 102).

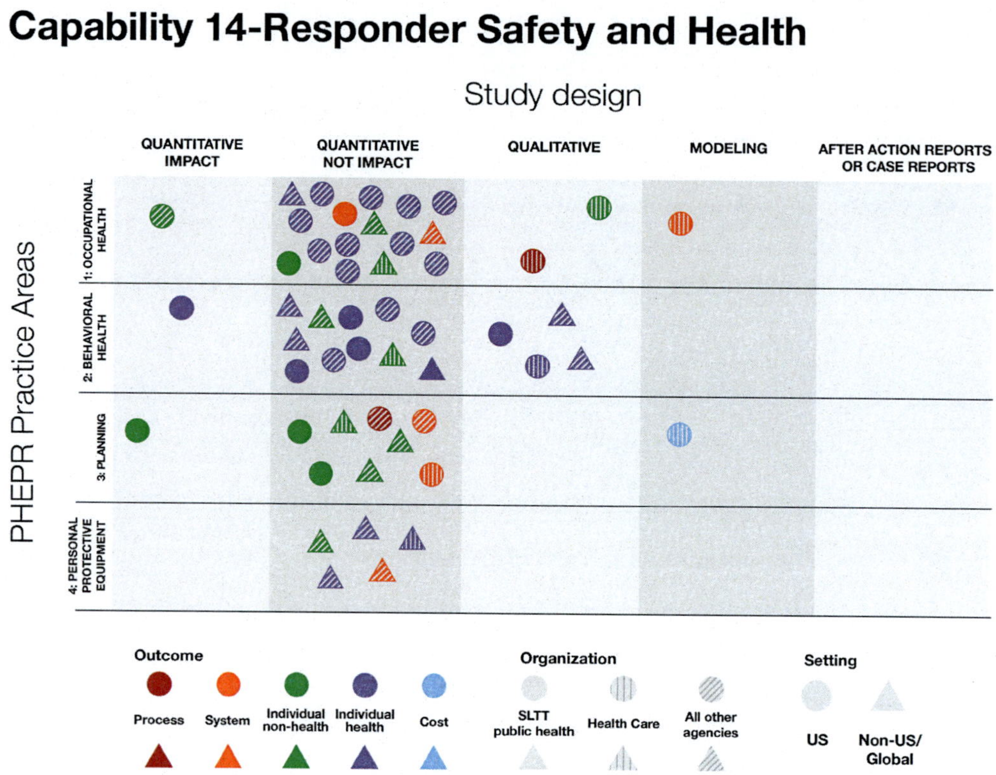

FIGURE D-24 Evidence map: Characteristics of studies for Responder Safety and Health (N = 51).

Capability 15-Volunteer Management

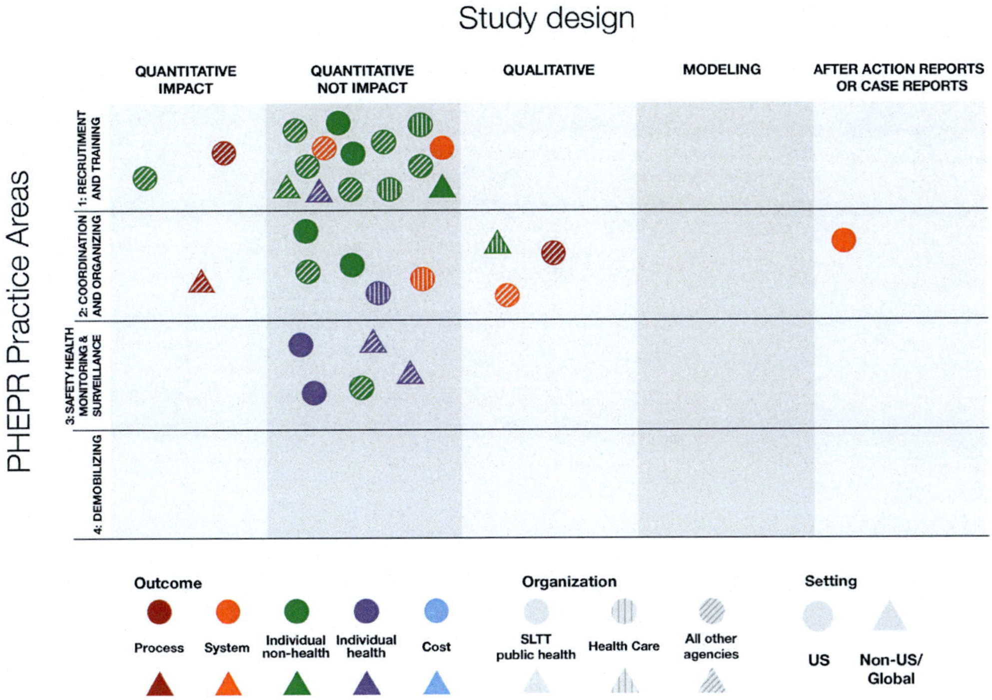

FIGURE D-25 Evidence map: Characteristics of studies for Volunteer Management (N = 55).

E

Public Committee Meeting Agendas and Proceedings of a Workshop—in Brief

The committee held 10 in-person meetings from January 2018 through March 2020; portions of 4 of these meetings were open to the public as part of the committee's information gathering for this study:

- The committee's first in-person meeting, held in January 2018, included an open session at which the sponsors of the study provided their perspectives on the charge to the committee, and state and local public health emergency preparedness and response (PHEPR) practitioners provided additional background information and context for the study.
- The committee's second in-person meeting, held in April 2018, included a public session at which the committee heard from researchers who have conducted similar reviews and grading of PHEPR practices to understand the nature of the evidence base, as well as the methods used and challenges experienced, and to hear from experts whose input helped inform the committee's prioritization of PHEPR Capabilities for this review.
- The committee's July 2018 in-person meeting included a public session at which researchers and practitioners discussed existing evidence-grading frameworks used to evaluate the effectiveness of practices in health and nonhealth fields, the potential application of those frameworks for assessing the effectiveness of PHEPR practices, and the potential role of evidence gleaned from sources other than controlled trials and quasi-experimental studies in an evidence review methodology for PHEPR practices. A summary of this discussion is captured in a Proceedings of a Workshop—in Brief.[1]
- The committee's January 2019 in-person meeting included a public session at which the committee engaged with PHEPR practitioners to identify knowledge gaps that matter to them, and to assess the relative priority, from their perspective, of potential

[1] Available at https://www.nap.edu/catalog/25510 (accessed June 18, 2020).

evidence review topics encompassed within the 15 Centers for Disease Control and Prevention (CDC) PHEPR Capabilities (see Appendix A for the results of this activity).

PUBLIC COMMITTEE MEETING AGENDAS

Monday, January 29, 2018

Keck Center of the National Academies
Room 208
500 Fifth Street, NW
Washington, DC 20001

OPEN SESSION

SESSION III: **Sponsor Briefing: Discussion of the Committee's Charge**
Objective: To hear from the sponsors of the study regarding their perspectives on the charge to the committee.

1:30 p.m. **Welcome and Introductions**
NED CALONGE, *Committee Chair*
President and Chief Executive Officer
The Colorado Trust

1:45 p.m. **Sponsor Perspective on Charge to the Committee**
ERIC CARBONE, *Study Sponsor*
Director, Office of Applied Research
Office of Public Health Preparedness and Response
Centers for Disease Control and Prevention

2:15 p.m. **Discussion with Committee**

3:15 p.m. **Break**

SESSION IV: **Additional Context for the Study—Defining the Problem**
Objective: To obtain additional background information and context for the study.

3:30 p.m. **Local Perspective**
SETH FOLDY
Director, Epidemiology, Informatics, and Preparedness
Denver Public Health

MAC MCCLENDON
Director, Office of Public Health Preparedness and Response
Harris County Public Health

State Perspective
PAUL PETERSEN
Director, Emergency Preparedness Program
Tennessee Department of Health

Marissa Levine
State Health Commissioner
Virginia Department of Health

4:00 p.m. **Discussion with Committee**

5:15 p.m. **ADJOURN OPEN SESSION**

Tuesday, April 24, 2018

National Academy of Sciences Building
Lecture Room
2101 Constitution Avenue, NW
Washington, DC 20418

OPEN SESSION

1:00 p.m. **Welcome and Introductions**
Ned Calonge, *Committee Chair*
President and Chief Executive Officer
The Colorado Trust

SESSION III: **Researcher Session**
Objectives:
1. To hear from researchers who have conducted similar reviews and grading of preparedness and response practices in the past to understand the nature of the evidence base as well as the methods used and the challenges experienced.
2. To hear from experts who can inform the prioritization of the public health preparedness capabilities.

1:05 p.m. Michael Stoto
Professor of Health Systems Administration and Population Health
Georgetown University

1:50 p.m. Yasmin Khan
Consultant Physician
Public Health Ontario

2:35 p.m. Valerie Yeager
Associate Professor for Health Policy and Management
Indiana University Fairbanks School of Public Health

3:20 p.m. **Break**

3:30 p.m. Marcia Testa
Senior Lecturer on Biostatistics
Harvard T.H. Chan School of Public Health

4:15 p.m. GLEN MAYS
Scutchfield Endowed Professor of Health Services and Systems Research
University of Kentucky College of Public Health

5:00 p.m. JENNIFER HORNEY
Department Head and Associate Professor of Epidemiology and Biostatistics
Texas A&M University Health Science Center School of Public Health

5:45 p.m. **Full Discussion with Committee**

6:00 p.m. **ADJOURN OPEN SESSION**

Thursday, July 26, 2018

National Academy of Sciences Building
Lecture Room
2101 Constitution Avenue, NW
Washington, DC 20418

OPEN SESSION

9:00 a.m. **Welcome and Introductions**
NED CALONGE, *Committee Chair*
President and Chief Executive Officer
The Colorado Trust

SESSION I: **Methodologies for Evaluating and Grading Evidence**
Objectives:
1. To examine similarities and differences between existing frameworks used to grade evidence of effectiveness for practices in health and nonhealth fields.
2. To discuss the potential application and adaptation of existing evidence-grading frameworks for assessing the effectiveness of public health preparedness and response practices.
3. To explore the potential role of evidence generated from sources other than randomized controlled trials and quasi-experimental studies in an evidence review methodology for public health preparedness and response practices.

9:05 a.m. **Panel 1: Evidence-Grading Frameworks in Health and Nonhealth Fields**
GUIDE TO COMMUNITY PREVENTIVE SERVICES
RANDY ELDER
Health Scientist, Guidelines and Recommendations Activity
Office of Science Quality, Office of the Associate Director for Science
Centers for Disease Control and Prevention

GRADE and GRADE-CERQual

Holger Schünemann (via Teleconference)
GRADE Co-Chair
Co-Director, World Health Organization Collaborating Centre for Evidence Informed Policy
Professor and Chair of the Department of Clinical Epidemiology and Biostatistics, Professor of Medicine
McMaster University

Jane Noyes
Professor in Health and Social Services Research and Child Health
Bangor University

What Works Clearinghouse

Jeffrey Valentine
Professor and Program Coordinator, Educational Psychology, Measurement, and Evaluation
College of Education and Human Development
University of Louisville

Clearinghouse for Labor Evaluation and Research

Demetra Nightingale
Institute Fellow
Urban Institute

Countermeasures That Work

Kristie Johnson
Research Psychologist, Office of Behavioral Safety Research
National Highway Traffic Safety Administration

11:05 a.m. **Break**

11:15 a.m. **Full Panel Discussion with Committee**

12:15 p.m. **Working Lunch**

1:00 p.m. **Panel 2: Additional Evidence Evaluation Methods for Assessing the Effectiveness of Interventions and Practices**

Jeff Marcus
Aviation Safety Recommendation Specialist, Safety Recommendations Division
National Transportation Safety Board

Jennifer Bishop
Chief, Writing and Editing Division, Office of Aviation Safety
National Transportation Safety Board

J. D. Polk
Chief Health and Medical Officer
National Aeronautics and Space Administration

Michael Woolcock
Lead Social Scientist, Development Research Group
The World Bank

1:45 p.m. **Full Panel Discussion with Committee**

2:30 p.m. **Break *(Committee Convenes in Closed Session)***

3:00 p.m. **Discussion with Panels 1 and 2**

4:00 p.m. **ADJOURN OPEN SESSION**

Thursday, January 10, 2019

Beckman Center of the National Academies
Huntington Room
100 Academy Way
Irvine, CA 92617

OPEN SESSION

SESSION V: **Practitioner Input on Review Topic Priorities**
Objective: 1. To identify priority topics for future evidence reviews based on practitioner input on critical knowledge gaps for PHEPR practices.

1:00 p.m. **Welcome and Introductions**
Ned Calonge, *Committee Chair*
President and Chief Executive Officer
The Colorado Trust

1:15 p.m. **In-Person PHEPR Practitioner Prioritization Activity**
- Review the intended use for the results from this activity
- Review activities and results from January 7 web-based meeting
- Review and rate priority level for each practice

6:00 p.m. **ADJOURN OPEN SESSION**

F Committee Member Biosketches

Bruce (Ned) Calonge, M.D., M.P.H. (*Chair*), is president and chief executive officer of The Colorado Trust, a private grant-making foundation dedicated to achieving health equity for all Coloradans. He is associate professor of family medicine at the Colorado School of Medicine, University of Colorado Denver, and associate professor of epidemiology at the Colorado School of Public Health. Nationally, he serves on the Centers for Disease Control and Prevention's (CDC's) Community Preventive Services Task Force. He also serves on the National Academies of Sciences, Engineering, and Medicine's Board on Population Health and Public Health Practice, as well as on the Roundtable on the Promotion of Health Equity. In 2016, he participated on two National Academies committees, supporting the release of two publications: *Communities in Action: Pathways to Health Equity* and *An Evidence Framework for Genetic Testing*. Dr. Calonge is past chair of the U.S. Preventive Services Task Force, past chair of CDC's Evaluating Genomic Applications in Practice and Prevention Working Group, past co-chair of the National Academies' Genomics in Public Health Action Collaborative, and ongoing consultant for and past member of the Secretary's Advisory Committee on Heritable Disorders in Newborns and Children. Dr. Calonge serves as a board member for Delta Dental of Colorado and is a board member and treasurer for the Colorado Association of Funders. Prior to coming to The Colorado Trust, he was chief medical officer of the Colorado Department of Public Health and Environment. He also served as chief of the Department of Preventive Medicine for the Colorado Permanente Medical Group and as a family physician for 10 years. He is past president of the Colorado Medical Board, the state physician-licensing board. Dr. Calonge received his B.A. in chemistry from The Colorado College, M.D. from the University of Colorado, and M.P.H. from the University of Washington. He was elected to the National Academy of Medicine in 2011.

David M. Abramson, Ph.D., M.P.H., is founding director of New York University's (NYU's) Program on Population Impact, Recovery and Resilience, faculty member of NYU's School of Global Public Health, and associate faculty member of the NYU Grossman School of Medicine's Department of Population Health. Prior to joining the NYU faculty in 2014,

Dr. Abramson was deputy director at Columbia University's National Center for Disaster Preparedness at the Earth Institute. He has led a number of major research studies examining the long-term impacts of disasters on communities and on vulnerable populations, including children. These studies include the longitudinal Gulf Coast Child and Family Health study, post–Hurricane Katrina, which recently received funding from the National Institutes of Health (NIH) to look at recovery 10 years after the storm, and the Sandy Child and Family Health study, currently being conducted in partnership with Rutgers University with funding from the New Jersey Department of Health. Dr. Abramson is also co-investigator of the NIH-funded Women's and Their Children's Health study, exploring the impact of the *Deepwater Horizon* oil spill on children's long-term health, in collaboration with Louisiana State University. Among his research-to-action initiatives, he is co-founder and co-director of the SHORE-line youth empowerment project with Colorado State University's Dr. Lori Peek, a curricular project-based learning program presently operating in a number of Gulf Coast and New York City high schools. In addition to disaster recovery work related to Hurricanes Katrina and Sandy and the *Deepwater Horizon* oil spill, he has studied short-term post-tornado community recovery in Joplin, Missouri; disaster recovery planning in four mid-sized U.S. cities; risk communication strategies; and organizational and attitudinal aspects of disaster preparedness. Dr. Abramson received his Ph.D. in sociomedical sciences from Columbia University, with a specialization in political science, and an M.P.H. from Columbia University. Over the past 25 years, he has conducted research on HIV/AIDS, public health systems, and civic engagement policy and practice. Prior to entering the field of public health, Dr. Abramson spent a decade as a national magazine journalist, having worked at or written for such publications as *Rolling Stone, Esquire,* and *Outside* magazines, among others.

Julie Casani, M.D., M.P.H., is medical director of Student Health Services at North Carolina State University, where she oversees the delivery of primary care, women's services, physical therapy, nutrition services, and pharmacy to students, faculty, and staff. She is an adjunct associate professor in biological sciences, providing instruction in global public health, agriculture security, and One Health, and mentors prehealth students. Until June 2017, she was director of public health preparedness and response in the North Carolina Division of Public Health. This branch coordinates the preparedness system for 4 regional offices, as well as 85 local health departments for which it provides response and recovery coordination, subject-matter expertise, and support. From 1999 to 2006, Dr. Casani was preparedness director at the Maryland Department of Health and Mental Hygiene. She has been a policy and health practice consultant to several national workshops and committees on weapons of mass destruction for federal and state agencies, serving on three defense science boards. She also served three consecutive terms as a member of the Homeland Security Science and Technology Advisory Committee for the U.S. Department of Homeland Security. She recently co-authored the text *Disasters and Public Health: Planning and Response*. Dr. Casani practiced clinical emergency medicine in the Johns Hopkins system for 17 years. She has been actively involved in emergency medical services (EMS) since the 1970s, serving at every level from ambulance provider to an appointed member of the Maryland State EMS Board. Dr. Casani received her M.D. from the New York University School of Medicine and her M.P.H. from the Johns Hopkins Bloomberg School of Public Health.

David Eisenman, M.D., M.S.H.S., is professor in residence at the David Geffen School of Medicine and the Fielding School of Public Health at the University of California, Los Angeles (UCLA), where he is director of the Center for Public Health and Disasters. For more than 15 years, Dr. Eisenman has been funded by the National Institutes of Health, the National Science Foundation, the Centers for Disease Control and Prevention, the U.S. Department of Homeland Security, and other federal agencies to conduct studies in the field of public health and disasters. He is a committee member for the National Health Security Preparedness Index and co-chairs the Social and Economic Standing Committee, National Institute of Standards and Technology *Community Resilience Planning Guide for Buildings and Infrastructure Systems*. From 2012 to 2016, Dr. Eisenman served as preparedness science officer for the Emergency Preparedness and Response Program at the Los Angeles County Department of Public Health. He is also an associate natural scientist at RAND Corporation, where he is a member of the Human Subjects Protection Committee. Dr. Eisenman is a credentialed physician for the Los Angeles County Emergency System, Advance Registration of Volunteer Health Professionals Program. He holds a board certification in internal medicine and cares for patients at the UCLA Medical Center.

Francisco García, M.D., M.P.H., is deputy county administrator and chief medical officer of Pima County in Tucson, Arizona. Located on the U.S.–Mexico border, Pima County is a large government jurisdiction the size of the state New Hampshire, with more than 1 million inhabitants. In that capacity he oversees the departments of Public Health, Behavioral Health, Animal Care Center, Medical Examiner, and Community & Workforce Development. Dr. García is former chair of the Centers for Disease Control and Prevention's National Breast and Cervical Cancer Prevention Advisory Committee. He is a former member of the National Academies' Roundtable on Health Equity and the Elimination of Health Disparities, as well as the Institute of Medicine Committee on Preventive Services for Women. He is also a past member of the U.S. Preventive Services Task Force. Prior to joining Pima County, Dr. García was a distinguished outreach professor of public health and obstetrics and gynecology, and served in a variety of leadership roles at the University of Arizona, including director of the Center of Excellence in Women's Health, the Arizona Hispanic Center of Excellence, and the Cancer Disparities Institute of the Arizona Cancer Center.

Paul Halverson, Dr.P.H., is founding dean of the Indiana University Richard M. Fairbanks School of Public Health in Indianapolis. He came to Indiana University from the Arkansas Department of Health, where he served as state health officer and director. Prior to his appointment as state health officer, Dr. Halverson served in senior leadership roles at the Centers for Disease Control and Prevention (CDC), including as senior advisor in the Office of Strategy and Innovation, senior scientist and director of the Division of Public Health Systems Development and Research, director of CDC's World Health Organization's Collaborating Center for Public Health Practice, and director of the National Public Health Performance Standards program. Before joining CDC, he served as senior health policy advisor for the North Carolina Department of Environment, Health, and Natural Resources. Dr. Halverson began his career in health administration and has 15 years of experience as a hospital and health system executive, working in Michigan, Minneapolis, and Phoenix. He earned his doctorate in public health from the University of North Carolina, his master's degree in health services administration from Arizona State University, and is a fellow of the American College of Healthcare Executives.

Sean Hennessy, Pharm.D., Ph.D., is professor of epidemiology in biostatistics at the University of Pennsylvania. He conducts research in the field of pharmacoepidemiology, which is the study of the health effects of drugs and other medical products in populations. His team identified a survival benefit of potassium supplementation in users of loop diuretics, and studied serious health consequences of drug–drug interactions involving high-risk drugs including anticoagulants, antidiabetic agents, and antiplatelet agents. His research has produced crucial knowledge about the cardiovascular safety of many widely used drugs for mental health conditions, including attention deficit hyperactivity disorder, depression, and schizophrenia. Dr. Hennessy also evaluated an early approach to using medical insurance data to improve prescribing, finding it ineffective despite its federal mandate. This work contributed to the omission of a requirement for drug utilization review programs in Medicare Part D. Dr. Hennessy co-led a pair of studies demonstrating the effectiveness and safety of the SA14-14-2 vaccine for Japanese encephalitis (JE), which subsequently led to the immunization of millions of children annually in populous countries including Cambodia, India, Malaysia, Nepal, Sri Lanka, and Thailand. Use of that vaccine has been credited with reducing the incidence of JE. Dr. Hennessy co-developed the trend-in-trend research design for studying the effects of rapidly increasing or declining exposures. He was the senior author of one of two citizen petitions to the U.S. Food and Drug Administration that led to the relabeling of metformin, the best-proven oral drug for diabetes, to permit its use in persons with mild to moderate renal insufficiency.

Edbert Hsu, M.D., M.P.H., FACEP, joined the Department of Emergency Medicine faculty after completing an international emegency medicine fellowship at Johns Hopkins. Combining his international health background with a special interest in disaster medicine, he has worked on emergency medicine program development and public health preparedness around the world. Currently, he serves on the leadership group of the Office of Critical Event Preparedness and Response. Dr. Hsu has been a co-investigator with the U.S. Department of Homeland Security Center for the Study of Preparedness and Catastrophic Event Response at Johns Hopkins and is currently a co–principal investigator on a Centers for Disease Control and Prevention–sponsored project studying public health leadership training for crises. He has completed several systematic reviews supported by the Agency for Healthcare Research and Quality. In recent years, he has been interested in the topic of mass gatherings and crowd disasters. Dr. Hsu serves as associate editor for the American Medical Association journal *Disaster Medicine and Public Health Preparedness.* He holds an M.D. from the University of Pittsburgh School of Medicine and an M.P.H. from the Johns Hopkins Bloomberg School of Public Health.

Nathaniel Hupert, M.D., M.P.H., is an internal medicine physician and public health researcher focusing on health care operations research, with a special emphasis on public health emergencies and response logistics. He currently serves as associate attending physician at NewYork-Presbyterian Hospital/Weill Cornell Medical Center, where he is associate professor of health care policy and research and of medicine; in addition, since 2006 he has been co-director of the Cornell Institute for Disease and Disaster Preparedness. Using a variety of computational and data analytic methods, his research seeks to improve the effectiveness of care delivery in both conventional and crisis settings. Since September 2000, Dr. Hupert has collaborated with local, state, federal, and international public health officials in advancing clinical and health system preparedness for bioterrorism and other public health emergencies. Several of his computer models of mass antibiotic dispensing and hospital surge capacity have been widely downloaded and used by public health professionals worldwide. Dr. Hupert led the development of two U.S. health care planning documents: *The Community Guide for Public Health Preparedness* (2004) and the *Guidebook for Hospital Preparedness Exercises* (2010). He has served on the Anthrax Modeling Working Group of the U.S. Department of Health and Human Services (HHS) (2003–2009), was a member of the 2007 RAND Expert Panel on Defining Public Health Preparedness, was founding director of the Preparedness Modeling Unit at the Centers for Disease Control and Prevention (CDC) (2008–2010), and served on the Scientific Advisory Board of the National Institutes of Health's Modeling of Infectious Disease Agent Study (MIDAS) (2012–2014). Between 2011 and 2017, he served as medical advisor for CDC's Division of Preparedness and Emerging Infections; he also held similar appointments at the HHS Biomedical Advanced Research and Development Authority (2014–2015) and the HHS National Healthcare Preparedness Program (2016). Dr. Hupert trained at the Harvard Medical School, the University of Pittsburgh Medical Center, and the Harvard T.H. Chan School of Public Health.

Rebecca A. Maynard, Ph.D., is professor of education and social policy at the University of Pennsylvania. She is a leading expert in the design and conduct of randomized controlled trials in the areas of education and social policy. She has conducted influential methodological research, including co-developing PowerUP! to support efficient sample designs for causal inference studies, and has been influential in advancing the development and application of research synthesis methods. In 2016, she stepped down from a 12-year tenure as director of the University of Pennsylvania's Predoctoral Training Program in Interdisciplinary Methods for Field-based Education Research, which has served more than 75 Ph.D. students from arts and sciences, business, and education. From 2010 through 2012, Dr. Maynard served as commissioner of the National Center for Education Evaluation and Regional Assistance at the Institute of Education Sciences. In this role, she oversaw the Institute's evaluation initiatives, the What Works Clearinghouse, the Regional Education Laboratories, and the National Library of Education (including ERIC). Prior to joining the faculty at the University of Pennsylvania in 1993, she was senior vice president at Mathematica Policy Research, Inc. Dr. Maynard holds a Ph.D. in economics from the University of Wisconsin–Madison.

Suzet McKinney, Dr.P.H., M.P.H., currently serves as chief executive officer and executive director of the Illinois Medical District, a 24/7/365 environment that includes 560 acres of hospitals, medical research facilities, laboratories, a biotech business incubator, universities, raw land development areas, and more than 40 health care–related facilities and is one of the largest urban medical districts in the United States. Dr. McKinney is former deputy commissioner of the Bureau of Public Health Preparedness and Emergency Response at the Chicago Department of Public Health, where she oversaw emergency preparedness efforts and coordinated those efforts within the broader spectrum of the City of Chicago's Public Safety activities, in addition to overseeing the Department's Division of Women and Children's Health. Dr. McKinney previously served as senior advisor for public health and preparedness at the Tauri Group, where she provided strategic and analytical consulting services to the U.S. Department of Homeland Security's (DHS's) BioWatch Program. Dr. McKinney serves on numerous boards, committees, and advisory boards. Current board memberships include the Board of Directors for Susan G. Komen Chicago, Thresholds, and the African-American Legacy of the Chicago Community Trust. Dr. McKinney is co-chair of the National Academies' Forum on Medical and Public Health Preparedness for Disasters and Emergencies and is a member of the Standing Committee on Health Threats Resilience. She also serves on the Science and Security Board for the Bulletin of the Atomic Scientists, the Board of Scientific Counselors for the Centers for Disease Control and Prevention, and the Office of Public Health Preparedness and Response, as well as the Federal Emergency Management Agency's National Advisory Council. She has served as an Incident Commander for the Chicago Department of Public Health and was a member of Chicago's Incident Management Team. She has been responsible for leading multiple emergency response efforts, including Chicago's 2014–2015 Ebola response; the operational response to the 2009 H1N1 outbreak, which was successful in vaccinating nearly 100,000 residents over a 6-week period; and the Chicago Department of Public Health's participation in the 2012 NATO Summit response and the 2010 Haiti Earthquake response. Dr. McKinney has earned a reputation as an experienced, knowledgeable public health official with exceptional communication skills. She has also supported the U.S. Department of Defense's Defense Threat Reduction Agency, providing subject-matter expertise in biological terrorism preparedness to the country of Poland. In academia, Dr. McKinney serves as instructor in the Division of Translational Policy and Leadership Development at the Harvard T.H. Chan School of Public Health and adjunct assistant professor of environmental and occupational health sciences at the University of Illinois at Chicago School of Public Health. Additionally, she serves as a mentor for the Biomedical Sciences Careers Project, also at Harvard University. She is author of the text *Public Health Emergency Preparedness: Practical Solutions for the Real World* (2018). Dr. McKinney received her doctorate from the University of Illinois at Chicago School of Public Health, with a focus on preparedness planning, leadership, and workforce development. She received a B.A. in biology from Brandeis University, where she was also a Howard Hughes Medical Institute fellow. She received her M.P.H. degree (health care administration) and certificates in managed care and health care administration from Benedictine University.

Jane P. Noyes, D.Phil., M.Sc., is professor of health and social services research and child health in the School of Health Sciences, Bangor University, United Kingdom. She is a clinical academic who completed health services research training with three competitive fellowships: Smith and Nephew 1-year predoctoral fellowship, UK Medical Research Council Health Services Research and Health of the Public 4-year doctoral fellowship, and UK Department of Health postdoctoral fellowship. She used these fellowship opportunities to develop and test methods for the new and emerging disciplines of mixed-method and qualitative evidence synthesis and the development, implementation, testing, and costing of complex interventions in complex health systems. Dr. Noyes is co-lead of the Wales National Centre for Population Health & Wellbeing Research and the Wales Kidney Research Unit. She is former co-chair and now member of the Cochrane Methods Executive, member of the Cochrane Scientific Committee, lead convenor of the Cochrane Qualitative and Implementation Methods Group, honorary visiting professor in child health at University College Dublin, and editor of the *Journal of Advanced Nursing*. She is a methodologist, systematic reviewer, and primary researcher with a particular interest in complex health and social interventions. Dr. Noyes is one of the founding members of the group that developed Grading of Recommendations Assessment, Development and Evaluation-Confidence in the Evidence from Reviews of Qualitative Research for assessing the confidence in findings of synthesized qualitative research. She also served as the methodologist on the World Health Organization team that developed the 2017 guideline for risk communication in public health emergencies. Dr. Noyes received her D.Phil. from York University in the United Kingdom.

Douglas K. Owens, M.D., M.S., is the Henry J. Kaiser Jr. Professor and director of the Center for Health Policy in the Freeman Spogli Institute for International Studies (FSI) and the Center for Primary Care and Outcomes Research (PCOR) in the Department of Medicine and School of Medicine at Stanford University. He is a general internist and associate director of the Center for Innovation to Implementation, a health services research center of excellence, at the U.S. Department of Veterans Affairs (VA) Palo Alto Health Care System. Dr. Owens is professor of medicine and, by courtesy, professor of health research and policy and professor of management science and engineering at Stanford University; he is also senior fellow at FSI. His research focuses on technology assessment, cost-effectiveness analysis, evidence synthesis, and methods for clinical decision making and guideline development. Dr. Owens served for 4 years as chair of the Clinical Guidelines Committee of the American College of Physicians, which develops clinical guidelines used widely and published regularly in the *Annals of Internal Medicine.* He is chair of the U.S. Preventive Services Task Force. He also directed the Stanford–University of California, San Fransisco (UCSF), Evidence-based Practice Center and the Program on Clinical Decision Making and Guideline Development at PCOR. He co-directs two training programs in health services research: the VA Postdoctoral Fellowship in Health Services Research and the VA Postdoctoral Informatics Fellowship Program. Dr. Owens received a B.S. and an M.S. from Stanford University and an M.D. from UCSF. He completed a residency in internal medicine at the University of Pennsylvania and a fellowship in health research and policy at Stanford University. He is past president of the Society for Medical Decision Making. He received the VA Under Secretary's Award for Outstanding Achievement in Health Services Research and the Eisenberg Award for Leadership in Medical Decision Making from the Society for Medical Decision Making. He was elected to the American Society for Clinical Investigation and the Association of American Physicians.

Sandra Quinn, Ph.D., is professor and chair in the Department of Family Science and senior associate director of the Maryland Center for Health Equity, School of Public Health, University of Maryland. She is currently co–principal investigator on a National Institute of General Medical Sciences/National Institutes of Health (NIH) grant on Supplementing Survey-Based Analyses of Group Vaccination Narratives and Behaviors Using Social Media. She was co–principal investigator on a National Institute on Minority Health and Health Disparities (NIMHD)/NIH Center of Excellence in Race, Ethnicity and Health Disparities Research. In recent years she was principal investigator on two U.S. Food and Drug Administration (FDA)-funded studies: (1) Public Attitudes toward Medical Countermeasures, and (2) Investigating Factors Associated with Participation of Racial and Ethnic Minority Populations in FDA Regulated Research. Dr. Quinn was co–principal investigator of a Grand Opportunity grant from the Office of the Director, NIH and NIMHD, on Bioethics Research Infrastructure Initiative: Building Trust between Minorities and Researchers. As principal investigator of a Centers for Disease Control and Prevention (CDC)-funded study on Public Attitudes Toward H1N1 Influenza, she led two national surveys during the H1N1 influenza pandemic, becoming the first to examine public attitudes toward emergency use authorizations for drugs and vaccines and to test an empirical model of disparities in exposure, susceptibility, and access to care during a pandemic. She was also funded by CDC to study communication between postal workers and public health professionals during the anthrax attacks. Her research interests include vaccine acceptance in routine and emergency situations; the impact of social media on vaccine attitudes and behaviors; racial disparities in vaccine uptake; crisis and emergency risk communication, with a specific focus on minority populations; and engagement of minority and marginalized communities in research.

Paul Shekelle, M.D., Ph.D., M.P.H., spent 20 years as director of the Southern California Evidence-Based Practice Center site at RAND Corporation. He is consultant in health sciences at RAND; professor of medicine at the University of California, Los Angeles (UCLA), School of Medicine; and staff physician at the U.S. Department of Veterans Affairs Medical Center in West Los Angeles. He received his M.D. from Duke University, M.P.H. from UCLA, and Ph.D. from the UCLA School of Public Health. His scholarly interests are in the areas of evidence-based medicine, practice guidelines, and quality of care.

Andy Stergachis, Ph.D., B.Pharm., is professor of pharmacy and global health and adjunct professor of health services and epidemiology; associate dean, School of Pharmacy; and director of the Global Medicines Program, University of Washington (UW). He is the author of 165 peer-reviewed publications in such areas as drug safety, pharmaceutical outcomes, emergency preparedness and response, and clinical epidemiology and served as editor-in-chief of the *Journal of the American Pharmacists Association.* He is an elected member of the National Academy of Medicine. He is a fellow of the International Society for Pharmacoepidemiology and the American Pharmacists Association. He has been a member of the Drug Safety and Risk Management Advisory Committee for the U.S. Food and Drug Administration and was chair of the Malaria in Pregnancy Consortium Safety Working Group. He served as chair, Emergency Pharmaceutical Distribution Collaborative Group, Centers for Public Health Preparedness, Association of Schools of Public Health; was a member of the State of Washington Joint Advisory Committee for Public Health and Hospital Emergency Preparedness and Response; and served as coordinator for the Strategic National Stockpile for King County, Washington. Through his affiliation with the UW Northwest Center for Public Health Practice, he works with the public health community on workforce development and research in emergency preparedness. Dr. Stergachis has received numerous honors, including Pharmacist of the Year from the Washington State Pharmacy Association and the Martin Luther King, Jr. Community Volunteer Recognition Award from UW.

Mitch Stripling, M.P.A., is currently national director of emergency preparedness and response at the Planned Parenthood Federation of America. In this capacity, he works across the Planned Parenthood Federation to develop emergency preparedness programs that include planning, training, and exercises to prepare for likely threats, as well as building out an incident command system to deal with crises as they occur. He also coordinates contingency planning around such critical issues as the future of abortion access. Previously, Mr. Stripling oversaw the agency preparedness and response efforts at the New York City Department of Health and Mental Hygiene, including units for planning, training and exercises, risk analysis, intelligence, and evaluations. He coordinated citywide planning for the 2009 H1N1 pandemic and served as a planning section chief at the department for the responses to Hurricanes Irene and Sandy, the Ebola crisis, and the recent outbreaks of *Legionella* and Zika. His unit has developed nationally recognized threat response guides for 21 of the highest-risk scenarios that could impact New York City, a data- and consensus-driven risk assessment methodology, a principal scientific advisor model for public health incident command systems, and a strategic planning directive model for civilian use. Previously, he worked for the Florida Department of Health, where he helped plan and implement the responses to six federally declared disasters, including the 2004 record-breaking hurricane season and Florida's response in southern Mississippi after Hurricane Katrina. During that time, he developed, rostered, and trained environmental health and other public health strike teams; built national training standards in collaboration with the Centers for Disease Control and Prevention; and focused on making communities more resilient in the face of environmental threats. Before working in public health, Mr. Stripling spent several years providing strategic consulting for Fortune 500 companies and government agencies. He began his career working at the United Nations Global Teaching and Learning Project on human rights issues.

Steven M. Teutsch, M.D., M.P.H., is an independent consultant; adjunct professor at the Fielding School of Public Health, University of California, Los Angeles; and senior fellow, Leonard D. Schaeffer Center for Health Policy and Economics, University of Southern California. Until 2014 he was chief science officer, Los Angeles County Public Health, where

he continued his work on evidence-based public health and policy. Previously, he worked at Merck, where he was responsible for scientific leadership in developing evidence-based clinical management programs, conducting outcomes research studies, and improving outcomes measurement to enhance quality of care. Prior to joining Merck, he was director of the Division of Prevention Research and Analytic Methods (DPRAM) at the Centers for Disease Control and Prevention (CDC), where he was responsible for assessing the effectiveness, safety, and cost-effectiveness of disease and injury prevention strategies. DPRAM developed comparable methodology for studies of the effectiveness and economic impact of prevention programs, provided training in these methods, developed CDC's capacity for conducting necessary studies, and provided technical assistance for conducting economic and decision analysis. The Division also evaluated the impact of interventions in urban areas, developed *The Guide to Community Preventive Services,* and provided support for CDC's analytic methods. Dr. Teutsch has served as a member of the Community Preventive Services Task Force and the U.S. Preventive Services Task Force, as well as the Americas Health Information Community Personalized Health Care Workgroup and the Evaluation of Genomic Applications in Prevention and Practice Workgroup. He has chaired and served on a number of expert committees. Dr. Teutsch joined CDC in 1977, where he served in various capacities, focusing on parasitic diseases, kidney donation and kidney diseases, diabetes control, epidemiology, disease monitoring, and prevention effectiveness. He received his undergraduate degree in biochemical sciences at Harvard University, an M.P.H. in epidemiology from the University of North Carolina School of Public Health, and his M.D. from the Duke University School of Medicine. He completed his residency training in internal medicine at The Pennsylvania State University. He was certified by the American Board of Internal Medicine in 1977 and the American Board of Preventive Medicine in 1995, and is a fellow of the American College of Physicians and American College of Preventive Medicine. Dr. Teutsch has published more than 200 articles and 8 books in a broad range of fields in epidemiology, including parasitic diseases, diabetes, technology assessment, health services research, and surveillance.

Tener Goodwin Veenema, Ph.D., M.P.H., M.S., R.N., FAAN, is professor of nursing and public health at the Johns Hopkins University School of Nursing and the Johns Hopkins Bloomberg School of Public Health. As an internationally recognized expert in disaster nursing and public health emergency preparedness, she has served as senior scientist to the U.S. Department of Health and Human Services Office of Human Services Emergency Preparedness and Response, the U.S. Department of Homeland Security, the Federal Emergency Management Agency, and the Veterans Affairs Emergency Management Evaluation Center. An accomplished researcher, Dr. Veenema is a member of the American Red Cross National Scientific Advisory Board and is an elected fellow in the American Academy of Nursing; the National Academies of Practice; and the Royal College of Surgeons, Dublin, Ireland. She is editor of *Disaster Nursing and Emergency Preparedness for Chemical, Biological and Radiological Terrorism and Other Hazards,* 4th ed., the leading textbook in the field, and developer of Disaster Nursing, an innovative technology app. Dr. Veenema received master's degrees in nursing administration (1992), pediatrics (1993), and public health (1999) and a Ph.D. in health services research and policy (2001) from the University of Rochester School of Medicine and Dentistry. She was awarded the Florence Nightingale Medal of Honor (International Red Crescent, 2013), the highest international award in nursing, for her professional service in disasters and public health emergencies and was the recipient of a Fulbright U.S. Scholar Award (2017). Dr. Veenema previously served on the National Academies' Standing Committee for the Strategic National Stockpile. She currently serves as the 2017–2018 National Academy of Medicine Distinguished Nurse Scholar-in-Residence.

Matthew Wynia, M.D., M.P.H., is director of the Center for Bioethics and Humanities, University of Colorado, and professor of medicine at the University of Colorado School of Medicine. His training is in internal medicine, infectious diseases, public health, and health services research. From 1997 to 2015, Dr. Wynia worked at the American Medical Association (AMA), where he developed a research institute and training programs focused on bioethics, professionalism, and policy issues (the AMA Institute for Ethics) and founded the AMA's Center for Patient Safety. He also practiced at the University of Chicago. His research has focused on understanding and improving the practical management of ethical issues in medicine and public health. He has led projects on a wide variety of issues related to ethics and professionalism. He has served on committees and expert panels and as a reviewer for the Health and Medicine Division of the National Academies, the Joint Commission, federal agencies, the Hastings Center, the American Board of Medical Specialties, and other organizations, and has delivered and held more than two dozen named lectures and visiting professorships nationally and internationally. Dr. Wynia is the author of more than 140 published articles, chapters, and essays. His work has been published in numerous leading medical and ethics journals, and he is a contributing editor for the *American Journal of Bioethics*. He is past president of the American Society for Bioethics and Humanities and has chaired the Ethics Forum of the American Public Health Association and the Ethics Committee of the Society for General Internal Medicine. He holds current board certifications in internal medicine and infectious diseases.

NATIONAL ACADEMY OF MEDICINE FELLOW

Mahshid Abir, M.D., M.Sc., was the National Academy of Medicine fellow supporting this study. Dr. Abir is an emergency physician and health services researcher with a joint appointment at the University of Michigan and RAND Corporation. She is director of the Acute Care Research Unit at the University of Michigan's Institute for Healthcare Policy and Innovation. Her research evaluates strategies for improving acute care delivery in the United States along the care delivery continuum, including the prehospital, emergency, inpatient, ambulatory care, and community settings. Her work focuses on addressing policy-related issues pertaining to utilization, quality, efficiency, outcomes, and costs of acute care delivery in these settings.